HUMAN EMBRYOLOGY & DEVELOPMENTAL BIOLOGY

Second Edition

HUMAN EMBRYOLOGY & DEVELOPMENTAL BIOLOGY

Bruce M. Carlson, MD, PhD

Professor and Chairman
Department of Anatomy and Cell Biology
University of Michigan
Ann Arbor, Michigan

with 502 illustrations

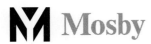 Mosby

St. Louis Baltimore Boston Carlsbad Chicago Minneapolis New York Philadelphia Portland
London Milan Sydney Tokyo Toronto

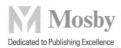

Mosby

Dedicated to Publishing Excellence

A Times Mirror Company

Publisher: Richard Furn
Editor: Beverly Copland
Senior Developmental Editor: Linda Caldwell
Project Manager: Carol Sullivan Weis
Project Specialist: Pat Joiner
Designer: Jen Marmarinos
Manufacturing Manager: Betty Mueller
Illustrators: Mike Saiz, Marion Tasker, Jenni Miller

Second Edition
Copyright © 1999 by Mosby, Inc.

Previous edition copyrighted 1994

Printed in the United States of America
Composition by Accu-Color, Inc.
Lithography/color film by Accu-Color, Inc.
Printing/binding by Von Hoffmann Press, Inc.

Mosby, Inc.
11830 Westline Industrial Drive
St. Louis, Missouri 63146

Library of Congress Cataloging-in-Publication Data

Carlson, Bruce M.
    Human embryology and developmental biology / Bruce M. Carlson.—2nd ed.
    p. cm.
    Includes bibliographical references and index.
    ISBN 0-8151-1458-3
    1. Embryology, Human.   2. Developmental biology.   3. Human growth.
I. Title.
    [DNLM: 1. Abnormalities—embryology.   2. Developmental Biology.
3. Fetal Development—physiology.   QS 604 C284h 1998]
QM601.C29 1998
612.6' 4—dc21
DNLM/DLC
For Library of Congress   98-29769
                                                                                                  CIP

98 99 00 01 02/9 8 7 6 5 4 3 2 1

Reviewers

DEBORAH J. ANDREW, PhD

Associate Professor, Department of Cell Biology and Anatomy
The Johns Hopkins University School of Medicine
Baltimore, Maryland

JO ANN CAMERON, PhD

Associate Professor, Department of Cell and Structural Biology
University of Illinois College of Medicine
Urbana, Illinois

RAYMOND F. GASSER, PhD

Professor, Department of Anatomy
Louisiana State University Medical Center
New Orleans, Louisiana

REV. JOSEPH C. GREGOREK, PhD

Professor, Department of Biology
Gannon University
Erie, Pennsylvania

GERALD D. MEETZ, PhD

Professor, Department of Anatomy
University of Osteopathic Medicine and Health Sciences
Des Moines, Iowa

ALEXANDER SANDRA, PhD

Professor, Department of Anatomy and Cell Biology
University of Iowa College of Medicine
Iowa City, Iowa

MIKEL SNOW, PhD

Professor, Department of Cell and Neurobiology
University of Southern California School of Medicine
Los Angeles, California

PREFACE

The past decade has seen the revolutionary transformation of human embryology from an almost wholly morphologically oriented discipline to one in which morphology can be related to an underlying molecular blueprint. Although many of the steps between the localization of specific regulatory molecules and the emergence of form and function remain to be filled in, the importance of molecular embryology is so great that not to present the basic elements of this aspect of development would cheat the student from exposure to one of the most exciting and rapidly advancing fields in the biomedical sciences.

The time allotted to a typical medical embryology course does not permit a detailed exposition of molecular embryology, but in an attempt to balance desirability with reality, I have included in the text those aspects of molecular embryology that are of major importance in understanding how the basic pattern of an organ or a part of the body is laid down. For many of these, examples of malformations caused by absent or inappropriate gene expression are known in the mouse or human. Because this aspect of embryology is changing so rapidly, I have tried to err on the conservative side and introduce material that is likely to stand the test of time, but experience has shown that the discovery of new molecules can often bump the current molecular "star" into the rank of also-rans.

The organization of this second edition continues to be integrative because I strongly feel that a real working understanding of how our bodies are put together can best be attained by seeing how molecular and morphological processes work in concert during development. Not only does this approach lead to a better appreciation of normal development, but it also allows a deeper understanding of why development can go awry when certain links in the developmental chain are missing or disturbed.

My experience in using this text for the medical class at the University of Michigan has led to a number of modifications in the second edition. Important among these are the following:

- A new section in Chapter 5 that introduces general features of the major classes of developmentally important molecules
- A table of these key molecules, located inside the cover
- Clinical Vignette and Clinical Correlation features providing additional clinical examples
- New multiple-choice review questions at the end of each chapter
- A significant number of new or extensively modified illustrations
- More tabular or summary material in the text
- Much greater use of full-color in the illustration program
- The addition of the developmental time frame to many of the morphological illustrations

Last, some comments on feedback. All textbook authors need feedback to be sure that their books are meeting the needs of the instructors and students. After having written textbooks for nearly 30 years, I have ceased to be amazed at how little feedback typically reaches authors. I learned several valuable lessons from my organic chemistry professor in college, who offered his students a point for every mistake that they found in our textbook. Not only did it help the author, but more important, it taught the students that mistakes abound in the printed word. Students in my classes have been very helpful in his regard, but I would encourage readers with comments on any aspect of the text to contact me at brcarl@umich.edu.

ACKNOWLEDGMENTS

Thanks are due to many people whose help was invaluable in getting the second edition put together:

Emma Underdown, Developmental Editor of the first edition, for the existence of the second edition

Linda Caldwell, Developmental Editor of the second edition, for a very pleasant and effective working relationship

Pat Joiner, Project Specialist, for guiding the manuscript through the production process

Margaret Croup Brudon, who was once again wonderful in transforming my preliminary sketches into first class artwork

Mason Barr, MD, of the Department of Pediatrics at the University of Michigan for continuing access to his large collection of photographs of fetuses with congenital malformations; Adrienne Noe, PhD, Director of the Human Developmental Anatomy Center at the National Museum of Health and Medicine for access to and permission to use photographs from its collections in this edition; and Donald MacCallum, PhD, of the Department of Anatomy and Cell Biology at the University of Michigan for original slides of endometrial tissue

Jim Beals for his help in digitizing original photographs

Danny Pyne and his crew of illustrators who digitized and colorized much of the original artwork

Pam Taylor for efficient secretarial work and keeping track of my various disks and drafts of chapters

My teaching partner, Pamela Raymond, PhD, for excellent reviews of parts of the manuscript, and the manuscript reviewers designated by the publisher for their comments and criticisms

Bruce M. Carlson

CONTENTS

DEVELOPMENTAL TABLES

Carnegie Stages of Early Human Embryonic Development (Weeks 1-8)

Age (days)	External features	Carnegie stage	Crown-rump length (mm)	Pairs of somites
1	Fertilized oocyte	1	0.1	
2-3	Morula (4-16 cells)	2	0.1	
4	Free blastocyst	3	0.1	
5-6	Attachment of blastocyst to endometrium	4	0.1	
7-12	Implantation, bilaminar embryo with primary yolk sac	5	0.1-0.2	
13-15	Trilaminar embryo with primitive streak, chorionic villi	6	0.2-0.3	
16	Gastrulation, formation of notochordal process	7	0.4	
18	Hensen's node and primitive pit, notochord and neurenteric canal, appearance of neural plate, neural folds, and blood islands	8	1.0-1.5	
20	Appearance of first somites, deep neural groove, elevation of cranial neural folds, early heart tubes	9	1.5-2.5	1-3
22	Beginning of fusion of neural folds, formation of optic sulci, presence of first two pharyngeal arches, beginning heart beat, curving of embryo	10	2.0-3.5	4-12
24	Closure of cranial neuropore, formation of optic vesicles, rupture of oropharyngeal membrane	11	2.5-4.5	13-20
26	Closure of caudal neuropore, formation of pharyngeal arches 3 and 4, appearance of upper limb buds and tail bud, formation of otic vesicle	12	3-5	21-29
28	Appearance of lower limb buds, lens placode, separation of otic vesicle from surface ectoderm	13	4-6	30+
32	Formation of lens vesicle, optic cup, and nasal pits	14	5-7	
33	Development of hand plates, primary urogenital sinus, prominent nasal pits, evidence of cerebral hemispheres	15	7-9	
37	Development of foot plates, visible retinal pigment, development of auricular hillocks, formation of upper lip	16	8-11	
41	Appearance of finger rays, rapid head enlargement, six auricular hillocks, formation of nasolacrimal groove	17	11-14	
44	Appearance of toe rays and elbow regions, beginning of formation of eyelids, tip of nose distinct, presence of nipples	18	13-17	
48	Elongation and straightening of trunk, beginning of herniation of midgut into umbilical cord	19	16-18	
51	Bending of arms at elbows, distinct but webbed fingers, appearance of scalp vascular plexus, degeneration of anal and urogenital membranes	20	18-22	
52	Longer and free fingers, distinct but webbed toes, indifferent external genitalia	21	22-24	
54	Longer and free toes, better development of eyelids and external ear	22	23-28	
57	More rounded head, fusion of eyelids	23	27-31	

Data taken largely from O'Rahilly R, Müller F: *Developmental stages in human embryos,* Pub 637, Washington, DC, 1987, Carnegie Institution of Washington.

Major Developmental Events During the Fetal Period

External features	Internal features
8 WEEKS	
Head is almost half the total length of fetus.	Midgut herniation into umbilical cord occurs.
Cervical flexure is about 30 degrees.	Extraembryonic portion of allantois has degenerated.
Indifferent external genitalia are present.	Ducts and alveoli of lacrimal glands form.
Eyes are converging.	Paramesonephric ducts begin to regress in males.
Eyelids are unfused.	Recanalization of lumen of gut tube occurs.
Tail disappears.	Lungs are becoming glandlike.
Nostrils are closed by epithelial plugs.	Diaphragm is completed.
	First ossification begins in skeleton.
	Definitive aortic arch system takes shape.
9 WEEKS	
Neck develops and chin rises from thorax.	Intestines are herniated into umbilical cord.
Cranial flexure is about 22 degrees.	Early muscular movements occur.
Chorion is divided into chorion laeve and chorion frondosum.	ACTH and gonadotropins are produced by pituitary.
Eyelids meet and fuse.	Corticosteroids are produced by adrenal cortex.
External genitalia begin to become gender specific.	Semilunar valves in heart are completed.
	Fused paramesonephric ducts join vaginal plate.
	Urethral folds begin to fuse in males.
10 WEEKS	
Cervical flexure is about 15 degrees.	Intestines return into body cavity from umbilical cord.
Gender differences are apparent in external genitalia.	Bile is secreted.
Fingernails appear.	Blood islands are established in spleen.
Eyelids are fused.	Thymus is infiltrated by lymphoid stem cells.
	Prolactin production by pituitary occurs.
	First permanent tooth buds form.
	Deciduous teeth are in early bell stage.
	Epidermis has three layers.
11 WEEKS	
Cervical flexure is about 8 degrees.	Urine is excreted into amniotic fluid.
Nose begins to develop bridge.	Stomach musculature can contract.
	T lymphocytes emigrate into bloodstream.
	Colloid appears in thyroid follicles.
12 WEEKS	
Head is erect.	Ovaries descend below pelvic rim.
Neck is almost straight and well defined.	Parathyroid hormone is produced.
External ear is taking form and has moved close to its definitive position in the head.	Blood can coagulate.
Yolk sac has shrunk.	
Fetus swallows amniotic fluid.	
Fetus can respond to skin stimulation.	

Major Developmental Events During the Fetal Period—cont'd

External features	Internal features
4 MONTHS	
Skin is thin; blood vessels can easily be seen through it.	Seminal vesicle forms.
Nostrils are almost formed.	Transverse grooves appear on dorsal surface of cerebellum.
Fetus may begin to suck its thumb.	Bile is produced by liver and stains meconium green.
Eyes have moved to front of face.	Gastric glands bud off from gastric pits.
Legs are longer than arms.	Brown fat begins to form.
Fine lanugo hairs appear on head.	Pyramidal tracts begin to form in brain.
Fingernails are well formed; toenails are forming.	Hematopoiesis begins in bone marrow.
Epidermal ridges appear on fingers and palms of hand.	Ovaries contain primordial follicles.
Enough amniotic fluid is present to permit amniocentesis.	
Mother can feel fetal movements.	
5 MONTHS	
Epidermal ridges form on toes and soles of feet.	Myelination of spinal cord begins.
Vernix caseosa begins to be deposited on skin.	Sebaceous glands begin to function.
Abdomen begins to fill out.	Thyroid-stimulating hormone is released by pituitary.
Eyelids and eyebrows develop.	Testes begin to descend.
Lanugo hairs cover most of body.	
6 MONTHS	
Skin is wrinkled and red.	Surfactant begins to be secreted.
Decidua capsularis degenerates because of reduced blood supply.	Tip of spinal cord is at S1 level.
Lanugo hairs darken.	
7 MONTHS	
Eyelids begin to open.	Sulci and gyri begin to appear on brain.
Eyelashes are well developed.	Subcutaneous fat storage begins.
Scalp hairs are lengthening (longer than lanugo).	Testes are descending into scrotum.
Skin is slightly wrinkled.	Termination of splenic erythropoiesis occurs.
8 MONTHS	
Skin is pink and smooth.	Regression of hyaloid vessels from lens occurs.
Eyes are capable of pupillary light reflex.	Testes enter scrotum.
Fingernails have reached tip of fingers.	
9 MONTHS	
Toenails have reached tip of toes.	Larger amounts of pulmonary surfactant are secreted.
Most lanugo hairs are shed.	Ovaries are still above brim of pelvis.
Skin is covered with vernix caseosa.	Testes have descended into scrotum.
Attachment of umbilical cord becomes central in abdomen.	Tip of spinal cord is at L3.
About 1 L of amniotic fluid is present.	Myelination of brain begins.
Placenta weighs about 500 g.	
Fingernails extend beyond fingertips.	
Breasts protrude and secrete "witches' milk."	

PART I

EARLY DEVELOPMENT AND THE FETAL-MATERNAL RELATIONSHIP

1

GETTING READY FOR PREGNANCY

Human pregnancy begins with the fusion of an egg and a sperm, but a great deal of preparation precedes this event. First, both male and female sex cells must pass through a long series of changes (**gametogenesis**) that convert them genetically and phenotypically into mature **gametes**, which are capable of participating in the process of fertilization. Next, the gametes must be released from the gonads and make their way to the upper part of the uterine tube, where fertilization normally takes place. Finally, the fertilized egg, now properly called an **embryo,** must enter the uterus, where it sinks into the uterine lining (**implantation**) to be nourished by the mother. All these events involve interactions between the gametes or embryo and the adult body in which they are housed, and most of them are mediated or influenced by parental hormones. This chapter focuses on gametogenesis and the hormonal modifications of the body that enable reproduction to occur.

GAMETOGENESIS

Gametogenesis is typically divided into four phases: (1) the extraembryonic origin of the germ cells and their migration into the gonads, (2) an increase in the number of germ cells by mitosis, (3) a reduction in chromosomal number by meiosis, and (4) structural and functional maturation of the eggs and spermatozoa. The first phase of gametogenesis is identical in both males and females, whereas distinct differences exist between the male and female patterns in the last three phases.

Phase 1: Origin and Migration of Germ Cells

Primordial germ cells, the earliest recognizable precursors of gametes, arise outside the gonads and migrate into the gonads during early embryonic development. Human primordial germ cells first become readily recognizable at 24 days after fertilization in the endodermal layer of the yolk sac (Figure 1-1, A) by their large size and high content of the enzyme alkaline phosphatase. In the mouse, their origin has been traced even earlier in development (p. 376). Germ cells exit from the yolk sac into the hindgut epithelium and then

migrate through the dorsal mesentery until they reach the primordia of the gonads (Figure 1-1, B). In the mouse, an estimated 100 cells leave the yolk sac, and through mitotic multiplication (six to seven rounds of cell division), about 4000 primordial germ cells enter the primitive gonads.

Misdirected primordial germ cells that lodge in extragonadal sites usually die, but if such cells survive, they may develop into **teratomas.** Teratomas are bizarre growths that contain scrambled mixtures of highly differentiated tissues, such as skin, hair, cartilage, and even teeth (Figure 1-2). They are found in the mediastinum, the sacrococcygeal region, and the oral region.

Phase 2: Increase in the Number of Germ Cells by Mitosis

Once they arrive in the gonads, the primordial germ cells begin a phase of rapid mitotic proliferation. In a mitotic division, each germ cell produces two **diploid** progeny that are genetically equal. Through several series of mitotic divisions, the number of primordial germ cells increases exponentially from hundreds to millions. The pattern of mitotic proliferation differs markedly between male and female germ cells. **Oogonia,** as mitotically active germ cells in the female are called, go through a period of intense mitotic activity in the embryonic ovary from the second through the fifth month of pregnancy in the human. During this period the population of germ cells increases from only a few thousand to nearly 7 million (Figure 1-3). This number represents the maximum number of germ cells that is ever found in the ovaries. Shortly thereafter, large numbers of oogonia undergo a natural degeneration called **atresia.** Atresia of germ cells is a continuing feature of the histological landscape of the human ovary until menopause.

Spermatogonia in the male, which are the counterparts of oogonia, follow a pattern of mitotic proliferation that differs greatly from that in the female. Mitosis also begins early in the embryonic testes, but in contrast to female germ cells, male germ cells maintain the ability to divide throughout life. The seminiferous tubules of the testes are lined with a germinative population of spermatogonia. Beginning at puberty, subpopulations of spermatogonia undergo periodic waves of

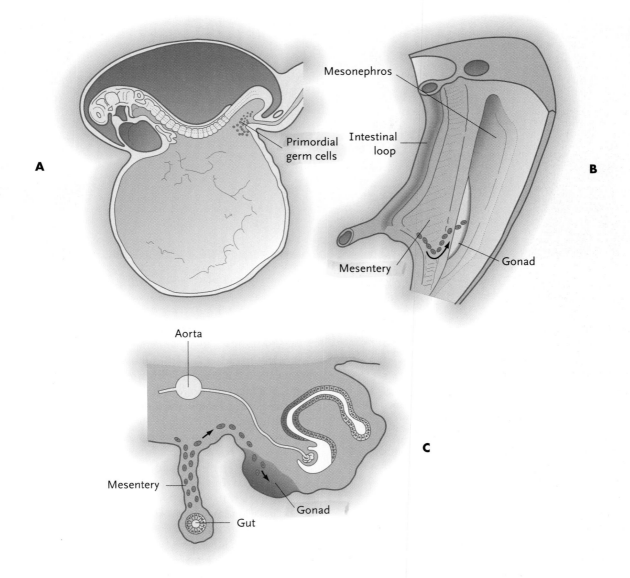

A

B

C

Figure 1-1 Origin and migration of primordial germ cells in the human embryo. **A,** Location of primordial germ cells in the 16-somite human embryo. **B,** Pathway of migration (*arrow*) through the dorsal mesentery. **C,** Cross section showing the pathway of migration (*arrows*) through the dorsal mesentery and into the gonad.

mitosis. The progeny of these divisions enter meiosis as synchronous groups. This pattern of spermatogonial mitosis continues throughout life.

Phase 3: Reduction in Chromosomal Number by Meiosis

Stages of meiosis

The biological significance of meiosis in the human is similar to that in other species. Of primary importance are (1) reduction of the number of chromosomes from the diploid (2n) to the **haploid** (1n) number so that the species number of

chromosomes can be maintained from generation to generation, (2) independent reassortment of maternal and paternal chromosomes for better mixing of genetic characteristics, and (3) further redistribution of maternal and paternal genetic information through the process of crossing-over during the first meiotic division.

Meiosis involves two sets of divisions (Figure 1-4). Before the first meiotic division, deoxyribonucleic acid (DNA) replication has already occurred, so at the beginning of meiosis, the cell is 2n, 4c. (In this designation, **n** is the species number of chromosomes and **c** is the amount of DNA in a single set [n] of chromosomes before DNA replication has occurred.) The cell contains the normal number (2n) of chromosomes,

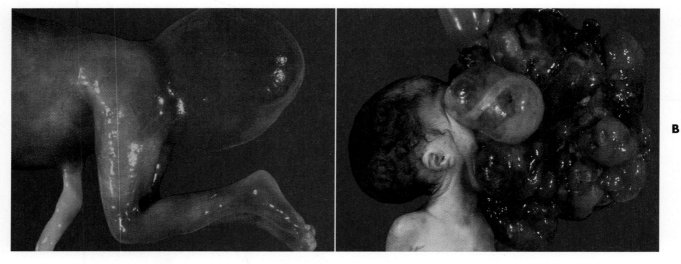

Figure 1-2 A, Sacrococcygeal teratoma in a fetus. **B,** Massive oropharyngeal teratoma. (Courtesy M. Barr, Ann Arbor, Michigan.)

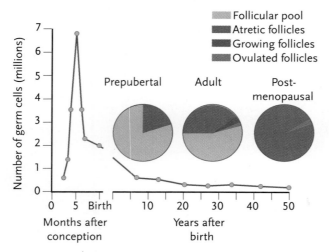

Figure 1-3 Changes in the number of germ cells and proportions of follicle types in the human ovary with increasing age. (Based on studies by Baker TG. In Austin CR, Short RV: *Germ cells and fertilization (reproduction in mammals),* vol 1, Cambridge, England, 1970, Cambridge University Press, p 20; and Goodman AL, Hodgen GD: *Recent Progr Hormone Res* 39:1-73,1983.)

but as the result of replication, its DNA content (4c) is double the normal amount (2c).

In the first meiotic division, often called the **reductional division,** a prolonged prophase (see Figure 1-4) results in the pairing of homologous chromosomes and frequent **crossing-over,** resulting in the exchange of segments between members of the paired chromosomes. During metaphase of the first meiotic division, the chromosome pairs (tetrads) line up at the metaphase (equatorial) plate so that at anaphase I, one chromosome of a homologous pair moves toward one pole of the spindle and the other chromosome moves toward the opposite pole. This represents one of the principal differences between a meiotic and mitotic division. In a mitotic anaphase, the centromere between the sister chromatids of each chro-

mosome splits after the chromosomes have lined up at the metaphase plate, and one chromatid from each chromosome migrates to each pole of the mitotic spindle. This results in genetically equal daughter cells after a mitotic division, whereas the daughter cells are genetically unequal after the first meiotic division. Each daughter cell of the first meiotic division contains the haploid (1n) number of chromosomes, but each chromosome still consists of two chromatids (2c) connected by a centromere. No new duplication of chromosomal DNA is required between the first and second meiotic divisions because each haploid daughter cell resulting from the first meiotic division already contains chromosomes in the replicated state.

The second meiotic division, called the **equational division,** is similar to an ordinary mitotic division, except that before division the cell is haploid (1n, 2c). When the chromosomes line up along the equatorial plate at metaphase II, the centromeres between sister chromatids divide, allowing the sister chromatids of each chromosome to migrate to opposite poles of the spindle apparatus during anaphase II. Each daughter cell of the second meiotic division is truly haploid (1n, 1c).

Meiosis in females

The period of meiosis involves other cellular activities in addition to the redistribution of chromosomal material. As the oogonia enter the first meiotic division late in the fetal period, they are called **primary oocytes.**

Meiosis in the human female is a very leisurely process. As the primary oocytes enter the diplotene stage of the first meiotic division in the early months after birth, the first of two blocks in the meiotic process occurs (Figure 1-5). The suspended diplotene phase of meiosis is the period when the primary oocyte prepares for the needs of the embryo. In oocytes of amphibians and other lower vertebrates, which must develop outside the mother's body and often in a hostile environment, it is highly advantageous for the early stages of de-

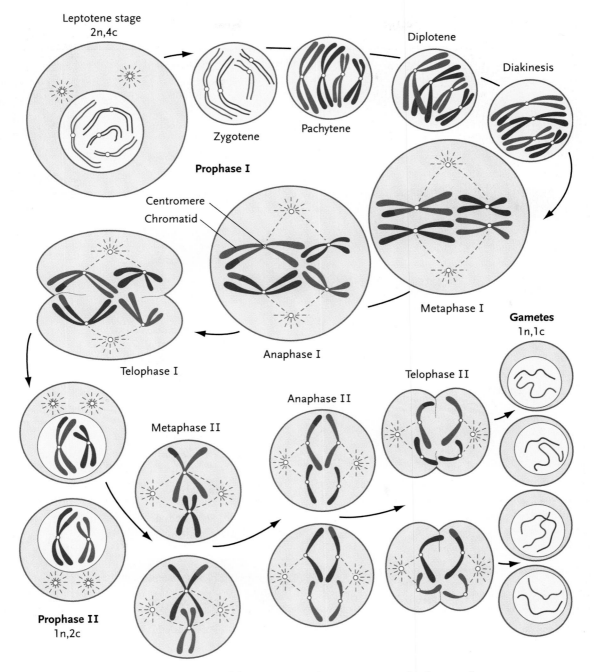

Figure 1-4 Summary of the major stages of meiosis in a generalized germ cell.

velopment to occur very rapidly so that the stage of independent locomotion and feeding is attained as soon as possible. These conditions necessitate a strategy of storing up the materials needed for early development well in advance of ovulation and fertilization because normal synthetic processes would not be rapid enough to produce the materials required for the rapidly cleaving embryo. In such species, yolk is accumulated, the genes for producing ribosomal ribonucleic acid (rRNA) are amplified, and many types of RNA molecules are synthesized and stored in an inactive form for later use.

The morphological substrate for ribonucleic acid (RNA) synthesis in the amphibian oocyte is represented by the lampbrush chromosomes, which are characterized by many prominent loops of spread-out DNA on which messenger RNA (mRNA) molecules are synthesized. The amplified genes for producing rRNA are manifested by the presence of 600 to 1000 nucleoli within the nucleus. Primary oocytes also prepare for fertilization by producing several thousand cortical granules, which are of great importance during the fertilization process (see Chapter 2).

Age	Follicular histology		Meiotic events in ovum	Chromosomal complement
Fetal period	No follicle		Oogonium	2n,2c
			Mitosis	
Before or at birth	Primordial follicle		Primary oocyte	2n,4c
			Meiosis in progress	
After birth	Primary follicle		Primary oocyte	2n,4c
			Arrested in diplotene stage of first meiotic division	
After puberty	Secondary follicle		Primary oocyte	2n,4c
			First meiotic division completed, start of second meiotic division	
	Tertiary follicle		Secondary oocyte + Polar body I	1n,2c
			Ovulation	
	Ovulated ovum		Secondary oocyte + Polar body I	1n,2c
			Arrested at metaphase II	
			Fertilization — second meiotic division completed	
	Fertilized ovum		Fertilized ovum + Polar body II	1n,1c + sperm

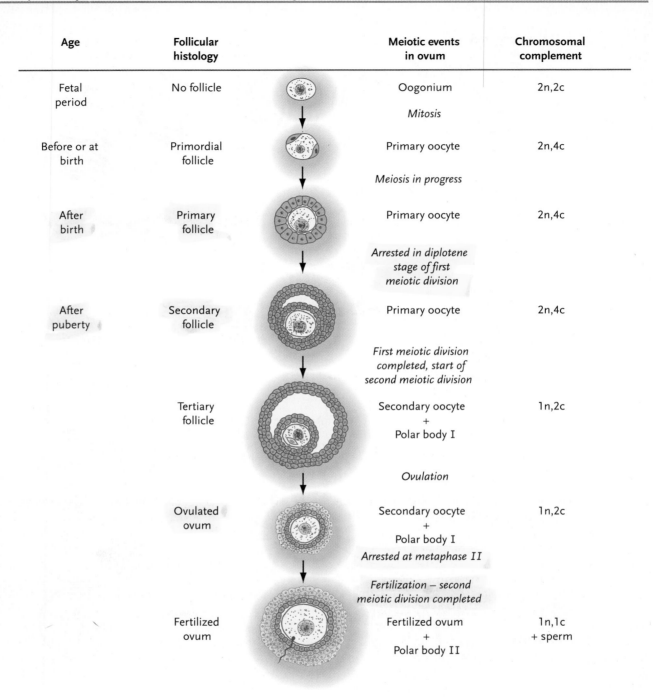

Figure 1-5 Summary of the major events in human oogenesis and follicular development.

The mammalian oocyte prepares for an early embryonic period that is more prolonged than that of amphibians and that takes place in the nutritive environment of the maternal reproductive tract. Therefore it is not faced with the need to store as great a quantity of materials as are the eggs of lower vertebrates. As a consequence, the buildup of yolk is negligible. However, some evidence indicates a low level of ribosomal DNA (rDNA) amplification (2 to 3 times) in diplotene human oocytes, suggesting that some degree of molecular advance planning is also required to support early cleavage in the human. The presence of 2 to 40 small (2 μm) RNA-containing micronuclei (miniature nucleoli) per oocyte nucleus correlates with the molecular data.

Analysis of RNA accumulation in mammalian oocytes is based principally on results obtained in the mouse, in which some RNA accumulation begins during the diplotene stage.

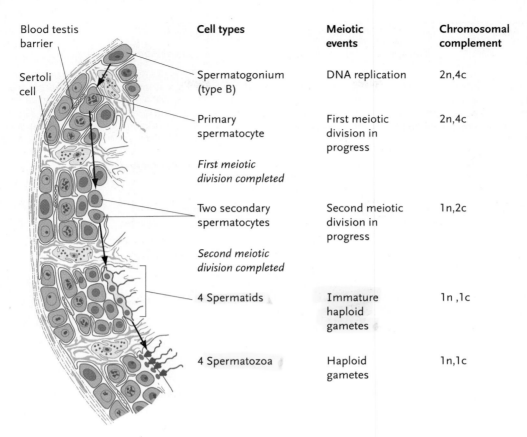

Cell types	Meiotic events	Chromosomal complement
Spermatogonium (type B)	DNA replication	2n,4c
Primary spermatocyte	First meiotic division in progress	2n,4c
First meiotic division completed		
Two secondary spermatocytes	Second meiotic division in progress	1n,2c
Second meiotic division completed		
4 Spermatids	Immature haploid gametes	1n,1c
4 Spermatozoa	Haploid gametes	1n,1c

Labels: Blood testis barrier; Sertoli cell

Figure 1-6 Summary of the major events in human spermatogenesis.

Human diplotene chromosomes do not appear to be arranged in a true lampbrush configuration, and massive amounts of RNA synthesis seem unlikely. The developing mammalian (mouse) oocyte produces 10,000 times less rRNA and 1000 times less mRNA than does its amphibian counterpart. Nevertheless, there is a steady accumulation of mRNA and a proportional accumulation of rRNA. These amounts of maternally derived RNA seem to be enough to take the fertilized egg through the first couple of cleavage divisions, after which the embryonic genome takes control of macromolecular synthetic processes.

Because cortical granules play an important role in preventing the entry of excess spermatozoa during fertilization in human eggs (see p. 32), the formation of cortical granules (mainly from the Golgi apparatus) continues to be one of the functions of the diplotene stage that is preserved in humans. Roughly 4500 cortical granules are produced in the mouse oocyte. A somewhat higher number is likely in the human oocyte.

Unless they degenerate, all primary oocytes remain arrested in the diplotene stage of meiosis until puberty. During the reproductive years, small numbers (10 to 30) of primary oocytes complete the first meiotic division with each menstrual cycle and begin to develop further. The other primary oocytes remain arrested in the diplotene stage, some for as long as 50 years.

With the completion of the first meiotic division shortly before ovulation, two unequal cellular progeny result. One is a large cell, called the **secondary oocyte**. The other is a small, nonfunctional cell called the **first polar body** (see Figure 1-5). The secondary oocytes begin the second meiotic division, but again the meiotic process is arrested, this time at metaphase. The stimulus for the release from this meiotic block is fertilization by a spermatozoon. Unfertilized secondary oocytes fail to complete the second meiotic division. The second meiotic division is also unequal; one of the daughter cells is again relegated to becoming a small, nonfunctional second polar body. The first polar body may also divide during the second meiotic division.

Meiosis in males

Meiosis in the male does not begin until after puberty. In contrast to the primary oocytes in the female, not all spermatogonia enter meiosis at the same time. In fact, large numbers of spermatogonia remain in the mitotic cycle throughout much of the reproductive lifetime of males. Once the progeny of a spermatogonium have entered the meiotic cycle as **primary spermatocytes**, they spend several weeks passing through the first meiotic division (Figure 1-6). The result of the first meiotic division is the formation of two **secondary**

CLINICAL CORRELATION 1-1
Meiotic Disturbances Resulting in Chromosomal Aberrations

Chromosomes sometimes fail to separate during meiosis, a phenomenon known as **nondisjunction.** As a result, one haploid daughter gamete contains both members of a chromosomal pair for a total of 24 chromosomes, whereas the other haploid gamete contains only 22 chromosomes (Figure 1-7). When such gametes combine with normal gametes of the opposite sex (with 23 chromosomes), the resulting em-

bryos contain 47 chromosomes (with a **trisomy** of one chromosome) or 45 chromosomes (**monosomy** of one chromosome). (Specific syndromes associated with the nondisjunction of chromosomes are summarized in Chapter 7.) The generic term given to a condition characterized by an abnormal number of chromosomes is **aneuploidy.**

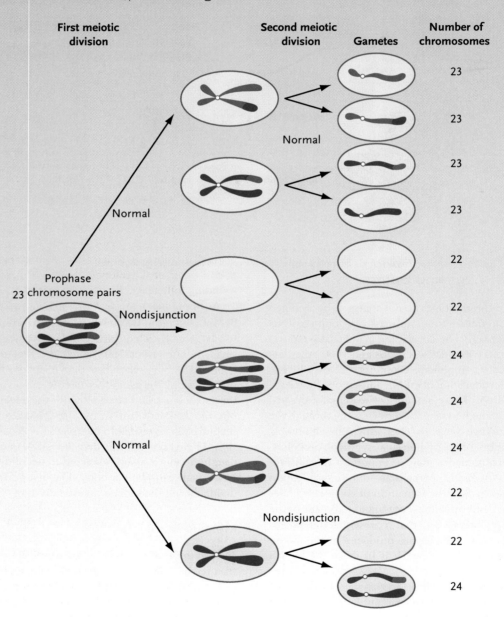

Figure 1-7 Possibilities for nondisjunction. *Top arrow,* Normal meiotic divisions; *middle arrow,* nondisjunction during the first meiotic division; *bottom arrow,* nondisjunction during the second meiotic division.

In other cases, part of a chromosome can be **translocated** to another chromosome during meiosis, or part of a chromosome can be **deleted.** Similarly, duplications or inversions of parts of chromosomes occasionally occur during meiosis. These conditions may result in syndromes similar to those seen after the nondisjunction of entire chromosomes. Under some circumstances (e.g., simultaneous fertilization by two spermatozoa, failure of the second polar body to separate from the oocyte during the second meiotic division), the cells of the embryo contain more than two multiples of the haploid number of chromosomes **(polyploidy).**

Chromosomal abnormalities are the underlying cause of a high percentage of spontaneous abortions during the early weeks of pregnancy. Over 75% of the spontaneous abortions occurring before the second week and over 60% of those occurring during the first half of pregnancy contain chromosomal abnormalities ranging from trisomies of individual chromosomes to overall polyploidy. Although the incidence of chromosomal anomalies declines with stillbirths occurring after the fifth month of pregnancy, it is close to 6%, a tenfold higher incidence over the 0.5% of living infants who are born with chromosomal anomalies. In counseling patients who have had a stillbirth or a spontaneous abortion, it can be useful to mention that this is often nature's way of handling an embryo destined to be highly abnormal.

spermatocytes, which immediately enter the second meiotic division. About 8 hours later, the second meiotic division is completed, and four haploid (1n, 1c) **spermatids** remain as progeny of the single primary spermatocyte. The total length of human spermatogenesis is 64 days.

Disturbances that can occur during meiosis and result in chromosomal aberrations are discussed in Clinical Correlation 1-1.

Phase 4: Final Structural and Functional Maturation of Eggs and Sperm

Oogenesis

Of the roughly 2 million primary oocytes present in the ovaries at birth, only about 40,000—all of which are arrested in the diplotene stage of the first meiotic division—survive until puberty. From this number, approximately 400 (one per menstrual cycle) are actually ovulated. The rest of the primary oocytes degenerate without leaving the ovary, but many of them undergo some further development before becoming atretic.

The egg along with its surrounding cells is called a **follicle.** Maturation of the egg is intimately bound with the development of its cellular covering. Because of this, considering the development of the egg and its surrounding follicular cells as an integrated unit is a useful approach in the study of oogenesis.

In the embryo, oogonia are naked, but after meiosis begins, cells from the ovary partially surround the primary oocytes to form **primordial follicles** (see Figure 1-5). By birth, the primary oocytes are invested with one or two complete layers of follicular cells, and the complex of primary oocyte and the follicular (granulosa) cells is called a **primary follicle** (Figure 1-8). Both the oocyte and the surrounding follicular cells develop prominent microvilli and gap junctions that connect the two cell types.

The gap junctions permit the exchange of amino acids and glucose metabolites that are required for growth of the oocyte. Considerable evidence indicates that the follicular cells secrete a **meiotic inhibitory factor** responsible for maintaining the first arrest of meiosis in the diplotene stage. The inhibitory factor is transferred from the follicular cells to the oocyte via the gap junctions that connect them. The release of meiotic inhibition shortly before ovulation is associated with the luteinizing hormone surge and the subsequent disruption of the gap junction connections. The oocyte also appears to influence the development of the surrounding follicular cells, especially in mature follicles. Follicular functions that depend on interactions between the oocyte and surrounding follicular cells are summarized in Box 1-1.

As the primary follicle takes shape, a prominent, translucent, noncellular membrane called the **zona pellucida** forms between the primary oocyte and its enveloping follicular cells (Figure 1-9). The microvillous connections between the oocyte and follicular cells are maintained through the zona pellucida. In rodents, the characterized components of the zona pellucida (three glycoproteins and glycosaminoglycans) are synthesized almost entirely by the egg, but in some mammals, follicular cells may also contribute materials to the zona. The zona pellucida contains sperm receptors and other components that are important in fertilization and early postfertilization development. (The functions of these molecules are discussed more fully in Chapter 2.)

In the prepubertal years, many of the primary follicles enlarge, mainly because of an increase in the size of the oocyte and the number of follicular cells. A basement membrane called the **membrana granulosa** surrounds the epithelial **granulosa cells** of the primary follicle. The membrana granulosa forms a barrier to capillaries, and, as a result, both the oocyte and the granulosa cells depend on the diffusion of oxygen and nutrients for their survival.

An additional set of cellular coverings, derived from the ovarian connective tissue (**stroma**), begins to form around the developing follicle after it has become two to three cell layers thick. Known initially as the **theca folliculi,** this covering ul-

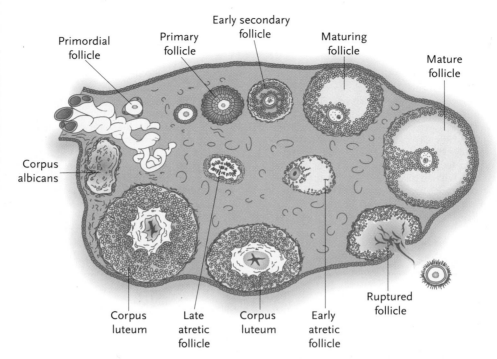

Figure 1-8 The sequence of maturation of follicles within the ovary, starting with the primordial follicle and ending with the formation of a corpus albicans.

BOX 1-1   Functional Processes in Ovarian Follicles that Depend on Factors Exchanged Between Oocytes and Follicular Cells

OOCYTE FUNCTIONS DEPENDENT ON FACTORS FROM GRANULOSA CELLS

Metabolism
Growth
Meiotic arrest
Maturation

GRANULOSA CELL FUNCTIONS DEPENDENT ON FACTORS FROM OOCYTES

Proliferation
Differentiation
Follicle organization
Cumulus expansion

From Eppig JJ: *Bioessays* 13:569-574, 1991.

---

timately differentiates into two layers: a highly vascularized and glandular **theca interna** and a more connective tissue–like outer capsule called the **theca externa.** The early thecal cells appear to secrete an **angiogenesis factor,** which stimulates the growth of blood vessels in the thecal layer. This nutritive support facilitates growth of the follicle.

Early development of the follicle occurs without the significant influence of hormones, but as puberty approaches, continued follicular maturation requires the action of the pituitary gonadotrophic hormone **follicle-stimulating hor-**

mone (**FSH**) on the granulosa cells, which have by this time developed FSH receptors on their surfaces (see Figure 1-9). After blood-borne FSH is bound to the FSH receptors, the stimulated granulosa cells produce small amounts of **estrogens.** The most obvious indication of the further development of some of the follicles is the formation of an **antrum,** a cavity filled with a fluid called **liquor folliculi.** Initially formed by secretions of the follicular cells, the antral fluid is later formed mostly as a transudate from the capillaries on the outer side of the membrana granulosa. With the appearance of the antrum, the follicle is called a **secondary follicle.**

Enlargement of the follicle results in large part from the proliferation of the granulosa cells. The direct stimulus for granulosa cell proliferation is a signaling protein, **activin,** a member of the **transforming growth factor-β (TGF-β)** family of signaling molecules (see Table 5-2). The local action of activin is enhanced by the actions of FSH.

Responding to the stimulus of pituitary hormones, secondary follicles produce significant amounts of steroid hormones. The cells of the theca interna possess receptors for **luteinizing hormone (LH),** also secreted by the anterior pituitary (see Figure 1-14). The theca interna cells produce **androgens** (e.g., testosterone), which pass through the membrana granulosa to the granulosa cells. The influence of FSH induces the granulosa cells to synthesize the enzyme (**aromatase**) that converts the theca-derived androgens into estrogens (mainly 17β-estradiol). Not only does the estradiol leave the follicle to exert important effects on other parts of the body, but it also stimulates the formation of LH receptors on the granulosa cells. Through this mechanism, the follic-

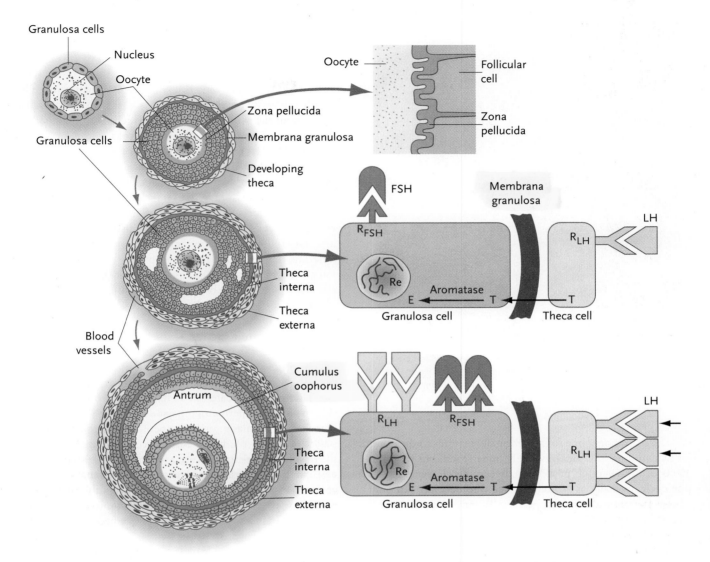

Figure 1-9 Growth and maturation of a follicle along with major endocrine interactions in the theca cells and granulosa cells. *E,* Estrogen; *R,* receptor; *T,* testosterone.

ular cells are able to respond to the large LH surge that immediately precedes ovulation (see Figure 1-15).

Under multiple hormonal influences, the follicle enlarges rapidly (Figs. 1-9 and 1-10) and presses against the surface of the ovary. At this point, it is called a **tertiary (graafian) follicle.** About 10 to 12 hours before ovulation, meiosis resumes.

The egg, now a secondary oocyte, is located in a small mound of cells known as the **cumulus oophorus,** which lies on one side of the greatly enlarged antrum. The oocyte appears to secrete a factor or factors that pass through the gap junctions into the surrounding cumulus cells. The factor enables the cumulus cells to respond to gonadotrophic hormones and to secrete hyaluronic acid, which results in an expansion of the cumulus oophorus. In keeping with the hormonally induced internal changes, the diameter of the follicle increases from about 6 mm early in the second week to almost 2 cm at ovulation.

The tertiary follicle protrudes from the surface of the ovary like a blister. The granulosa cells contain large numbers of both FSH and LH receptors, and LH receptors are abundant in the cells of the theca interna. The follicular cells secrete large amounts of estradiol (see Figure 1-15), which prepares many other components of the female reproductive tract for gamete transport. Within the antrum, the follicular fluid contains (1) a complement of proteins similar to that seen in serum but in a lower concentration; (2) as many as 20 enzymes; (3) dissolved hormones, including FSH, LH, and steroids; and (4) proteoglycans. The strong negative charge of the proteoglycans attracts water molecules, and with greater amounts of secreted proteoglycans, the volume of antral fluid increases correspondingly. The follicle is now poised for ovulation and awaits the stimulus of the preovulatory surge of FSH and LH released by the anterior pituitary gland.

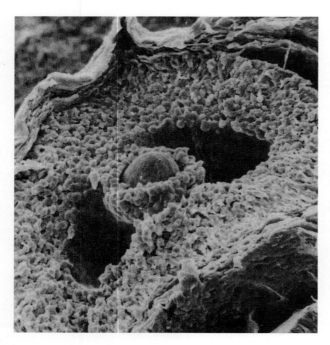

Figure 1-10 Scanning electron micrograph of a mature follicle in the rat ovary. The spherical oocyte (*center*) is surrounded by smaller cells of the corona radiata, which projects into the antrum. (×840.) (Courtesy P. Bagavandoss, Ann Arbor, Michigan.)

The reason only one follicle normally matures to the point of ovulation is still not completely understood, but some aspects of the selection process are becoming clearer. Early in the cycle, as many as 50 follicles begin to develop, but only about 3 attain a diameter as great as 8 mm. Initial follicular growth is gonadotropin independent, but continued growth depends on a minimum "tonic" level of gonadotropins, principally FSH. During the phase of gonadotropin-induced growth, one dominant enlarging follicle becomes independent of FSH and secretes large amounts of **inhibin** (see pp. 19-20). Inhibin suppresses the secretion of FSH by the pituitary, and when the FSH levels fall below the tonic threshold, the other developing follicles, which are still dependent on FSH for maintenance, become atretic. The dominant follicle acquires its status about 7 days before ovulation. It may also secrete an inhibiting substance that acts directly on the other growing follicles.

Spermatogenesis

Spermatogenesis begins in the seminiferous tubules of the testes after the onset of puberty. In the broadest sense, the process begins with mitotic proliferation of the spermatogonia. At the base of the **seminiferous epithelium** are several populations of spermatogonia. **Type A spermatogonia** represent the stem cell population that mitotically maintains proper numbers of spermatogonia throughout life. Type A spermatogonia give rise to **type B spermatogonia**, which are destined to leave the mitotic cycle and enter meiosis. Many spermatogonia and

their cellular descendants are connected by intercellular cytoplasmic bridges, which may be instrumental in maintaining the synchronous development of large clusters of sperm cells.

All spermatogonia are sequestered at the base of the seminiferous epithelium by interlocking processes of **Sertoli cells**, which are very complex cells that are regularly distributed throughout the periphery of the seminiferous epithelium and that occupy about 30% of its volume (see Figure 1-6). As the progeny of the type B spermatogonia (called *primary spermatocytes*) complete the leptotene stage of the first meiotic division, they pass through the Sertoli cell barrier to the interior of the seminiferous tubule. This translocation is accomplished by the formation of a new layer of Sertoli cell processes beneath these cells and slightly later, the dissolution of the original layer that was between them and the interior of the seminiferous tubule. The Sertoli cell processes are very tightly joined and form an immunological barrier (**blood-testis barrier**) [see Figure 1-6]) between the forming sperm cells and the rest of the body, including the spermatogonia. Once they have begun meiosis, developing sperm cells are immunologically different from the rest of the body. Autoimmune infertility can arise if the blood-testis barrier is broken down.

The progeny of the type B spermatogonia, which have entered the first meiotic division, are the **primary spermatocytes** (see Figure 1-6). Located in a characteristic position just inside the layer of spermatogonia and still deeply embedded in Sertoli cell cytoplasm, primary spermatocytes spend 24 days passing through the first meiotic division. During this time, the developing sperm cells use a strategy similar to that of the egg: namely, producing in advance molecules that are needed at later periods when changes occur very rapidly. Such preparation involves the production of mRNA molecules and their storage in an inactive form until they are needed to produce the necessary proteins.

A well-known example of preparatory mRNA synthesis involves the formation of **protamines**, which are small, arginine- and cysteine-rich proteins that displace the lysine-rich nuclear histones and allow the high degree of compaction of nuclear chromatin required during the final stages of sperm formation. Protamine mRNAs are first synthesized in primary spermatocytes but are not translated into proteins until the spermatid stage. In the meantime, the protamine mRNAs are complexed with proteins and are inaccessible to the translational machinery.

After completion of the first meiotic division, the primary spermatocyte gives rise to two **secondary spermatocytes**, which remain connected by a cytoplasmic bridge. The secondary spermatocytes enter the second meiotic division without delay. This phase of meiosis is very rapid, typically completed in approximately 8 hours. Each secondary spermatocyte produces two immature haploid gametes, the **spermatids**. The four spermatids produced from a primary spermatocyte progenitor are still connected to one another and typically to as many as 100 other spermatids as well. In mice, some genes are transcribed as late as the spermatid stage.

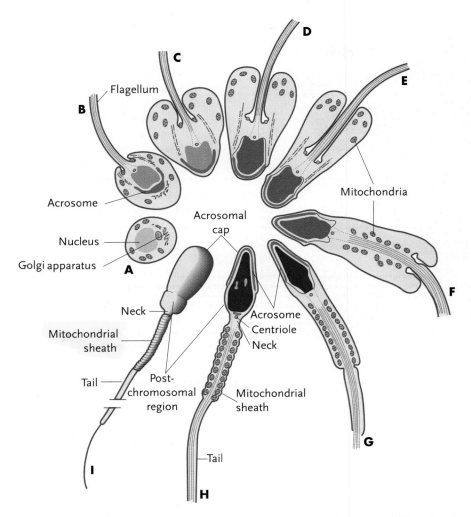

Figure 1-11 Summary of the major stages in spermiogenesis, starting with a spermatid (**A**) and ending with a mature spermatozoon (**I**).

Spermatids do not divide further, but they undergo a series of profound changes that transform them from relatively ordinary looking cells to highly specialized **spermatozoa** (singular, **spermatozoon**). The process of transformation from spermatids to spermatozoa is called **spermiogenesis** or **spermatid metamorphosis.**

Several major categories of change occur during spermiogenesis (Figure 1-11). One is the progressive reduction in the size of the nucleus and tremendous condensation of the chromosomal material, which is associated with the replacement of histones by protamines. Along with the changes in the nucleus, a profound reorganization of the cytoplasm occurs. Cytoplasm streams away from the nucleus, but a condensation of the Golgi apparatus at the apical end of the nucleus ultimately gives rise to the **acrosome.** The acrosome is an enzyme-filled structure that plays a very important role in the fertilization process. At the other end of the nucleus, a prominent **flagellum** grows out of the centriolar region. **Mitochondria** are arranged in a spiral around the proximal part of the flagellum.

During spermiogenesis, the plasma membrane of the head of the sperm is partitioned into a number of antigenically distinct molecular domains. These domains undergo numerous changes as the sperm cells mature in the male and at a later point when the spermatozoa are traveling through the female reproductive tract. As spermiogenesis continues, the remainder of the cytoplasm (**residual body**) moves away from the nucleus and is shed along the developing tail of the sperm cell. The residual bodies are phagocytosed by Sertoli cells.

For many years, gene expression in postmeiotic (haploid) spermatids was considered to be impossible. However, molecular biological research on mice has shown that gene expression in postmeiotic spermatids is not only possible but common. Nearly 100 proteins that are produced only after the completion of the second meiotic division have been identified, and many additional proteins are synthesized both during and after meiosis (Figure 1-12).

After spermiogenesis (approximately 64 days after the start of spermatogenesis), the **spermatozoon** is a highly specialized

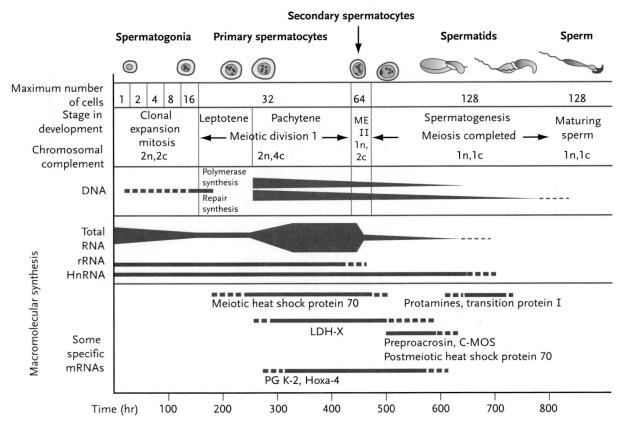

Figure 1-12 Summary of the major events in spermatogenesis in the mouse, with specific examples of macromolecular synthesis superimposed. The solid lines represent qualitative periods of known synthesis. Broken segments in the lines represent uncertainty about the onset or duration of the activity. Bars with varying thicknesses represent relative amounts of the gene product that is represented. *LDH-X,* Lactic dehydrogenase; *ME II,* second meiotic division. (Modified from Erickson RP: *Trends Genet* 6:264-269, 1990.)

cell well adapted for motion and the delivery of its packet of DNA to the egg. The sperm cell consists of a head (2 to 3 μm wide and 4 to 5 μm long) containing the nucleus and acrosome; a midpiece containing the centrioles, the proximal part of the flagellum, and the mitochondrial helix; and the tail (about 50 μm long), which consists of a highly specialized flagellum (see Figure 1-11). (Specific functional properties of these components of the sperm cell are discussed in Chapter 2.)

Although spermatozoa in the seminiferous tubules appear to be mature by morphological criteria, they are nonmotile and incapable of fertilizing an egg. From the testis, they are carried to the **epididymis** via fluid currents that originate in the seminiferous tubules. While in transit through the epididymis, the spermatozoa undergo biochemical maturation, becoming covered with a glycoprotein coating and experiencing other surface modifications. The glycoprotein coating is removed in the female reproductive tract through the **capacitation** reaction, thus rendering the spermatozoa capable of fertilizing an egg. Final biochemical maturation and provision of the spermatozoa with an external energy source occur when the ejaculated sperm are mixed with secretions of the **prostate gland** and **seminal vesi-**

cles during ejaculation. At this point, the spermatozoa are provided with an environment conducive to independent motion.

Abnormal Spermatozoa. Substantial numbers (up to 10%) of mature spermatozoa are grossly abnormal. The spectrum of anomalies ranges from double heads or tails to defective flagella or variability in head size. Such defective sperm cells are highly unlikely to fertilize an egg. If the percentage of defective spermatozoa rises above 20% of the total, reduced fertility may result.

PREPARATION OF THE FEMALE REPRODUCTIVE TRACT FOR PREGNANCY

Structure

The structure and function of the female reproductive tract are well adapted for the transport of gametes and maintenance of the embryo. Many of the subtler features of this adaptation are under hormonal control and are cyclic. This section briefly reviews the aspects of female reproductive structure

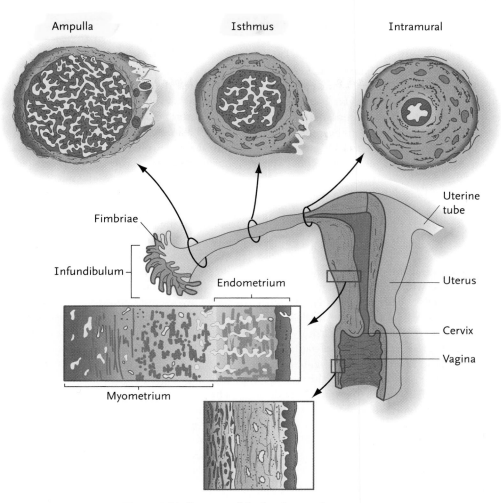

Figure 1-13 Structure of the female reproductive tract.

that are of greatest importance in understanding gamete transport and embryonic development.

Ovaries and uterine tubes

The **ovaries** and **uterine** (or **fallopian**) **tubes** form a functional complex devoted to the production and transport of eggs. The almond-shaped ovaries, located on either side of the uterus, are positioned very near the open, funnel-shaped ends of the uterine tubes. Numerous small, fingerlike projections called **fimbriae** (Figure 1-13) project from the open **infundibulum** of the uterine tube toward the ovary and are involved in directing the ovulated egg into the tube. The uterine tube is characterized by a very complex internal lining with a high density of prominent longitudinal folds in the upper **ampulla** and a simpler lining nearer to the uterus. The lining epithelium of the uterine tubes contains a mixture of ciliated cells that assist in gamete transport and secretory cells that produce a fluid supporting early development of the embryo. Layers of smooth muscle throughout the uterine tubes provide the basis for peristaltic contrac-

tions. The amount and function of many of these components are under cyclic hormonal control, and the overall effect of these changes is to facilitate the transport of gametes and the fertilized egg.

Uterus

The principal functions of the uterus are to receive and maintain the embryo during pregnancy and to expel the fetus at the termination of pregnancy. The first function is carried out by the uterine mucosa (endometrium) and the second by the muscular wall (myometrium). Under the cyclic effect of hormones, the uterus undergoes a series of prominent changes throughout the course of each menstrual cycle.

The **uterus** is a pear-shaped organ with thick walls of smooth muscle (**myometrium**) and a complex mucosal lining (see Figure 1-13). The mucosal lining, called the **endometrium**, has a structure that changes daily throughout the menstrual cycle. The endometrium can be subdivided into two layers: a **functional layer** that is shed with each menstrual period or after parturition and a **basal layer** that remains intact. The general structure of the endometrium consists of (1) a columnar **surface epithelium**, (2) **uterine glands**, (3) a specialized connective tissue stroma, and (4) **spiral arteries** that coil from the basal layer toward the surface of the endometrium. All these structures participate in the implantation and nourishment of the embryo.

The lower outlet of the uterus is the **cervix**. The mucosal surface of the cervix is not typical uterine endometrium but is studded with a variety of irregular crypts. The cervical epithelium produces a glycoprotein-rich cervical mucus, the composition of which varies considerably throughout the menstrual cycle. The differing physical properties of cervical mucus make it easier or more difficult for spermatozoa to penetrate through the cervix and find their way into the uterus.

Vagina

The **vagina** is a channel for sexual intercourse and also serves as the birth canal. It is lined with a stratified squamous epithelium, but the epithelial cells contain deposits of **glycogen**, which vary in amount throughout the menstrual cycle. Glycogen breakdown products contribute to the acidity (pH, 4.3) of the vaginal fluids. The low pH of the upper vagina appears to serve a bacteriostatic function and prevents infectious agents from entering the upper genital tract through the cervix and ultimately spreading to the peritoneal cavity through the open ends of the uterine tubes.

Hormonal Control of the Female Reproductive Cycle

Reproduction in the human female is governed by a complex series of interactions between hormones and the tissues that they influence. The hierarchy of cyclic control begins with input to the **hypothalamus** of the brain (Figure 1-14). The hypothalamus influences hormone production by the anterior lobe of the pituitary gland. The pituitary hormones are spread via the blood throughout the entire body and act on the ovaries, which are in turn stimulated to produce their own sex steroid hormones. During pregnancy, the placenta exerts a powerful effect on the mother by producing a number of hormones. The final level of hormonal control of female reproduction is that exerted by the ovarian or placental hormones on other reproductive target organs (e.g., uterus, uterine tubes, vagina, breasts).

Hypothalamic control

The first level of hormonal control of reproduction resides in the hypothalamus. Various inputs stimulate neurosecretory cells in the hypothalamus to produce **gonadotropin-releasing hormone (GnRH)** along with releasing factors for other pituitary hormones. Releasing factors as well as an inhibiting factor are carried to the anterior lobe of the pituitary gland by blood vessels of the **hypothalamohypophyseal portal system**, where they stimulate the secretion of pituitary hormones (Table 1-1).

Pituitary gland (hypophysis)

Producing its hormones in response to stimulation by the hypothalamus, the **pituitary gland** constitutes a second level of hormonal control of reproduction. The pituitary gland consists of two components: the **anterior pituitary (adenohypophysis)**, an epithelial glandular structure that produces various hormones in response to factors carried to it by the hypothalamohypophyseal portal system, and the **posterior pituitary (neurohypophysis)**, a neural structure that releases hormones by a neurosecretory mechanism.

Under the influence of GnRH and direct feedback by steroid hormone levels in the blood, the anterior pituitary secretes two polypeptide **gonadotrophic hormones**, FSH and LH, from the same cell type (see Table 1-1). In the absence of an inhibiting factor (**dopamine**) from the hypothalamus, the anterior pituitary also produces **prolactin**, which acts on the mammary glands.

The only hormone from the posterior pituitary that is directly involved in reproduction is **oxytocin**, an oligopeptide involved in childbirth and the stimulus for milk let-down from the mammary glands in lactating women.

Ovaries and placenta

The ovaries and, during pregnancy, the placenta constitute a third level of hormonal control. Responding to blood levels of the anterior pituitary hormones, the granulosa cells of the ovarian follicles convert androgens (**androstenedione** and **testosterone**) synthesized by the theca interna into estrogens (mainly **estrone** and the tenfold more powerful **17β-estradiol**), which then pass into the bloodstream. After ovulation, **progesterone** is the principal secretory product of the follicle after its conversion into the corpus luteum (see Chapter 2). During later pregnancy, the placenta supplements the production of ovarian steroid hormone by synthesizing its own estrogens and progesterone. It also produces two polypeptide hormones (see Table 1-1). **Human chorionic gonadotropin (HCG)** acts on the ovary to maintain the activity of the corpus luteum during pregnancy. **Human placental lactogen (somatomammotropin)** acts on the corpus luteum; it also promotes breast development by enhancing the effects of estrogens and progesterone and stimulates the synthesis of milk constituents.

Reproductive target tissues

The last level in the hierarchy of reproductive hormonal control constitutes the target tissues, which ready themselves both structurally and functionally for gamete transport or pregnancy in response to ovarian and placental hormones binding to specific cellular receptors. Changes in the number of ciliated cells and in smooth muscle activity in the uterine tubes, the profound changes in the endometrial lining of the uterus, and the cyclic changes in the glandular tissues of the breasts are some of the more prominent examples of hormonal effects on target tissues. These changes are described more fully later.

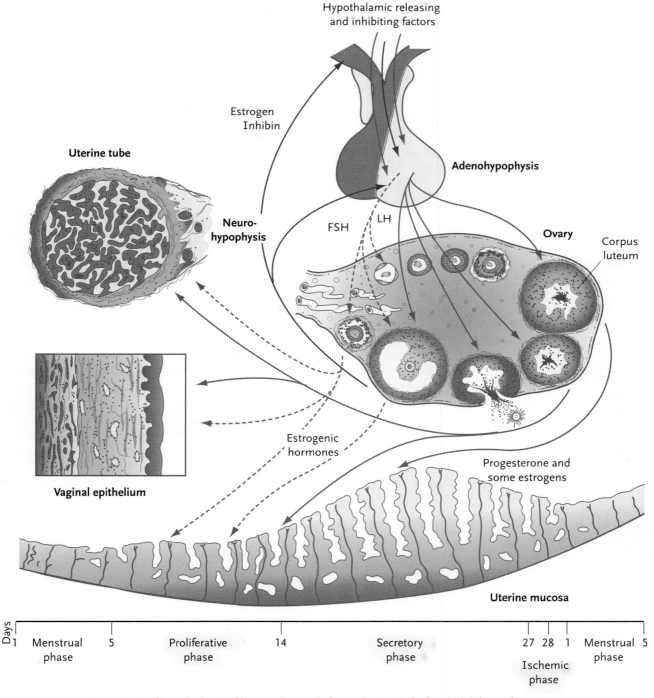

Figure 1-14 General scheme of hormonal control of reproduction in the female. Inhibitory factors are represented by purple arrows. Stimulatory factors are represented by red arrows. Hormones involved principally in the proliferative phase of the menstrual cycle are represented by dashed arrows; those involved principally in the secretory phase are solid.

TABLE 1-1   Major Hormones Involved in Mammalian Reproduction

Hormone	Chemical nature	Function
HYPOTHALAMUS		
Gonadotropin-releasing hormone (GnRH, LHRH)	Decapeptide	Stimulates release of LH and FSH by anterior pituitary
Prolactin-inhibiting factor	Dopamine	Inhibits release of prolactin by anterior pituitary
ANTERIOR PITUITARY		
Follicle-stimulating hormone (FSH)	Glycoprotein (α and β subunits) (MW, ~35,000)	Male: Stimulates Sertoli cells to produce androgen-binding protein Female: Stimulates follicle cells to produce estrogen
Luteinizing hormone (LH)	Glycoprotein (α and β subunits) (MW, ~28,000)	Male: Stimulates Leydig cells to secrete testosterone Female: Stimulates follicle cells and corpus luteum to produce progesterone
Prolactin	Single-chain polypeptide (198 amino acids)	Promotes lactation
POSTERIOR PITUITARY		
Oxytocin	Oligopeptide (MW, ~1100)	Stimulates ejection of milk by mammary gland
OVARY		
Estrogens	Steroid	Has multiple effects on reproductive tract, breasts, body fat, and bone growth
Progesterone	Steroid	Has multiple effects on reproductive tract and breast development
Testosterone	Steroid	Is precursor for estrogen biosynthesis, induces follicular atresia
Inhibin	Protein (MW, ~32,000)	Inhibits FSH secretion, has local effects on ovaries
Activin	Protein (MW, ~28,000)	Stimulates granulosa cell proliferation
TESTIS		
Testosterone	Steroid	Has multiple effects on male reproductive tract, hair growth, and other secondary sexual characteristics
Inhibin	Protein (MW, ~32,000)	Inhibits FSH secretion, has local effects on testis
PLACENTA		
Estrogens	Steroid	Has same functions as ovarian estrogens
Progesterone	Steroid	Has same functions as ovarian progesterone
Human chorionic gonadotrophin (HCG)	Glycoprotein (MW, ~30,000)	Maintains activity of corpus luteum during pregnancy
Human placental lactogen (somatomammotropin)	Polypeptide (MW, ~20,000)	Promotes development of breasts during pregnancy

LHRH, Luteinizing hormone–releasing hormone; *MW*, molecular weight.

A general principle recognized some time ago is the efficacy of first priming reproductive target tissues with estrogen so that progesterone can exert its full effects. Estrogen induces the target cells to produce large quantities of progesterone receptors, which must be in place for progesterone to act on these same cells.

Hormonal Interactions with Tissues during Female Reproductive Cycles

All tissues of the female reproductive tract are influenced by the reproductive hormones. In response to the hormonal environment of the body, they undergo cyclic modifications that improve the chances for successful reproduction.

Knowledge of the changes the ovaries undergo is necessary to understand hormonal interactions and tissue responses during the female reproductive cycle. Responding to both FSH and LH secreted by the pituitary just before and during a menstrual period, a set of secondary ovarian follicles begins to mature and secrete 17β-estradiol. By ovulation, all of these follicles except one have undergone atresia, their main contribution having been to produce part of the supply of estrogens needed to prepare the body for ovulation and gamete transport.

During the preovulatory, or **proliferative, phase** (days 5 to 14) of the menstrual cycle, estrogens produced by the ovary act on the female reproductive tissues (see Figure 1-14). The uterine lining becomes reepithelialized from the just-completed menstrual period. Then, under the influence of estrogens, the endometrial stroma progressively thickens, the uterine glands elongate, and the spiral arteries begin to grow toward the surface of the endometrium. The mucous glands of the cervix secrete a glycoprotein-rich but relatively watery mucus, which facilitates the passage of spermatozoa through the cervical canal. As the proliferative phase progresses, a higher percentage of the epithelial cells lining the uterine tubes becomes ciliated, and smooth muscle activity in the tubes increases. In the days preceding ovulation, the fimbriated ends of the uterine tubes move closer to the ovaries.

Toward the end of the proliferative period, a pronounced increase in the levels of estradiol secreted by the developing ovarian follicle acts on the hypothalamohypophyseal system, causing increased responsiveness of the anterior pituitary to GnRH and a surge in the hypothalamic secretion of GnRH. Approximately 24 hours after the level of 17β-estradiol reaches its peak in the blood, a preovulatory surge of LH and FSH is sent into the bloodstream by the pituitary gland (Figure 1-15). The **LH surge** is not a steady increase in gonadotropin secretion; rather, it constitutes a series of sharp pulses of secretion that appear to be responding to a hypothalamic timing mechanism.

The LH surge leads to ovulation, and the graafian follicle becomes transformed into a **corpus luteum** (yellow body). The basal lamina surrounding the granulosa of the follicle breaks down and allows blood vessels to grow into the layer of granulosa cells. Through proliferation and hypertrophy, the granulosa cells undergo major structural and biochemical changes and now produce progesterone as their primary secretory product. Some estrogen is still secreted by the corpus luteum. After ovulation, the menstrual cycle, which is now dominated by the secretion of progesterone, is said to be in the **secretory phase** (days 14 to 28 of the menstrual cycle).

After the LH surge and with the increasing concentration of progesterone in the blood, the basal body temperature rises (see Figure 1-15). Because of the link between a rise in basal body temperature and the time of ovulation, accurate temperature records are the basis of the **rhythm method** of birth control.

Around the time of ovulation, the combined presence of estrogen and progesterone in the blood causes the uterine tube to engage in a rhythmic series of muscular contractions designed to promote transport of the ovulated egg. Progesterone prompts epithelial cells of the uterine tube to secrete fluids that provide nutrition for the cleaving embryo. Later during the secretory phase, high levels of progesterone induce regression of some of the ciliated cells in the tubal epithelium.

In the uterus, progesterone prepares the estrogen-primed endometrium for implantation of the embryo. The endometrium, which has thickened under the influence of estrogen during the proliferative phase, undergoes further changes. The straight uterine glands begin to coil and accumulate glycogen and other secretory products in the ep-

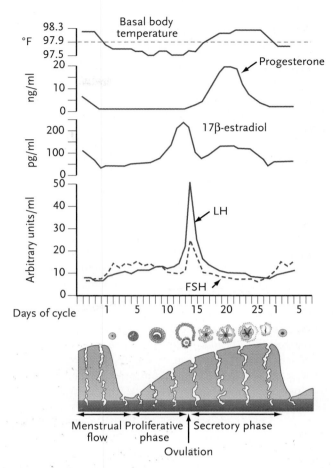

Figure 1-15 Comparison of curves representing daily serum concentrations of gonadotropins and sex steroids and basal body temperature in relation to events in the human menstrual cycle. (Redrawn from Midgley AR and others. In Hafez ES, Evans TN, eds: *Human reproduction,* New York, 1973, Harper & Row.)

ithelium. The spiral arteries grow farther toward the endometrial surface, but mitosis in the endometrial epithelial cells decreases. Through the action of progesterone, the cervical mucus becomes highly viscous and acts as a protective block, inhibiting the passage of materials into or out of the uterus. During the secretory period, the vaginal epithelium becomes thinner.

In the mammary glands, progesterone furthers the estrogen-primed development of the secretory components and causes water retention in the tissues. However, more extensive development of the lactational apparatus awaits its stimulation by placental hormones.

Midway through the secretory phase of the menstrual cycle, the epithelium of the uterine tubes has already undergone considerable regression from its midcycle peak, whereas the uterine endometrium is at full readiness to receive a cleaving embryo. If pregnancy does not occur, a series of hormonal interactions bring the menstrual cycle to a close. One of the early feedback mechanisms is the production of the protein **inhibin**

TABLE 1-2   Homologies between Hormone-Producing Cells in Male and Female Gonads

Parameter	Granulosa cells (female)	Sertoli cells (male)	Theca cells (female)	Leydig cells (male)
Origin	Rete ovarii	Rete testis	Stromal mesenchyme	Stromal mesenchyme
Major receptors	FSH	FSH	LH	LH
Major secretory products	Estrogens, progesterone, inhibin	Estrogen, inhibin, androgen-binding protein	Androgens	Testosterone

by the granulosa cells. Inhibin is carried by the bloodstream to the anterior pituitary, where it directly inhibits the secretion of gonadotropins, especially FSH. Through mechanisms that are still unclear, the secretion of LH is also reduced. This inhibition results in regression of the corpus luteum and marked reduction in the secretion of progesterone by the ovary.

Some of the main consequences of the regression of the corpus luteum are the infiltration of the endometrial stroma with leukocytes, the loss of interstitial fluid, and the spasmodic constriction and breakdown of the spiral arteries, causing local ischemia. The ischemia results in local hemorrhage and the loss of integrity of areas of the endometrium. These changes initiate menstruation (by convention, constituting days 1 to 5 of the menstrual cycle). Over the next few days, the entire functional layer of the endometrium is shed in small bits, along with the attendant loss of about 30 ml of blood. By the time the menstrual period is over, only a raw endometrial base interspersed with the basal epithelium of the uterine glands remains as the basis for the healing and reconstitution of the endometrium during the next proliferative period.

HORMONAL INTERACTIONS INVOLVED WITH REPRODUCTION IN MALES

Along with the homologies of certain structures between the testis and ovary, some strong parallels exist between the hormonal interactions involved in reproduction in males and females. The most important homologies are between granulosa cells in the ovarian follicle and Sertoli cells in the seminiferous tubule of the testis and between theca cells of the ovary and Leydig cells in the testis (Table 1-2).

The hypothalamic secretion of GnRH stimulates the anterior pituitary to secrete FSH and LH. The LH binds to the nearly 20,000 LH receptors on the surface of each Leydig (interstitial) cell, and through a cascade of second messengers involving cyclic adenosine monophosphate and protein phosphorylation, LH stimulates the synthesis of testosterone from cholesterol. Testosterone is released into the blood and is taken to the Sertoli cells and throughout the body, where it affects a variety of secondary sexual tissues, often after it has been locally converted to dihydrotestosterone.

BOX 1-2   Major Functions of Sertoli Cells

Maintenance of the blood-testis barrier
Secretion of tubular fluid (10 to 20 μL/gm of testis/hr)
Secretion of androgen-binding protein
Secretion of inhibin
Secretion of a wide variety of other proteins (e.g., growth factors, transferrin, retinal-binding protein, metal-binding proteins)
Maintenance and coordination of spermatogenesis
Phagocytosis of residual bodies of sperm cells

CLINICAL VIGNETTE

A 33-year-old woman has had both ovaries removed because of large bilateral ovarian cysts. The next year she is on an extended expedition in northern Canada, and her canoe tips, sending her replacement hormonal medication to the bottom of the lake. More than 6 weeks elapse before she is able to obtain a new supply of medication.

Which of the following would be least affected by the loss of the woman's medication?
  A. Blood levels of FSH and LH
  B. Ciliated cells of the uterine tube
  C. Mass of the heart
  D. Glandular tissue of the breasts
  E. Thickness of the endometrium

Sertoli cells are stimulated by pituitary FSH via surface FSH receptors and by testosterone from the Leydig cells via cytoplasmic receptors. After FSH stimulation, the Sertoli cells convert some of the testosterone to estrogens (as the granulosa cells in the ovary do). Some of the estrogen diffuses back to the Leydig cells along with a **Leydig cell stimulatory factor**, which is produced by the Sertoli cells and reaches the Leydig cells by a **paracrine** (non–blood-borne) mode of secretion (Figure 1-16). The FSH-stimulated Sertoli cell produces **androgen-binding protein**, which binds testosterone and is carried into the fluid compartment of the seminiferous

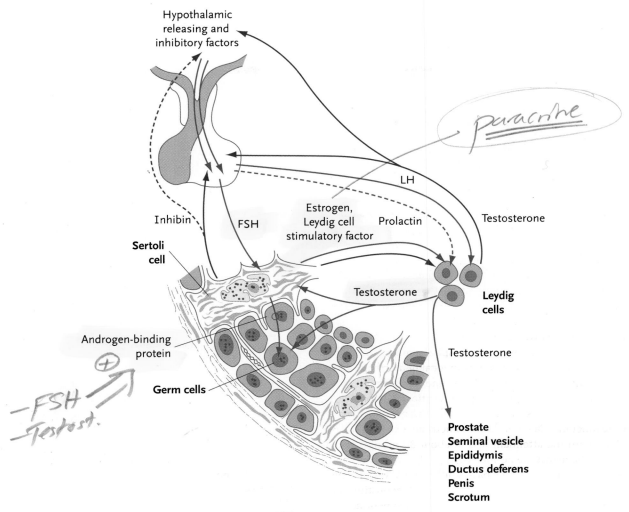

Figure 1-16 General scheme of hormonal control in the male reproductive system. Red arrows represent stimulatory influences. Purple arrows represent inhibitory influences. Suspected interactions are represented by dashed arrows.

tubule, where it exerts a strong influence on the course of spermatogenesis. Like their granulosa cell counterparts in the ovary, the hormone-stimulated Sertoli cells produce inhibin, which is carried by the blood to the anterior pituitary and possibly the hypothalamus. There inhibin acts by negative feedback to inhibit the secretion of FSH. In addition to inhibin and androgen-binding protein, the Sertoli cells have a wide variety of other functions, the most important of which are summarized in Box 1-2.

SUMMARY

- Gametogenesis is divided into four phases:
    1. Extraembryonic origin of germ cells and their migration into the gonads
    2. An increase in the number of germ cells by mitosis
    3. A reduction in chromosomal material by meiosis
    4. Structural and functional maturation

- Primordial germ cells are first readily recognizable in the yolk sac endoderm. They then migrate through the dorsal mesentery to the primordia of the gonads.
- In the female, oogonia undergo intense mitotic activity in the embryo only. In the male, spermatogonia are capable of mitosis throughout life.
- Meiosis involves a reduction in chromosome number from diploid to haploid, independent reassortment of paternal and maternal chromosomes, and further redistribution of genetic material through the process of crossing-over.
- In the oocyte, there are two meiotic blocks—in diplotene of prophase I and in metaphase II. In the female, meiosis begins in the 5-month embryo; in the male, meiosis begins at puberty.
- Failure of chromosomes to separate properly during meiosis results in nondisjunction, which is associated with multiple anomalies depending on which chromosome is affected.
- Developing oocytes are surrounded by layers of follicular cells and interact with them through gap junctions. When stimulated

CLINICAL CORRELATION 1-2
Dating of Pregnancy

Two different systems for dating pregnancies have evolved. One, used by embryologists, dates pregnancy from the time of fertilization **(fertilization age)**, so that a 6-week-old embryo is 6 weeks (42 days) from the day of fertilization. The other system, used by obstetricians and many clinicians, dates pregnancy from the woman's last menstrual period **(menstrual age)** because this is a convenient reference point from the standpoint of a history taken from a patient. The menstrual age of a human embryo is 2 weeks greater than the fertilization age because usually 2 weeks elapse between the start of the last menstrual period and fertilization. Thus an embryo with a fertilization age of 6 weeks is assigned a menstrual age of 8 weeks, and the typical duration of pregnancy is 38 weeks' fertilization age and 40 weeks' menstrual age (Figure 1-17; see also Figure 17-16).

For valid clinical reasons, obstetricians subdivide pregnancy into three equal **trimesters,** whereas em-bryologists divide pregnancy into unequal periods corresponding to major developmental events.

0-3 weeks   Early development (cleavage, gastrulation)
4-8 weeks   Period of embryonic organogenesis
9-38 weeks   Fetal period

A recognition of the existence of different systems for dating pregnancy is essential. In a courtroom case involving a lawsuit about a birth defect, a 2-week misunderstanding about the date of a pregnancy could make the difference between winning or losing the case. In a case involving a cleft lip or cleft palate (see p. 303), the difference in development of the face between 6 and 8 weeks (see Figure 13-6) would make some scenarios impossible. For example, an insult at 6 weeks could potentially be the cause of a cleft lip, whereas by 8 weeks, the lips have formed, so a cleft would be most unlikely to form at that time.

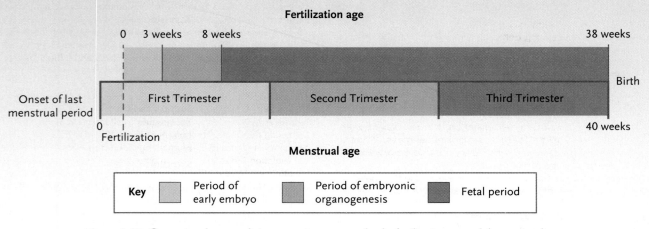

Figure 1-17 Comparison between dating events in pregnancy by the fertilization age and the menstrual age.

by pituitary hormones (e.g., FSH, LH), the follicular cells produce steroid hormones (estrogens and progesterone). The combination of oocyte and follicular (granulosa) cells is called a *follicle.* Under hormonal stimulation, certain follicles greatly increase in size, and each month, one of these follicles undergoes ovulation.

- Spermatogenesis occurs in the testis and involves successive waves of mitosis of spermatogonia, meiosis of primary and secondary spermatocytes, and final maturation (spermiogenesis) of postmeiotic spermatids into spermatozoa. Functional maturation of spermatozoa occurs in the epididymis.
- Female reproductive tissues undergo cyclic, hormonally induced preparatory changes for pregnancy. In the uterine tubes, this involves the degree of ciliation of the epithelium and smooth muscle activity of the wall. Under the influence of estrogens and then progesterone, the endometrium of the uterus builds up in prepa-ration to receive the embryo. In the absence of fertilization and with the subsequent withdrawal of hormonal support, the endometrium breaks down and is shed (menstruation). Cyclic changes in the cervix involve thinning of the cervical mucus at the time of ovulation.

- Hormonal control of the female reproductive cycle is hierarchical, with releasing or inhibiting factors from the hypothalamus acting on the adenohypophysis, causing the release of pituitary hormones (e.g., FSH, LH). The pituitary hormones sequentially stimulate the ovarian follicles to produce estrogens and progesterone, which act on the female reproductive tissues. In pregnancy, the remains of the follicle (corpus luteum) continue to produce progesterone, which maintains the early embryo until the placenta begins to produce sufficient hormones to maintain pregnancy.
- In the male, LH stimulates the Leydig cells to produce testosterone, and FSH acts on the Sertoli cells, which support sper-

matogenesis. In both the male and the female, feedback inhibition decreases the production of pituitary hormones.

- There are two systems for dating pregnancy:
  1. Fertilization age: dates the age of the embryo from the time of fertilization.
  2. Menstrual age: dates the age of the embryo from the start of the mother's last menstrual period. The menstrual age is 2 weeks greater than the fertilization age.

REVIEW QUESTIONS

1. During spermatogenesis, histone is replaced by what to allow better packing of the condensed chromatin in the head of the spermatozoon?
    - A. Inhibin
    - B. Prostaglandin E
    - C. Testosterone
    - D. Protamine
    - E. Androgen-binding protein
2. Which cell type is located outside the blood-testis barrier?
    - A. Spermatozoon
    - B. Secondary spermatocyte
    - C. Spermatid
    - D. Primary spermatocyte
    - E. Spermatogonium
3. Which of the following cells normally participates in mitotic divisions?
    - A. Primary oocyte
    - B. Oogonium
    - C. Primary spermatocyte
    - D. Spermatid
    - E. Secondary spermatocyte
4. In a routine chest x-ray examination, the radiologist sees what appears to be teeth in a mediastinal mass. What is the likely diagnosis, and what is a probable embryological explanation for its appearance?
5. When does meiosis begin in the female and in the male?
6. At what stages of oogenesis is meiosis arrested in the female?
7. What is the underlying cause of most spontaneous abortions during the early weeks of pregnancy?
8. What is the difference between spermatogenesis and spermiogenesis?
9. The actions of what hormones are responsible for the changes in the endometrium during the menstrual cycle?
10. Sertoli cells in the testis are stimulated by what two major reproductive hormones?

REFERENCES

Browder LW, ed: *Developmental biology*, vol 1, *Oogenesis*, New York, 1985, Plenum.

Clermont Y: The cycle of the seminiferous epithelium in man, *Am J Anat* 112:35-51, 1963.

Dym M: Spermatogonial stem cells of the testis, *Proc Natl Acad Sci USA* 91:11287-11289, 1994.

Eddy EM and others: Origin and migration of primordial germ cells in mammals, *Gamete Res* 4:333-362, 1981.

Eppig JJ: Intercommunication between mammalian oocytes and companion somatic cells, *Bioessays* 13:569-574, 1991.

Erickson RP: Post-meiotic gene expression, *Trends Genet* 6(8):264-269, 1990.

Fawcett DW: *A textbook of histology*, Philadelphia, 1986, WB Saunders.

Gilbert EF, Opitz JM: Developmental and other pathological changes in syndromes caused by chromosome anomalies, *Perspect Pediatr Pathol* 7:1-63, 1982.

Gougeon A: *Dynamics of follicular growth.* In Adashi EY, Leung PCK, eds: *The ovary*, New York, 1993, Raven, pp 21-39.

Halvorson LM, DeCherney AH: Inhibin, activin, and follistatin in reproductive medicine, *Fertil Steril* 65:459-469, 1996.

Kerr JB: Functional cytology of the human testis, *Bailleres Clin Endocrinol Metab* 6(2):235-250, 1992.

Knobil E, Neill JD, eds: *The physiology of reproduction*, ed 2, New York, 1994, Raven.

Larson WJ and others: Expansion of the cumulus-oocyte complex during the preovulatory period: possible roles in oocyte maturation, ovulation, and fertilization. In Familiari G, Makabe S, Motta PM, eds: *Ultrastructure of the ovary*, Boston, 1991, Kluwer Academic, pp 45-61.

Mather JP, Moore A, Li R-H: Activins, inhibins, and follistatins: further thoughts on a growing family of regulators, *Proc Soc Exp Biol Med* 215:209-222, 1997.

Moodbidri SB, Garde SV, Sheth AR: Inhibin: unity in diversity, *Arch Androl* 28:149-157, 1992.

Salustri A and others: Oocyte-granulosa cell interactions. In Adashi EY, Leung PCK, eds: *The ovary*, New York, 1993, Raven, pp 209-225.

Shoham Z and others: The luteinizing hormone surge: the final stage in ovulation induction: modern aspects of ovulation triggering, *Fertil Steril* 64:237-251, 1995.

Taieb F, Thibier C, Jessus C: On cyclins, oocytes and eggs, *Mol Reprod Devel* 48:397-411, 1997.

Verhoeven G: Local control systems within the testis, *Bailleres Clin Endocrinol Metab* 6(2):313-333, 1992.

Willard HF: Centromeres of mammalian chromosomes, *Trends Genet* 6(12):410-416, 1990.

Wynn RM: *Biology of the uterus*, New York, 1977, Plenum.

Zamboni L: Physiology and pathophysiology of the human spermatozoon: the role of electron microscopy, *J Electron Microsc Tech* 17:412-436, 1991.

2

TRANSPORT OF GAMETES
AND FERTILIZATION

Chapter 1 describes the origins and maturation of male and female gametes and the hormonal conditions that make such maturation possible. It also describes the cyclic, hormonally controlled changes in the female reproductive tract that ready it for fertilization and the support of embryonic development. This chapter first explains the way the egg and sperm cells come together in the female reproductive tract so that fertilization can occur. It also outlines the complex set of interactions involved in fertilization of the egg by a sperm.

OVULATION AND EGG AND SPERM TRANSPORT

Ovulation

Toward the midpoint of the menstrual cycle, the mature graafian follicle, containing the egg that has been arrested in prophase of the first meiotic division, has moved to the surface of the ovary. Under the influence of follicle-stimulating hormone (FSH) and luteinizing hormone (LH), the follicle expands dramatically. The first meiotic division is completed, and the second meiotic division proceeds until the metaphase stage, at which the second meiotic arrest occurs. After the first meiotic division, the first polar body is expelled. By this point, the follicle bulges from the surface of the ovary. The apex of the protrusion is the **stigma.**

The stimulus for ovulation is the surge of LH secreted by the anterior pituitary at the midpoint of the menstrual cycle. Within minutes after the sharp rise in LH concentration in the blood, local blood flow increases in the outer layers of the follicular wall and throughout the ovary as well. Along with increased blood flow, plasma proteins leak into the tissues through the postcapillary venules, resulting in local edema. The edema and the release of a number of pharmacologically active compounds, such as prostaglandins, histamine, and vasopressin, provide the starting point for a series of reactions that results in the local production of

collagenase (Figure 2-1). At the same time, the secretion of hyaluronic acid by the granulosa cells results in loosening of the granulosa layers. The collagen degradation, the ischemia, and the death of some of the overlying cells cause a weakness of the outer follicular wall. The weakened follicular wall, with possible contributions by the steady pressure of the antral fluid (about 15 to 20 mm Hg), and the contraction of local smooth muscle–like elements lead to rupture of the outer follicular wall about 28 to 36 hours after the LH surge.

Ovulation results in the expulsion of both antral fluid and the ovum from the ovary into the peritoneal cavity. The ovum, however, is not ovulated as a single naked cell but as a complex consisting of (1) the ovum, (2) the zona pellucida, (3) the two- to three-cell-thick corona radiata, and (4) a sticky matrix containing surrounding cells of the cumulus oophorus. By convention, the adhering cells are designated as **corona radiata** after ovulation has occurred. Normally, one egg is released at ovulation. The release and fertilization of two eggs can result in fraternal twinning.

Some women experience mild to pronounced pain at the time of ovulation. Often called **Mittelschmerz** (German for "middle pain"), such pain may accompany slight bleeding from the ruptured follicle. Another sign of ovulation is a slight rise in basal body temperature. This has often been used as a reference point in rhythm methods of contraception.

Egg Transport

The first step in egg transport is capture of the ovulated egg by the uterine tube. Shortly before ovulation, the epithelial cells of the uterine tube become more highly ciliated, and smooth muscle activity in the tube and its suspensory ligament increases as the result of hormonal influences. By ovulation, the fimbriae of the uterine tube move closer to the ovary and seem to rhythmically sweep over its surface. This action, plus the currents set up by the cilia, efficiently captures the ovulated egg complex. Experimental studies on rab-

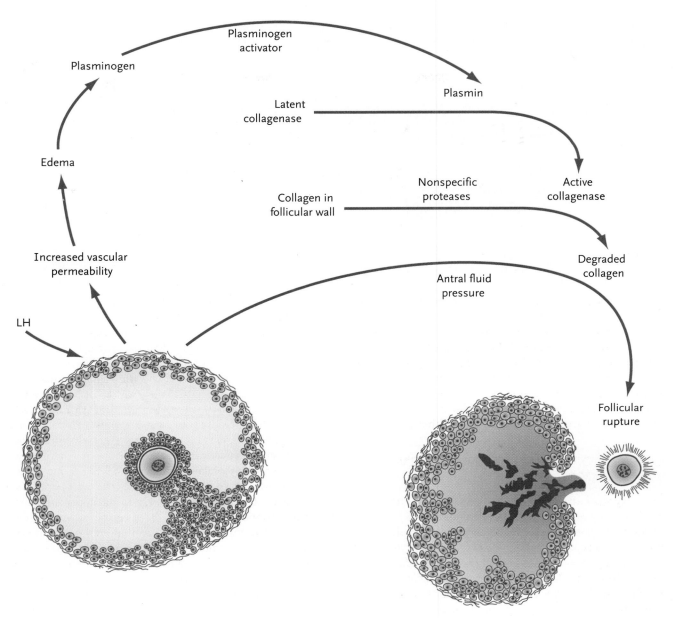

Figure 2-1 Factors involved in mammalian ovulation. (Based on Lipner H. In Knobil E, Neill J, eds: *The physiology of reproduction*, vol 1, New York, 1988, Raven, pp 447-488.)

bits have shown that the bulk provided by the cellular coverings of the ovulated egg is important in facilitating the egg's capture and transport by the uterine tube. Denuded ova or inert objects of that size are not so readily transported. Some evidence suggests that the human egg may rely less on its cellular coverings for transport than the egg of a rabbit.

Even without these types of natural adaptations, the ability of the uterine tubes to capture eggs is remarkable. If the fimbriated end of the tube has been removed, egg capture occurs remarkably often, and pregnancies have occurred in women who have had one ovary and the contralateral uterine tube removed. In such cases, the ovulated egg would

have to travel free in the pelvic cavity for a considerable distance before entering the ostium of the uterine tube on the other side, or an extra long tube could possibly swing to reach the contralateral ovary.

Once inside the uterine tube, the egg is transported toward the uterus, mainly as the result of contractions of the smooth musculature of the tubal wall. Although the cilia lining the tubal mucosa may also play a role in egg transport, their action is not obligatory because women with **immotile cilia syndrome** are normally fertile.

While in the uterine tube, the egg is bathed in **tubal fluid,** which is a combination of secretion by the tubal epithelial

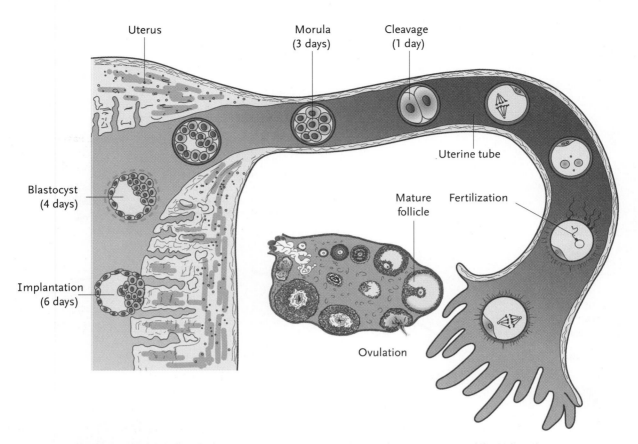

Figure 2-2 Follicular development in the ovary, ovulation, fertilization, and transport of the early embryo down the uterine tube and into the uterus.

cells and transudate from capillaries just below the epithelium. In some mammals, exposure to oviductal secretions is important to the survival of the ovum, but the role of tubal fluid in humans is less clear.

Tubal transport of the egg usually takes 3 to 4 days, regardless of whether fertilization occurs (Figure 2-2). Egg transport typically occurs in two phases: slow transport in the ampulla (approximately 72 hours) and a more rapid phase (8 hours) during which the egg or embryo passes through the isthmus and into the uterus (see p. 38). By a poorly understood mechanism, possibly local edema or reduced muscular activity, the egg is temporarily prevented from entering the isthmic portion of the tube, but under the influence of progesterone, the uterotubal junction relaxes and permits entry of the ovum.

By roughly 80 hours after ovulation, the ovulated egg or embryo has passed from the uterine tube into the uterus. If fertilization has not occurred, the egg degenerates and is phagocytized. (Implantation of the embryo is discussed in Chapter 3.)

Sperm Transport

Sperm transport occurs in both the male and the female. In the male, transport of spermatozoa is closely connected with their structural and functional maturation, whereas in the female reproductive tract, it is important for as many spermatozoa as possible to pass quickly to the upper uterine tube, where they can meet the ovulated egg.

After spermiogenesis in the seminiferous tubules, the spermatozoa are morphologically mature but are nonmotile and incapable of fertilizing an egg (Figure 2-3). Spermatozoa are passively transported via testicular fluid from the seminiferous tubules to the caput (head) of the epididymis through the rete testis and the efferent ductules. They are propelled by fluid pressure generated in the seminiferous tubules and are assisted by smooth muscle contractions and ciliary currents in the efferent ductules. Spermatozoa spend about 12 days in the highly convoluted duct of the epididymis, during which time they undergo biochemical maturation. This period of maturation is associated with changes in the glycoproteins in the plasma membrane of the sperm head. By the time the spermatozoa have reached the cauda (tail) of the epididymis, they are capable of fertilizing an egg.

On ejaculation, the spermatozoa rapidly pass through the **ductus deferens** and become mixed with fluid secretions from the **seminal vesicles** and **prostate gland**. Prostatic fluid is rich in citric acid, acid phosphatase, zinc, and magnesium ions, whereas fluid of the seminal vesicle is rich in fructose (the principal energy source of spermatozoa) and prostaglandins. The 2 to 6 ml of ejaculate (**semen,** or **seminal fluid**) typically consists of 40 to 250 million spermatozoa mixed with alka-

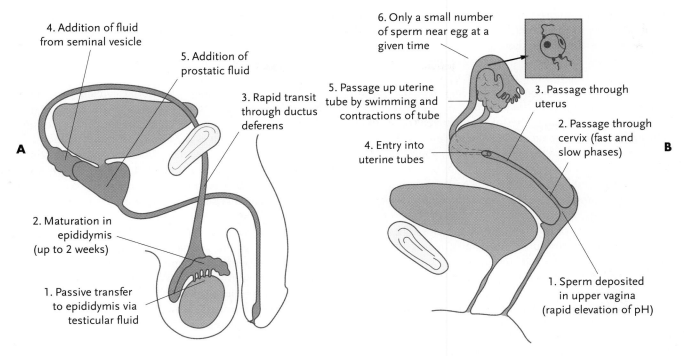

Figure 2-3 Sperm transport in (**A**) the male and (**B**) the female reproductive tract.

line fluid from the seminal vesicles (60% of the total) and acid secretion (pH, 6.5) from the prostate (30% of the total). The pH of normal semen is typically between 7.2 and 7.8. Despite the large number of spermatozoa normally present in an ejaculate, a number as small as 25 million per ejaculate may be compatible with normal fertility.

In the female, sperm transport begins in the upper vagina and ends in the ampulla of the uterine tube, where the spermatozoa make contact with the ovulated egg. During copulation, the seminal fluid is normally deposited in the upper vagina (see Figure 2-3), where its composition and buffering capacity immediately protect the spermatozoa from the acid fluid found in the upper vaginal area. The acidic vaginal fluid normally serves a bacteriocidal function in protecting the cervical canal from pathogenic organisms. Within about 10 seconds, the pH of the upper vagina is raised from 4.3 to as much as 7.2. The buffering effect lasts only a few minutes in humans but provides enough time for the spermatozoa to approach the cervix in an environment (pH, 6.0 to 6.5) optimal for sperm motility.

The next barrier that the sperm cells must overcome is the cervical canal and the cervical mucus that blocks it. Changes in intravaginal pressure may suck spermatozoa into the cervical os, but swimming movements also appear to be important for most spermatozoa in penetrating the cervical mucus.

The composition and viscosity of cervical mucus vary considerably throughout the menstrual cycle. Composed of **cervical mucin** (a glycoprotein with a high carbohydrate composition) and soluble components, cervical mucus is not

readily penetrable. However, between days 9 and 16 of the cycle, its water content increases, which facilitates the passage of sperm through the cervix around the time of ovulation; such mucus is sometimes called **E mucus**. After ovulation, under the influence of progesterone, the production of watery cervical mucus ceases, and a new type of sticky mucus, which has a much decreased water content, is produced. This progestational mucus, sometimes called **G mucus**, is almost completely resistant to sperm penetration. Knowledge of the properties of cervical mucus has been used as a highly effective method of natural family planning.

There are two main modes of sperm transport through the cervix. One is a phase of initial rapid transport, by which some spermatozoa can reach the uterine tubes within 5 to 20 minutes of ejaculation. Such rapid transport relies more on muscular movements of the female reproductive tract than on the motility of the spermatozoa themselves. The second, slow phase of sperm transport involves the swimming of spermatozoa through the cervical mucus (traveling at a rate of 2 to 3 mm/hr), their storage in cervical crypts, and their final passage through the cervical canal as much as 2 to 4 days later.

Relatively little is known about the passage of spermatozoa through the uterine cavity, but the contraction of uterine smooth muscle, rather than sperm motility, seems to be the main intrauterine transport mechanism. At this point the spermatozoa enter one of the uterine tubes. Although there have been suggestions that follicular fluid or something associated with the ovulated egg may exert a chemoattractive influence on mammalian spermatozoa, this has not been proved, and it remains highly likely that chance determines which uterine tube a given sperm enters. Once inside the uterine tube, spermatozoa collect in the isthmus until some signal associated with ovulation stimulates their further migration up the uterine tube. At the time of their release, the spermatozoa enter a temporary **period of hyperactivity** consisting of exaggerated swimming movements that may free them from temporary binding sites in the isthmus.

A surprisingly small number of spermatozoa (only about 200) are found in the upper uterine tube at a given time. With muscular movements of the tube and some swimming movements, sperm cells work their way up the tube and even out through the infundibulum and into the peritoneal cavity. The simultaneous transport of an egg down the tube and spermatozoa up the tube is currently explained on the basis of peristaltic contractions of the uterine tube muscles. These contractions subdivide the tube into compartments. Within a given compartment, the gametes are caught up in churning movements that over 1 or 2 days, bring the egg and spermatozoa together.

The most recent estimates suggest that spermatozoa can retain their function in the female reproductive tract for about 80 hours. During their passage through the reproductive tract, the spermatozoa undergo the capacitation reaction. **Capacitation**, which is the alteration of the glycoprotein surface of spermatozoa under the influence of secretions of the tissues of the female reproductive tract, is required for spermatozoa to be able to fertilize an egg. Fertilization of the egg typically occurs in the ampullary portion of the uterine tube.

Formation and Function of the Corpus Luteum of Ovulation and Pregnancy

While the ovulated egg is passing through the uterine tubes, the ruptured follicle from which it arose undergoes a series of striking changes that are essential for the progression of events leading to and supporting pregnancy (see Figure 1-8).

Soon after ovulation, the basement membrane that separates the granulosa cells from the theca interna breaks down, allowing thecal blood vessels to grow into the cavity of the ruptured follicle. The granulosa cells simultaneously undergo a series of major changes in form and function (**luteinization**). Within 30 to 40 hours of the LH surge, these cells, now called **granulosa lutein cells**, begin secreting increasing amounts of progesterone along with some estrogen. This pattern of secretion provides the hormonal basis for the changes in the female reproductive tissues during the last half of the menstrual cycle. During this period, the follicle continues to enlarge. Because of its yellow color, it is known as the **corpus luteum**. The granulosa lutein cells are terminally differentiated. They have stopped dividing, but they continue to secrete progesterone for 10 days.

In the absence of fertilization and a hormonal stimulus provided by the early embryo, the corpus luteum begins to deteriorate (**luteolysis**) late in the menstrual cycle. Luteolysis appears to involve both the preprogramming of the luteal cells to **apoptosis** (cell death) and **uterine luteolytic factors**, such

as **prostaglandin F$_2$**. Regression of the corpus luteum and the accompanying reduction in progesterone production cause the hormonal withdrawal that results in the degenerative changes of the endometrial tissue during the last days of the menstrual cycle.

During the regression of the corpus luteum, the granulosa lutein cells degenerate and are replaced with collagenous scar tissue. Because of its white color, the former corpus luteum now becomes known as the **corpus albicans** ("white body").

If fertilization occurs, the production of the protein hormone **chorionic gonadotropin** by the future placental tissues maintains the corpus luteum in a functional condition and even causes an increase in its size and hormone production. Because the granulosa lutein cells are unable to divide and also cease producing progesterone after 10 days, the large **corpus luteum of pregnancy** is composed principally of theca lutein cells. The corpus luteum of pregnancy remains functional for the first few months of pregnancy. After the second month, the placenta produces enough estrogens and progesterone to maintain pregnancy on its own. At this point the ovaries can be removed, and pregnancy will continue.

FERTILIZATION

Fertilization is a series of processes rather than a single event. Viewed in the broadest sense, these processes begin when spermatozoa start to penetrate the corona radiata that surrounds the egg and end with the intermingling of the maternal and paternal chromosomes after the spermatozoon has entered the egg.

Penetration of the Corona Radiata

When the spermatozoa first encounter the ovulated egg in the ampullary part of the uterine tube, they are confronted by the corona radiata and possibly some remnants of the cumulus oophorus, which represents the outer layer of the egg complex (Figure 2-4). The corona radiata is a highly cellular layer with an intercellular matrix consisting of proteins and a high concentration of carbohydrates, especially hyaluronic acid.

Although it has been widely believed that hyaluronidase emanating from the sperm head plays a major role in penetration of the corona radiata, the evidence is not unequivocal. The active swimming movements of the spermatozoa appear to play a significant role in penetration.

Attachment to and Penetration of the Zona Pellucida

The **zona pellucida**, which is 13 μm thick in humans, consists principally of three glycoproteins—ZP1, ZP2, and ZP3—with molecular weights of 200,000, 120,000, and 83,000 daltons. ZP2 and ZP3 combine to form basic units that polymerize into long filaments. These filaments are periodi-

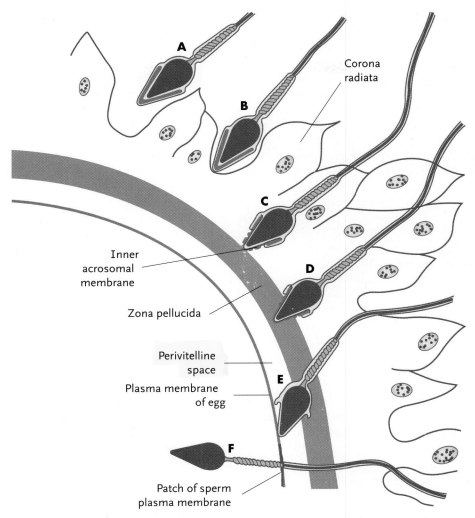

Corona
radiata

Inner
acrosomal
membrane

Zona pellucida

Perivitelline
space

Plasma membrane
of egg

Patch of sperm
plasma membrane

Figure 2-4 The sequence of events in penetration of the coverings and plasma membrane of the egg. A and B, Penetration of the corona radiata. C and D, Attachment to the zona pellucida and acrosomal reaction. E and F, Binding to plasma membrane and entry into the egg.

cally linked by cross-bridges of ZP1 molecules (Figure 2-5). The zona pellucida of the unfertilized mouse egg is estimated to contain over a billion copies of the ZP3 protein.

After they have penetrated the corona radiata, spermatozoa bind tightly to the zona pellucida by means of the plasma membrane of the sperm head (see Figure 2-4). The ZP3 molecule, specifically the O-linked oligosaccharides attached to the polypeptide core, acts as the sperm receptor in the zona in the mouse. Molecules on the surface of the sperm head act as specific binding sites for the ZP3 sperm receptors on the zona pellucida. Several molecules have been proposed; a likely candidate is a galactosyl transferase.

On binding to the zona pellucida, mammalian spermatozoa undergo the **acrosomal reaction**. The essence of the acrosomal reaction is the fusion of parts of the outer acrosomal membrane with the overlying plasma membrane and the pinching off of fused parts as small vesicles. This results

in the liberation of the multitude of enzymes that are stored in the acrosome (Box 2-1).

The acrosomal reaction in mammals appears to be stimulated by the ZP3 molecule (see Figure 2-5). In contrast to the sperm receptor function of ZP3, a large segment of the polypeptide chain of the ZP3 molecule must be present to induce the acrosomal reaction. One of the initiating events of the acrosomal reaction is a massive influx of Ca^{++} through the plasma membrane of the sperm head. This process, accompanied by an influx of Na^+ and an efflux of H^+, raises the intracellular pH. Fusion of the outer acrosomal membrane with the overlying plasma membrane soon follows. As the vesicles of the fused membranes are shed, the enzymatic contents of the acrosome are freed and can assist the spermatozoa in making its way through the zona pellucida.

After the acrosomal reaction, the inner acrosomal membrane forms the outer surface covering of most of the sperm

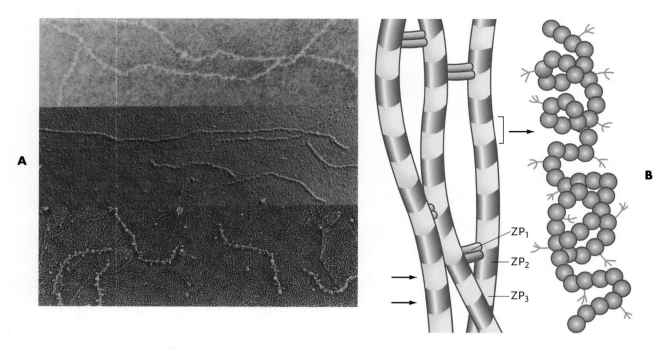

Figure 2-5 A, Filamentous components of the mammalian (mouse) zona pellucida. **B,** Molecular organization of the filaments in the zona pellucida. *Far right,* Structure of the ZP3 glycoprotein. (**A** and **B** from Wasserman PM: *Sci Am* 259(6):82, 1988.)

BOX 2-1	Some Major Mammalian Acrosomal Enzymes

Acid proteinase	β-Galactosidase
Acrosin	β-Glucuronidase
Arylaminidase	Hyaluronidase
Arylsulfatase	Neuraminidase
Collagenase	Phospholipase C
Esterase	Proacrosin

head (see Figure 2-4, *D*). Toward the base of the sperm head (in the equatorial region), the inner acrosomal membrane fuses with the remaining **postacrosomal plasma membrane** to maintain membrane continuity around the sperm head.

Only after completing the acrosomal reaction can the spermatozoon successfully begin to penetrate the zona pellucida. Penetration of the zona is accomplished by a combination of mechanical propulsion by movements of the sperm's tail and digestion of a pathway through the action of acrosomal enzymes. Although the action of several acrosomal enzymes may be involved in initiating penetration through the zona, the most important enzyme is **acrosin,** a serine proteinase that is bound to the inner acrosomal membrane. Many investigators feel that the well-defined tunnel marking the pathway of the sperm through the zona can be attributed to the fact that acrosin is membrane bound rather than diffusible. Once the sperm has made its way through the zona and into the **perivitelline space** (the space between the egg's plasma membrane and the zona pellucida), it can make direct contact with the plasma membrane of the egg.

Binding and Fusion of Spermatozoon and Egg

After a brief transit period through the perivitelline space, the spermatozoon makes contact with the egg. In two distinct steps, the spermatozoon first binds to and then fuses with the plasma membrane of the egg. Binding between the spermatozoon and egg occurs at the **equatorial region** of the sperm head, where the inner acrosomal membrane has previously fused with the remaining plasma membrane of the spermatozoon, and the microvilli surrounding most of the egg. Molecules on the plasma membrane of the sperm head bind to $\alpha6\beta1$ **integrin** molecules on the surface of the egg. The acrosomal reaction seems to cause some change in the membrane properties of the spermatozoon because if the acrosomal reaction has not occurred, the spermatozoon is unable to fuse with the egg. Actual fusion between spermatozoon and egg brings their plasma membranes into continuity. After initial fusion, the contents of the spermatozoon (the head, midpiece, and usually the tail) sink into the egg (Figure 2-6), whereas the sperm's plasma membrane, which is antigenically distinct from that of the egg, becomes incorporated into the egg's plasma membrane and remains recognizable at least until

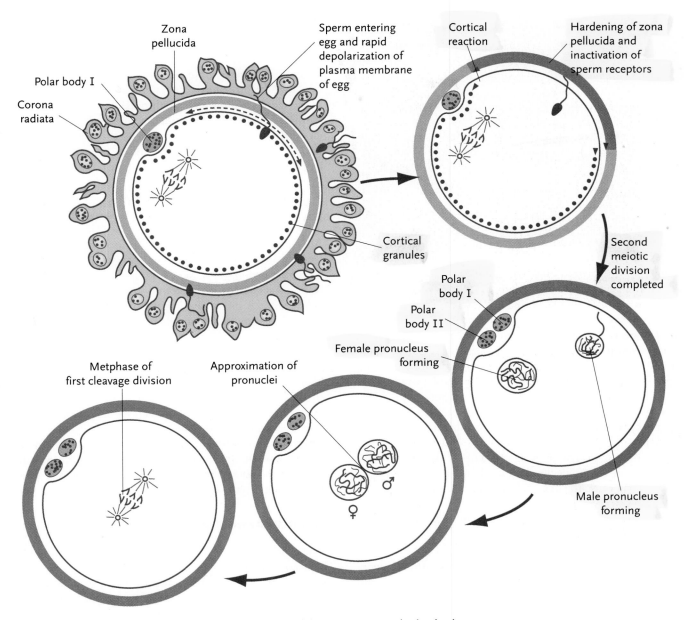

Figure 2-6 Summary of the main events involved in fertilization.

the start of cleavage. Although mitochondria located in the sperm neck enter the egg, they do not seem to contribute to the functional mitochondrial complement of the zygote.

Prevention of Polyspermy

Once a spermatozoon has fused with an egg, the entry of other spermatozoa into the egg (**polyspermy**) must be prevented or abnormal development will likely result. Two blocks to polyspermy, fast and slow, are typically present in vertebrate fertilization.

The **fast block to polyspermy,** which has been best studied in sea urchins, consists of a rapid electrical depolarization of the plasma membrane of the egg. The resting membrane potential of the egg changes from about -70 mV to $+10$ mV within 2 to 3 seconds after fusion of the spermatozoon with the egg. This change in membrane potential prevents other spermatozoa from adhering to the egg's plasma membrane. Little is known about the fast block to polyspermy in the human egg, but because there are no more than a few spermatozoa in the vicinity of the mammalian egg at the moment of fertilization, the need for an effective fast block appears to be less than in the sea urchin. The fast block is short lived, usually lasting only about a minute in sea urchins and 5 minutes in mammals. This time is sufficient for the egg to mount the permanent slow block.

The **slow block to polyspermy** begins with the propagation of a wave of Ca^{++} from the site of sperm-egg fusion. Within a couple of minutes, the Ca^{++} wave has passed through the egg, sequentially acting on the cortical granules as it passes by them. Exposure to Ca^{++} causes the cortical granules to fuse with the plasma membrane and to release their contents (hydrolytic enzymes and polysaccharides) into the perivitelline space. The polysaccharides released into the perivitelline space become hydrated and swell, causing the zona pellucida to elevate from the surface of the egg.

The secretory products of the cortical granules diffuse into the porous zona pellucida and hydrolyze the sperm receptor molecules (ZP3 in the mouse) in the zona. This reaction, called the **zona reaction**, essentially eliminates the ability of spermatozoa to adhere to and penetrate the zona. The zona reaction has been visually observed in human eggs that have undergone in vitro fertilization.

Interspecies molecular differences in the sperm-binding regions of the ZP3 molecule may serve as the basis for the inability of spermatozoa of one species to fertilize an egg of another species. In mammals, there is less species variation in the composition of ZP3; this may explain the reason that penetration of the zona pellucida by spermatozoa of closely related mammalian species is sometimes possible, whereas it is rare among lower animals. The specificity between the ZP3 receptor site and binding sites on the spermatozoon could be used as the basis for an immunologically based mode of contraception.

In addition to changes in the zona pellucida, alterations in sperm receptor molecules on the plasma membrane of the human egg cause the egg itself to become refractory to penetration by other spermatozoa.

Metabolic Activation of the Egg

One of the significant changes brought about by the penetration of a sperm is a rapid intensification of the egg's respiration and metabolism. The mechanisms underlying these changes are not fully understood even in the best-studied systems, but the early release of Ca^{++} from internal stores is believed to be the initiating event. In some species, Ca^{++} release is shortly followed by an exchange of extracellular Na^+ for intracellular H^+ through the plasma membrane. This results in a rise in intracellular pH, which precedes an increase in oxidative metabolism.

Decondensation of the Sperm Nucleus

In the mature spermatozoon, the nuclear chromatin is very tightly packed, due in large part to the —SS— (disulfide) cross-linking that occurs among the protamine molecules complexed with the deoxyribonucleic acid (DNA) during spermatogenesis. Shortly after the head of the sperm enters the cytoplasm of the egg, the permeability of its nuclear mem-

brane begins to increase, allowing cytoplasmic factors within the egg to affect the nuclear contents of the sperm. After reduction of the —SS— crosslinks of the protamines to sulfhydryl (—SH) groups by reduced glutathione in the ooplasm, the protamines are rapidly lost from the chromatin of the spermatozoon, and the chromatin begins to spread out within the nucleus (now called a **pronucleus**) as it moves closer to the nuclear material of the egg. After a short period during which the male chromosomes are naked, histones begin to associate with the chromosomes.

Completion of Meiosis and the Development of Pronuclei in the Egg

After penetration of the egg by the spermatozoon, the nucleus of the egg, which had been arrested in metaphase of the second meiotic division, completes the last division, releasing a **second polar body** into the perivitelline space (see Figure 2-6). A pronuclear membrane, derived largely from the endoplasmic reticulum of the egg, forms around the female chromosomal material. Cytoplasmic factors appear to control the growth of both the female and the male pronuclei. DNA replication occurs in the developing haploid pronuclei, and each chromosome forms two chromatids as the pronuclei approach each other. When the male and female pronuclei come into contact, their membranes break down, and the chromosomes intermingle. The maternal and paternal chromosomes quickly become organized around a mitotic spindle in preparation for an ordinary mitotic division. At this point, the process of fertilization can be said to be complete and the fertilized egg is called a **zygote**.

What Is Accomplished by Fertilization?

The process of fertilization ties together a number of biological loose ends:

1. It stimulates the egg to complete the second meiotic division.
2. It restores to the zygote the normal diploid number of chromosomes (46 in the human).
3. The sex of the future embryo is determined by the chromosomal complement of the spermatozoon. (If the sperm contains 22 autosomes and an X chromosome, the embryo will be a genetic female, and if it contains 22 autosomes and a Y chromosome, the embryo will be a male. See Chapter 15 for further details.)
4. Through the mingling of maternal and paternal chromosomes, the zygote is a genetically unique product of chromosomal reassortment, which is important for the viability of any species.
5. The process of fertilization causes metabolic activation of the egg, which is necessary for cleavage and subsequent embryonic development to occur.

CLINICAL CORRELATION 2-1
Treatment of Infertility by In Vitro Fertilization and Embryo Transfer

Certain types of infertility caused by inadequate numbers or mobility of spermatozoa or by obstruction of the uterine tubes are now treatable by fertilizing an ovum in vitro and then transferring the cleaving embryo into the reproductive tract of the woman. Accomplishing this requires the sequential application of various techniques that were initially developed for the assisted reproduction of domestic animals, such as cows and sheep. The relevant techniques are (1) stimulating gamete production, (2) obtaining male and female gametes, (3) storing gametes, (4) fertilizing eggs, (5) culturing cleaving embryos in vitro, (6) preserving embryos, and (7) introducing embryos into the uterus (Figure 2-7).

STIMULATION OF GAMETE PRODUCTION

Ovulation is stimulated by altering existing hormonal relationships. For women who are **anovulatory** (do not ovulate), these techniques alone may be sufficient to allow conception.

Three types of therapy have been commonly used to stimulate gamete production. The first consists of the administration of **clomiphene citrate**, a nonsteroidal antiestrogen that competes with estrogens for binding sites in the pituitary and possibly the hy-

pothalamus and ovaries. Clomiphene acts to suppress the normal negative feedback by estrogens on the pituitary (see Figure 1-14), resulting in an increase in the serum concentrations of LH and FSH. This typically results in multiple ovulation, a desired outcome for artificial fertilization because fertilizing more than one egg at a time is more efficient. Sometimes, however, a woman who has used clomiphene for the induction of ovulation produces multiple offspring, with a number of cases of quintuplet to septuplet births having been recorded.

Other methods of inducing ovulation are the application of **human menopausal gonadotropins (hMGs)** or the pulsatile administration of gonadotropin-releasing hormone (GnRH). These techniques are more expensive than the administration of clomiphene.

OBTAINING GAMETES

For artificial insemination in vivo or artificial fertilization in vitro, spermatozoa are typically collected by masturbation. The collection of eggs, however, requires technological assistance. Ongoing monitoring of the course of induced ovulation is accomplished by the application of imaging techniques, especially diagnostic ultrasound.

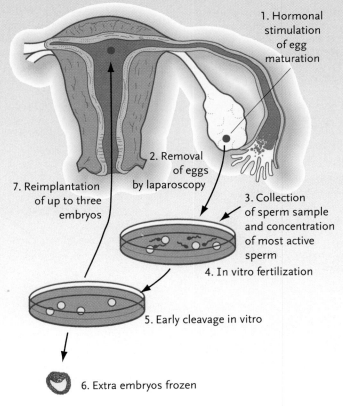

1. Hormonal stimulation of egg maturation

2. Removal of eggs by laparoscopy

7. Reimplantation of up to three embryos

3. Collection of sperm sample and concentration of most active sperm

4. In vitro fertilization

5. Early cleavage in vitro

6. Extra embryos frozen

Figure 2-7 Schematic representation of a typical in vitro fertilization and embryo transfer procedure in humans.

Continued

CLINICAL CORRELATION 2-1
Treatment of Infertility by In Vitro Fertilization and Embryo Transfer—cont'd

The actual recovery of oocytes involves their aspiration from ripe follicles. Although originally accomplished by **laparoscopy** (direct observation by inserting a laparoscope through a small slit in the woman's abdominal wall), visualization is now done with the assistance of ultrasound. An aspiration needle is inserted into each mature follicle, and the ovum is gently sucked into the needle and then placed into culture medium in preparation for fertilization in vitro.

STORING GAMETES

Although eggs and sperm are usually placed together shortly after they are obtained, in some circumstances the gametes (especially spermatozoa) are stored for various periods of time before use. By bringing glycerinated preparations of spermatozoa down to the temperature of liquid nitrogen, spermatozoa can be kept for years without losing their normal fertilizing power. The freezing of eggs is possible, but much more problematic.

IN VITRO FERTILIZATION AND EMBRYO CULTURE

Three ingredients for successful in vitro fertilization are (1) mature eggs; (2) normal, active spermatozoa; and (3) an appropriate culture environment.

One of the most important factors in obtaining successful in vitro fertilization is having oocytes that are properly mature. The eggs aspirated from a woman are sometimes at different stages of maturity. Immature eggs are cultured for a short time to become more fertilizable. The aspirated eggs are surrounded by the zona pellucida, the corona radiata, and a varying amount of cumulus oophorus tissue.

Spermatozoa, either fresh or frozen, are prepared by separating them as much as possible from the seminal fluid. Seminal fluid reduces their fertilizing capacity, in part because it contains decapacitating factors. After capacitation, which in the human can be accomplished by exposing spermatozoa to certain ionic solutions, a defined number of spermatozoa are added to the culture in concentrations from 10,000 to 500,000/ml. Rates of fertilization in vitro vary from one center to another, but 75% represents a realistic average.

In cases of infertility caused by **oligospermia** (too few spermatozoa) or excessively high percentages of abnormal sperm cells, multiple ejaculates may be obtained over an extended period. These are frozen and pooled to obtain adequate numbers of viable spermatozoa. In some cases, small numbers of spermatozoa are microinjected into the **perivitelline space** inside the zona pellucida. Although this procedure can compensate for very small numbers of viable spermatozoa, it introduces the risk of polyspermy because the normal gating function of the zona is bypassed. A recent variant on in vitro fertilization is direct injection of a spermatozoon into an oocyte (Figure 2-8). This technique has been used in cases of severe sperm impairment.

The initial success of in vitro fertilization is determined the next day by examination of the egg. If two pronuclei are evident (Figure 2-9), fertilization is assumed to have taken place.

Fortunately, the cleavage in vitro of human embryos is more successful than that of most other

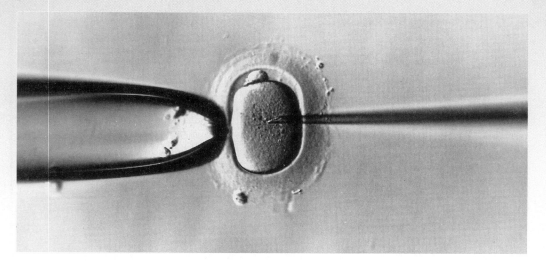

Figure 2-8 Microinjection of a spermatozoon into a human oocyte. The micropipette containing the spermatozoon is entering the oocyte from the right side. (From Veeck LL: *Atlas of the human oocyte and early conceptus,* vol 2, Baltimore, 1991, Williams & Wilkins.)

CLINICAL CORRELATION 2-1
Treatment of Infertility by In Vitro Fertilization and Embryo Transfer—cont'd

mammalian species. The embryos are usually allowed to develop to the two- to eight-cell stage before they are considered ready to implant into the uterus.

Typically, all the eggs obtained from the multiple ovulations of the woman are fertilized in vitro during the same period. Very practical reasons exist for doing this. One is that because of the low success rate of embryo transfer, implanting more than one embryo (commonly up to three) into the uterus at a time is advisable. Another reason is financial and also relates to the low success rate of embryo transfer. Embryos other than those used during the initial procedure are stored for future use if the first embryo transfer proves unsuccessful. Such stockpiling saves a great deal of time and thousands of dollars for the patient.

EMBRYO PRESERVATION

Embryos preserved for potential future use are treated with cryoprotectants (usually glycerol or dimethyl sulfoxide) to reduce ice crystal damage. They are slowly brought to very low temperatures (usually below −100° C) to halt all metabolic activity. The length of time frozen embryos should be kept and the procedure for handling them if the first implantation attempt is successful are questions with both technical and ethical aspects.

EMBRYO TRANSFER INTO THE MOTHER

Transfer of the embryo into the mother is technically simple; yet this is the step in the entire operation that is subject to the greatest failure rate. Typically only 10% to 25% of the embryo transfer attempts result in a viable pregnancy.

Embryo transfer is commonly accomplished by introducing a catheter through the cervix into the uterine cavity and then expelling the embryo or embryos from the catheter. The patient remains quiet, preferably lying down for several hours after embryo transfer.

The reasons for the low success rate of embryo transfers are poorly understood, but the number of completed pregnancies after normal fertilization in vivo is also likely to be only about one third. If normal implantation does occur, the remainder of the pregnancy is typically uneventful and is followed by a normal childbirth.

INTRAFALLOPIAN TRANSFER

Certain types of infertility are caused by factors such as hostile cervical mucus and pathological or anatomical abnormalities of the upper ends of the uterine tubes. A somewhat simpler method for dealing with these conditions is to introduce both male and female gametes directly into the lower end of a uterine tube (often at the junction of its isthmic and ampullary regions). Fertilization occurs within the tube, and the early events of embryogenesis occur naturally. The method of **gamete intrafallopian transfer (GIFT)** has resulted in slightly higher percentages of pregnancies than the standard in vitro fertilization and embryo transfer methods.

A variant on this technique is **zygote intrafallopian transfer (ZIFT)**. In this case a cleaving embryo that has been produced by in vitro fertilization is implanted into the uterine tube.

SURROGACY

In some circumstances a woman can produce fertile eggs but cannot become pregnant. An example would be the woman whose uterus has been removed but who still possesses functioning ovaries. One option in this case is in vitro fertilization and embryo transfer, but the embryo is transferred into the uterus of another woman **(surrogate mother)**. From the biological perspective, this procedure differs little from embryo transfer into the uterus of the biological mother, but it introduces a host of social, ethical, and legal issues.

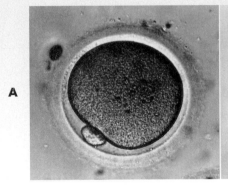 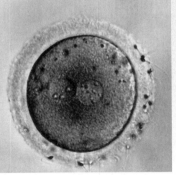

Figure 2-9 A, Photomicrograph of a mature human oocyte arrested at metaphase II. This oocyte will be fertilized in vitro. B, Photomicrograph of a human oocyte newly fertilized in vitro. Two pronuclei are visible. (From Veeck LL: *Atlas of the human oocyte and early conceptus*, vol 2, Baltimore, 1991, Williams & Wilkins.)

CLINICAL VIGNETTE

A 33-year-old woman who has had her uterus surgically removed desperately wants her own child. She is capable of producing eggs because her ovaries remain functional. She and her extremely wealthy husband want to attempt in vitro fertilization and embryo transfer. They find a woman who, for $10,000, is willing to allow the couple's embryo to be transferred to her uterus and will serve as a surrogate mother during the pregnancy. Induction of superovulation is very successful, and the physicians are able to fertilize eight eggs in vitro. Three embryos are implanted into the surrogate mother. The remaining embryos are frozen for possible future use. The embryo transfer is successful, and the surrogate mother becomes pregnant with twins. The twins are born, but the surrogate mother feels that she has bonded with them so much that she should have the right to raise them. The genetic parents take the case to court, but before the case comes to trial they are both killed in an airplane accident. The surrogate mother now claims that she should get the large inheritance in the name of her twins, but the father's sister, equally aware of the financial implications, claims that she should care for the twins. The issue of what to do with the remaining five frozen embryos also comes up.

This case is fictitious, but all of its elements have occurred on an isolated basis. How would you deal with the following legal and ethical issues?
  A. To whom should the twins be awarded?
  B. What should be done with the remaining frozen embryos?

SUMMARY

- Ovulation is stimulated by a surge of LH and FSH in the blood. Expulsion of the ovum from the graafian follicle involves local edema, ischemia, and collagen breakdown, with a possible contribution by fluid pressure and smooth muscle activity in rupturing the follicular wall.
- The ovulated egg is swept into the uterine tube and transported through it by ciliary action and smooth muscle contractions as it awaits fertilization by a sperm cell.
- Sperm transport in the male involves a slow exit from the seminiferous tubules, maturation in the epididymis, and rapid expulsion at ejaculation, where the spermatozoa are joined by secretions from the prostate and seminal vesicles to form semen.
- In the female, sperm transport involves entry into the cervical canal from the vagina, passage through the cervical mucus, and transport through the uterus into the uterine tubes, where capacitation occurs. The meeting of egg and sperm typically occurs in the upper third of the uterine tube.
- The fertilization process consists of several sequential events:
  1. Penetration of the corona radiata
  2. Attachment to the zona pellucida
  3. Acrosomal reaction and penetration of the zona pellucida
  4. Binding and fusion of sperm and egg
  5. Prevention of polyspermy
  6. Metabolic activation of the egg
  7. Decondensation of the sperm nucleus
  8. Completion of meiosis in the egg
  9. Development and fusion of male and female pronuclei
- Attachment of the spermatozoon to the zona pellucida is mediated by the ZP3 protein, which also stimulates the acrosomal reaction.
- The acrosomal reaction involves fusion of the outer acrosomal membrane with the plasma membrane of the sperm call and the fragmentation of the fused membranes, leading to the release of the acrosomal enzymes. One of the acrosomal enzymes, acrosin, is a serine proteinase, which digests components of the zona pellucida and assists the penetration of the swimming spermatozoa through the zona.
- After fusion of the spermatozoa to the egg membrane, a rapid electrical depolarization produces the first block to polyspermy in the egg. This is followed by a wave of Ca^{++} that causes the cortical granules to release their contents into the perivitelline space and ultimately inactivate the sperm receptors in the zona pellucida.
- Sperm penetration stimulates a rapid intensification of respiration and metabolism of the egg.
- Within the egg, the nuclear material of the spermatozoon decondenses and forms the male pronucleus. At the same time, the egg completes the second meiotic division, and the remaining nuclear material becomes surrounded by a membrane, thereby forming the female pronucleus.
- After DNA replication, the male and female pronuclei join, and their chromosomes become organized for a mitotic division. Fertilization is then complete, and the fertilized egg is properly called a *zygote*.
- Treatment of infertility by in vitro fertilization and embryo transfer is a multistage process involving stimulating gamete production by drugs such as clomiphene citrate, obtaining eggs by laparoscopic techniques in the female, storing gametes by freezing, performing in vitro fertilization and culture of embryos, preserving the embryo, and transferring the embryo to the mother.
- Other techniques used for the treatment of infertility are GIFT, the transfer of gametes directly into the uterine tube, and ZIFT, the transfer of zygotes into the uterine tube. These techniques can be used with both biological and surrogate mothers.

REVIEW QUESTIONS

1. Of the barriers to sperm survival and transport within the female reproductive tract, low pH is most important in the:
   A. Upper uterine tube
   B. Lower uterine tube
   C. Uterine cavity
   D. Cervix
   E. Vagina
2. The principal energy source for ejaculated spermatozoa is:
   A. Prostatic acid phosphatase
   B. Internal glucose
   C. Prostatic citric acid
   D. Fructose in seminal vesicle fluid
   E. Glycogen released from the vaginal epithelium
3. What is the principal hormonal stimulus for ovulation?
4. What is capacitation?
5. Where does fertilization take place?
6. Name two functions of the ZP3 protein of the zona pellucida.

7. What is polyspermy, and how is it prevented after a spermatozoon enters the egg?
8. A woman gives birth to septuplets. What is the likely reason for the multiple births?
9. When multiple oocytes obtained by laparoscopy are fertilized in vitro, why are up to three embryos implanted into the woman's uterus and why are the other embryos commonly frozen?
10. Why do some reproductive technology centers insert spermatozoa under the zona pellucida or even directly into the oocyte?

REFERENCES

American Fertility Society: Guidelines for human embryology and andrology laboratories, *Fertil Steril* 19(suppl 58):1S-16S, 1992.

Austin CR: *Human embryos: the debate on assisted reproduction*, Oxford, England, 1989, Oxford University.

Austin CR, Short RV, eds: *Reproduction in mammals*, book 1, ed 2, Cambridge, England, 1982, Cambridge University.

Braden TD, Belfiore CJ, Niswender GD: Hormonal control of luteal function. In Findlay JK, ed: *Molecular biology of the female reproductive system*, New York, 1994, Academic, pp 259-287.

Chang MC: Experimental studies of mammalian fertilization, *Zool Sci* 1:349-364, 1984.

Dietl J, ed: *The mammalian egg coat: structure and function*, Berlin, 1989, Springer-Verlag.

Eisenbach M, Ralt D: Precontact mammalian sperm-egg communication and role in fertilization, *Am J Physiol* 262(3):C1095-C1101, 1992.

Espey LL, Lipner H: Ovulation. In Knobil E, Neill JD, eds: *The physiology of reproduction*, ed 2, New York, 1994, Raven, pp 725-780.

Familiari G, Makabe S, Motta PM: The ovary and ovulation: a three-dimensional study. In Van Blerkom J, Motta PM, eds: *Ultrastructure of human gametogenesis and early embryogenesis*, Boston, 1989, Kluwer Academic, pp 85-124.

Gaunt SJ: Spreading of the sperm surface antigen within the plasma membrane of the egg after fertilization in the rat, *J Embryol Exp Morph* 75:257-270, 1983.

Geerling JH: Natural family planning, *Am Fam Physician* 52:1749-1756, 1995.

Gwatkin RBL: *Fertilization mechanisms in man and mammals*, New York, 1977, Plenum.

Harper MJK: Gamete and zygote transport. In Knobil E, Neill JD, eds: *The physiology of reproduction*, vol 1, New York, 1988, Raven, pp 103-134.

Hartmann JF, ed: *Mechanism and control of animal fertilization*, New York, 1983, Academic.

Hoodbhoy T, Talbot P: Mammalian cortical granules: contents, fate, and function, *Mol Reprod Devel* 39:439-448, 1994.

Jones GS: Corpus luteum: composition and function, *Fertil Steril* 54:21-26, 1990.

Jones HW and others, eds: *In vitro fertilization*, Baltimore, 1986, Williams & Wilkins.

Jones R: Identification and functions of mammalian sperm-egg recognition molecules during fertilization, *J Reprod Fertil* 42(suppl):89-105, 1990.

Klemm U, Muller-Esterl W, Engel W: Acrosin, the peculiar sperm-specific serine protease, *Hum Genet* 7:635-641, 1991.

Kopf GS: Zona pellucida-mediated signal transduction in mammalian spermatozoa, *J Reprod Fertil* 42(suppl):33-49, 1990.

McLeskey SB and others: Molecules involved in mammalian sperm-egg interaction, *Int Rev Cytol* 177:57-113, 1998.

Metz CB, Monroy A, eds: *Biology of fertilization*, vols 1-3, New York, 1985, Academic.

Myles DG, Koppel DE, Primakoff P: Defining sperm surface domains. In Alexander NJ and others, eds: *Gamete interaction: prospects for immunocontraception*, New York, 1990, Wiley-Liss, pp 1-11.

Niswender GD, Nett TM: The corpus luteum and its control. In Knobil E, Neill JD, eds: *The physiology of reproduction*, vol 1, New York, 1988, Raven, pp 489-526.

Phillips DM: Structure and function of the zona pellucida. In Familiari G, Makabe S, Motta PM, eds: *Ultrastructure of the ovary*, Boston, 1991, Kluwer Academic, pp 63-72.

Saling PM: How the egg regulates sperm function during gamete interaction: facts and fantasies, *Biol Reprod* 44:246-251, 1991.

Snell WJ, White JM: The molecules of mammalian fertilization, *Cell* 85:629-637, 1996.

Töpfer-Peterson E and others: Sperm acrosin and binding to the zona pellucida. In Alexander NJ and others, eds: *Gamete interaction: prospects for immunocontraception*, New York, 1990, Wiley-Liss, pp 197-212.

Veeck LL: *Atlas of the human oocyte and early conceptus*, vols 1 and 2, Baltimore, 1986, 1991, Williams & Wilkins.

Wassarman PM: The biology and chemistry of fertilization, *Science* 235:553-560, 1987.

Wasserman PM: Profile of a mammalian sperm receptor, *Development* 108:1-17, 1990.

Wood C, Trounson A, eds: *Clinical in vitro fertilization*, ed 2, London, 1989, Springer-Verlag.

Yanagimachi R: Mammalian fertilization. In Knobil E, Neill J, eds: *The physiology of reproduction*, ed 2, New York, 1994, Raven, pp 189-317.

Zaneveld LJD, DeJonge CJ: Mammalian sperm acrosomal enzymes and the acrosome reaction. In Dunbar BS, O'Rand MB, eds: *A comparative overview of mammalian fertilization*, New York, 1991, Plenum, pp 63-79.

3

Cleavage and Implantation

The act of fertilization releases the ovulated egg from a depressed metabolism and prevents its ultimate disintegration within the female reproductive tract. Immediately after fertilization, the zygote undergoes a pronounced shift in metabolism and begins several days of **cleavage**. During this time, the embryo, still encased in its zona pellucida, is transported down the uterine tube and into the uterus. Roughly 6 days later, the embryo sheds its zona pellucida and attaches to the uterine lining.

With intrauterine development and a placental connection between the embryo and mother, higher mammals, including humans, have evolved greatly differing modes of early development from those found in most invertebrates and lower vertebrates. The eggs of lower animals, which are typically laid outside the body, must contain all the materials required for the embryo to attain the stage of independent feeding. Two main strategies have evolved. One is to complete early development as rapidly as possible, a strategy that has been adopted by *Drosophila*, the sea urchin, and many amphibians. This strategy involves storing a moderate amount of yolk in the oocyte and also preproducing much of the molecular machinery necessary for the embryo to move rapidly through cleavage to the start of gastrulation. The oocytes of such species typically produce and store huge amounts of ribosomes, messenger ribonucleic acid (mRNA) and transfer RNA (tRNA). These represent maternal gene products, and it means that early development in these species is controlled predominantly by the maternal genome. The other strategy of independent development, adopted by birds and reptiles, consists of producing a very large egg containing enough yolk that early development can proceed at a slower pace. This eliminates the need for the oocyte to synthesize and store large amounts of RNAs and ribosomes before fertilization.

Mammalian embryogenesis uses some fundamentally different strategies from those used by the lower vertebrates. Because the placental connection to the mother obviates the need for the developing oocyte to store large amounts of yolk, the eggs of mammals are very small. However, because mammalian development is internal and the embryo receives nourishment from the mother, cleavage is a prolonged process that typically coincides with the time required to transport the early embryo from the site of fertilization in the uterine tube to the place of implantation in the uterus. One of the prominent innovations in early mammalian embryogenesis is the formation of the **trophoblast**, the specialized tissue that forms the trophic interface between the embryo and the mother, during the cleavage period. The placenta represents the ultimate manifestation of the trophoblastic tissues.

CLEAVAGE

Morphology

In comparison with most other species, mammalian cleavage is a leisurely process measured in days rather than hours. Development proceeds at the rate of roughly one cleavage division per day for the first 3 or 4 days (Figures 3-1 and 3-2). After the two-cell stage, mammalian cleavage is asynchronous, with one of the two cells (**blastomeres**) dividing to form a three-cell embryo. When the embryo consists of approximately 16 cells, it is sometimes called a **morula** (derived from Greek and Latin words meaning "mulberry").

After several cleavage divisions, the embryos of placental mammals enter into a phase called **compaction**, during which the individual outer blastomeres tightly adhere through gap and tight junctions and lose their individual identity when viewed from the surface. Through the activity of a Na$^+$,K$^+$-ATPase-based Na$^+$ transport system, Na$^+$ and H$_2$O move across the epithelium-like outer blastomeres and accumulate in spaces among the inner blastomeres. This process, which occurs about 4 days after fertilization, is called **cavitation**, and the fluid-filled space is known as the **blastocoele**. At this stage, the embryo as a whole is known as a **blastocyst**.

At the blastocyst stage, the embryo consists of two types of cells: an outer superficial layer (the **trophoblast**) that surrounds a small inner group of cells called the **inner cell mass**.

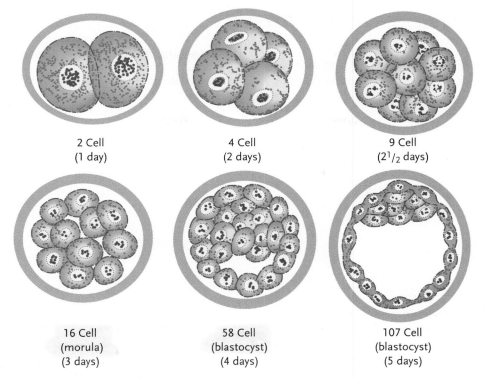

2 Cell
(1 day)

4 Cell
(2 days)

9 Cell
(2¹/₂ days)

16 Cell
(morula)
(3 days)

58 Cell
(blastocyst)
(4 days)

107 Cell
(blastocyst)
(5 days)

Figure 3-1 Drawings of early cleavage stages in human embryos. The drawings of the 58- and 107-cell stages represent sections made through the embryos.

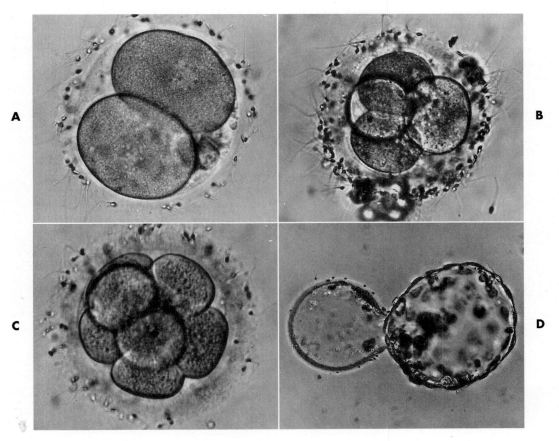

Figure 3-2 Photomicrographs of cleavage stages of human eggs fertilized in vitro. **A,** Two blastomeres 39 hours after fertilization. A polar body is seen to the right of the boundary between the blastomeres. **B,** Four blastomeres 42 hours after fertilization. **C,** Eight blastomeres 49 hours after fertilization. **D,** Hatching blastocyst 123 hours after fertilization. The empty zona pellucida is on the left. In **A** to **C,** numerous spermatozoa can be seen clinging to the zona pellucida. (From Veeck LL: *Atlas of the human oocyte and early conceptus,* vol 2, Baltimore, 1991, Williams & Wilkins.)

The appearance of these two cell types reflects major organizational changes that have occurred within the embryo and represents the specialization of the blastomeres into two distinct cell lineages. Cells of the inner cell mass give rise to the body of the embryo itself plus a number of extraembryonic structures, whereas cells of the trophoblast form only extraembryonic structures, including the outer layers of the placenta. Box 3-1 describes control of the cell cycle during cleavage.

Molecular Biology and Genetics

Most studies of the molecular biology and genetics of early mammalian development have been performed on the mouse. Until more information on early primate embryogenesis becomes available, results obtained from experimentation on mice must be used as a guide.

The consequence of the lack of advance storage of ribosomes and RNAs during mammalian oogenesis is that the zygote must rely on embryonic gene products very early during

---

BOX 3-1 Control of the Cell Cycle during Cleavage

The hallmark of the cleavage period is the successive waves of mitosis that sweep through the embryo. Each mitotic division is under the control of proteins so basic that their structures and functions have been preserved for almost a billion years. Such an interpretation is based on their presence in organisms as diverse as humans and yeasts.

Early research on frog eggs suggested the presence of a *maturation-promoting factor* (**MPF**), now often referred to as mitosis-promoting factor, that induces meiosis in early oocytes. MPF was found to be a regulator of both meiosis and mitosis. Further research showed that active MPF is a complex of two proteins, **cdc2** (cell division cycle 2) and **cyclin**, which guide a cell through its mitotic cycle.

The normal mitotic cycle is divided into four phases (Figure 3-3). **Interphase** (often called the G_1 **phase**) is the period during which the cell typically carries out its assigned functions. As it prepares for mitosis, the cell moves into the **S phase**, during which its nuclear DNA is replicated. DNA synthesis is followed by a usually brief G_2 (gap 2) **phase**, which precedes actual mitosis (**M phase**).

The cdc2 protein is present throughout the mitotic cycle. Cyclin (actually cyclin B) is synthesized and accumulates in the cell during interphase, but it combines with

cdc2 to form a prematuration-promoting factor (pre-MPF) before mitosis (see Figure 3-3). Enzymatic modification converts this complex to an active form of MPF that initiates mitosis. Among the specific actions of MPF are the initiation of the breakdown of the nuclear envelope and the stimulation of assembly of the mitotic spindle. Many of the actions of MPF involve the phosphorylation of proteins. For example, breakdown of the nuclear envelope results from the phosphorylation of **nuclear lamins**, or envelope proteins. Phosphorylation causes the lamins to dissociate, leading to disintegration of the nuclear envelope. Active MPF also activates enzymes that abruptly break down cyclin.

When cyclin levels fall below a certain threshold, the cdc protein of MPF loses its activity, thus ending mitosis. The loss of MPF activity allows cellular phosphatase enzymes to remove phosphate groups that were added to proteins under the influence of MPF. One effect of this is reformation of the nuclear envelope as the nuclear lamins become dephosphorylated. The phosphatases also inactivate the enzymes that break down cyclin, allowing the cyclin to again accumulate in the cell during interphase. This sets the stage for a repetition of the mitotic cycle.

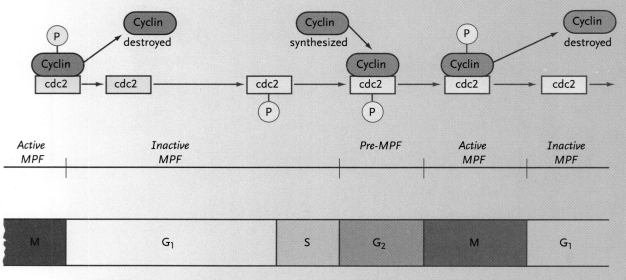

Figure 3-3 Cell cycle and its control. G_1 (gap 1), S (DNA synthesis), G_2 (gap 2), and M (mitosis) are stages of the cell cycle (see text). *P*, Phosphate.

cleavage, typically by the two- or four-cell stage (four to eight cells in the human). There does not appear, however, to be a sharp transition between the cessation of reliance on purely maternal gene products and the initiation of transcription from the embryonic genome. For example, paternal gene products (e.g., isoforms of β-glucuronidase and β$_2$-microglobulin) appear in the embryo very early, while maternal actin and histone mRNAs are still being used for the production of corresponding proteins. As an indication of the extent to which the early embryo relies on its own gene products, development past the two-cell stage does not take place in the mouse if mRNA transcription is inhibited. In contrast, similar treatment of amphibian embryos does not disrupt development until late cleavage, at which time the embryos begin to synthesize the mRNAs required to control morphogenetic movements and gastrulation.

An important gene in early development is **oct-3**, a specific transcription factor that binds the octamer ATTTGCAT on deoxyribonucleic acid (DNA). There is a close relationship between the expression of the *oct-3* gene and the highly undifferentiated state of cells. In the mouse, maternally derived oct-3 protein is found in developing oocytes and is active in the zygote. After the experimentally induced loss of oct-3 protein, development is arrested at the one-cell stage. Such studies indicate that maternally derived oct-3 protein is required to permit development to proceed to the two-cell stage, when the transcription of embryonic genes begins.

Oct-3 gene is expressed in all blastomeres up to the morula stage. As various differentiated cell types begin to emerge in the embryo, the level of *oct-3* gene expression decreases until it is no longer detectable. Such a decrease is first noted in cells that become committed to forming extraembryonic structures and finally in cells of the specific germ layers as they emerge from the primitive streak (see Chapter 4). Even after virtually all cells of the embryo have ceased to express the *oct-3* gene, it is still detectable in the primordial germ cells as they migrate from the region of the allantois to the genital ridges. Because of its patterns of distribution, oct-3 protein is suspected of playing a regulatory role in early determination or differentiation decisions by cells.

Along with a small amount of preformed maternal mRNAs in mammalian embryos is a correspondingly low capacity for translation of mRNAs. Various injection experiments suggest that the factor limiting translational efficiency may be the small number of ribosomes stored in the egg.

Even at an early stage the blastomeres of a cleaving embryo are not homogeneous. Simple staining methods reveal pronounced differences among cells in human embryos as early as the seven-cell stage (Figure 3-4). Autoradiographic studies have shown that all blastomeres of four-cell human embryos have low levels of extranucleolar and no nucleolar RNA synthesis. By the eight-cell stage, some blastomeres have very high levels of RNA synthesis, but other blastomeres still show the pattern seen in blastomeres of four-cell embryos. Morphological studies show corresponding differences between transcriptionally active and inactive blastomeres.

Once cleavage begins, transcription products from both maternally and paternally derived chromosomes are active in guiding development. Haploid embryos commonly die during cleavage or just after implantation. However, there is

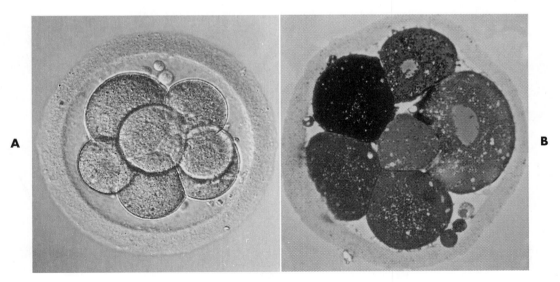

Figure 3-4 Seven-cell human embryo recovered from the uterine tube. Three small polar bodies are seen in the lower part of each photograph. The zona pellucida surrounds the blastomeres and polar bodies. **A**, Photograph of the intact embryo before fixation. **B**, Photomicrograph of a section through the embryo stained with toluidine blue. Two blastomeres stain differently (metachromatically) from the others. (Modified from Avendaño S and others: *Fertil Steril* 26:1167-1172, 1975.)

increasing evidence that the control of early development involves more than simply having a diploid set of chromosomes in each cell.

Parental imprinting

Experimentation, coupled with observations on some unusual developmental disturbances in mice and humans, has shown that the expression of certain genes derived from the egg differs from the expression of the same genes derived from the spermatozoon. Called **parental imprinting**, the effects are manifest in different ways. It is possible to remove a pronucleus from a newly inseminated mouse egg and replace it with a pronucleus taken from another inseminated egg at a similar stage of development (Figure 3-5). If a male or female pronucleus is removed and replaced with a corresponding male or female pronucleus, development is normal. However, if a male pronucleus is removed and replaced with a female pronucleus (resulting in a zygote with two female pronuclei), the embryo itself develops fairly normally, but the placenta and yolk sac are poorly developed. Conversely, a zygote with two male pronuclei produces a severely stunted embryo, whereas the placenta and yolk sac are nearly normal.

Paternal imprinting selectively turns off certain genes involved in the development of the embryo itself, whereas maternal imprinting turns off some genes involved in the formation of extraembryonic structures such as the placenta. Parental imprinting occurs during gametogenesis through the methylation of certain bases (especially cytosines in CpG sequences). This methylation results in the differential expression of paternal and maternal alleles of the imprinted genes during embryonic development. The imprinted genes operate

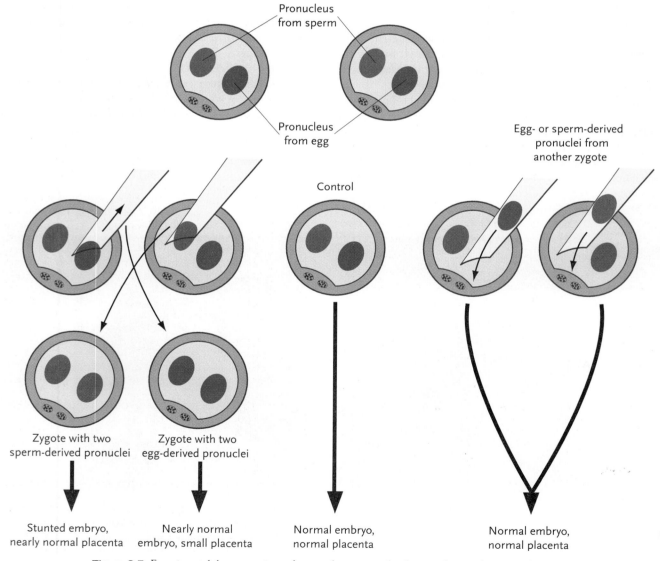

Figure 3-5 Experimental demonstrations of parental imprinting by the use of pronuclear transplants.

during development and possibly into adulthood, but a given imprint is not passed on to that individual's progeny. Instead, the parental imprints on the genes in the gametes are erased and new imprints, corresponding to the sex of that individual, are established in the eggs or sperm during gametogenesis.

Not all genes are parentally imprinted. As of this writing, fewer than two dozen imprinted genes have been identified, but estimates suggest that up to 500 of the roughly 100,000 human genes may be affected by imprinting (Table 3-1). Clinical Correlation 3-1 discusses some conditions and syndromes associated with parental imprinting.

X-chromosome inactivation

Another example of the inequality of genetic expression during early development is the pattern of X-chromosome inactivation in female embryos. It is well known from cytogenetic studies that one of the two X chromosomes in the cells of females is inactivated by extreme condensation. This is the basis for the **sex chromatin** or **Barr body** that can be demonstrated in cells of females but not those of normal males. The purpose of X-chromosome inactivation is dosage compensation, or preserving the cells from an excess of X-chromosomal gene products.

Studies of levels of enzymes encoded in the DNA of the X chromosome in mice have shown that both X chromosomes are transcriptionally active during early cleavage of female embryos. After differentiation of the blastomeres into either trophoblast or inner cell mass, the pattern changes (Figure 3-6). Both X chromosomes continue to be active in cells of the inner cell mass, whereas in all cells of the trophoblast (**trophectoderm**), the paternally derived X chromosome is selectively inactivated. As the cells of the inner cell mass become subdivided into other lineages, differential X-chromosomal inactivation also occurs. X inactivation ultimately occurs in all cells, and only during oogenesis do both X chromosomes of the oocytes become active again. The selective inactivation of

the paternal X chromosome in the trophoblast is another example of parental genetic imprinting, although the mechanism of inactivation may be different.

A recently discovered gene, X-inactive specific transcript (**XIST**), is involved in the inactivation of an X chromosome. Its RNA transcripts remain in the nucleus and do not form proteins. Through a counting mechanism that is not yet understood, one X chromosome breaks down its XIST mRNAs. The remaining X chromosome accumulates stabilized XIST mRNA and subsequently undergoes inactivation. X-chromosomal inactivation occurs when cells undergo restriction and begin to differentiate, rather than remaining **totipotent** (capable of forming all types of progeny). Paternal imprinting on the *XIST* gene accounts for the selective inactivation of the paternal X chromosome in the extraembryonic trophectoderm and extraembryonic endoderm during cleavage (see Figure 3-6). Because they retain their totipotency longer, cells of the inner cell mass do not undertake X-chromosomal inactivation until later, but why random inactivation of either a maternally or a paternally derived X chromosome occurs in these cells is not understood.

TABLE 3-1 Differential Effects of Paternally and Maternally Expressed Genes

Function	Paternal imprinting	Maternal imprinting
Overall growth	Stimulated (IGF-2)	Reduced (H-19)
Stem cell behavior	Proliferation	Differentiation
Enhanced differentiation	Muscle	Epidermis
Localization of activity in brain	Hypothalamus	Neocortex
Effect on behavior	Hyperkinetic	Hypokinetic

Modified from Reik W: *Exp Physiol* 81:163, 1996.

CLINICAL CORRELATION 3-1
Conditions and Syndromes Associated with Parental Imprinting

A striking example of paternal imprinting in the human is a **hydatidiform mole** (see Figure 6-17), which is characterized by the overdevelopment of trophoblastic tissues and the extreme underdevelopment of the embryo. This condition can result from the fertilization of an egg by two spermatozoa and the consequent failure of the maternal genome of the egg to participate in development or from the duplication of a sperm pronucleus in an "empty" egg. This form of highly abnormal development is consistent with the hypothesis that paternal imprinting favors the development of the trophoblast at the expense of the embryo.

Several other syndromes are also based on parental imprinting. The **Beckwith-Wiedemann syndrome**, characterized by fetal overgrowth and an increased incidence of childhood cancers, has been mapped to the imprinted region on chromosome 11, which contains the genes for insulin-like growth factor-2 (IGF-2, which promotes cell proliferation) and H19 (a growth suppressor). It occurs when both alleles of the *IGF-2* gene express a paternal imprinting pattern. Another instructive example involves deletion of the long arm of chromosome 15. Children of either sex who inherit the maternal deletion develop **Angelman's syndrome**, which includes severe mental retardation, seizures, and ataxia. A child who inherits a paternal deletion of the same region develops the **Prader-Willi syndrome**, characterized by obesity, short stature, hypogonadism, a bowed upper lip, and mild mental retardation.

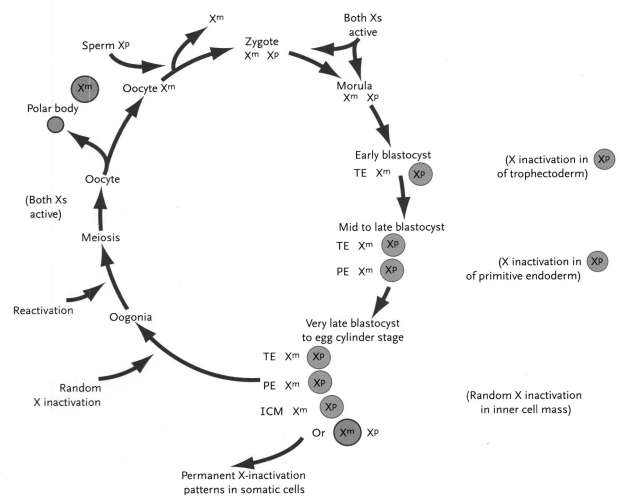

Figure 3-6 X-chromosomal inactivation and reactivation during the mammalian life cycle. The red and green circles refer to inactivated paternally and maternally derived X chromosomes, respectively. *ICM*, Inner cell mass; *PE*, primitive (extraembryonic) endoderm; *TE*, trophectoderm; *X^m*, maternal X chromosome; *X^p*, paternal X chromosome. (Based on Gartler SM, Riggs HD: *Annu Rev Genet* 17:155-190, 1983.)

Developmental Properties of Cleaving Embryos

Early mammalian embryogenesis is considered to be a highly regulative process. **Regulation** is the ability of an embryo or organ primordium to produce a normal structure if parts have been removed or added.* At the cellular level, it means that the fates of cells in a regulative system are not irretrievably fixed and that the cells can still respond to environmental cues. Because the assignment of blastomeres into different cell

*Opposed to regulative development is **mosaic development,** which is characterized by the inability to compensate for defects or to integrate extra cells into a unified whole. In a mosaic system, the fates of cells are rigidly determined, and removal of cells results in an embryo or a structure missing the components that the removed cells were destined to form. Most regulative systems have an increasing tendency to exhibit mosaic properties as development progresses.

lineages is one of the principal features of mammalian development, identifying the environmental factors that are involved is important.

Of the experimental techniques used to demonstrate regulative properties of early embryos, the simplest is to separate the blastomeres of early cleavage–stage embryos and determine whether each one can give rise to an entire embryo. This method has been used to demonstrate that single blastomeres from two- and sometimes four-cell embryos can form normal embryos, although blastomeres from later stages cannot do so. In mammalian studies, a single cell is more commonly taken from an early cleavage–stage embryo and injected into the blastocoele of a genetically different host. Such injected cells become incorporated into the host embryo, forming cellular **chimeras** or **mosaics.** When genetically different donor blastomeres are injected into host embryos, the donor cells can be

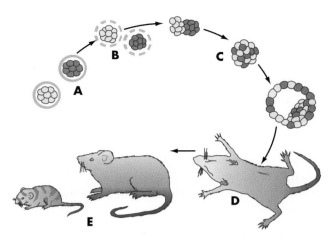

Figure 3-7 Procedure for producing tetraparental embryos. A, Cleavage stages of two different strains of mice. B, Removal of the zona pellucida. C, Fusion of the two embryos. D, Implantation of embryos into a foster mother. E, Chimeric offspring obtained from the implanted embryos.

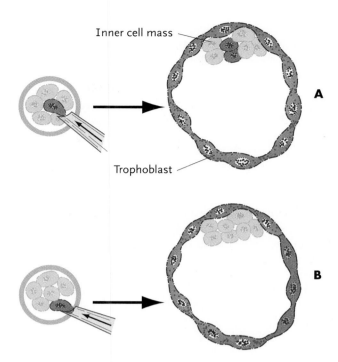

Figure 3-8 Experiments illustrating the inside-outside hypothesis of cell determination in early mammalian embryos. A, If a marked blastomere is inserted into the interior of a morula, it and its progeny become part of the inner cell mass. B, If a marked blastomere is placed on the outside of a host morula, it and its descendants contribute to the trophoblast.

identified by histochemical or cytogenetic analysis, and their fate (the tissues that they form) can be determined. **Fate mapping** experiments are important in embryology because they allow one to follow the pathways along which a particular cell can differentiate. Fate mapping experiments, which involve different isozymes of the enzyme **glucose phosphate isomerase,** have shown that all blastomeres of an eight-cell mouse embryo remain **totipotent;** that is, they retain the ability to form any cell type in the body. Even at the 16-cell stage of cleavage, some blastomeres are capable of producing progeny that are found in both the inner cell mass and the trophoblastic lineage.

Another means of demonstrating the regulative properties of early mammalian embryos is to dissociate mouse embryos into separate blastomeres and then to combine the blastomeres of two or three embryos (Figure 3-7). The combined blastomeres soon aggregate and reorganize to become a single large embryo, which then goes on to become a normal-appearing **tetraparental** or **hexaparental mouse.** By various techniques of making chimeric embryos, it is even possible to combine blastomeres to produce interspecies chimeras (e.g., a sheep-goat).

One of the most important steps in early mammalian development is the decision that results in the appearance of two separate lines of cells—the trophoblast and the inner cell mass—from the early blastomeres. Up to the eight-cell stage in mice, all blastomeres are virtually identical in their developmental potential. Shortly thereafter, differences are noted between cells that have at least one surface situated on the outer border of the embryo and those that are completely enclosed by other blastomeres.

The relationship between the position of the blastomeres and their ultimate developmental fate was incorporated into the **inside-outside hypothesis.** The outer blastomeres ulti-

mately differentiate into the trophoblast, whereas the inner blastomeres form the inner cell mass, from which the body of the embryo arises. Although this hypothesis has been supported by various experiments, the mechanisms by which the blastomeres recognize their positions and then differentiate accordingly have remained elusive and are still little understood. If marked blastomeres from disaggregated embryos are placed on the outside of another early embryo, they typically contribute to the formation of the trophoblast. Conversely, if the same marked cells are introduced into the interior of the host embryo, they participate in the formation of the inner cell mass (Figure 3-8). Outer cells in the early mammalian embryo are linked by tight and gap junctions, but whether this morphological characteristic is a cause or an effect of their differentiation into trophoblast is not known. Experiments of this type demonstrate that the **developmental potential or potency** (the types of cells that a precursor cell can form) of many cells is greater than their normal **developmental fate** (the types of cells that a precursor cell normally forms).

Another characteristic of cleavage-stage mammalian embryos is the absence of rigidly fixed body axes. In many lower vertebrates the dorsoventral axis is fixed in the egg before fertilization, and the anteroposterior axis is determined at fertilization by the site of penetration of the egg by the sperm. Avian and mammalian embryos, on the other hand, do not show evidence of axial fixation until considerably later during cleavage. In the 4- to 5-day-old human blastocyst with a well-defined inner cell mass, the dorsal surface is the part of the inner cell mass that abuts the outer trophoblast, and the ventral surface is the part that faces the blastocyst cavity. Not until almost 2 weeks after fertilization can the longitudinal axis be identified. Recognizing the cranial from the caudal end of the embryo (longitudinal axis) is possible only after the appearance of the primitive streak early in the third week.

Experimental Manipulations of Cleaving Embryos

Much of the knowledge about the developmental properties of early mammalian embryos is the result of recently devised techniques for experimentally manipulating them. Typically, the use of these techniques must be combined with other techniques that have been designed for in vitro fertilization, embryo culture, and embryo transfer (see Chapter 2).

Classic strategies for investigating the developmental properties of embryos are (1) removing a part and determining the way that the remainder of the embryo compensates for the loss (such experiments are called **deletion** or **ablation experiments**) and (2) adding a part and determining the way that the embryo integrates the added material into its overall body plan (such experiments are called **addition**

experiments). Although some deletion experiments have been done, the strategy of addition experiments has proved to be most fruitful in elucidating mechanisms controlling mammalian embryogenesis.

Blastomere deletion and addition experiments (Figure 3-9) have convincingly demonstrated the regulative nature (i.e., the strong tendency for the system to be restored to wholeness) of early mammalian embryos. Such knowledge is important in understanding why the exposure of early human embryos to unfavorable environmental influences typically results in either death or a normal embryo.

One of the most powerful experimental techniques of the last two decades has been the injection of genetically or artificially labeled cells into the blastocyst cavity of a host embryo (see Figure 3-9, *B*). This technique has been used to show that the added cells become normally integrated into the body of the host embryo, providing additional evidence for embryonic regulation. An equally powerful use of this technique has been in the study of cell lineages in the early embryo. By identifying the progeny of the injected marked cells, investigators have been able to determine the developmental potency of the donor cells.

A technique that is providing new insight into the genetic control mechanisms of mammalian development is the production of **transgenic embryos.** Transgenic embryos (com-

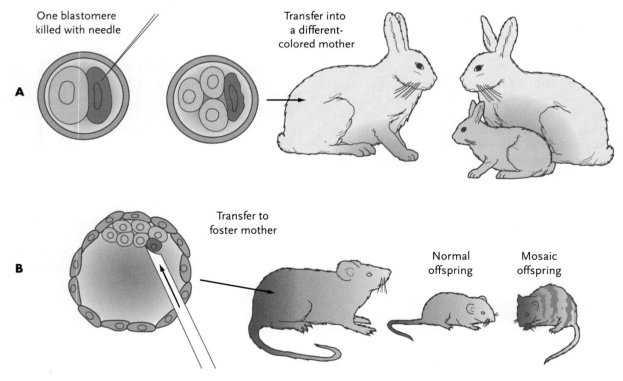

Figure 3-9 Blastomere addition and deletion experiments. **A,** If one blastomere is killed with a needle and the embryo is transferred into a different-colored mother, a normal offspring of the color of the experimentally damaged embryo is produced. **B,** If a blastomere of a different strain is introduced into a blastocyst, a mosaic offspring with color markings characteristic of the strain of the introduced blastomere is produced.

monly mice) are produced by directly injecting foreign DNA into the pronuclei of zygotes (Figure 3-10, *A*). The DNA, typically recombinant DNA for a specific gene, can be fused with a different regulatory element that can be controlled by the investigator. For example, transgenic mice have been created by injecting the rat growth hormone gene coupled with a metallothionein promoter region (*MT-I*) into the pronuclei of mouse zygotes. The injected zygotes are transplanted into the uteri of foster mothers, which give birth to normal-looking transgenic mice. Later in life, when these transgenic mice are fed a diet rich in zinc, which stimulates the MT-I promoter region, the rat growth hormone gene is activated, causing the liver to produce large amounts of the polypeptide growth hormone. The function of the transplanted gene is obvious; under the influence of the rat growth hormone that they were producing, the transgenic mice grew to a much larger size than their normal littermates (Figure 3-11). The

technique of producing transgenic embryos is being increasingly used both to examine factors regulating the expression of specific genes in embryos and to disrupt genes in the host embryos. In addition, the efficacy of this technique to correct known genetic defects is being increasingly explored in mice.

An important technological advance is the creation of lines of embryo-derived stem cells (**ES cells**). ES cells are originally derived from inner cell masses and can be propagated in vitro as lines of pluripotential cells that can be either maintained in an undifferentiated condition or stimulated to undergo specific lines of differentiation. It is now possible to genetically engineer specific genes in ES cells. When such genetically manipulated cells are introduced into blastocysts, they can become incorporated into the host embryo (see Figure 3-10, *B*). If the progeny of a genetically engineered ES cell become incorporated into the germ line, the genetic trait can be passed to succeeding generations.

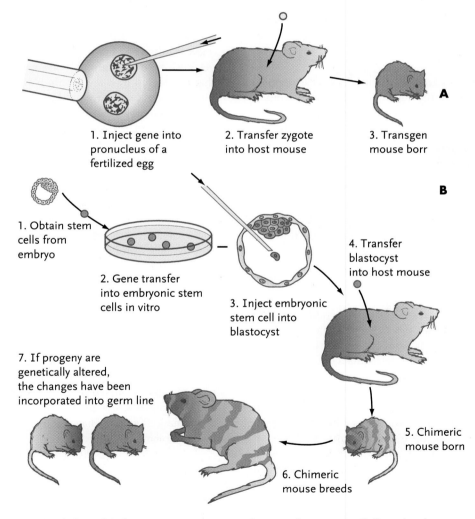

Figure 3-10   A, Procedure for creating transgenic mice by pronuclear injection. **B,** Procedure for inserting genes into mice by first introducing them into embryonic stem cells and then inserting the transfected stem cells into an otherwise normal blastocyst.

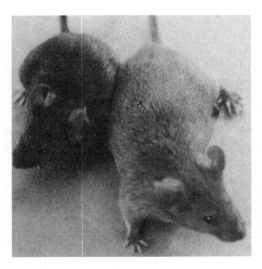

Figure 3-11 Photograph of two 10-week-old mice. The one on the left (normal mouse) weighs 21.2 gm. The one on the right (a transgenic littermate of the normal mouse) carries a rat gene coding for growth hormone. It weighs 41.2 gm. (From Palmiter RD and others: *Nature* 300:611-615, 1982.)

Some types of twinning represent a natural experiment that demonstrates the highly regulative nature of early human embryos, as described in Clinical Correlation 3-2.

EMBRYO TRANSPORT AND IMPLANTATION

Transport Mechanisms by the Uterine Tube

The entire period of early cleavage takes place while the embryo is being transported from the place of fertilization to its implantation site in the uterus (see Figure 2-2). It is increasingly apparent that the early embryo and the female reproductive tract influence one another during this period of transport, but knowledge is still fragmentary.

At the beginning of cleavage, the zygote is still encased in the zona pellucida and the cells of the corona radiata. The corona radiata is lost within 2 days of the start of cleavage. The zona pellucida, however, remains intact until the embryo reaches the uterus.

The embryo remains in the ampullary portion of the uterine tube for approximately 3 days. It then traverses the isthmic portion of the tube in as little as 8 hours. Under the influence of progesterone, the uterotubal junction relaxes, allowing the embryo to enter the uterine cavity. A couple of days later (6 to 8 days after fertilization), the embryo implants into the midportion of the posterior wall of the uterus.

Zona Pellucida

During the entire period from ovulation until its entry into the uterine cavity, the ovum and then the embryo are sur-

rounded by the zona pellucida. After the embryo reaches the uterine cavity, it sheds the zona pellucida in preparation for implantation. The blastocyst "hatches" from the zona by digesting a hole through it by means of a trypsin-like enzyme that is secreted by a few trophoblastic cells. The blastocyst then extrudes itself through the hole. Very few specimens of human embryos have been taken in vivo from the period just preceding implantation, but in vitro studies on human embryos suggest a similar mechanism, which probably occurs 1 to 2 days before implantation (see Figure 3-2, *D*). Box 3-2 summarizes the functions of the zona pellucida.

Implantation into the Uterine Lining

Approximately 6 to 7 days after fertilization, the embryo begins to make a firm attachment to the epithelial lining of the endometrium. Soon thereafter, it sinks into the endometrial stroma, and its original site of penetration into the endometrium becomes closed over by the epithelium, much like a healing skin wound.

Successful implantation requires a high degree of preparation and coordination by both the embryo and the endometrium (Table 3-2). The complex hormonal preparations of the endometrium that began at the close of the previous menstrual period are all aimed at providing a suitable cellular and nutritional environment for the embryo. Dissolution of the zona pellucida signals the readiness of the embryo to begin implantation.

The first stage in implantation consists of attachment of the expanded blastocyst to the endometrial epithelium. The apical surfaces of the hormonally conditioned endometrial epithelial cells express a variety of adhesion molecules (integrin subunits) that allow implantation to occur in the narrow window of 20 to 24 days in the ideal menstrual cycle. Correspondingly, the trophoblastic cells of the preimplantation blastocyst also express integrins on their surfaces. According

---

BOX 3-2   Summary of Functions of the Zona Pellucida

1. The zona pellucida serves as a barrier that normally allows only sperm of the same species access to the egg.
2. After fertilization, the modified zona prevents any additional spermatozoa from reaching the zygote.
3. During the early stages of cleavage, it acts as a porous filter through which certain substances secreted by the uterine tube can reach the embryo.
4. Because it lacks histocompatibility (HLA) antigens, it serves as an immunological barrier between the mother and the antigenically different embryo.
5. It prevents the blastomeres of the early cleaving embryo from dissociating.
6. It normally prevents premature implantation of the cleaving embryo into the wall of the uterine tube.

CLINICAL CORRELATION 3-2
Twinning

Some types of twinning represent a natural experiment that demonstrates the highly regulative nature of early human embryos. In the United States, roughly one pregnancy in 90 results in twins, and one in 8000 results in triplets. Of the total number of twins born, approximately two thirds are **fraternal**, or **dizygotic**, twins and one third are **identical**, or **monozygotic**, twins. Dizygotic twins are the product of the fertilization of two ovulated eggs, and the mechanism of their formation involves the endocrine control of ovulation. Monozygotic twins and some triplets, on the other hand, are the product of one fertilized egg. They arise by the subdivision and splitting of a single embryo. Although monozygotic twins could theoretically arise by the splitting of a two-cell embryo, it is commonly accepted that most arise by the subdivision of the inner cell mass in a blastocyst (Figure 3-12). Because the majority of monozygotic twins are perfectly normal, the early human embryo can obviously be subdivided and each component regulated to form a normal embryo. Inferences on the origin and relations of multiple births can be made from the arrangement of the extraembryonic membranes at the time of birth (see Chapter 6).

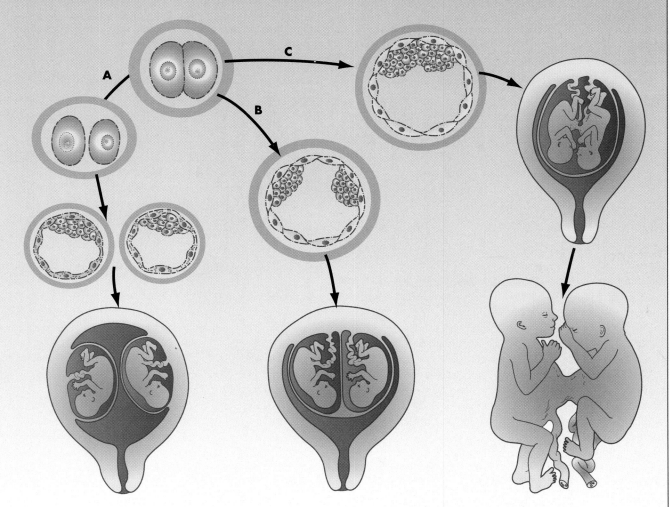

Figure 3-12 Modes of monozygotic twinning. **A,** Cleavage of an early embryo, with each half developing as a completely separate embryo. **B,** Splitting of the inner cell mass of a blastocyst and the formation of two embryos enclosed in a common trophoblast. This is the most common mode of twinning. **C,** If the inner cell mass does not completely separate or if separated portions of the inner cell mass secondarily rejoin, conjoined twins may result.

Continued

CLINICAL CORRELATION 3-2
Twinning—cont'd

Quadruplets or higher orders of multiple births occur very rarely. In previous years, these could be combinations of multiple ovulations and splitting of single blastocysts. In the modern era of reproductive technology, the majority of multiple births, sometimes up to septuplets, can be attributed to the side effects of fertility drugs taken by the mother.

The separation of portions of the inner cell mass in an embryo is sometimes incomplete, and although two embryos take shape, they are joined by a tissue bridge of varying proportions. When this occurs, the twins are called **conjoined twins** (sometimes colloquially called *Siamese twins*). The extent of bridging between the twins varies from a relatively thin connection in the chest or back to massive fusions along much of the body axis. Examples of the wide va-

riety of types of conjoined twins are illustrated in Figures 3-13 and 3-14. With the increasing sophistication of surgical techniques, twins with more complex degrees of fusion can be separated. A much less common variety of conjoined twin is a **parasitic twin,** in which a much smaller but often remarkably complete portion of a body protrudes from the body of an otherwise normal host twin (Figure 3-15). Common attachment sites of parasitic twins are the oral region, the mediastinum, and the pelvis. The mechanism of conjoined twinning has not been directly demonstrated experimentally, but possible theoretical explanations are the partial secondary fusion of originally separated portions of the inner cell mass or the formation of two primitive streaks in a single embryo (see Chapter 4).

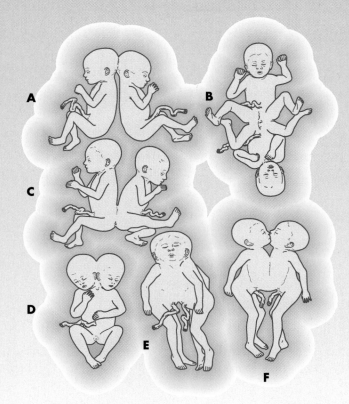

Figure 3-13 Types of conjoined twins. **A,** Head-to-head fusion (cephalopagus). **B** and **C,** Rump-to-rump fusion (pygopagus). **D,** Massive fusion of head and trunk, resulting in a reduction in the number of appendages and a single umbilical cord. **E,** Fusion involving both head and thorax (cephalothoracopagus). **F,** Chest-to-chest fusion (thoracopagus).

CLINICAL CORRELATION 3-2
Twinning—cont'd

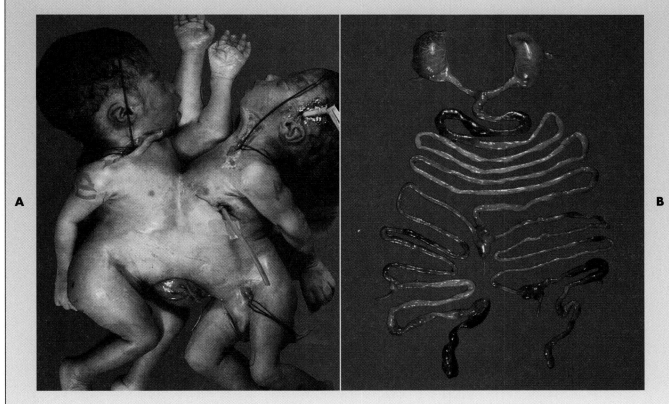

Figure 3-14 A, Conjoined twins with broad truncal attachment (thoracopagus). **B,** Dissected intestinal tracts from the same twins showing partial fusion of the small intestine and mirror image symmetry of the stomachs. (Courtesy M. Barr, Ann Arbor, Michigan.)

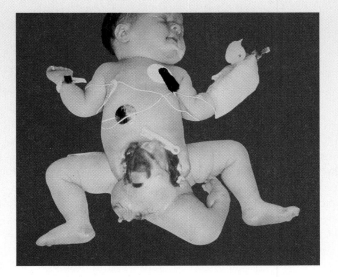

Figure 3-15 Parasitic twin arising from the pelvic region of the host twin. One well-defined leg and some hair can be seen on the parasitic twin. (Courtesy M. Barr, Ann Arbor, Michigan.)

Continued

CLINICAL CORRELATION 3-2
Twinning—cont'd

One phenomenon often encountered in conjoined twins is a reversal of symmetry of the organs of one of the pair (see Figure 3-14, *B*). Such reversals of symmetry are common in duplicated organs or entire embryos. Over a century ago, this phenomenon was recorded in a large variety of biological situations and was incorporated into what is now called **Bateson's rule,** which states that when duplicated structures are joined during critical developmental stages, one structure is the mirror image of the other. Despite the long recognition of this phenomenon, only in recent years has there been any understanding of the mechanism behind the reversal of symmetry.

Reversal of symmetry, called **situs inversus,** is also seen in roughly one in 10,000 superficially normal individuals born from single births (Figure 3-16). Such an individual is often not recognized until examined relatively late in life by an astute diagnostician. The basis for the normal asymmetry of the body (e.g., stomach on left, liver on right) has only recently begun to be understood. With the discovery of a recessive mutation that consistently produces situs inversus in mice, a genetic basis for the normal asymmetry of the body has been established. A molecular basis for body asymmetry is also being pieced together, with certain key signaling molecules being expressed on either the right or the left side of the organizing region during gastrulation (see p. 69).

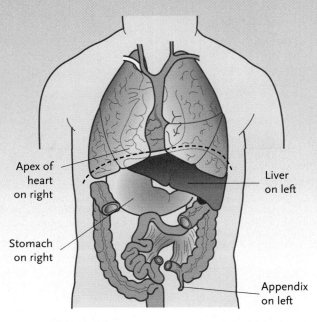

Apex of heart on right

Liver on left

Stomach on right

Appendix on left

Figure 3-16   Complete situs inversus in an adult.

to a contemporary model, the blastocyst attaches to the endometrial epithelium through the mediation of bridging ligands that connect with the integrins on their surfaces. Both in vivo and in vitro studies have shown that attachment of the blastocyst occurs at the area above the inner cell mass (**embryonic pole**), suggesting that the surfaces of the trophoblast are not all the same.

The next stage of implantation is penetration of the uterine epithelium. In primates, the cellular trophoblast undergoes a further stage in its differentiation just before it contacts the endometrium. In the area around the inner cell mass, cells derived from the cellular trophoblast (**cytotrophoblast**) fuse to

form a multinucleated **syncytiotrophoblast.** Although only a small area of syncytiotrophoblast is evident at the start of implantation, this structure (sometimes called the **syntrophoblast**) soon surrounds the entire embryo. Small projections of syncytiotrophoblast insert themselves between uterine epithelial cells. They then spread along the epithelial surface of the basal lamina that underlies the endometrial epithelium to form a somewhat flattened **trophoblastic plate.** Within a day or so, syncytiotrophoblastic projections from the small trophoblastic plate begin to penetrate the basal lamina (Figure 3-17, *A* and *B*). The early syncytiotrophoblast is a highly invasive tissue, and it quickly expands and erodes

TABLE 3-2   Stages in Human Implantation

Age (days)	Developmental event in embryos
5	Maturation of blastocyst
5	Loss of zona pellucida from blastocyst
6?	Attachment of blastocyst to uterine epithelium
6-7	Epithelial penetration
7½-9	Trophoblastic plate formation and invasion of uterine stroma by blastocyst
9-11	Lacuna formation along with erosion of spiral arteries in endometrium
12-13	Primary villus formation
13-15	Secondary placental villi, secondary yolk sac formation
16-18	Branching and anchoring villus formation
18-22	Tertiary villus formation

Modified from Enders AC. In *Encyclopedia of human biology,* vol 4, New York, 1991, Academic.

CLINICAL VIGNETTE

Within a week, two young women in their 20s come to the emergency room of a large city hospital, each complaining of acute pain in her lower left abdominal quadrant. On physical examination, both are exquisitely sensitive to mild pressure in that area.

Further questioning of the first woman revealed that she had had a menstrual period 2 weeks previously. Emergency surgery was performed, and it was found that the woman had a ruptured appendix. During the surgical procedure a major anatomical abnormality was found and confirmed with subsequent study.

What is a likely explanation for this?

The second young woman gave a history of gonorrhea and had been treated for pelvic inflammation. Her last menstrual period was 9 weeks previously. During emergency surgery, her left uterine tube was removed.

What was the likely reason for doing so?

its way into the endometrial stroma. Although the invasion of the syncytiotrophoblast into the endometrium is obviously enzymatically mediated, the biochemical basis in humans is little understood. By 10 to 12 days after fertilization, the embryo is completely embedded in the endometrium. The site of initial penetration is first marked by a bare area or a noncellular plug and is later sealed by migrating uterine epithelial cells (Figure 3-17, C and D).

As early implantation continues, projections from the invading syncytiotrophoblast envelop portions of the maternal endometrial blood vessels. They erode into the vessel walls, and maternal blood begins to fill the isolated lacunae that have been forming in the trophoblast (see Figure 3-17, C and D). Trophoblastic processes enter the blood vessels and even share junctional complexes with the endothelial cells. By the time blood-filled lacunae have formed, the trophoblast changes character, and it is not as invasive as it was during the first few days of implantation.

While the embryo burrows into the endometrium and some cytotrophoblastic cells fuse into syncytiotrophoblast, the fibroblast-like stromal cells of the somewhat edematous endometrium swell, with the accumulation of glycogen and lipid droplets (see Figure 6-6). These cells, called **decidual cells,** are tightly adherent and form a massive cellular matrix that first surrounds the implanting embryo and later occupies most of the endometrium. Concurrent with the **decidual reaction,** as this transformation is called, the leukocytes that have infiltrated the endometrial stroma during the late progestational phase of the endometrial cycle secrete **interleukin-2,** which prevents maternal recognition of the embryo as a foreign body during the early stages of implantation. An embryo is antigenically different from the mother and con-

sequently should be rejected by a cellular immune reaction similar to the type that rejects an incompatible heart or kidney transplant. It appears that a primary function of the decidual reaction is to provide an immunologically privileged site to protect the developing embryo from being rejected, but a real understanding of how this is accomplished has resisted years of intensive research.

Not infrequently, a blastocyst fails to attach to the endometrium, and implantation does not occur. Failure of implantation is a particularly vexing problem in in vitro fertilization and embryo transfer procedures, for which the success rate of implantation of transferred embryos remains at about 20% (Clinical Correlation 3-3).

Embryo Failure and Spontaneous Abortion

A high percentage of fertilized eggs (over 50%) do not develop to maturity and are spontaneously aborted. Most spontaneous abortions (**miscarriages**) occur during the first 3 weeks of pregnancy. Because of the small size of the embryo at that time, spontaneous abortions are often not recognized by the mother, who may equate the abortion and attendant hemorrhage with a late and unusually heavy menstrual period.

Examinations of early embryos obtained after spontaneous abortion or from uteri removed by hysterectomy during the early weeks of pregnancy have shown that many of the aborted embryos are highly abnormal. Chromosomal abnormalities represent the most common category of abnormality in abortuses (about 50% of the cases). When viewed in the light of the accompanying pathological conditions, spontaneous abortion can be viewed as a natural mechanism for reducing the incidence of severely malformed infants.

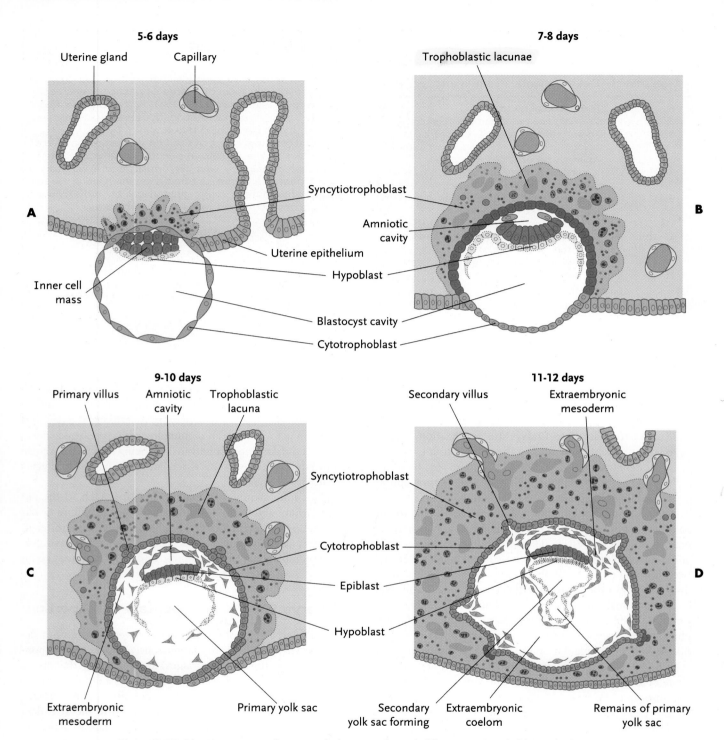

5-6 days

Uterine gland

Capillary

A

Inner cell mass

7-8 days

Trophoblastic lacunae

Syncytiotrophoblast

Amniotic cavity

Uterine epithelium

Hypoblast

Blastocyst cavity

Cytotrophoblast

B

9-10 days

Primary villus   Amniotic cavity   Trophoblastic lacuna

C

Extraembryonic mesoderm

Primary yolk sac

Syncytiotrophoblast

Cytotrophoblast

Epiblast

Hypoblast

11-12 days

Secondary villus   Extraembryonic mesoderm

D

Secondary yolk sac forming

Extraembryonic coelom

Remains of primary yolk sac

Figure 3-17 Major stages in implantation of a human embryo. **A,** The syncytiotrophoblast is just beginning to invade the endometrial stroma. **B,** Most of the embryo is embedded in the endometrium; there is early formation of the trophoblastic lacunae. The amniotic cavity and yolk sac are beginning to form. **C,** Implantation is almost complete, primary villi are forming, and the extraembryonic mesoderm is appearing. **D,** Implantation is complete; secondary villi are forming.

CLINICAL CORRELATION 3-3
Ectopic Pregnancy

The blastocyst typically implants into the posterior wall of the uterine cavity, but in a low percentage (0.25% to 1.0%) of cases, implantation occurs in an abnormal site. Such a condition is known as an **ectopic pregnancy.**

Tubal pregnancies are by far the most common type of ectopic pregnancy. Although most tubal pregnancies are found in the ampullary portion of the tube, they can be located anywhere from the fimbriated end to the uterotubal junction (Figure 3-18). Tubal pregnancies (Figure 3-19) are most commonly seen in women who have had **endometriosis** (a condition characterized by the presence of endometrium-like tissue in abnormal locations), prior surgery, or **pelvic inflammatory disease.** Scarring from inflammation or sometimes anatomical abnormalities result in blind pockets among the mucosal folds of the uterine tube; these can trap a blastocyst. Typically, the woman shows the normal signs of early pregnancy, but at about 2 to 2½ months, the implanted embryo and its associated trophoblastic derivatives have grown to the point where the stretching of the tube causes acute abdominal pain. If untreated, a tubal pregnancy typically ends with rupture of the tube and hemorrhage, often severe enough to be life threatening to the mother.

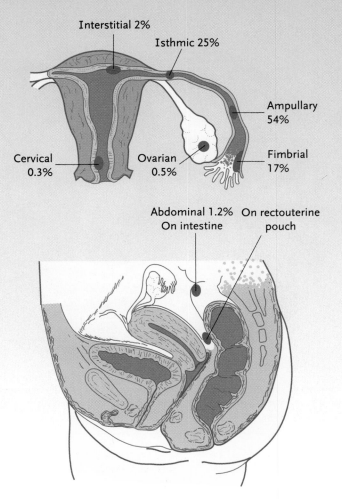

Figure 3-18 Sites of ectopic pregnancy (indicated by red dots) and the frequency of their occurrence.

Continued

CLINICAL CORRELATION 3-3
Ectopic Pregnancy—cont'd

Very rarely an embryo implants in the ovary **(ovarian pregnancy)** or in the abdominal cavity **(abdominal pregnancy).** Such instances can be the result of fertilization of an ovum before it enters the tube, the reflux of a fertilized egg from the tube, or very rarely, the penetration of a tubal pregnancy through the wall of the tube. The most common implantation site for an abdominal pregnancy is in the **rectouterine pouch (pouch of Douglas),** which is located behind the uterus. Implantation on the intestinal wall or mesentery is very dangerous because of the likelihood of severe hemorrhage as the embryo grows. In some instances, an embryo has developed to full term in an abdominal location. If not delivered, such an embryo can calcify, forming a **lithopedion.**

Within the uterus, an embryo can implant close to the cervix. Although embryonic development is likely to be normal, the placenta typically forms a partial covering over the cervical canal. This condition, called **placenta previa,** can result in hemorrhage during late pregnancy and if untreated, would likely cause the death of the fetus, the mother, or both persons because of premature placental detachment with accompanying hemorrhage. Implantation directly within the cervical canal is extremely rare.

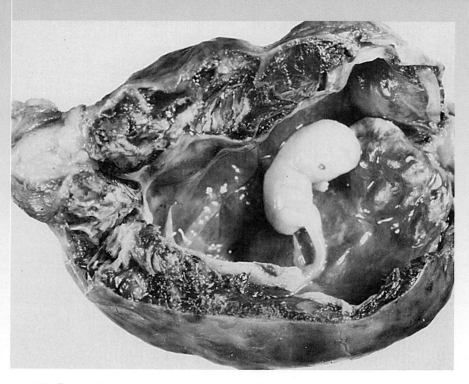

Figure 3-19 Ruptured ectopic pregnancy in a 34-year-old woman. Because of the increasing size of the fetus and associated membranes, the uterine tube ruptured during the third month of pregnancy. (From Rosai J: *Ackerman's surgical pathology,* vol 2, ed 8, St Louis, 1996, Mosby.)

SUMMARY

- Early human cleavage is slow, with roughly one cleavage division occurring per day for the first 3 to 4 days. The cleaving embryo passes through the morula stage (16 cells) and enters a stage of compaction. By day 4, a fluid-filled blastocoele forms within the embryo, and the embryo becomes a blastocyst with an inner cell mass surrounded by a trophoblast.

- The zygote relies on maternal mRNAs, but by the two-cell stage, the embryonic genome becomes activated. The *oct-3* gene is important in very early development, and its expression is associated with the undifferentiated state of cells.

- Cleavage divisions (and all cell divisions) are regulated by a maturation-promoting factor, which is a complex of cdc2 and cyclin proteins. After mitosis, cyclin is broken down. Before the next cell division, cyclin is built up and complexes with cdc2. This complex becomes activated to become maturation-promoting factor, which initiates mitosis.

- Through parental imprinting, specific homologous chromosomes derived from the mother and father exert different effects on embryonic development. In female embryos, one X chromosome per cell becomes inactivated through the action of the *XIST* gene, forming the sex chromatin body. The early embryo has distinct patterns of X-chromosomal inactivation.

- The early mammalian embryo is highly regulative. It can compensate for the loss or addition of cells to the inner cell mass and still form a normal embryo. According to the inside-outside hypothesis, the position of a blastomere determines its developmental fate (i.e., whether it will become part of the inner cell mass or the trophoblast).

- Transgenic embryos are produced by injecting recombinant DNA into the pronuclei of zygotes. Such embryos are used to study the effects of specific genes on development.

- Monozygotic twinning, usually caused by the complete separation of the inner cell mass, is possible because of the regulative properties of the early embryo. Incomplete splitting of the inner cell mass can lead to the formation of conjoined twins.

- After fertilization, the embryo spends several days in the uterine tube before entering the uterus. During this time, it is still surrounded by the zona pellucida, which prevents premature implantation.

- Implantation of the embryo into the uterine lining involves several stages: apposition of the expanded (hatched) blastocyst to the endometrial epithelium, penetration of the uterine epithelium, invasion into the tissues underlying the epithelium, and erosion of the maternal vascular supply. Connective tissue cells of the endometrium undergo the decidual reaction in response to the presence of the implanting embryo. Implantation is accomplished through the invasive activities of the syncytiotrophoblast, which is derived from the cytotrophoblast.

- Implantation of the embryo into a site other than the upper uterine cavity results in an ectopic pregnancy. Ectopic pregnancy is most often encountered in the uterine tube.

- A high percentage of fertilized eggs and early embryos do not develop and are spontaneously aborted. Many of these embryos contain major chromosomal abnormalities.

REVIEW QUESTIONS

1. What is the most common condition associated with spontaneously aborted embryos?
   A. Maternal imprinting
   B. Paternal imprinting
   C. Ectopic pregnancy
   D. Chromosomal abnormalities
   E. Lack of X-chromosomal inactivation
2. What tissue from the implanting embryo directly interfaces with the endometrial connective tissue?
   A. Corona radiata
   B. Inner cell mass
   C. Extraembryonic mesoderm
   D. Epiblast
   E. Syncytiotrophoblast
3. Identical twinning is made possible by what process or property of the early embryo?
   A. Regulation
   B. Aneuploidy
   C. Paternal imprinting
   D. Maternal imprinting
   E. X-chromosomal inactivation
4. The zona pellucida:
   A. Aids in penetration of the endometrial epithelium
   B. Serves as a source of nutrients for the embryo
   C. Prevents premature implantation of the cleaving embryo
   D. All of the above
   E. None of the above
5. What is the importance of the inner cell mass of the cleaving embryo?
6. What intracellular event stimulates mitosis?
7. Parental imprinting is a phenomenon demonstrating that certain homologous maternal and paternal chromosomes have somewhat different influences on the development of the embryo. Excess paternal influences result in the abnormal development of what type of tissue at the expense of development of the embryo itself?
8. What property of cleaving mammalian embryos is responsible for the production of normal monozygotic twins and the repair of damage to the embryo?
9. What is the cellular origin of the syncytiotrophoblast of the implanting embryo?
10. A woman who is 2 to 3 months pregnant suddenly develops severe lower abdominal pain. In the differential diagnosis, the physician must include the possibility of what condition?

REFERENCES

Aplin JD: The cell biology of human implantation, *Placenta* 17:269-275, 1996.

Avendaño S and others: A seven-cell human egg recovered from the oviduct, *Fertil Steril* 26:1167-1172, 1975.

Baltz JM: Intracellular pH regulation in the early embryo, *BioEssays* 15:523-530, 1993.

Barlow DP: Genetic imprinting in mammals, *Science* 270:1610-1613, 1995.

Bateson W: *Materials for the study of variation*, London, 1894, Macmillan.

Coucouvanis E, Martin GR: Signals for death and survival: a two-step mechanism for cavitation in the vertebrate embryo, *Cell* 83:279-287, 1995.

Cruz YP: Role of ultrastructural studies in the analysis of cell lineage in the mammalian pre-implantation embryo, *Microsc Res Tech* 22:103-125, 1992.

Denker HW: Trophoblast-endometrial interactions at embryo implantation: a cell biological paradox. In Denker HW, Aplin JD, eds: *Trophoblast research*, vol 4, New York, 1990, Plenum, pp 3-29.

Enders AC: Implantation. In *Encyclopedia of human biology*, vol 4, New York, 1991, Academic, pp 423-430.

Enders AC: Trophoblast differentiation during the transition from trophoblastic plate to lacunar stage of implantation in the rhesus monkey and human, *Am J Anat* 186:85-98, 1989.

Gardner RL: Clonal analysis of early mammalian development, *Philos Trans R Soc Lond [Biol]* 312:163-178, 1985.

Gartler SM, Riggs HD: Mammalian X-chromosome inactivation, *Annu Rev Genet* 17:155-190, 1983.

Gualtieri R, Santella L, Dale B: Tight junctions and cavitation in the human pre-embryo, *Mol Reprod Dev* 32:81-87, 1992.

Kidder GM, Watson AJ: Gene expression required for blastocoele formation in the mouse. In Heyner S, Wiley LM, eds: *Early embryo development and paracrine relationships*, New York, 1990, Liss, pp 97-107.

King T, Brown NA: The embryo's one-sided genes, *Curr Biol* 5:1364-1366, 1995.

Kuroda MI, Meller VH: Transient XIST-ence, *Cell* 91:9-11, 1997.

Latham KE: X chromosome imprinting and inactivation in the early mammalian embryo, *Trends Genet* 12:134-138, 1996.

Latham KE, McGrath J, Solter D: Mechanistic and developmental aspects of genetic imprinting in mammals, *Int Rev Cytol* 160:53-98, 1995.

Leese HJ: The energy metabolism of the preimplantation embryo. In Heyner S, Wiley LM, eds: *Early embryo development and paracrine relationships*, New York, 1990, Liss, pp 67-78.

Levin M and others: A molecular pathway determining left-right asymmetry in chick embryogenesis, *Cell* 82:803-814, 1995.

Monk M, Surani A, eds: Genomic imprinting, *Development* 1990(suppl):1-155, 1990.

Moore T, Haig D: Genomic imprinting in mammalian development: a parental tug-of-war, *Trends Genet* 7:45-49, 1991.

Nakao M, Sasaki H: Genomic imprinting: significance in development and diseases and the molecular mechanisms, *J Biochem* 120:467-473.

Palmiter RD and others: Dramatic growth of mice that develop from eggs microinjected with metallothionein-growth hormone fusion genes, *Nature* 300:611-615, 1982.

Pederson RA, Burdsal CA: Mammalian embryogenesis. In Knobil E, Neill J, eds: *The physiology of reproduction*, ed 2, New York, 1988, Raven, pp 319-390.

Reik W: Genetic imprinting: the battle of the sexes rages on, *Exp Physiol* 81:161-172, 1996.

Rosner MH and others: *Oct-3* and the beginning of mammalian development, *Science* 253:144-145, 1991.

Sapienza C: Parental imprinting of genes, *Sci Am* 263:52-60, 1990.

Sheardown SA and others: Stabilization of XIST RNA mediates initiation of X chromosome inactivation, *Cell* 91:99-107, 1997.

Spencer R: Conjoined twins: theoretical embryologic basis, *Teratology* 45:591-602, 1992.

Spencer R: Rachipagus conjoined twins: they really do occur, *Teratology* 52:346-356, 1995.

Splitt MP, Burn J, Goodship J: Defects in the determination of left-right asymmetry, *J Med Genet* 33:498-503, 1996.

Tarkowski AK, Wroblewska J: Development of blastomeres of mouse eggs isolated at the 4- and 8-cell stage, *J Embryol Exp Morphol* 18:155-180, 1967.

Tesarik J and others: Early morphological signs of embryonic genome expression in human preimplantation development as revealed by quantitative electron microscopy, *Dev Biol* 128:15-20, 1988.

Thie M, Fuchs P, Denker H-W: Epithelial cell polarity and embryo implantation in mammals, *Int J Devel Biol* 40:389-393, 1996.

Uchida IA: Twinning in spontaneous abortions and developmental abnormalities, *Issues Rev Teratol* 5:155-180, 1990.

Weitlauf HM: Biology of implantation. In Knobil E, Neill J, eds: *The physiology of reproduction*, New York, 1988, Raven, pp 231-262.

Wilding M: Calcium and cell cycle control in early embryos, *Zygote* 4:1-6, 1996.

Yokoyama T and others: Reversal of left right symmetry: a situs inversus mutation, *Science* 260:679-682, 1993.

Yost HJ: Vertebrate left-right development, *Cell* 82:689-692.

4

FORMATION OF GERM LAYERS AND EARLY DERIVATIVES

As it is implanting into the uterine wall, the embryo undergoes profound changes in its organization. Up to the time of implantation, the blastocyst consists of the inner cell mass, from which the body of the embryo proper arises, and the outer trophoblast, which represents the future tissue interface between the embryo and mother. Both components of the blastocyst serve as the precursors of other tissues that appear in subsequent stages of development. Chapter 3 discusses the way that the cytotrophoblast gives rise to an outer syncytial layer, the syncytiotrophoblast, shortly before attaching to uterine tissue (see Figure 3-17). Not long thereafter, the inner cell mass begins to give rise to other tissue derivatives as well. The subdivision of the inner cell mass ultimately results in an embryonic body that contains the three primary embryonic germ layers: the **ectoderm** (outer layer), **mesoderm** (middle layer), and **endoderm** (inner layer). The process by which the germ layers are formed through cell movements is called **gastrulation.**

After the germ layers have been laid down, the continued progression of embryonic development depends on a series of signals called **embryonic inductions** that are exchanged between the germ layers or other tissue precursors. In an inductive interaction, one tissue (the **inductor**) acts on another (**responding tissue**) so that the developmental course of the latter is different from what it would have been in the absence of the inductor.

The developments that can be seen with a microscope during this period are tangible reflections of profound changes in gene expression and cellular properties of implanting embryos. In recent years a virtual explosion of molecular information on early development in *Drosophila* flies has been translated to studies on early development in amphibians and mammals. Some of the major findings are introduced in this chapter and in Chapter 5.

TWO-GERM-LAYER STAGE

Just before the embryo implants into the endometrium early in the second week, significant changes begin to occur in the inner cell mass as well as in the trophoblast. As the cells of the inner cell mass rearrange into an epithelial configuration, a thin layer of cells appears ventral to the main cellular mass (see Figure 3-17). The main upper layer of cells is known as the **epiblast,** and the lower layer is called the **hypoblast,** or **primitive endoderm** (Figure 4-1).

How the hypoblast forms in human embryos is not understood, but comparative embryological data suggest that cells of this layer arise by **delamination** (a separation or dropping down) from the inner cell mass. The hypoblast is considered an **extraembryonic endoderm,** and it ultimately gives rise to the endodermal lining of the **yolk sac** (see Figure 3-17). After the hypoblast has become a well-defined layer and the epiblast has taken on an epithelial configuration, the former inner cell mass is transformed into a **bilaminar disk,** with the epiblast on the dorsal surface and the hypoblast on the ventral surface.

The epiblast contains the cells that will make up the embryo itself, but extraembryonic tissues also arise from this layer. The next layer to appear after the hypoblast is the **amnion,** a layer of extraembryonic ectoderm that ultimately encloses the entire embryo in a fluid-filled chamber called the **amniotic cavity** (see Chapter 6). Because of the paucity of specimens, the earliest stages in the formation of the amnion and amniotic cavity are not completely understood. Studies on primate embryos indicate that a primordial amniotic cavity first arises by **cavitation** (formation of an internal space) within the preepithelial epiblast; it is covered by cells derived from the inner cell mass (Figure 4-2). According to some investigators, the roof of the amnion then opens, exposing the primordial amniotic cavity to the overlying cytotrophoblast. Soon thereafter (by about 8 days after fertilization), the original amniotic epithelium re-forms a solid roof over the amniotic cavity.

While the early embryo is still sinking into the endometrium (about 9 days after fertilization), cells of the hypoblast begin to spread, lining the inner surface of the cytotrophoblast with a continuous layer of extraembryonic

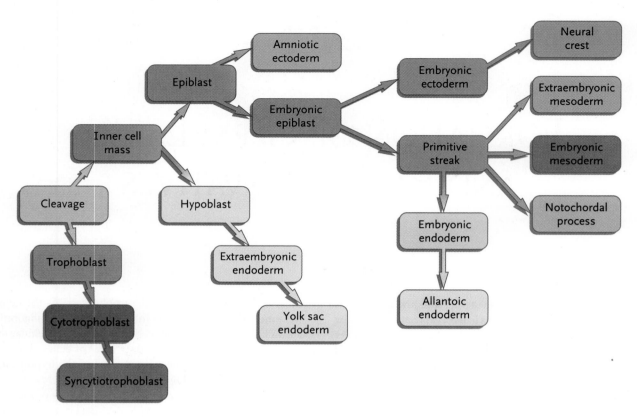

Figure 4-1 Cell and tissue lineages in the mammalian embryo. (The colors in the boxes are found in all illustrations involving the embryonic and extraembryonic germ layers.)

endoderm called **parietal endoderm** (see Figure 4-2). When the endodermal spreading is completed, a vesicle called the **primary yolk sac** has taken shape (see Figure 3-17, C). At this point (roughly 10 days after fertilization), the embryo complex constitutes the bilaminar germ disk, which is located between the primary yolk sac on its ventral surface and the amniotic cavity on its dorsal surface. Shortly after it forms, the primary yolk sac becomes constricted, forming a secondary yolk sac and leaving behind a remnant of the primary yolk sac (see Figures 3-17, D, and 4-2, E).

Starting at about 12 days after fertilization, another extraembryonic tissue, the **extraembryonic mesoderm,** begins to appear (see Figure 4-2). The first extraembryonic mesodermal cells seem to arise from a transformation of parietal endodermal cells. These cells are later joined by extraembryonic mesodermal cells that have originated from the primitive streak. The extraembryonic mesoderm becomes the tissue that supports the epithelium of the amnion and yolk sac as well as the **chorionic villi,** which arise from the trophoblastic tissues (see Chapter 6). The support supplied by the extraembryonic mesoderm is not only mechanical but also trophic, since the mesoderm serves as the substrate through which the blood vessels supply oxygen and nutrients to the various epithelia.

GASTRULATION AND THE THREE EMBRYONIC GERM LAYERS

At the end of the second week the embryo consists of two flat layers of cells, the epiblast and the hypoblast. As the third week of pregnancy begins, the embryo enters the period of gastrulation, during which the three embryonic germ layers become clearly established. The morphology of human gastrulation follows the pattern seen in birds. Because of the large amount of yolk in birds' eggs, the avian embryo forms the primary germ layers as three overlapping flat disks that rest on the yolk much like a stack of pancakes. Only later do the germ layers fold to form a cylindrical body. Although the mammalian egg is essentially devoid of yolk, the morphological conservatism of early development still constrains the human embryo to follow a pattern of gastrulation similar to that seen in reptiles and birds. Because of the scarcity of material, even the morphology of gastrulation in human embryos is not known in detail. Nevertheless, extrapolation from avian and mammalian gastrulation can provide a reasonable working model of human gastrulation.

All embryonic germ layers originate from the epiblast (see Figure 4-1). The first evidence of gastrulation is the forma-

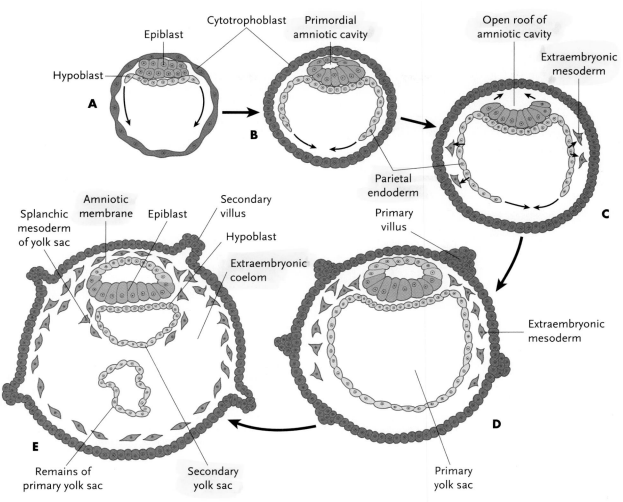

Figure 4-2 Origins of the major extraembryonic tissues. The syncytiotrophoblast is not shown.
A, Beginning of implantation at **6 days.** B, Implanted blastocyst at 7½ **days.** C, Implanted blastocyst at
8 days. D, Embryo at **9 days.** E, Beginning of **third week.**

tion of the **primitive streak,** which appears first as a thick-ening and then as a short line on the dorsal surface of the epi-blast (Figure 4-3). The early primitive streak is a condensa-tion caused by the converging of epiblastic cells toward that area. With the appearance of the primitive streak, the an-teroposterior (craniocaudal) and right-left axes of the embryo can be readily identified (Figures 4-4 and 4-5).

Recognition of the cellular dynamics associated with the primitive streak makes it easier to understand the detailed structure of this area. As cells of the epiblast reach the prim-itive streak, they change shape and pass through it on their way to forming new cell layers beneath (ventral to) the epi-blast (see Figure 4-4). The movement of cells through the primitive streak results in the formation of a groove (the **prim-itive groove**) along the midline of the primitive streak. At the end of the primitive streak is a small but well-defined accu-mulation of cells called the **primitive node,** or **Hensen's**

node.* This structure is of great developmental significance because it is the area through which migrating epiblastic cells are channeled into a rodlike mass of mesenchymal cells called the **notochord.** (The notochord and its functions in the early embryo are discussed on p. 63.)

The movements of the cells passing through the primitive streak are accompanied by major changes in their structure and organization (Figure 4-6). While in the epiblast, the cells have the properties of typical epithelial cells, with well-defined apical and basal surfaces, and they are associated with a basal lamina that underlies the epiblast. As they enter the primitive streak, these cells elongate, lose their basal lamina,

*Strictly speaking, *Hensen's node* is the designation for the primitive node in avian embryos, but this term is sometimes used in the mammalian embry-ological literature as well. This structure is the structural and functional equiv-alent of the dorsal lip of the blastopore in amphibians

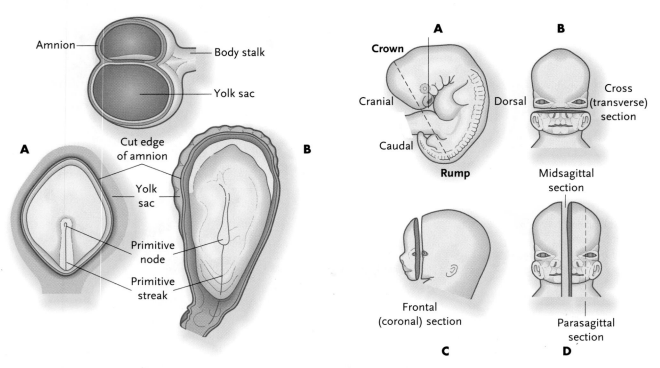

Figure 4-3 Dorsal views of **16-day** (A) and **18-day** (B) human embryos. *Top*, Sagittal section through an embryo and its extraembryonic membranes during early gastrulation.

Figure 4-5 Various planes, sections, and other descriptive terms used in descriptions of embryonic material. **A**, Lateral view of **6-week-old** embryo. The dashed line indicates the crown-rump length, one of the standard ways of measuring human embryos. The crown-rump length is the greatest straight-line distance between the apex of the head and the caudal end of the trunk. **B** through **D**, Heads of **8-week-old** embryos, illustrating common planes of section.

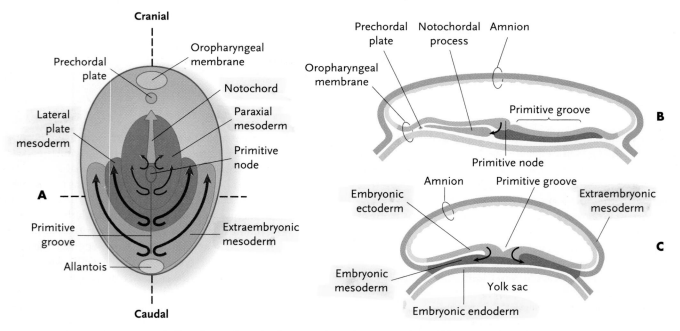

Figure 4-4 **A**, Dorsal view through a human embryo during gastrulation. The arrows show the directions of cellular movements across the epiblast toward, through, and away from the primitive streak as newly formed mesoderm. The illustrated fates of the cells that have passed through the primitive streak are based on studies of mouse embryos. **B**, Sagittal section through the craniocaudal axis of the same embryo. The curved arrow indicates cells passing through the primitive node into the notochord. **C**, Cross section through the level of the primitive streak in **A** (*dashed lines*).

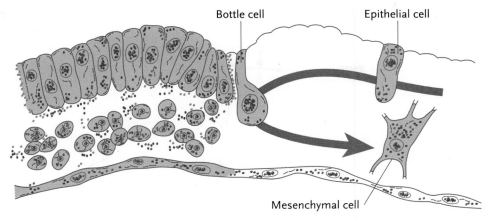

Bottle cell   Epithelial cell

Mesenchymal cell

Figure 4-6 Changes in the shape of a cell as it migrates along the epiblast (epithelium), through the primitive streak (bottle cell), and away from the groove as a mesenchymal cell that will become part of the mesodermal germ layer. The same cell can later assume an epithelial configuration as part of a somite.

and take on a characteristic morphology that has led to their being called **bottle cells.** When they become free of the epiblastic layer in the primitive groove, the bottle cells assume the morphology and characteristics of mesenchymal cells, which are able to migrate as individual cells if provided with the proper extracellular environment (see Figure 4-6). Included in this transformation is the loss of specific cell adhesion molecules (see p. 72) as the cells convert from an epithelial to a mesenchymal configuration.

In birds, the first cells to leave the primitive streak enter the hypoblast layer, displacing some of the extraembryonic endodermal cells to form the definitive **embryonic endoderm.** This process has not been confirmed in the human embryo, but the morphology of human gastrulation is comparable to that seen in birds.

The most prominent feature of human gastrulation is the formation of mesoderm. Some cells that migrate through the primitive streak form extraembryonic mesoderm. Much of the extraembryonic mesoderm forms the **body stalk,** which connects the caudal part of the embryo to the extraembryonic tissues that surround it (Figures 4-7 and 6-1). The body stalk later becomes the umbilical cord.

After the primitive streak is well established, the majority of cells passing through it spread out between the epiblast and the hypoblast to form the **embryonic mesoderm** (see Figure 4-4). Tracing studies have shown that cells leaving the node and primitive streak at given craniocaudal levels are destined to form specific types of mesoderm. For example, cells passing through the primitive node become either notochord or paraxial mesoderm, whereas cells leaving the primitive streak form paraxial mesoderm (see p. 88), lateral plate mesoderm (see p. 92), or extraembryonic mesoderm, depending on the craniocaudal level at which they exit the primitive streak (see Figure 4-4). The transformations of morphology and the behavior of the cells passing through the primitive streak are associated with profound changes not only in their

adhesive properties and internal organization but also in the way that they relate to their external environment.

Starting in early gastrulation, cells of the epiblast produce **hyaluronic acid,** which enters the space between the epiblast and hypoblast. Hyaluronic acid, a polymer consisting of repeating subunits of **D-glucuronic acid** and **N-acetylglucosamine,** is frequently associated with cell migration in developing systems. The molecule has a tremendous capacity to bind water (up to 1000 times its own volume), and it functions to keep mesenchymal cells from aggregating during cell migrations. Although after leaving the primitive streak the mesenchymal cells of the embryonic mesoderm find themselves in a hyaluronic acid–rich environment, hyaluronic acid alone is not enough to support their migration from the primitive streak. In all vertebrate embryos that have been investigated to date, the spread of mesodermal cells away from the primitive streak or the equivalent structure is found to depend on the presence of **fibronectin** associated with the basal lamina beneath the epiblast. The embryonic mesoderm ultimately spreads laterally as a thin sheet of mesenchymal cells between the epiblast and hypoblast layers (see Figure 4-4). By the time the mesoderm has formed a discrete layer in the human embryo, the upper germ layer (remains of the former epiblast) is called the **ectoderm,** and the lower germ layer, which has displaced the original hypoblast, is called the **endoderm.** This terminology is used for the remainder of this text.

Regression of the Primitive Streak

After its initial appearance at the extreme caudal end of the embryo, the primitive streak expands cranially until about 18 days after fertilization (see Figure 4-3). Thereafter, it regresses caudally (see Figure 4-13), stringing out the notochord in its wake. Vestiges remain into the fourth week. During that time, the formation of mesoderm continues by means of cells migrating from the epiblast through the primitive groove.

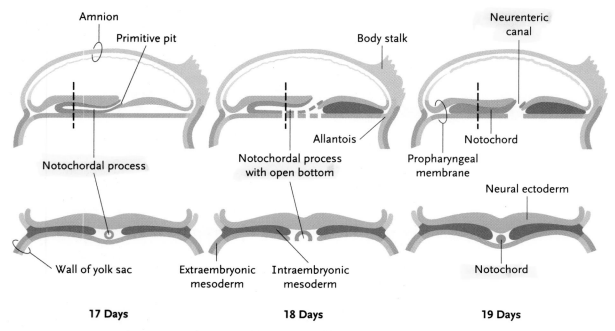

Figure 4-7 Later stages in formation of the notochord. *Top,* Sagittal sections. *Bottom,* Cross sections at the level of the vertical line in the upper figure. In the upper row, the cranial end is on the left. The function of the neurenteric canal (C) remains obscure.

The primitive streak normally disappears without a trace, but in rare instances, large tumors called **teratomas** appear in the sacrococcygeal region (see Figure 1-2, *A*). Teratomas often contain bizarre mixtures of many different types of tissue, such as cartilage, muscle, fat, hair, and glandular tissue. Because of this, sacrococcygeal teratomas are thought to arise from remains of the primitive streak (which can form all germ layers). Teratomas are also found in the gonads and the mediastinum. These tumors are thought to originate from germ cells.

Notochord and Prechordal Plate

The **notochord,** the structure that is the basis for giving the name *Chordata* to the phylum to which all vertebrates belong, is a cellular rod running along the longitudinal axis of the embryo just ventral to the central nervous system. Although both phylogenetically and ontogenetically it serves as the original longitudinal support for the body, the notochord also plays an extremely important role as a prime mover in a series of signaling episodes (inductions) that transform unspecialized embryonic cells into definitive tissues and organs. In particular, inductive signals from the notochord (1) stimulate the conversion of overlying surface ectoderm into neural tissue, (2) specify the identity of certain cells (floor plate) within the early nervous system, (3) transform certain mesodermal cells of the somites into vertebral bodies, and (4) stimulate the earliest steps in the development of the dorsal pancreas.

The notochord arises from the ingression of a population of epiblastic cells through the primitive node as a loose cylin-

drical cellular aggregation called the **notochordal process** (see Figure 4-4). In mammals, shortly after ingression, the cells of the notochordal process temporarily spread out and fuse with the embryonic endoderm (Figure 4-7, *B*), resulting in the formation of a transitory **neurenteric canal** that connects the emerging amniotic cavity with the yolk sac. Later, the cells of the notochord separate from the endodermal roof of the yolk sac and form the definitive notochord, a solid rod of cells in the midline between the embryonic ectoderm and endoderm (Figure 4-7, C).

Cranial to the notochord is a small region where embryonic ectoderm and endoderm abut without any intervening mesoderm. Called the **oropharyngeal membrane** (see Figure 4-4), this structure marks the site of the future oral cavity. Between the cranial tip of the notochordal process and the oropharyngeal membrane is a small aggregation of mesodermal cells closely apposed to endoderm, called the **prechordal plate** (see Figure 4-4). The prechordal plate emits molecular signals that are instrumental in stimulating the formation of the forebrain (see p. 66).

INDUCTION OF THE NERVOUS SYSTEM

Neural Induction

The inductive relationship between the notochord (**chordamesoderm**) and the overlying ectoderm in the genesis of the nervous system was recognized in the early 1900s. Although the original experiments were done on amphibians,

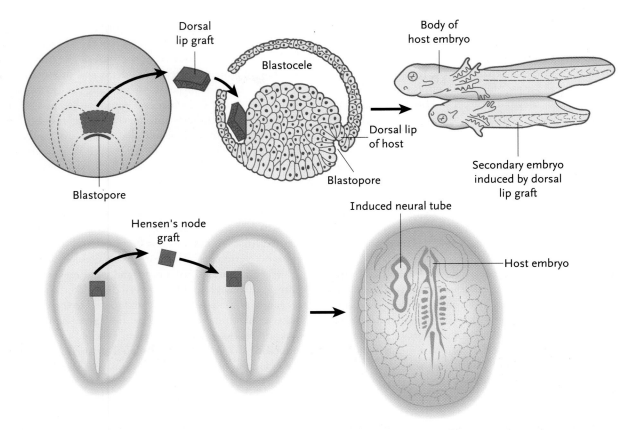

Figure 4-8 Early experiments demonstrating neural induction. *Top,* Graft of the dorsal lip of the blastopore in a salamander embryo induces a secondary embryo to form. *Bottom,* Graft of Hensen's node from one chick embryo to another induces the formation of a secondary neural tube. (*Top* based on studies by Spemann H: *Embryonic development and induction,* New York, 1938, Hafner; *bottom* based on studies by Waddington C: *J Exp Biol* 10:38-46, 1933.)

similar experiments in higher vertebrates have shown that the essential elements of **neural** (or **primary**) **induction** are the same in all vertebrates.

Deletion and transplantation experiments in amphibians set the stage for the present understanding of neural induction. (See Chapters 5 and 10 for further details on the formation of the nervous system.) In the absence of chordamesoderm moving from the dorsal lip of the blastopore (the amphibian equivalent of the primitive node), the nervous system, which is first represented by a thickened plate of transformed ectodermal cells situated along the dorsal midline of the embryo, does not form from the dorsal ectoderm. On the other hand, if the dorsal lip of the blastopore is grafted beneath the belly ectoderm of another host, a secondary nervous system and body axis form in the area of the graft (Figure 4-8). The dorsal lip has been called the **organizer** because of its ability to stimulate the formation of a secondary body axis. Subsequent research has shown that the interactions occurring in the region of the dorsal lip in amphibians are far more complex than a single induction between chordamesoderm and ectoderm.

Experiments of the type described have also been conducted on embryos of birds and mammals (see Figure 4-8);

clearly the primitive node and the notochordal process in birds and mammals are homologous in function to the dorsal lip and chordamesoderm in amphibians. This means that in higher vertebrates the primitive node and the notochordal process act as the neural inductor and the overlying ectoderm is the responding tissue. This fundamental relationship was established more than a half century ago. Since that time, embryologists have devoted an enormous amount of research to identifying the nature of the inductive signal that passes from the chordamesoderm to the ectoderm.

Early attempts to uncover the nature of the inductive stimulus were marked by a great deal of optimism. As early as the 1930s, various laboratories had proposed that molecules as diverse as proteins and steroids were the inductive stimulus. Soon thereafter came the discovery that an even wider variety of stimuli, such as inorganic ions or killed tissues, could elicit neural induction. With such a plethora of possible inductors, attention turned to the properties of the responding tissue (the dorsal ectoderm) and ways that it might react, through a final common pathway, to the inductive stimulus. The quest for the neural inductive molecules and their mode of action has been arduous and frustrating, with many blind alleys and wrong turns encountered along the way.

A number of laboratories found that isolated ectoderm could respond in vitro to inductive stimuli and become transformed into neural tissue. A very useful technique for studying induction in vitro involved separating the responding tissue from the inducing tissue by a filter with pores that permitted the passage of molecules but not cells. This technique has been used in the analysis of a variety of mammalian inductive systems.

Various experimental manipulations have clearly shown that neural induction is not a simple all-or-nothing process. Rather, considerable regional specificity exists. (For example, certain artificial inductors stimulate the formation of more anterior neural structures, and others stimulate the formation of more posterior ones.) In amphibian embryos, anterior chordamesoderm has different inducing properties from posterior chordamesoderm.

Recent research has identified specific molecules that bring about neural induction. In birds and mammals, two signaling molecules, **noggin** and **chordin,** given off by the notochord are the inductive agents. It was first thought that noggin and chordin directly stimulate uncommitted cells of the dorsal ectoderm to form neural tissue, but subsequent research on amphibians has shown that these inductors act by blocking the action of an inhibitor, **bone morphogenetic protein-4 (BMP-4),** in the dorsal ectoderm (see Figure 4-10). In the absence of BMP-4 activity, dorsal ectoderm forms neural tissue as a default state. This set of molecular interactions commits ectodermal cells over the notochord to becoming neural tissue, but it is only the first step in the formation of the nervous system. An important second step is regionalization of the central nervous system.

Regionalization refers to the subdivision of the central nervous system into broad craniocaudal regions. As already indicated, early experiments showed that certain inductors caused the formation of more cranial and others more caudal neural structures. It is now recognized that through the actions of noggin and chordin alone, more cranial neural structures form. However, if **fibroblast growth factor** is added to the mix, more caudal neural structures (hindbrain) form. In vivo, a yet unidentified factor secreted by the newly formed mesoderm exerts a caudalizing effect on the neural ectoderm. One of the recently discovered functions of the prechordal plate is to specify the formation of the forebrain region. The prechordal plate alone cannot induce dorsal ectoderm to become neural tissue, but once neural induction by noggin and chordin has occurred, the prechordal plate plays an important role in the forebrain regionalization of the central nervous system.

Mesodermal Induction

When initially described, neural induction was considered the first inductive process that takes place in the embryo, and it was often called *primary induction.* Subsequent experimentation conducted principally on amphibians has shown that other important inductions occur before neural induction. The best understood of these is the induction of mesoderm in the am-

phibian blastula. The mesoderm normally arises from a ring of cells around the equatorial region of the blastula (Figure 4-9). If the ectoderm located at the roof of the blastocoele is isolated, it remains general ectoderm and produces normal levels of **keratin** proteins, which are ectoderm-specific molecules. If the same piece of ectoderm is apposed to endoderm, it differentiates into mesoderm, as indicated by its producing α-**actin,** a molecule characteristic of muscle. In recent years, understanding of the nature of mesodermal induction has been greatly enhanced by the demonstration that certain specific proteins—**activin, noggin,** and **Vg1** (see Table 5-2)—are effectors of mesodermal induction.

Although most current research on induction in early embryos is being conducted on amphibians, many principles learned from amphibians can be transferred to the embryos of higher vertebrates. If an early avian epiblast is isolated and grown in culture, a notochord and axial mesoderm do not form. If an intact hypoblast or even dissociated and then reaggregated hypoblastic cells are juxtaposed to the cultured epiblast, axial structures form. Another experiment has shown that adding tissue culture medium exposed to a mesodermal inductor (XTC cells) to an isolated avian epiblast results in the induction of the epiblast to form axial mesodermal structures. Activin alone can induce axial structures in the avian epiblast. There is every reason to believe that these results also apply to mammalian embryos (Boxes 4-1 and 4-2).

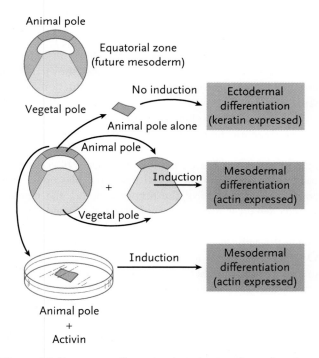

Figure 4-9 Experiments illustrating the induction of mesoderm in the amphibian blastula. The animal pole is the region of yolk-poor cells corresponding to the future rostral end of the amphibian embryo. The vegetal pole is the region of yolk-rich cells corresponding to the future caudal region of the amphibian embryo.

BOX 4-1   Molecular Aspects of Gastrulation

Although many decades of research have by now resulted in a reasonable understanding of the cellular aspects of gastrulation and germ layer formation in birds and mammals, knowledge of the molecular underpinnings of these events is based almost entirely on research conducted since 1990. Even though only the rudiments of the molecular basis for early development have been established to date, it is readily apparent that molecules and morphology must be linked for any real understanding of embryological development to occur. A general introduction to the major families of molecules currently known to control much of development is presented in Chapter 5. Figure 4-10 summarizes some of the genes whose expression is most important for early mammalian development to proceed. Products of these genes (or variants of them) have been identified during gastrulation in all classes of vertebrates, indicating their importance.

The primitive node, which is the focal point of early developmental events, is the site of expression of a number of important genes (see Figure 4-10). Some influence principally the development of the cranial part of the body, others act on caudal structures, and still others exert their effects along the entire body axis.

Not only is **HNF-3β** (hepatic nuclear factor) important for the formation of the node itself, but it is vital for the establishment of midline structures cranial to the node. *HNF-3β* is required for the initiation of notochord function. In its absence, not only the notochord but also the floor plate of the neural tube (see Chapter 10) fail to form. On the other hand, endoderm, the primitive streak, and intermediate mesoderm do develop.

The exact molecular action of **goosecoid** is poorly understood, but this gene is prominently expressed in the organizer (node) region of all vertebrates studied. If ectopically expressed, it stimulates the formation of a secondary body axis. More recently, *goosecoid* expression has also been associated with the prechordal plate.

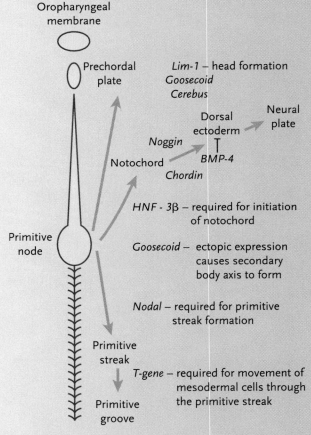

Figure 4-10 Summary of major genes involved in gastrulation and neural induction. Names of specific genes (*italics*) are placed by the structures in which they are expressed.

Continued

BOX 4-1   Molecular Aspects of Gastrulation—cont'd

Lim-1 is a homeobox gene (see Chapter 5) that is expressed in the primitive node and later in the prechordal plate. The Lim-1 protein is a vital regulator of head-organizing activity. Lim-1 null mutant mice develop without heads (Figure 4-11). Specifically, they lack structures anterior to rhombomere 3 (see Figure 5-12). The expression of *Lim-1* in prechordal mesoderm suggests that this structure is important in stimulating the formation of forebrain and cranial structures, whereas the notochord plays a vital role in stimulating the formation of the more posterior parts of the brain and spinal cord.

Expression of the **T** gene appears to be activated by products of the *HNF-3β* and *goosecoid* genes. In T mutants **(brachyury),** the notochord begins to form through the activities of *HNF-3β*, but it fails to complete development. Studies on T mutants have shown that activity of the *T* gene is necessary for normal movements of future mesodermal cells through the primitive streak during gastrulation. In brachyury (short-tail) mutant mice, mesodermal cells pile up at a poorly formed primitive streak, and the embryos show defective elongation of the body axis (including a short tail)

posterior to the forelimbs. *T* gene mutants may be responsible for certain gross caudal body defects in humans.

Nodal, a member of the TGF-β family of growth factor genes (see Table 5-2), is expressed throughout the epiblast before gastrulation, but its activity is concentrated at the primitive node during gastrulation. Like the *T* gene, the effects of *nodal* are more strongly seen in the caudal than in the cranial regions of the embryo. In the null mutant of *nodal,* the primitive streak fails to form and the embryo is deficient in mesoderm.

Two proteins that are strongly associated with the organizer region and neural induction are **sonic hedgehog** (Shh) and **noggin.** Both are secreted molecules that are not members of known large superfamilies of growth factor genes. Noggin, which has been most extensively studied in amphibians, has the ability to convert isolated pieces of general ectoderm into neurectoderm and is an excellent candidate for the main neural inductive agent. In amphibians, noggin is also known to influence the earlier process of mesodermal induction. Shh is a powerful molecule that exerts major influences on a number of developing systems (see Table 5-3).

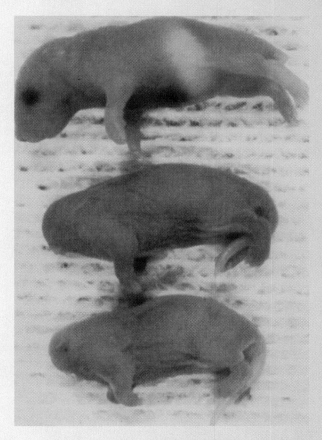

Figure 4-11 Newborn headless mice and a normal mouse. The headless mice have a null mutant of the *Lim-1* gene. (From Shawlot W, Behringer RR: *Nature* 374:425-430,1994.)

BOX 4-2 Molecular Basis for Left-Right Asymmetry

In the discussion of conjoined twins in Chapter 3, Bateson's rule of mirror image asymmetry in duplicated structures was mentioned (p. 52). Reversal of the normal left-right asymmetry of the body, called **situs inversus,** occurs in roughly one in 10,000 individuals born from single births (see Figure 3-16). Situs inversus is often not diagnosed until examined relatively late in life by an astute clinician, but in **Kartagener's syndrome,** situs inversus is associated with respiratory symptoms (paranasal sinusitis and bronchiectasis) that can be attributable to the absence of dynein arms in cilia (immotile cilia). The basis for the normal asymmetry of the body (e.g., heart and stomach on the left, liver on the right) has only recently begun to be understood. With the discovery of a recessive mutation that consistently produces situs inversus in mice (*inversus viscerum* gene), a genetic basis for the normal asymmetry of the body has been established. It has recently been demonstrated that the gene (*left/right-dynein*) associated with the respiratory symptoms in Kartagener's syndrome is mutated along with the *inversus viscerum* gene in mice. This would explain the connection between respiratory symptoms and situs inversus, but more important, there are indications that *dynein,* which acts as an intracellular motor, may be directly involved in the cellular mechanism of asymmetry.

Even more recently, a molecular basis for the structural asymmetry of the body has begun to be uncovered. Research on chick embryos has shown a sequence of asymmetrical expression of several developmentally important molecules in the region of Hensen's node (Figure 4-12). **Activin,** a powerful inducer of mesoderm in the frog and a stimulator of primitive streak formation in the chick, along with a receptor for activin (cAct-RIIa) are asymmetrically expressed on the right side of the primitive streak and Hensen's node. This inhibits the expression of Shh on the right side. In the absence of activin activity on the left side, Shh continues to be expressed on the left side of Hensen's node, and Shh stimulates the expression of a nodal-like gene in the same area. The **nodal** protein, a growth factor, may then stimulate the asymmetrical proliferation of mesodermal cells on the left through yet unknown pathways, leading to asymmetrical growth and bending of the heart tube and asymmetrical rotation of the body as a whole.

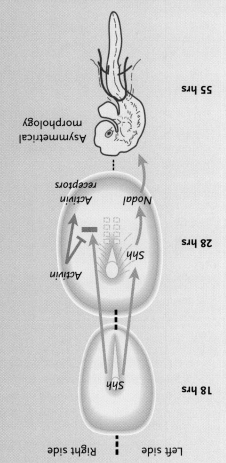

Figure 4-12 Currently known molecular basis for body asymmetry, based on studies of the chick embryo. At an early stage (top) sonic hedgehog is expressed on both sides of the embryo, but later an activin-like molecule on the right suppresses Shh on the right, leading to a cascade of asymmetrical gene expression on the left.

Early Formation of the Neural Plate

The first obvious morphological response of the embryo to neural induction is the transformation of the dorsal ectoderm overlying the notochordal process into an elongated patch of thickened epithelial cells called the **neural plate** (Figure 4-13). With the formation of the neural plate, the ectodermal germ layer becomes subdivided into two developmental lineages: neural and nonneural. This example illustrates several fundamental developmental concepts: restriction, determination, and differentiation. The zygote and blastomeres resulting from the first couple of cleavage divisions are **totipotent** (i.e., capable of forming any cell in the body). As development progresses, certain decisions are made that narrow the developmental options of cells (Figure 4-14). For example, at an early stage in cleavage, some cells become committed to the extraembryonic trophoblastic line and are no longer capable of participating in the formation of the embryo itself. At the decision point where cells become committed to becoming trophoblast, a **restriction** event has occurred. When a cell or group of cells has passed its last decision point (e.g., the transition from cytotrophoblast to syncytiotrophoblast), their fate is fixed, and they are said to be **determined**. These terms, which were coined in the early days of experimental embryology, are now understood to reflect limitations in gene expression as cell lineages follow their normal developmental course. The rare instances in which

cells or tissues strongly deviate from their normal developmental course, a phenomenon called **metaplasia**, are of considerable interest to pathologists and those who study the control of gene expression.

Restriction and determination signify the progressive limitation of the developmental capacities in the embryo. **Differentiation** describes the actual morphological or functional expression of the portion of the genome that remains available to a particular cell or group of cells. Differentiation commonly connotes the course of phenotypic specialization of cells. One example of differentiation occurs in spermatogenesis, when spermatogonia, relatively ordinary-looking cells, become transformed into highly specialized spermatozoa.

CELL ADHESION MOLECULES

In the early 1900s, researchers determined that suspended cells of a similar type have a strong tendency to aggregate. If different types of embryonic cells are mixed together, they typically sort according to tissue type. Their patterns of sorting even give clues to their properties and behavior in the mature organism. For example, if embryonic ectodermal and mesodermal cells are mixed, they come together into an aggregate with a superficial layer of ectodermal cells surrounding a central aggregate of mesodermal cells.

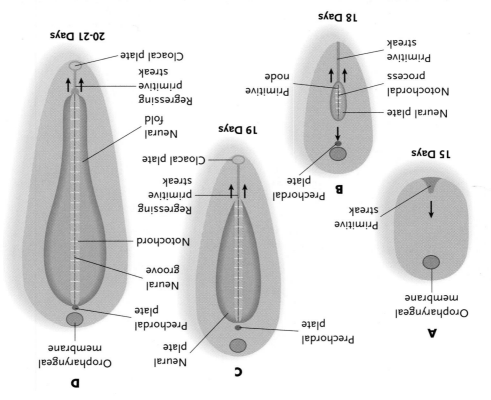

Figure 4-13 Relationships between the neural plate and primitive streak. A, Day 15. B, Day 18. C, Day 19. D, Days 20 to 21.

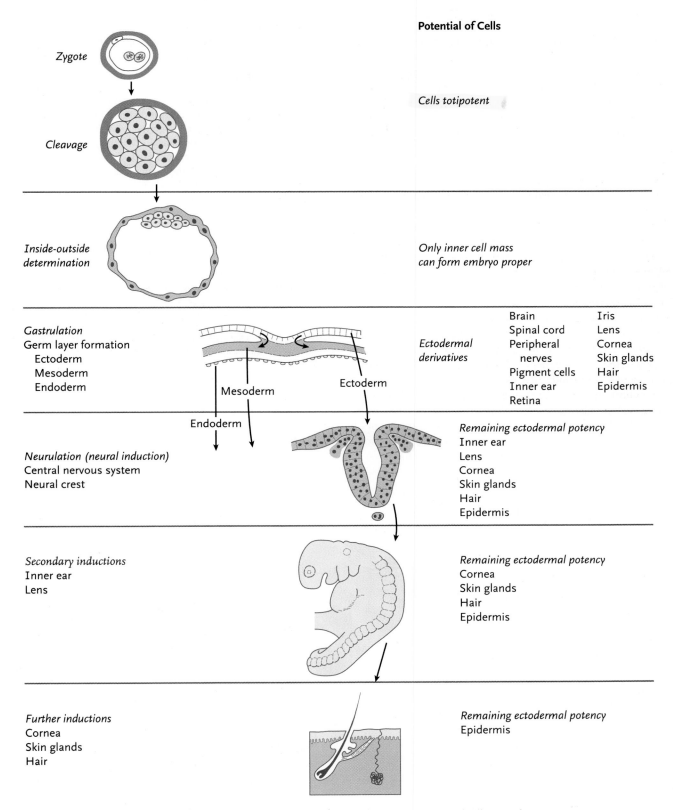

Potential of Cells

Zygote

Cells totipotent

Cleavage

Inside-outside determination

Only inner cell mass can form embryo proper

Gastrulation
Germ layer formation
  Ectoderm
  Mesoderm
  Endoderm

Mesoderm   Ectoderm

Ectodermal derivatives

Brain	Iris
Spinal cord	Lens
Peripheral	Cornea
nerves	Skin glands
Pigment cells	Hair
Inner ear	Epidermis
Retina	

Endoderm

Neurulation (neural induction)
Central nervous system
Neural crest

Remaining ectodermal potency
Inner ear
Lens
Cornea
Skin glands
Hair
Epidermis

Secondary inductions
Inner ear
Lens

Remaining ectodermal potency
Cornea
Skin glands
Hair
Epidermis

Further inductions
Cornea
Skin glands
Hair

Remaining ectodermal potency
Epidermis

Figure 4-14 Restriction during embryonic development. The labels on the right illustrate the progressive restriction of the developmental potential of cells that are in the line leading to the formation of the epidermis. On the left are developmental events that remove groups of cells from the epidermal track.

Contemporary research has begun to provide a molecular basis for many of the cell aggregation and sorting phenomena described by earlier embryologists. Several families of **cell adhesion molecules (CAMs)** have been characterized. CAMs have been extensively studied in relation to early developmental events. In pregastrulation avian embryos, cells of both epiblast and hypoblast contain two CAMs (N-CAM and L-CAM) on their surfaces. A significant change occurs when cells of the epiblast migrate through the primitive streak. They lose the expression of both CAMs during the migratory phase and while they are beginning to form an organized mesoderm. Later, certain mesodermal cell derivatives re-express CAMs. In general, when an epithelial cell type becomes transformed into a mesenchymal cell, its surface CAMs are lost.

The expression of CAMs is a sensitive indicator of primary induction in the early embryo. Before induction, the epiblast expresses both N-CAM and L-CAM (also called *E-cadherin*). After primary induction of the nervous system, the cells of the neural plate retain N-CAM but lose the expression of L-CAM. Conversely, in nonneural ectoderm, N-CAM expression is lost, but L-CAM expression is retained.

Some CAMs require the presence of Ca^{++} to function, whereas others are independent of Ca^{++}. N-CAM, a Ca^{++}-independent CAM, binds directly to other N-CAM molecules on neighboring cells of the same type (Figure 4-15). N-CAM is unusual in having a high concentration of **negatively charged sialic acid** groups in the carbohydrate component of the molecule, and embryonic forms of N-CAM have 3 times as much sialic acid as the adult form of the molecule.

SUMMARY

- Just before implantation, the inner cell mass becomes reorganized as an epithelium (epiblast), and a second layer (hypoblast) begins to form beneath it. Within the epiblast, the amniotic cavity forms by cavitation; outgrowing cells of the hypoblast give rise to the endodermal lining of the yolk sac. Extraembryonic mesoderm appears to form by an early transformation of parietal endodermal cells and cells migrating through the primitive streak.
- During gastrulation, a primitive streak forms in the epiblast at the caudal end of the bilaminar embryo. Cells migrating through the primitive streak form the mesoderm and endoderm, and the remaining epiblast becomes ectoderm.

CLINICAL VIGNETTE

A 35-year-old married man with a history of chronic respiratory infections is found on a routine x-ray examination to have dextrocardia. Further physical examination and imaging studies reveal that he has complete situs inversus. He has also been going to another clinic for a completely different problem, which is related to the same underlying defects.

Which is the most likely clinic?
A. Urology
B. Dermatology
C. Infertility
D. Orthopedic
E. Oncology

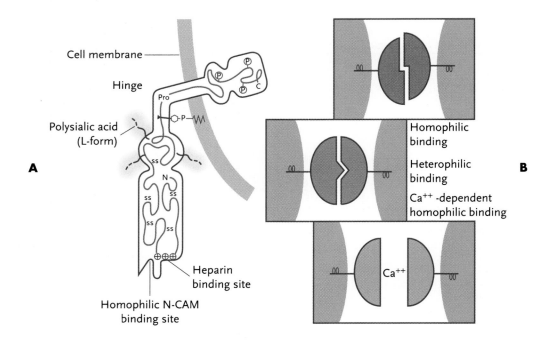

Figure 4-15 A, Structure of the neuronal cell adhesion molecule (N-CAM). **B,** Types of intercellular adhesion. *P,* Phosphate; *Pro,* proline; *ss,* disulfide.

- The primitive node, located at the cranial end of the primitive streak, is the source of the cells that become the notochord. It also functions as the organizer or primary inductor of the future nervous system.
- As they pass through the primitive streak, future mesodermal cells in the epiblast change in morphology from epithelial epiblastic cells to bottle cells and then to mesenchymal cells. Extraembryonic mesodermal cells form the body stalk. The migration of mesenchymal cells during gastrulation is facilitated by extracellular matrix molecules such as hyaluronic acid and fibronectin.
- Late in the third week after fertilization, the primitive streak begins to regress caudally. Normally the primitive streak disappears, but sacrococcygeal teratomas occasionally form in the area of regression.
- The essential elements of neural induction are the same in all vertebrates. In mammals, the primitive node and the notochordal process act as the primary inductor of the nervous system. Mesodermal induction occurs even earlier than neural induction. Growth factors such as Vg1 and activin are the effective agents in mesodermal induction. The hypoblast determines the origin and orientation of the primitive streak.
- A number of genes, expressed in the primitive node, are known to control various early developmental events, such as the formation of the notochord and primitive streak and the formation of the mesoderm. Some, such as *Lim-1*, control the organization of cranial structures, whereas others, such as *T*, guide the development of caudal regions of the body. Asymmetrical expression of certain genes (e.g., sonic hedgehog) around the node directs the normal asymmetrical development of organs, such as the heart, liver, and stomach.
- Early blastomeres are totipotent. As development progresses, cells pass through restriction points that limit their differentiation. When the fate of a cell is fixed, the cell is said to be determined. *Differentiation* refers to the actual expression of the portion of the genome that remains available to a determined cell, and the term connotes the course of phenotypic specialization of a cell.
- Embryonic cells of the same type adhere to one another and will reaggregate if separated. The molecular basis for cell aggregation and adherence is the presence of cell adhesion molecules (CAMs) on their surfaces. Among the several families of adhesion molecules, some are Ca^{++} dependent and some are Ca^{++} independent.

REVIEW QUESTIONS

1. The principal inductor in primary neural induction is the:
    - A. Hypoblast
    - B. Primitive streak
    - C. Extraembryonic mesoderm
    - D. Notochordal process
    - E. Embryonic ectoderm
2. Which of the following tissues arises from cells passing through the primitive streak?
    - A. Embryonic endoderm
    - B. Hypoblast
    - C. Cytotrophoblast
    - D. Primary yolk sac
    - E. Amnion

3. Cells of which germ layer are not present in the oropharyngeal membrane?
    - A. Ectoderm
    - B. Mesoderm
    - C. Endoderm
    - D. All are present
4. The prechordal plate plays an important role in regionalization of the:
    - A. Notochord
    - B. Forebrain
    - C. Embryonic mesoderm
    - D. Primitive node
    - E. Hindbrain
5. Brachyury, a deficiency in caudal tissues in the body, is caused by a mutation in what gene?
    - A. *Lim-1*
    - B. *Noggin*
    - C. *T*
    - D. *Sonic hedgehog*
    - E. *Activin*
6. Which layer of the bilaminar (two-layered) embryo gives rise to all of the embryonic tissue proper?
7. Of what importance is the primitive node in embryonic development?
8. The migration of mesodermal cells from the primitive streak is facilitated by the presence of what molecules of the extracellular matrix?
9. What molecules can bring about mesodermal induction in an early embryo?
10. At what stage in the life history of many cells are cell adhesion molecules lost?

REFERENCES

Boncinelli E, Mallamaci A: Homeobox genes in vertebrate gastrulation, *Curr Opin Genet Devel* 5:619-627, 1995.

Edelman GM: Cell adhesion molecules in the regulation of animal form and tissue pattern, *Annu Rev Cell Biol* 2:81-116, 1986.

Enders AC: Trophoblastic differentiation during the transition from trophoblastic plate to lacunar stage of implantation in the rhesus monkey and human, *Am J Anat* 186:85-98, 1989.

Enders AC, King BF: Formation and differentiation of extraembryonic mesoderm in the rhesus monkey, *Am J Anat* 181:327-340, 1988.

Foley AC, Storey KG, Stern CD: The prechordal region lacks neural inducing ability, but can confer anterior character to more posterior neuroepithelium, *Development* 124:2983-2996, 1997.

Fujinaga M: Development of sidedness of asymmetric body structures in vertebrates, *Int J Devel Biol* 41:153-186, 1997.

Hemmati-Brivanlou A, Melton D: Vertebrate embryonic cells will become nerve cells unless told otherwise, *Cell* 88:13-17, 1997.

Herrmann BG, ed: The *brachyury* gene, *Semin Devel Biol* 6:381-435, 1995.

Kavka AI, Green JBA: Tales of tails: brachyury and the T-box genes, *Biochem Biophys Acta* 1333:F73-F84, 1997.

Lemaire L, Kessel M: Gastrulation and homeobox genes in chick embryos, *Mech Devel* 67:3-16, 1997.

Levin M and others: A molecular pathway determining left-right asymmetry in chick embryogenesis, *Cell* 82:803-814, 1995.

Luckett WP: The development of primordial and definitive amniotic cavities in early rhesus monkey and human embryos, *Am J Anat* 144:149-168, 1975.

Luckett WP: Origin and differentiation of the yolk sac and extraembryonic mesoderm in presomite human and rhesus monkey embryos, *Am J Anat* 152:59-98, 1978.

Melloy PG and others: No turning, a mouse mutation causing left-right and axial patterning defects, *Devel Biol* 193:77-89, 1998.

Mitrani E, Shimoni Y: Induction by soluble factors of organized axial structures in chick epiblasts, *Science* 247:1092-1094, 1990.

Mitrani E and others: Activin can induce the formation of axial structures and is expressed in the hypoblast of the chick, *Cell* 63:495-501, 1990.

Muhr J, Jessell TM, Edlund T: Assignment of early caudal identity to neural plate cells by a signal from caudal paraxial mesoderm, *Neuron* 19:487-502, 1997.

Pera EM, Kessel M: Patterning of the chick forebrain anlage by the prechordal plate, *Development* 124:4153-4162, 1997.

Shawlot W, Behringer RR: Requirement for *Lim1* in head organizer function, *Nature* 374:425-430, 1994.

Spemann H: *Embryonic development and induction*, New York, 1938, Hafner.

Spemann H, Mangold H: Ueber Induktion von Embryonenanlagen durch Implantation ortfremder Organisatoren, *Arch Microskop Anat Entw-Mech* 100:599-638, 1924.

Sulik K and others: Morphogenesis of the murine node and notochordal plate, *Devel Dynam* 201:260-278, 1994.

Supp DM and others: Mutation of an axonemal dynein affects left-right asymmetry in inversus viscerum mice, *Nature* 389:963-966, 1997.

Takeichi M: The cadherins: cell-cell adhesion molecules controlling animal morphogenesis, *Development* 102:639-655, 1988.

Tam PL, Williams EA, Chan WY: Gastrulation in the mouse embryo: ultrastructural and molecular aspects of germ layer morphogenesis, *Microscop Res Tech* 26:301-328, 1993.

Townes PL, Holtfreter J: Directed movements and selective adhesion of embryonic amphibian cells, *J Exp Zool* 128:53-120, 1955.

Weinstein DC and others: The winged-helix transcription factor *HNF-3β* is required for notochord development in the mouse embryo, *Cell* 78:575-588, 1994.

Zhou X and others: Nodal is a novel TGF-beta-like gene expressed in the mouse node during gastrulation, *Nature* 361:543-547, 1993.

5

ESTABLISHMENT OF THE BASIC EMBRYONIC BODY PLAN

After gastrulation is complete, the embryo proper consists of a flat, three-layered disk containing the ectodermal, mesodermal, and endodermal germ layers. Its cephalocaudal axis is defined by the location of the primitive streak. Because of the pattern of cellular migration through the primitive streak and the regression of the streak toward the caudal end of the embryo, a strong **cephalocaudal gradient** of maturity is established. This gradient is marked initially by the formation of the notochord and later by the appearance of the neural plate, which results from the primary induction of the dorsal ectoderm by the notochord.

Despite the relatively featureless morphological appearance of the early postgastrulation embryo during the third week, evidence is increasing that during this period and even earlier, the basic body plan is being established by patterned expression of specific genes. One of the earliest morphological manifestations of this pattern is the regular segmentation that becomes evident along the craniocaudal axis of the embryo. Such a segmental plan, which is a dominant characteristic of all early embryos, becomes less obvious as development progresses. Nonetheless, even in the adult the regular arrangement of the vertebrae, ribs, and spinal nerves persists as a reminder of humans' highly segmented phylogenetic and ontogenetic past. Only recently have embryologists begun to understand the molecular and cellular controls that underlie the process of segmentation.

Another major change critical in understanding the fundamental organization of the body plan is the lateral folding of the early embryo from three essentially flat, stacked, pancakelike disks of cells (the primary embryonic germ layers) to a cylinder, with the ectoderm on the outside, the endoderm on the inside, and the mesoderm between them. The cellular basis for lateral folding still remains better described than understood.

This chapter concentrates on the establishment of the basic overall body plan. In addition, it charts the appearance of the primordia of the major organ systems of the body from the undifferentiated primary germ layers (see Figure 5-32).

MOLECULAR BASIS FOR ORGANIZATION OF THE VERTEBRATE BODY PLAN

Since 1990 the application of new techniques in molecular biology has revolutionized the understanding of the mechanisms of both normal and abnormal embryonic development. It is not possible to have a contemporary understanding of embryonic development without integrating fundamental molecular and morphological aspects of embryology. This section serves as a general introduction to the most important families of molecules known to direct embryonic development. With new developmentally active genes being reported almost weekly, the approach used in this text is to introduce important examples illustrating molecular correlates or control of developing systems rather than to attempt completeness in any way.

One of the most important realizations of the past decade is the conservatism of the genes that guide development. Sequencing studies have shown remarkably few changes in the nucleotide bases of many developmentally regulated genes that are represented in species ranging from worms to *Drosophila* to humans. Because of this phylogenetic conservatism, it has been possible to identify mammalian counterparts of genes that are known from genetic studies to have important developmental functions in species (Box 5-1). It is also becoming clear that the same gene may have different functions at different periods of development and in different organs. Both before and after birth, specific genes can be expressed in normal and abnormal processes. One of the principal themes in contemporary cancer research is the role of mutant forms of developmentally important genes (e.g., protooncogenes) in converting normal cells to tumor cells.

Fundamental Molecular Processes in Development

From a functional standpoint, many of the important molecules that guide embryonic development can be grouped into a relatively small number of categories. Some

BOX 5-1 Early Developmental Genetics in *Drosophila*

Despite the discovery and characterization of many developmentally important genes in mammals, the basic framework for understanding the molecular basis of embryonic development still rests largely on studies of developmental genetics in *Drosophila*. Although the very earliest stages of human development occur under less rigid genetic control than those of *Drosophila*, an exposure to the fundamental aspects of early *Drosophila* development nevertheless sets the stage for a deeper understanding of molecular embryogenesis in mammals.

Embryonic development of *Drosophila* is under tight genetic control. In the earliest stages the dorsoventral and anteroposterior axes of the embryo are established by the ac-

tions of batteries of **maternal effect genes** (Figure 5-1). Once these broad parameters have been established, the oval-shaped embryo undergoes a series of three sequential steps that result in the segmentation of the entire embryo along its anteroposterior axis. The first step in segmentation, under the control of what are called **gap genes**, subdivides the embryo into broad regional domains. Loss-of-function gap mutants result in loss of structure, or gaps, in the body pattern several segments in width. In the second step, a group of **pair-rule genes** is involved in the formation of seven pairs of stripes along the craniocaudal axis of the embryo. The third level in the segmentation process is controlled by the **segment-polarity genes**, which work

Genetic hierarchy	Functions	Representative genes	Effects of mutation
Maternal effect genes 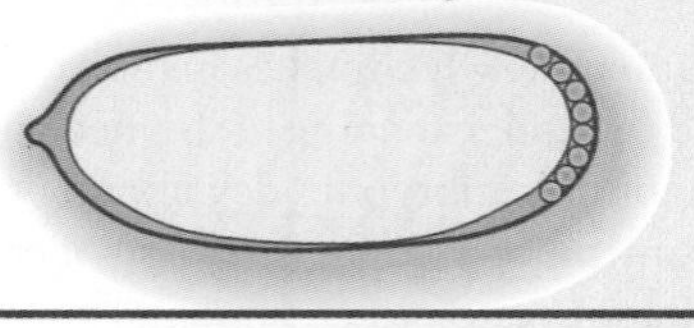	Establish gradients from anterior and posterior poles of the egg	Bicoid Swallow Oskar Caudal Torso Trunk	Major disturbances in anteroposterior organization
Segmentation genes 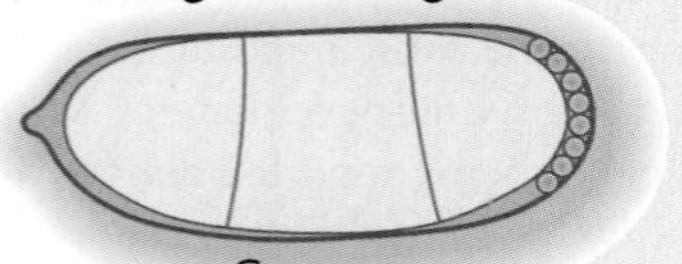 Gap genes	Define broad regions in the egg	Empty spiracles Hunchback Krüppel Knirps Tailless	Adjacent segments missing in a major region of the body
Pair-rule genes 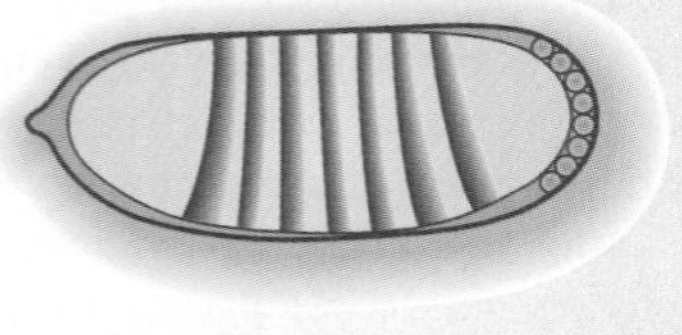	Define 7 segments	Hairy Even skipped Runt Fushi tarazu Odd paired Odd skipped Paired	Part of pattern deleted in every other segment
Segment polarity genes 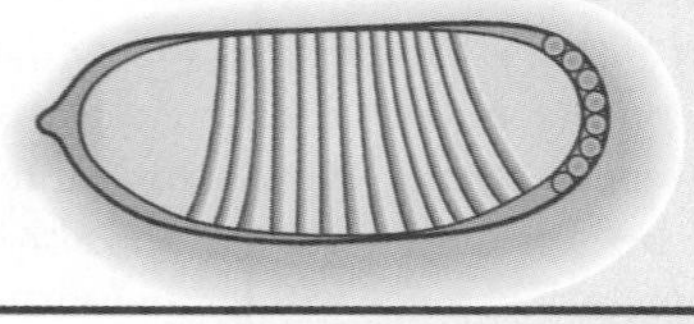	Define 14 segments	Engrailed Gooseberry Hedgehog Patched Wingless	Segments replaced by their mirror images
Homeotic genes 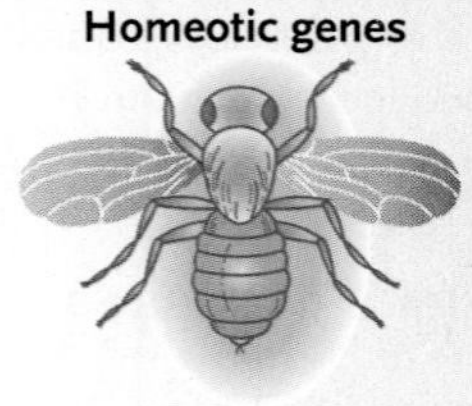	Determine regional characteristics	Antennapedia complex Bithorax complex	Inappropriate structures form for a given segmental level

Figure 5-1 Sequence of genetic control of early development in *Drosophila*. Within each level of genetic control are listed representative genes.

BOX 5-1   Early Developmental Genetics in *Drosophila*—cont'd

at the level of individual segments and are involved in their anteroposterior organization.*

The segmentation process results in a regular set of subdivisions along the anteroposterior axis of the early *Drosophila* embryo, but none of the previously mentioned developmental controls imparts specific or regional characteristics to the newly formed segments. This function is relegated to two large clus-

ters of **homeotic genes** found in the **antennapedia** complex and the **bithorax** complex. The specific genes in these two complexes determine the morphogenetic character of the body segments, such as segments bearing antennae, wings, or legs. Mutations of homeotic genes have long been known to produce bizarre malformations in insects, such as extra sets of wings or legs instead of antennae (hence the term *antennapedia*).

*In *Drosophila*, each stripe (segment) is subdivided into anterior and posterior halves. The posterior half of one segment and the anterior half of the next are collectively known as a **parasegment**. The genetics and developmental aspects of insect parasegments are beyond the scope of this text, but later in this chapter, when formation of the vertebral column is discussed, a similar set of divisions of the basic body segments in vertebrate embryos is introduced.

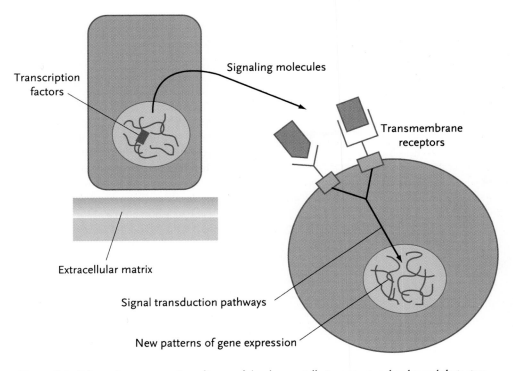

Figure 5-2 Schematic representation of types of developmentally important molecules and their sites of action.

of them remain in the cells that produced them and act as **transcription factors** (Figure 5-2). Transcription factors are proteins possessing domains that bind to the deoxyribonucleic acid (DNA) of promoter or enhancer regions of specific genes. They also possess a domain that interacts with ribonucleic acid (RNA) polymerase II or other transcription factors and consequently regulates the amount of messenger ribonucleic acid that gene produces. Other molecules act as intercellular **signaling molecules**. Such molecules leave the cells that produce them and exert their effects on other cells, which may be neighboring cells or cells located at greater distances from those that produce the signaling molecules. Many signaling molecules are members of large families of related proteins, called **growth factors**. To exert their effect, signaling molecules typically

bind to **receptor molecules** that are often transmembrane proteins protruding through the plasma membrane of the cells that they affect. When these receptor molecules form complexes with signaling molecules, they set off a cascade of events in a **signal transduction** pathway that transmits the molecular signal to the nucleus of the responding cell. This signal influences the nature of the gene products produced by that cell and often the cell's future course of development. In the past decade, many new, developmentally important molecules have been identified and their expression patterns during development described. Much effort is being expended toward understanding the molecular cascades that control developmental processes (e.g., the molecular events that stimulate the production of a developmentally important molecule and the pathway by

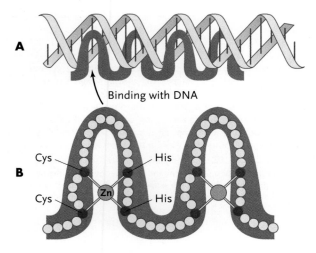

Figure 5-3 A, Binding to DNA of a zinc finger. **B,** Structure of a zinc finger DNA-binding sequence.

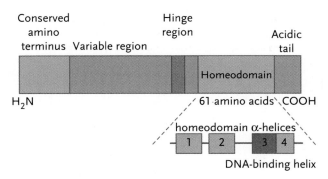

Figure 5-4 Structure of a typical homeodomain protein.

TABLE 5-1	Types of Specific Transcription Factors Mentioned in This Text

Type of factor	Examples
Basic helix-loop-helix	Myogenic regulatory factors
Zinc finger	WT-1, Krox-20, steroid-binding transcription factors
Homeodomain	Hox
POU	Pit-1, Oct-1, Oct-2
Paired box	Pax 1-9
Winged helix	Hepatocyte nuclear factor-3

which that molecule in turn exerts a downstream effect on other synthetic processes).

Transcription factors

Many families of molecules act as transcription factors. Some transcription factors are general ones that are found in virtually all the cells of an organism. Other transcription factors are specific for certain types of cells and stages of development. Specific **transcription factors** (Table 5-1) are often very important in initiating patterns of gene expression that result in major developmental changes.

One class of transcription factors is the **basic helix-loop-helix protein,** which contains a short stretch of amino acids in which two α-helices are separated by an amino acid loop. This region, with an adjacent basic region, allows the regulatory protein to bind to specific DNA sequences. The basic regions of these proteins bind DNA, and the helix-loop-helix domain is involved in homodimerization or heterodimerization. This configuration is common in a number of the transcription factors that regulate myogenesis (see Figure 8-27).

Another family of transcription factors is the **zinc finger proteins.** In these proteins, regularly placed cystine and his-

tidine units are bound by zinc ions to cause the polypeptide chain to pucker into fingerlike structures (Figure 5-3). These "fingers" can be inserted into specific regions in the DNA helix.

One of the most important types of transcription factors is represented by the **homeodomain proteins.** These proteins contain a highly conserved **homeodomain** of 61 amino acids, which is a type of helix-loop-helix region (Figure 5-4). The 183 nucleotides that encode the homeodomain are collectively called a **homeobox.** Homeobox regions were first discovered in the homeotic genes of the *antennapedia* and *bithorax* complex in *Drosophila* (see Figure 5-1), hence their name. This designation is sometimes confusing to students because since their initial description, homeoboxes have been found in a number of more distantly related genes outside the homeotic gene cluster.

The *Drosophila antennapedia/bithorax* complex consists of eight homeobox-containing genes located in two clusters on one chromosome. Mice and humans possess at least 38 homologous homeobox genes (called *Hox* genes in vertebrates), which are found in four clusters on four different chromosomes (Figure 5-5). The *Hox* genes on the four mammalian chromosomes are arranged in 13 **paralogous groups.**

Vertebrate *Hox* genes are strongly implicated in the craniocaudal segmentation of the body, and their spatiotemporal expression proceeds according to some remarkably regular rules. The genes are both activated and expressed according to a strict sequence in the 3' to 5' direction, corresponding to their positions on the chromosomes. Consequently, in both *Drosophila* and mammals, 3' genes are expressed earlier and more anteriorly than the 5' genes (Figure 5-6). Mutations of *Hox* genes result in morphological transformations of the segmental structures in which a specific gene is normally expressed. In general, **loss of function mutations** result in posterior-to-anterior transformations (e.g., cells of a given segment form the structural equivalent of the next most anterior segment), and **gain of function mutations** result in anterior-to-posterior structural transforma-

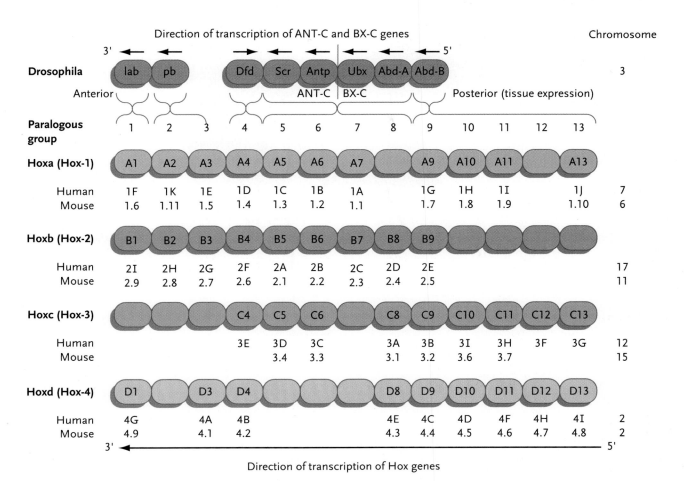

Figure 5-5 Comparison of mouse and human *Hox* complexes. The old terminology for human and mouse is given under the colored ovals. Genes on the 3' ends of the complexes are expressed earlier and more anteriorly than those on the 5' end (*right*). (Based on review by Scott MP: *Cell* 71:551-553, 1992.)

tions. Figure 5-7 illustrates an experiment in which injection of an antibody to a homeobox gene into an early frog embryo resulted in the transformation of the anterior spinal cord into an expanded hindbrain. The molecular events both upstream and downstream of *Hox* gene expression remain incompletely understood, but **fibroblast growth factor (FGF)** can selectively activate posterior homeobox-containing genes, whereas **transforming growth factor-β (TGF-β)** can selectively activate anterior *Hox* genes. Retinoic acid, a potent cause of birth defects in humans, can cause a posteriorization of *Hox* gene expression with attendant morphological abnormalities.

A number of other gene families contain not only a homeobox but also other conserved sequences (Figure 5-8). Some, such as *Engrailed* and *Lim* genes, consist of only a few members per group, but others, such as the *POU* and *paired (Pax)* genes, constitute large families, members of which are expressed in many developing structures.

The **POU gene family** gets its acronym from the first genes identified, namely, P*it-1*, a gene uniquely expressed in the pi-

tuitary, O*ct-1* and *Oct-2* (see p. 41), and U*nc-86*, a gene expressed in a nematode. Genes of the POU family contain, in addition to a homeobox, a region coding 75 amino acids, which also bind to DNA through a helix-loop-helix structure.

The **Pax gene family**, consisting of nine known members, is an important group of genes that are involved in many aspects of mammalian development (Figure 5-9). All Pax proteins contain a **paired domain** of 128 amino acids, which binds to DNA. Various members of the group also contain entire or partial homeobox domains and a conserved octapeptide sequence.

Signaling molecules

Signaling molecules, many of which are **peptide growth factors**, are mediators of most interactions, such as inductions, between groups of cells in embryos. Many of the signaling molecules that are most important in embryonic development are members of two large families: the **TGF-β** and **FGF** families. Members of another recently discovered family

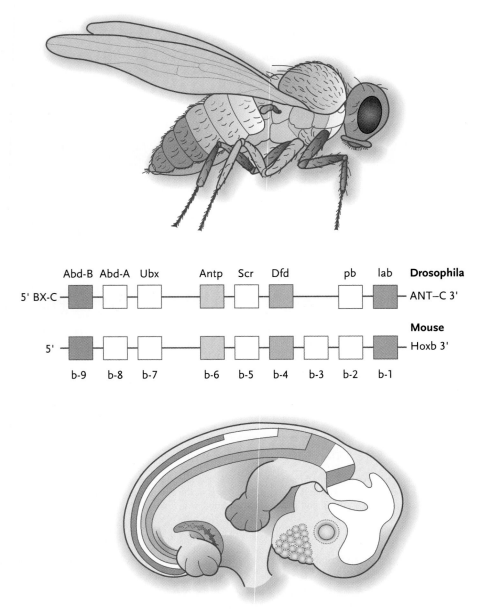

Figure 5-6 Organization of certain homeobox-containing genes of *Drosophila* and the mouse and their segmental expression in the body. (Based on review by DeRobertis EM, Oliver G, Wright CVE: *Sci Am* 263[1]:46-52, 1990.)

of signaling molecules, the **hedgehog proteins,** mediate of some of the most potent inductive interactions discovered to date. **Nerve growth factor,** which stimulates the growth of sensory and sympathetic neurons, was the first growth factor to be intensively investigated, with work starting in the 1950s.

The **TGF-β** family consists of a large number of molecules (up to 30 genes) that play a wide variety of roles during embryogenesis and postnatal life (Table 5-2). Members of the **FGF** family (FGF-1 to FGF-9) similarly fulfill various functions in embryogenesis, ranging from stimulation of mes-

enchymal cell proliferation to induction of elongation of the limb bud to stimulation of capillary growth to proliferation and survival of certain neurons.

One of the most influential families of embryonic signaling molecules is that of the hedgehog proteins, with **sonic hedgehog** playing a vital role as a chief secretory product produced by various organizing centers in the embryo (Table 5-3). The sonic hedgehog protein is unusual in that it undergoes proteolytic autocleavage, resulting in a 19-kDa N-terminal peptide and a 27-kDa C-terminal pep-

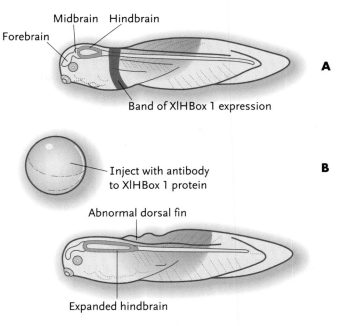

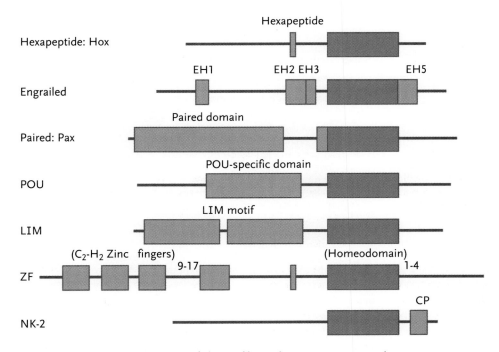

Figure 5-7 Effect of interference of *XlHbox 1* (~Hoxc-6) function on development in *Xenopus*. **A**, Normal larva, showing a discrete band (*green*) of *XlHbox 1* expression. **B**, Caudal expansion of the hindbrain after antibodies to *XlHbox 1*, protein are injected into the early embryo. (Based on studies by Wright CV and others: *Cell* 59:81-93, 1989.)

Figure 5-8 Schematic representation of classes of homeobox-containing genes also possessing conserved motifs outside the homeodomain. Names of the different classes of genes are listed on the left. The red boxes represent the homeodomain within each gene class. The other boxes represent conserved motifs specific to each class of genes. (Modified from Duboule D, ed: *Guidebook to the homeobox genes*, Oxford, 1994, Oxford University Press.)

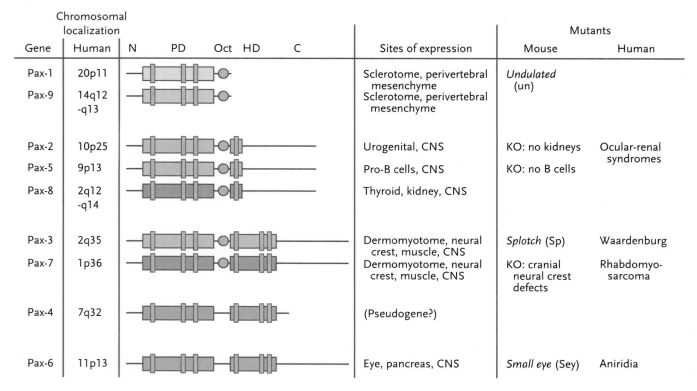

Gene	Chromosomal localization Human	N	PD	Oct	HD	C	Sites of expression	Mutants Mouse	Human
Pax-1	20p11						Sclerotome, perivertebral mesenchyme	*Undulated* (un)	
Pax-9	14q12 -q13						Sclerotome, perivertebral mesenchyme		
Pax-2	10p25						Urogenital, CNS	KO: no kidneys	Ocular-renal syndromes
Pax-5	9p13						Pro-B cells, CNS	KO: no B cells	
Pax-8	2q12 -q14						Thyroid, kidney, CNS		
Pax-3	2q35						Dermomyotome, neural crest, muscle, CNS	*Splotch* (Sp)	Waardenburg
Pax-7	1p36						Dermomyotome, neural crest, muscle, CNS	KO: cranial neural crest defects	Rhabdomyo-sarcoma
Pax-4	7q32						(Pseudogene?)		
Pax-6	11p13						Eye, pancreas, CNS	*Small eye* (Sey)	Aniridia

Figure 5-9 Summary diagram of the members of the *Pax* gene family, showing their location on human chromosomes, sites of expression, and known effects of mutants in both human and mouse. The structures of conserved elements of these genes are schematically represented. *CNS*, Central nervous system; *KO*, knockout. (Modified from Wehr R, Gruss P: *Int J Dev Biol* 40:369-377, 1996; and Epstein JC: *Trends Card Med* 6:255-260, 1996.)

TABLE 5-2   Members of the TGF-β Superfamily Mentioned in This Text

Member	Representative functions	Chapters
TGF-β_1 to TGF-β_5	Mesodermal induction	4
	Myoblast proliferation	8
	Invasion of cardiac jelly by atrioventricular endothelial cells	16
Activin	Granulose cell proliferation, mesodermal induction	1, 4
Inhibin	Inhibition of gonadotropin secretion by hypophysis	1
Müllerian inhibiting substance	Regression of paramesonephric ducts	15
Decapentaplegic	Signaling in limb development	9
Vg1	Mesodermal induction	4
Bone morphogenetic protein-1 to bone morphogenetic protein-9	Formation of the neural plate, skeletal differentiation, and other inductive interactions	4, 8
Nodal	Formation of primitive streak and left-right axis of embryo	4
Glial cell line–derived neurotrophic factor	Induction of outgrowth of ureteric bud	15

tide. The N-terminal peptide, which becomes covalently bound to cholesterol during proteolytic processing, is the portion of the cleaved molecule that appears to embody most of the important signaling properties of the molecule. To date, three forms of hedgehog (sonic, Indian, and desert), derived from three different genes, have been described in mammals. After binding with a receptor molecule in the target cell, the sonic hedgehog signal stimulates the target cell to produce new gene products or to undergo new pathways of differentiation.

TABLE 5-3   Sites in the Embryo Where Sonic Hedgehog Serves as a Signaling Molecule

Signaling center	Chapters
Primitive node	4
Notochord	5, 10
Floor plate (nervous system)	10
Intestinal portals	5
Zone of polarizing activity (limb)	9
Hair and feather buds	8
Ectodermal tips of facial processes	13
Apical ectoderm of second pharyngeal arch	13
Tips of epithelial buds in outgrowing lung	14

Receptor molecules

For intercellular signaling molecules to exert an effect on responding cells, they must normally interact with receptors in these cells. Most receptors are located on the cell surface, but some, especially those for lipid-soluble molecules, such as steroids, retinoids, and thyroid hormone, are intracellular.

Cell surface receptors are typically transmembrane proteins with **extracellular, transmembrane,** and **cytoplasmic domains** (see Figure 5-2). The extracellular domain contains a binding site for the **ligand,** which is typically a hormone, cytokine, or growth factor. When the ligand binds to a receptor, it effects a conformational change in the cytoplasmic domain of the receptor molecule. Cell surface receptors are of the following main types: those with intrinsic protein kinase activity and those that use a second messenger system to activate cytoplasmic protein kinases. An example of the first type is the family of receptors for FGFs, in which the cytoplasmic domain possesses **tyrosine kinase** activity. Receptors for growth factors of the TGF-β superfamily are also of this type, but in them the cytoplasmic domain contains **serine/threonine kinase** activity. In cell surface receptors of the second type, the protein kinase activity is separate from the receptor molecule itself. This type of receptor is also activated by binding with a ligand (e.g., neurotransmitter, peptide hormone, growth factor), but a series of intermediate steps is required to activate cytoplasmic protein kinases.

Signal transduction

Signal transduction is the process by which the signal provided by the **first messenger** (i.e., the growth factor or other signaling molecule) is translated into an intracellular response. Signal transduction begins when the first messenger, or ligand, binds to a receptor and changes its conformation. In the case of receptors that do not possess intrinsic protein kinase activity, binding of the ligand to the receptor stimu-

lates a chain reaction or **cascade,** leading to the production of a **second messenger,** which activates cytoplasmic protein kinases. A typical cascade (see Figure 5-2) consists of a series of steps by which the activated receptor, acting through **G proteins** (proteins that bind guanosine triphosphate and guanosine diphosphate), stimulates an **effector** enzyme (e.g., adenyl cyclase) to convert precursor molecules into second messengers. (Two important second messengers are cyclic adenosine monophosphate and inosine triphosphate plus diacylglycerol.) The second messenger then activates cytoplasmic protein kinases, which phosphorylate (add phosphate groups to) target proteins, either activating or inactivating them. After additional steps typically involving other kinases and the translocation of activated molecules to the nucleus, DNA transcription is affected. In this way the transduction cascade leads to a cellular response, which in embryonic development could be the transformation of cell type during differentiation or the production of a specific product by the target cell.

Molecules and Morphology

It has become almost axiomatic in studies of development that morphology is built on a molecular pattern. The pattern can be wide-reaching, as in the case of *Hox* gene expression in segmentation of the body axis, or it can have a very restricted domain, such as induction of the cornea by the lens. Many aspects of morphogenesis are still so poorly understood that the molecular blueprint remains to be discovered. Throughout the remainder of this text, instructive examples of the molecular control of cell differentiation or of morphogenesis are presented, especially when they offer clues to the disturbed mechanisms underlying abnormal development.

DEVELOPMENT OF THE ECTODERMAL GERM LAYER

Neurulation: Formation of the Neural Tube

The principal early morphological response of the embryonic ectoderm to neural induction is an increase in the height of the cells that are destined to become components of the nervous system. These transformed cells are evident as a thickened **neural plate** visible on the dorsal surface of the early embryo (Figures 5-10, *A*, and 5-11, *A*). Unseen but also important is the restricted expression of cell adhesion molecules (CAMs) from N-CAM and L-CAM/E-cadherin in the preinduced ectoderm to N-CAM and N-cadherin in the neural plate.

The first of four major stages in the formation of the neural tube is transformation of the general embryonic ectoderm into a thickened neural plate. The principal activity of the second stage is further shaping of the overall contours of the neural plate so that it becomes narrower and longer. Shaping of the neural plate is accomplished to a great extent by re-

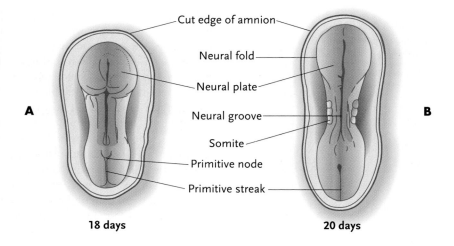

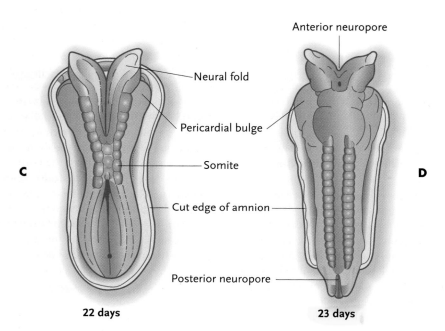

Figure 5-10 Early stages in the formation of the human central nervous system. A, At **18 days**. B, At **20 days**. C, At **22 days**, D, At **23 days**.

gion-specific changes in the shape of the neuroepithelial cells (e.g., an increase in height at the expense of basal surface area) and by rearrangements of these cells relative to one another.

The third major stage in the process of **neurulation** is the lateral folding of the neural plate, resulting in the elevation of each side of the neural plate along a midline **neural groove** (see Figures 5-10, B, and 5-11, B). Many explanations have been proposed for lateral folding of the neural plate and ultimate closure of the neural tube. Most have invoked a single or dominant mechanism, but it is now becoming apparent that lateral folding is the result of a number of region-specific mechanisms, both intrinsic and extrinsic to the neural plate.

The ventral midline of the neural plate, sometimes called the **median hinge point**, appears to act like an anchoring point about which the two sides become elevated at a sharp angle from the horizontal. At the median angle, bending can be largely accounted for by notochord-induced changes in the shape of the neuroepithelial cells of the neural plate. These cells become narrower at their apex and broader at their base (see Figure 5-11, C) through a combination of a basal position of the nuclei (causing a lateral expansion of the cell in that area) and a purse string-like contraction of a ring of actin-containing microfilaments in the apical cytoplasm. Throughout the lateral folding of the neural plate in the region of the spinal cord, much of the wall area of the neural plate remains flat

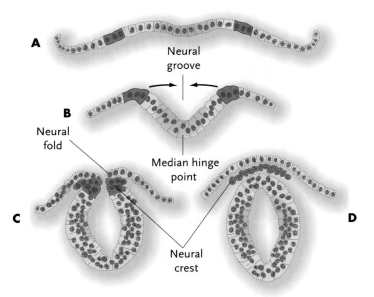

Figure 5-11 Cross sections through the forming neural tube. A, Neural plate. B, Neural fold. C, Neural folds apposed. D, Neural tube complete. (Neural crest before and after its exit from the neural epithelium is shown in green.)

(see Figure 5-11, *B*). Elevation of the **neural folds** appears to be accomplished largely by factors extrinsic to the neural epithelium, in particular pushing forces generated by the expanding surface epithelium lateral to the neural plate.

The fourth stage in the formation of the neural tube consists of apposition of the two most lateral apical surfaces of the neural folds, their fusion (mediated by cell surface glycoconjugates), and the separation of the completed segment of the neural tube from the overlying ectodermal sheet (see Figure 5-11, *C* and *D*). At the same time, cells of the **neural crest** begin to separate from the neural tube.

Closure of the neural tube begins almost midway along the craniocaudal extent of the nervous system of the 21- to 22-day-old embryo (see Figure 5-10, *C*). Over the next couple of days, closure extends both cephalically and caudally in a manner superficially resembling the closing of a double-headed zipper. The unclosed cephalic and caudal parts of the neural tube are called the **anterior** (cranial) and **posterior** (caudal) **neuropores.** The neuropores also ultimately close off so that the entire future central nervous system is organized in a way that is resembles an irregular cylinder sealed at both ends. Occasionally one or both neuropores remain open, resulting in serious birth defects (see p. 241).

Caudal to the posterior neuropore, the remaining neural tube (more prominent in animals with large tails) is formed by the process of **secondary neurulation.** Secondary neurulation in mammals appears to begin with the formation of a rodlike condensation of mesenchymal cells beneath the dorsal ectoderm of the tail bud. Within the mesenchymal rod, a central canal forms directly by **cavitation** (the formation of a space

within a mass of cells). This central canal becomes continuous with the one formed during primary neurulation by the lateral folding of the neural plate and closure of the posterior neuropore. Because of the poor development of the tail bud, secondary neurulation in humans is not a prominent process.

Segmentation in the Neural Tube

Soon after the neural tube has taken shape, the region of the future brain can be distinguished from the remaining spinal cord. The brain-forming region undergoes a series of subdivisions that constitute the basis for the fundamental gross organization of the adult brain. The first set of subdivisions results in a three-part brain, consisting of a forebrain (**prosencephalon**), midbrain (**mesencephalon**), and hindbrain (**rhombencephalon**). (The further subdivision and development of the brain are covered in Chapter 10 [see Figure 10-2].)

Various developmental mechanisms work in concert to subdivide the future brain into its structural and functional subdivisions. Very early in development, perhaps during or shortly after the induction of the neural plate, two broad regions of the developing brain are blocked out as a result of the influences of underlying tissues. Through the action of signaling molecules (e.g., Lim-1 and a recently identified secreted protein called **cerberus**), the mesodermal prechordal plate (see Figure 4-10) specifies the initial pattern for the forebrain within the neural plate as the rostral part of the head itself begins to be formed. More posteriorly, the hindbrain and spinal cord are specified by signals emanating from the underlying notochord and adjacent paraxial mesoderm.

Superimposed on the traditional gross morphological organization of the developing brain is another level of segmentation, the significance of which is just beginning to be understood. For over 150 years, some investigators have described transiently visible regular segments called **neuromeres** (Figure 5-12) in the posterior brain-forming regions of the neural tube, but only recently has their significance been appreciated. In the human embryo, neuromeres (often called **rhombomeres**) can be seen in the rhombencephalon from early in the fourth to late in the fifth week (see Figure 5-12, *B*). Individual cellular proliferation centers in the hindbrain give rise to the rhombomeres. The rhombomeres are arranged as odd and even pairs, and once established, they act like isolated compartments in insect embryos. Because of specific surface properties, cells from adjacent rhombomeres do not intermingle across boundaries between even and odd segments; however, marked cells from two even or two odd rhombomeres placed side by side do intermingle. During their brief existence, rhombomeres provide the basis for the fundamental organization of the hindbrain. In the adult, the segmental organization of the rhombomeres is manifested in the rhombomere-specific origin of many of the cranial nerves and parts of the reticular formation within the brainstem (see Figure 10-11).

Development of the rhombomeres is associated with highly regular patterns of expression of a large variety of

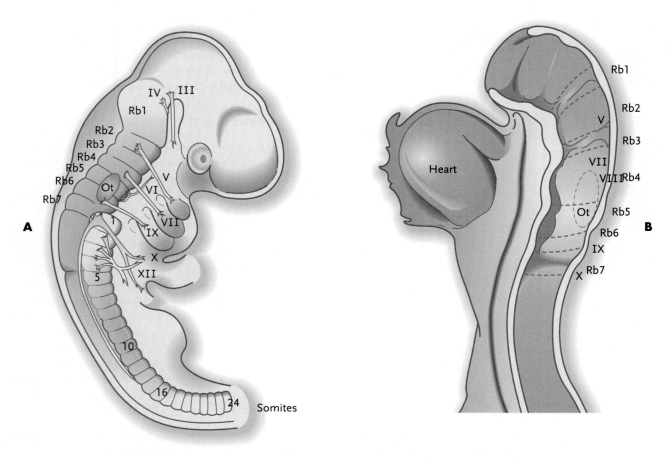

Figure 5-12 Neuromeres in 3-day-old chick brain (**A**) and **24-day-old** human (**B**) brain. *Ot,* Otic vesicle; *Rb,* rhombomeres (neuromeres in rhombencephalon); Roman numerals, cranial nerves; numbers, somites.

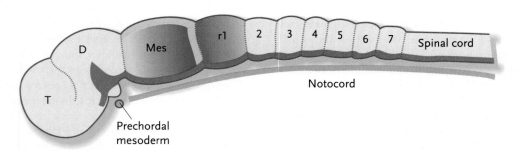

Figure 5-13 Molecular patterning of the midbrain and hindbrain region. The signaling molecules, FGF-8 (*green*) and Wnt-1 (*yellow*) are expressed at the midbrain/hindbrain boundary. This induces decreasing gradients of En-1 and En-2 (*blue*) on either side. Areas secreting sonic hedgehog are shown in red. *D,* Diencephalon; *Mes,* mesencephalon; *r,* rhombomere; *T,* telencephalon. (After Lumsden A, Krumlauf R: *Science* 274:1109-1115, 1996.)

genes, which work in concert in ways still poorly understood to specify the nature of the individual rhombomeres (see Figure 10-10). The *Hox* genes, in particular, appear to be instrumental in determining the segmental nature of the individual rhombomeres. Another gene important in the segmentation process of the hindbrain is the zinc finger transcription factor, **Krox-20,** which acts upstream of the *Hox* genes.

Another segmental boundary in the developing brain occurs at the junction between the midbrain and the hindbrain (Figure 5-13). This boundary is the site of production of two powerful signaling molecules, **FGF-8** and **Wnt-1** (a

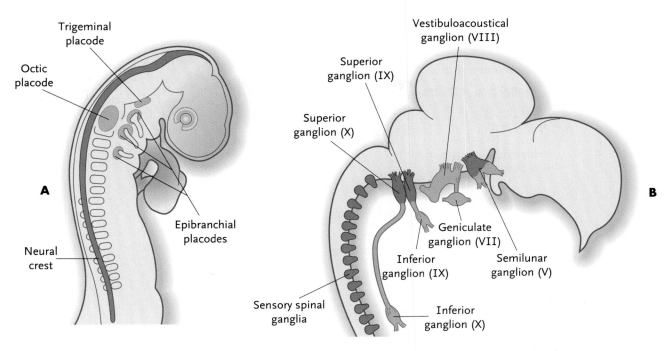

Figure 5-14 Ectodermal placodes and neural crest in the formation of sensory ganglia of cranial and spinal nerves in the chick embryo. **A,** At 2 days. **B,** At 8 days. Neural crest is shown in green, placodes in blue. (Modified from LeDouarin N and others: *Trends Neurosci* 9[4]:175-180, 1986.)

gene homologous with *wingless*, a segment polarity gene in *Drosophila* [see Figure 5-1]). These signals regulate a gradient of expression of two **Engrailed** genes (also segment polarity genes), transcription factors that are critical in organizing the development of both the midbrain and the cerebellum.

Both the fundamental organization and the developmental controls of the forebrain (telencephalon and diencephalon) continue to be debated, with some experts concluding that this region is organized on a transverse segmental basis, whereas others lean toward a more longitudinal organization. As stated earlier, the appearance of the forebrain along with the rostral part of the head depends on molecular signals emanating from the prechordal plate. Through the analysis of patterns of gene expression, some investigators have divided the forming diencephalon into four neuromeres, but it has been more difficult to demonstrate subdivisions in the early telencephalon.

Although neuromeres are not seen in the region of the neural tube that gives rise to the spinal cord, the regular arrangement of the exiting motor and sensory nerve roots is evidence of a fundamental segmental organization in this region of the body as well. In contrast to the brain, however, segmentation of the spinal cord appears to be imposed by signals emanating from the paraxial mesoderm rather than from molecular signals intrinsic to the neural tube. (The relationship between the spinal nerves and the mesodermal segments of the body [the somites and their derivatives] is illustrated in Figure 5-19.

Neural Crest

When the neural tube has just closed and is separating from the general cutaneous ectoderm, a population of cells called the **neural crest** leaves the dorsal part of the neural tube and begins to spread throughout the body of the embryo (see Figure 5-11). The neural crest produces an astonishing array of structures in the embryo (see Table 11-1), and its importance is such that the neural crest is sometimes called the *fourth germ layer of the body.* (Further consideration of the neural crest is presented in Chapter 11.)

Sensory Placodes and Secondary Inductions in the Cranial Region

As the cranial region begins to take shape, several series of ectodermal **placodes** (ectodermal thickenings) appear lateral to the neural tube. Most, if not all, result from secondary inductive processes between other tissues (in most cases, the neural tube or neural crest) and the overlying ectoderm. Among the prominent early placodes are the paired lens placodes, which ultimately form the lens of the eye (see Figure 12-1), and the otic placodes, which form the inner ear (see Figure 12-19). In the most rostral regions of the head, ectodermal placodes give rise to the olfactory sensory epithelium of the nose, and a similar invagination from the roof of the stomodeum gives rise to the anterior lobe of the pituitary gland. In the region of the hindbrain, several sets of placodes developing in concert with local neural crest share in the formation of the sensory ganglia of the cranial nerves (Figure 5-14).

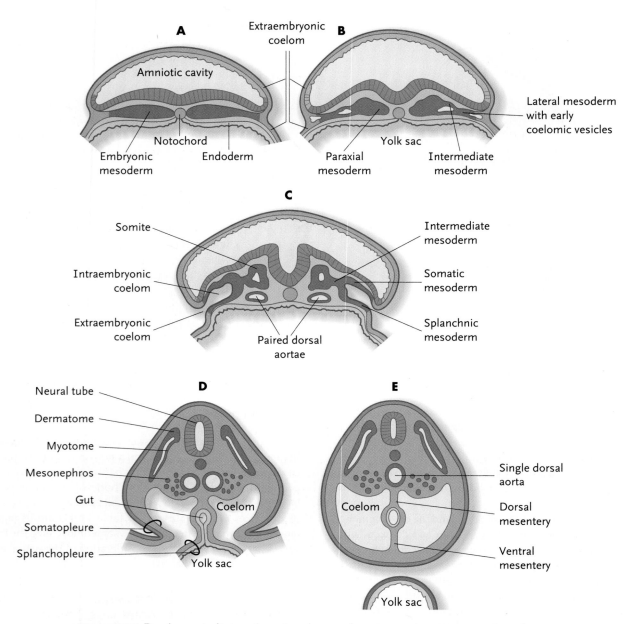

Figure 5-15 Development of intraembryonic and extraembryonic mesoderm in cross sections of human embryos.

DEVELOPMENT OF THE MESODERMAL GERM LAYER

Basic Plan of the Mesodermal Layer

After passing through the primitive streak, the mesodermal cells spread laterally between the ectoderm and endoderm as a continuous layer of mesenchymal cells (see Figure 4-6). Subsequently, three regions can be recognized in the mesoderm of cross-sectioned embryos (Figure 5-15, *B*). Nearest the neural tube is a thickened column of mesenchymal cells known as the **paraxial mesoderm**, or **segmental plate**. This tissue is soon organized into somites. Continuous with the

paraxial mesoderm is a compact region of **intermediate mesoderm**, which ultimately gives rise to the urogenital system. Beyond that, the **lateral mesoderm** ultimately splits into two layers and forms the bulk of the tissues of the body wall, the wall of the digestive tract, and the limbs (see Figure 5-32).

Paraxial Mesoderm

As the primitive node and the primitive streak regress toward the caudal end of the embryo, they leave behind the notochord and the induced neural plate. Lateral to the neural plate, the paraxial mesoderm appears to be a homogeneous

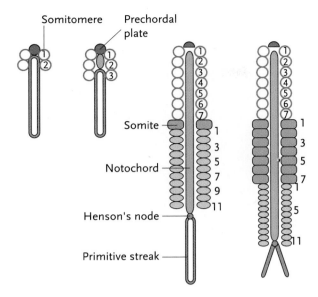

Figure 5-16 Relationship between somitomeres and somites in the early chick embryo. Cranial somitomeres (*open circles*) take shape along Hensen's node until seven pairs have formed. Caudal to the seventh somitomere, somites (*rectangles*) form from caudal somitomeres (*ovals*). As the most anterior of the caudal somitomeres transform into somites, additional caudal somitomeres take shape posteriorly. For a while, the equilibrium between transformation into somites anteriorly and new formation posteriorly keeps the number of caudal somitomeres at 11.

strip of closely packed mesenchymal cells. However, if scanning electron micrographs of this mesoderm are examined with stereoscopic techniques, a series of regular pairs of segments can be discerned. These segments, called **somitomeres**, have been most studied in avian embryos, but they are also found in mammals. New pairs of somitomeres form along the primitive node as it regresses toward the caudal end of the embryo (Figure 5-16). Not until almost 20 pairs of somitomeres have formed and the primitive node has regressed quite far caudally does the first pair of **somites** (brick-shaped masses of paraxial mesoderm) form behind the seventh pair of somitomeres.

After the first pair of somites has been established (approximately 20 days after fertilization), a regular relationship develops between the regression of the primitive streak and the formation of additional somites and somitomeres. The first 7 pairs of somitomeres in the cranial region do not undergo further separation or segmentation; the first pair of somites forms at the expense of the eighth pair of somitomeres. In the types of embryos studied to date, there is a constant relationship between the most caudal pair of definitive somites and the number of somitomeres (usually 10 to 11) that can be demonstrated behind them. Every few hours the pair of somitomeres located caudal to the last-formed somites becomes transformed into a new pair of somites, and a new pair of somitomeres is laid down at the caudal end of the paraxial mesoderm near the primitive node

(see Figure 5-16). Once the regression of the primitive node is complete, no more somitomeres are formed, but new somites continue to form until the last of the caudal somitomeres are obliterated.

Despite decades of research, the mechanisms underlying the initial formation of somites remain poorly understood, although it appears that segmentation is an intrinsic property of paraxial mesoderm. Recently, however, a tremendous amount has been learned about the biology of individual somites once they have formed (see next section). The way that somites and somitomeres stop forming is little better understood than the way they are generated, but one possibility is that genetically programmed cell death (apoptosis) in the tail disrupts the paraxial mesoderm or the late-forming somitomeres and acts as a stop signal.

Formation of individual somites

The formation of an individual somite involves the transformation of segmented blocks of cells with a mesenchymal morphology into a sphere of epithelial cells within the paraxial mesoderm (Figure 5-17, *A*). Although the segmentation of the paraxial mesoderm appears to be intrinsically controlled, epithelialization of the early somites depends on a yet unknown inductive signal from the overlying ectoderm. This signal stimulates the expression of a gene called **paraxis**, a basic helix-loop-helix transcription factor. Possibly because of the mediation of *paraxis*, the transformation from mesenchyme to epithelium is preceded by an increase in the intercellular adhesive properties of the presomitic cells. The cells of the epithelial somite are arranged so that their apical surfaces surround a small central lumen (which contains a small number of core cells) and their outer basal surfaces are surrounded by a basal lamina (containing laminin, fibronectin, and other components of the extracellular matrix).

Shortly after the formation of the epithelial somite, the cells of its ventromedial wall are subjected to an inductive stimulus in the form of the signaling molecule, **sonic hedgehog**, originating from the notochord and the ventral wall of the neural tube. The response is the expression of *Pax-1* and *Pax-9* in the ventral half of the somite, which is now called the **sclerotome** (Figure 5-18). This leads to a burst of mitosis, the loss of intercellular adhesion molecules (**N-cadherin**), the dissolution of the basal lamina in that region, and the transformation of the epithelial cells (and core cells) in that region back to a mesenchymal morphology (these cells are called **secondary mesenchyme**). These secondary mesenchymal cells migrate or are otherwise displaced medially from the remainder of the somite (Figure 5-17, *B*) and begin to produce **chondroitin sulfate proteoglycans** and other molecules characteristic of cartilage matrix as they aggregate around the notochord.

Under the influence of secreted products of *Wnt* genes produced by the dorsal neural tube, which counteract an inhibitory influence of sonic hedgehog, the dorsal half of the ep-

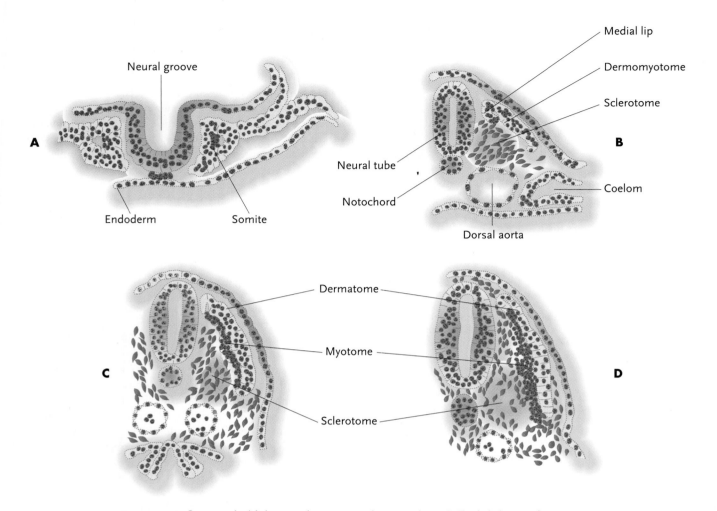

Figure 5-17 Stages in the life history of a somite in a human embryo. **A**, Epithelial stage of a somite in the preneural tube stage. **B**, Epitheliomesenchymal transformation of the ventromedial portion into the sclerotome. **C**, Appearance of a separate myotome from the original dermomyotome. **D**, Early stage of breakup of the epithelial dermatome into dermal fibroblasts.

ithelial somite becomes transformed into the **dermomyotome** (see Figure 5-17, *B*) and expresses its own characteristic genes (*Pax-3, Pax-7, paraxis*). Mesenchymal cells arising from the dorsomedial border of the dermomyotome form a separate layer, the **myotome**, beneath the remaining somitic epithelium, which is now called the **dermatome** (Figure 5-17, *C*). As their names imply, cells of the myotome produce muscle, and cells of the dermatome contribute to the dermis.

Organization of the somite and the basic segmental body plan

The epithelial somite can be subdivided into four cross-sectional quadrants, each of which gives rise to a different set of derivatives (Table 5-4). As described in the previous section, under the influence of sonic hedgehog secreted by the notochord, the ventral half of the somite becomes transformed into the sclerotome and goes on to form the vertebral

body. Two mouse mutants illustrate the importance of the interacting components in differentiation of the somite. In the **Danforth short tail** mutant, degeneration of the notochord (inducer of the sclerotome) is followed by poor formation of the vertebral bodies and intervertebral disks. A disruption of *Pax-1* expression in the sclerotome in the **undulated** mutant also leads to vertebral defects.

After the *Wnt*-mediated induction of the dorsal half of the somite to form the dermomyotome, a medial lip of cells forms from the dermomyotome (see Figure 5-17, *B*). The medial lip spreads out beneath the dermomyotome to form a separate muscle-forming layer, the **myotome** (see Figure 5-17, *C*). The medial portion of the myotome goes on to express several **myogenic regulatory factors** (see p. 174) as the cells prepare to form the intrinsic back muscles (see Table 5-4). Under the influence of **bone morphogenetic protein-4 (BMP-4)**, produced by the lateral mesoderm, the expression of myogenic regulatory factors in cells of the lateral dermomyotome is sup-

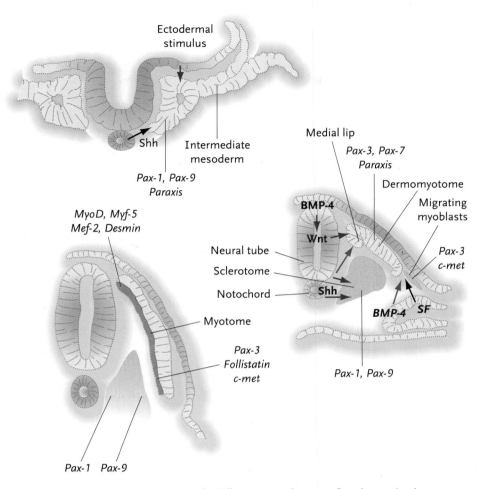

Figure 5-18 Molecular events involved in the differentiation of somites. Signaling molecules are represented by black arrows. Inhibitory signals are represented by red arrows. Genes expressed in responding tissues are indicated in italics. *SF*, Scatter factor. (Modified from Brand-Saberi B and others: *Int J Dev Biol* 40:411-420, 1996.)

TABLE 5-4   Subdivisions of the Epithelial Somite

	DORSAL		
	Dermatome Dermis **Myotome** Intrinsic back muscles (epaxial)	**Dermatome** Dermis **Myotome** Limb muscles Muscles of ventrolateral body wall (hypaxial)	
MEDIAL			LATERAL
	Sclerotome Vertebral body Intervertebral disk Proximal part of rib Connective tissue	**Sclerotome** Vertebral arch Pedicle of vertebra Distal part of rib Connective tissue around dorsal root ganglion	
	VENTRAL		

pressed, and they continue to express *Pax-3* and also a receptor molecule, **c-met**. A growth factor, **scatter factor** (also called **hepatic growth factor**), secreted in the region of the limb buds, binds to the c-met receptor of lateral dermomyotome cells. This stimulates these cells to migrate out of the somite and into the limb bud while they continue to express their myotomal marker, *Pax-3.*

As the cells of the sclerotome disperse around the notochord, cells of the anterior half of one somite aggregate with cells of the posterior half of the more cranial somite. Ultimately, this aggregate forms a single vertebra. Such an arrangement places the bony vertebrae out of phase with the myotomally derived segmental muscles of the trunk (Figure 5-19, C). This allows the contracting segmental muscles to move the vertebral column laterally. The relationship between the anterior half of one somite and the adjoining posterior half of its neighboring somite is reminiscent of the parasegments of *Drosophila* (similarly arranged subdivisions of the segments into two parts), but whether they are functionally similar in terms of genetic control is undetermined.

Intermediate Mesoderm

Connecting the paraxial mesoderm and the lateral plate mesoderm in the early embryo is a small cord of cells called the **intermediate mesoderm** that runs along the entire length of the trunk (see Figure 5-15, C). Possibly through a lack of receptors, the intermediate mesoderm does not appear to be influenced by the BMP-4 that is secreted by the lateral mesoderm, whereas somitic mesoderm exposed to high concentrations of BMP-4 assumes the characteristics of the lateral plate. The intermediate mesoderm is the precursor of the urogenital system. The earliest signs of differentiation of the intermediate mesoderm are in the most cranial regions, where vestiges of the earliest form of the kidney, the **pronephros**, briefly appear. In the lateral region of the intermediate mesoderm, a longitudinal **pronephric duct** appears on each side of the embryo. The pronephric duct is important in organizing the development of much of the adult urogenital system, which forms largely from cells of the caudal portions of the intermediate mesoderm (see Chapter 15).

Lateral Plate Mesoderm

Shortly after gastrulation, the ectoderm overlying the most lateral mesoderm produces BMP-4. Soon thereafter, the lateral mesoderm itself begins to produce BMP-4. Experimental studies have shown that this molecule has the ability to cause mesoderm, whether paraxial or lateral, to assume the molecular and cellular properties of lateral mesoderm. Whether early mesoderm develops the properties of paraxial or lateral mesoderm appears to depend on a balance between medializing influences emanating from the axial structures (neural tube and notochord) and lateralizing influences initially produced by lateral ectoderm.

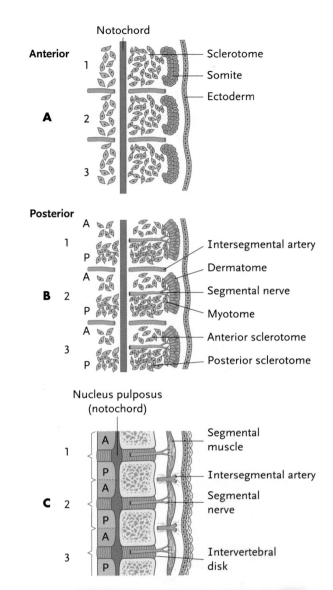

Figure 5-19 **A,** Early movement of seemingly homogeneous sclerotome from the somite. **B,** Breakup of the sclerotomal portions of the somites into anterior *(A)* and posterior *(P)* halves and the coalescence of the posterior portion of one somite with the anterior portion of the one caudal to it to form the body of a vertebra. **C,** With this rearrangement, the segmental muscles (derived from the myotomes) extend across intervertebral joints and are supplied by spinal nerves that grow out between the anterior and posterior halves of the somites.

The **lateral plate mesoderm** soon divides into two layers as the result of the formation and coalescence of coelomic (body cavity) spaces within it (see Figure 5-15, B and C). The dorsal layer, which is closely associated with the ectoderm, is called **somatic mesoderm**, and the combination of somatic mesoderm and ectoderm is called the **somatopleure** (see Figure 5-15, D). The ventral layer, called **splanchnic mesoderm**, is closely associated with the endoderm, and the combined endoderm and splanchnic mesoderm is called the **splanchnopleure**. The intraembryonic somatic and splanchnic mesodermal layers are continuous with the layers of extraembryonic mesoderm that line the amnion and yolk sac.

While the layers of somatic and splanchnic mesoderm are taking shape, the entire body of the embryo undergoes a lateral folding process that effectively transforms its shape from three flat germ layers to a cylinder, with a tube of endoderm (gut) in the center, an outer tubular covering of ectoderm (epidermis), and an intermediate layer of mesoderm. This transformation occurs before the appearance of the limbs.

Formation of the coelom

As the embryo undergoes lateral folding, the small coelomic vesicles that formed within the lateral mesoderm coalesce into the coelomic cavity (see Figure 5-15). Initially, the **intraembryonic coelom** is continuous with the **extraembryonic coelom,** but as folding is completed in a given segment of the embryo, the two coelomic spaces are separated. The last region of the embryo to undergo complete lateral folding is the area occupied by the yolk sac. In this area, small channels connecting the intraembryonic and extraembryonic coeloms persist until the ventral body wall is completely sealed.

In the cylindrical embryo, the somatic mesoderm constitutes the lateral and ventral body wall, and the splanchnic mesoderm forms the mesentery and the wall of the digestive tract. The somatic mesoderm of the lateral plate also forms the mesenchyme of the limb buds, which begin to appear late in the fourth week of pregnancy (see Figure 9-1).

Extraembryonic Mesoderm and the Body Stalk

The thin layers of extraembryonic mesoderm that line the ectodermal lining of the amnion and the endodermal lining of the yolk sac are continuous with the intraembryonic somatic and splanchnic mesoderm, respectively (see Figure 5-15, A and B). The posterior end of the embryo is connected with the trophoblastic tissues (future placenta) by the mesodermal **body stalk** (see Figure 6-1). As the embryo grows and a circulatory system becomes functional, blood vessels from the embryo grow through the body stalk to supply the placenta, and the body stalk itself becomes better defined as the **umbilical cord.** The extraembryonic mesoderm that lines the inner surface of the cytotrophoblast ultimately becomes the mesenchymal component of the placenta.

Early Stages in the Formation of the Circulatory System

As the embryo grows during the third week, it attains a size that does not permit simple diffusion to distribute oxygen and nutrients to all of its cells or efficiently remove waste products. The early development of the heart and circulatory system is an embryonic adaptation that permits the rapid growth of the embryo by providing an efficient means for the distribution of nutrients. The circulatory system faces the daunting task of having to grow and become continuously remodeled to keep pace with the embryo's overall growth while remaining fully functional in supplying the needs of the embryo's cells.

The earliest aspects of development of the circulatory system consist of the migration of heart-forming mesoderm through the primitive streak to form bilateral fields of precardiac splanchnic mesoderm. The cells in this field express genes for two sets of transcription factors (*Nkx2-5* and the MEF2 family) that are important for normal early heart development. The heart-forming cells that pass through the most cranial part of the primitive streak eventually contribute to the outflow tract of the heart, whereas those passing through the more posterior part of the streak contribute to the inflow tract. Of these fields of cardiogenic mesoderm, the heart and great vessels form from bilaterally paired vascular tubes that fuse in the midline beneath the foregut to produce a single tube. Blood has a different origin, with the first blood cells arising from **blood islands** in the mesodermal lining of the yolk sac. The definitive blood in adults arises from stem cells originating within the intraembryonic splanchnic mesoderm (see Chapter 16).

Heart and great vessels

The heart is derived from splanchnic mesoderm as bilateral tubular primordia located ventrolateral to the early pharynx (Figure 5-20). Experimental studies on lower vertebrates have traced the precardiac mesoderm to even earlier stages in development, where the heart-forming region constitutes a horseshoe-shaped region of mesoderm extending back on either side along the foregut (Figure 5-21). An inductive influence from the neighboring endoderm has been postulated to stimulate the early formation of the heart.

In human embryos the earliest recognizable precardiac mesoderm is a crescent-shaped zone of thickened mesoderm rostral to the embryonic disk of the gastrulating embryo early in the third week (Figure 5-22, A). As the mesoderm begins to split into the splanchnic and somatic layers, a **cardiogenic plate** is recognizable in the splanchnic mesoderm rostral to the oropharyngeal membrane (see Figure 5-22, B). In this area the space between the two layers of mesoderm is the forerunner of the **pericardial cavity.** The main layer of splanchnic mesoderm in the precardiac region thickens to become the **myocardial primordium.** Between this structure and the endoderm of the primitive gut, isolated mesodermal vesicles appear, which soon fuse to form the tubular **endocardial primordia** (see Figure 5-20, A and B). The endocardial primordia ultimately fuse and become the inner lining of the heart.

As the head of the embryo takes shape by both lateral and ventral folding, the bilateral cardiac primordia come together in the midline ventral to the gut and fuse to form a primitive single tubular heart. This structure consists of an inner **endocardial lining** surrounded by a loose layer of specialized extracellular matrix that has historically been called **cardiac**

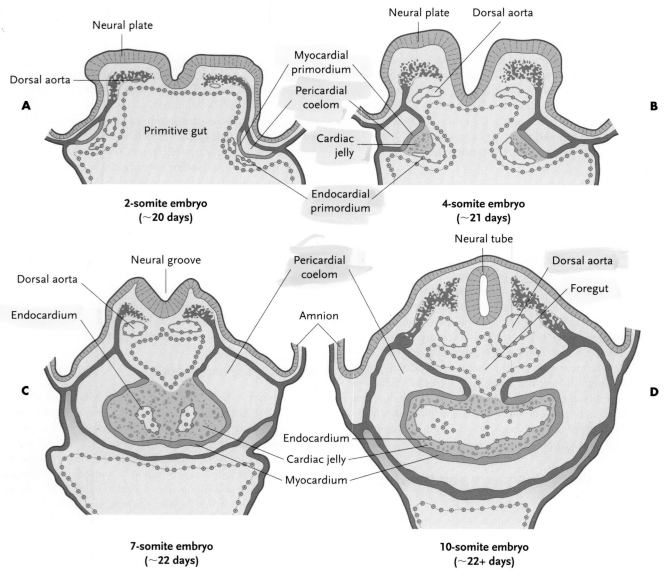

Neural plate

Dorsal aorta

Dorsal aorta

A

Primitive gut

2-somite embryo
(~20 days)

Neural plate   Dorsal aorta

Myocardial
primordium

Pericardial
coelom

Cardiac
jelly

B

Endocardial
primordium

4-somite embryo
(~21 days)

Neural groove

Dorsal aorta

Endocardium

Pericardial
coelom

Amnion

C

7-somite embryo
(~22 days)

Neural tube

Dorsal aorta

Foregut

D

Endocardium

Cardiac jelly

Myocardium

10-somite embryo
(~22+ days)

Figure 5-20 Cross sections through the level of the developing heart from **20 to 22 days. A,** Two-somite embryo. **B,** Four-somite embryo. **C,** Seven-somite embryo. **D,** Ten-somite embryo.

jelly (see Figure 5-20, C). Outside the cardiac jelly is the **my-ocardium**, which ultimately forms the muscular part of the heart. The outer lining of the heart, called the **epicardium**, is derived from the **proepicardial** primordium, which is located near the dorsal mesocardium. Cells migrating from the proepicardium cover the surface of the tubular heart. The entire tubular heart is located in the space known as the **pericardial coelom**. Shortly after the single tubular heart is formed, it begins to form a characteristic S-shaped loop that presages its eventual organization into the configuration of the adult heart (Figure 5-23). (Additional cellular and molecular aspects of early cardiogenesis are covered in Chapter 16.)

The early heart does not form in isolation. At its caudal end, the endocardial tubes do not fuse but rather extend to-

ward the posterior part of the body as the venous inflow tract of the heart (see Figure 5-23, A). Similarly, the endothelial tube leading out from the heart at its cranial end produces vascular arches that loop around the pharynx. Migrating neural crest cells form much of the walls of these vessels. By 21 or 22 days after fertilization, differentiation of cardiac muscle cells in the myocardium is sufficiently advanced to allow the heart to begin beating.

Blood and blood vessels

The formation of blood and blood vessels begins in the mesodermal wall of the yolk sac as well as in the wall of the chorion outside the embryo proper. Stimulated by an in-

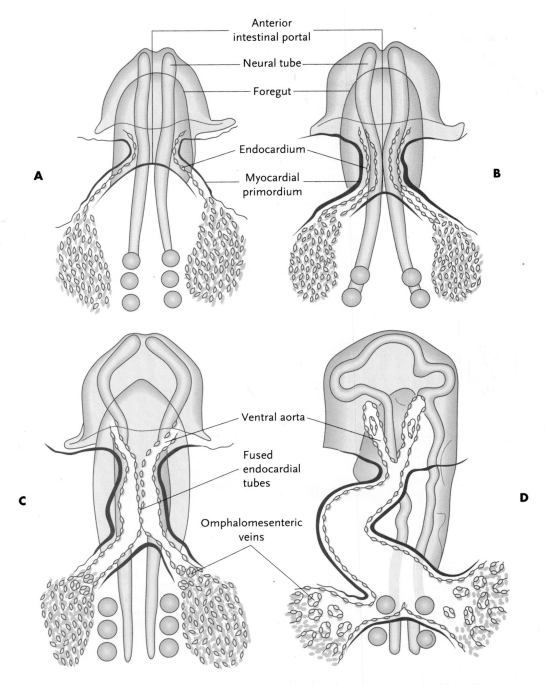

Figure 5-21 Formation of the tubular heart in the chick embryo from paired primordia. The embryo is viewed from the ventral side. **A**, Stage 8. **B**, Stage 9. **C**, Stage 10. **D**, Stage 11.

ductive interaction with the endoderm of the yolk sac, many small blood islands, consisting of stem cells called **hemangioblasts** appear in the extraembryonic splanchnic mesoderm of the yolk sac (Figure 5-24). As the result of a poorly understood mechanism, the central cells of the blood islands become blood-forming cells (**hemocytoblasts**), whereas those on the outside acquire the characteristics of **endothe-**

lial lining cells, which form the inner walls of blood vessels. As the vesicular blood islands in the wall of the yolk sac fuse, they form primitive vascular channels that extend toward the body of the embryo. Connections are made with the endothelial tubes associated with the tubular heart and major vessels, and the primitive plan of the circulatory system begins to take shape.

heart tube cranial to oro. memb.

longitudinal folding

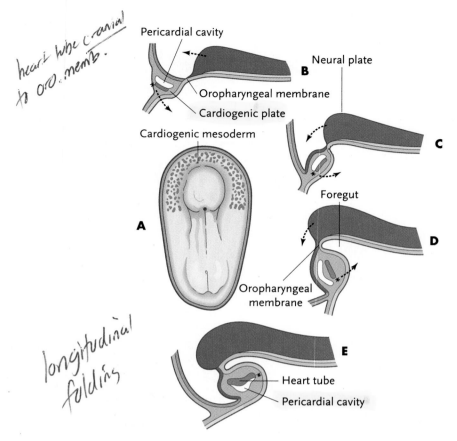

Figure 5-22 Formation of the heart from precardiac mesoderm in the human embryo. **A,** Dorsal view of an **18-day-old** embryo. **B** to **E,** Sagittal sections through the cranial ends of **18- to 22-day-old** embryos showing the roughly 180-degree rotation of the primitive heart tube and pericardium with the expansion of the cranial end of the embryo.

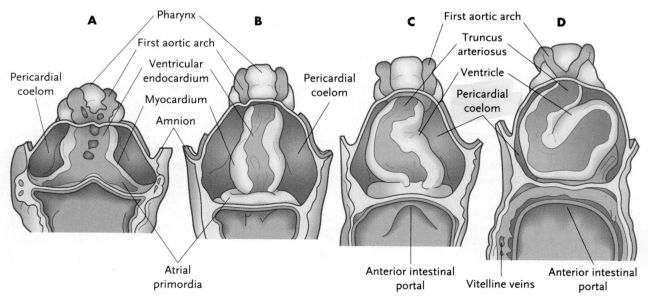

Figure 5-23 Formation of the S-shaped heart from fused cardiac tubes in the human embryo at about **21 to 23 days. A,** Four-somite embryo. **B,** Eight-somite embryo. **C,** Ten- to eleven-somite embryo. **D,** Twelve-somite embryo.

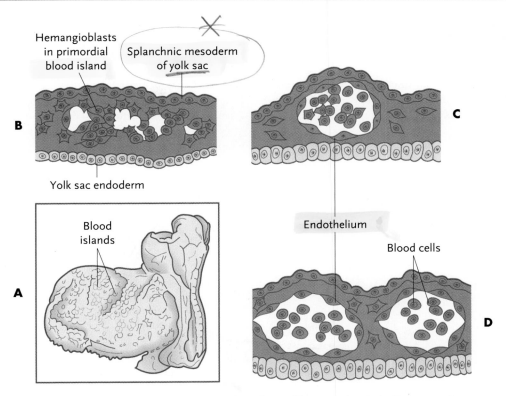

Hemangioblasts in primordial blood island

Splanchnic mesoderm of yolk sac

B

C

Yolk sac endoderm

Blood islands

Endothelium

Blood cells

A

D

Figure 5-24 Development of blood islands in the yolk sac of human embryos. **A,** Gross view of a 10-somite human embryo showing the location of blood islands on the yolk sac. **B to D,** Successive stages in the formation of blood islands. (From Corner GW: *Carnegie Contr Embryol* 20:81-102, 1929.)

DEVELOPMENT OF THE ENDODERMAL GERM LAYER

Development of the endodermal germ layer continues with the transformation of the flat intraembryonic endodermal sheet into a tubular gut as a result of the lateral folding of the embryonic body and the ventral bending of the cranial and caudal ends of the embryo into a roughly C-shaped structure (Figures 5-15 and 5-25). A major morphological consequence of these folding processes is the sharp delineation of the yolk sac from the digestive tube.

Early in the third week, when the three embryonic germ layers are first laid down, the intraembryonic endoderm constitutes the roof of the roughly spherical yolk sac (see Figure 5-25). Expansion of either end of the neural plate, particularly the tremendous growth of the future brain region, results in the formation of the **head fold** and **tail fold** along the sagittal plane of the embryo. This process, along with concomitant lateral folding, results in the formation of the beginnings of the tubular **foregut** and **hindgut**. This process also begins to delineate the yolk sac from the gut proper. The sequence of steps in the formation of the tubular gut can be likened to a purse string constricting the ventral region of the embryo, although the actual mechanism is more related to the overall growth of the embryo than to a real constriction. The region of the imaginary purse string becomes the **yolk**

stalk (also called the **omphalomesenteric** or **vitelline duct**), with the embryonic gut above and the yolk sac below (see Figures 5-15, *D*, and 5-25, *D*). The portion of the gut that still opens into the yolk sac is called the **midgut**, and the points of transition between the open-floored midgut and the tubular anterior and posterior regions of the gut are called the **anterior** and **posterior intestinal portals** (see Figure 5-25, *B*).

The endodermal edges of the anterior and posterior intestinal portals are also sites of expression of the signaling molecule **sonic hedgehog**. In the posterior intestinal portal, the appearance of sonic hedgehog in the endoderm is followed shortly by the expression of another signaling molecule, BMP-4 (see Table 5-2). This in turn is followed by the appearance of a gradient of mesodermal expression of paralogous groups 9-13 of the *Hox* genes (see Figure 5-5 for an illustration of paralogous groups), with *Hoxa-d-9* being expressed most cranially and *Hoxa-d-13* being expressed most caudally, near the cloaca. This distribution of *Hox* gene expression associated with hindgut formation is reminiscent of that already described for the early hindbrain region (see p. 86). It is likely that this gradient is instrumental in guiding the regional differentiation of the gut because later in development the gut-associated mesoderm is able to induce undifferentiated endoderm to form structures specific to the craniocaudal level of the mesoderm.

The anterior end of the foregut remains temporarily sealed off by an ectodermal-endodermal bilayer called the **oropha-**

ryngeal membrane (see Figure 5-25, *B*). This membrane separates the future mouth (**stomodeum**), which is lined by ectoderm, from the **pharynx**, the endodermally lined anterior part of the foregut. Without an intervening layer of mesoderm, this bilayer of two epithelial sheets is inherently unstable and eventually breaks down. The rapid bulging of the

cephalic region, in conjunction with the constriction of the ventral region, has a major topographic effect on the rapidly developing cardiac region. In the early embryo the cardiac primordia are located cephalic to the primitive gut. The forces that shape the tubular foregut, however, cause the bilateral cardiac primordia to turn 180 degrees in the craniocaudal di-

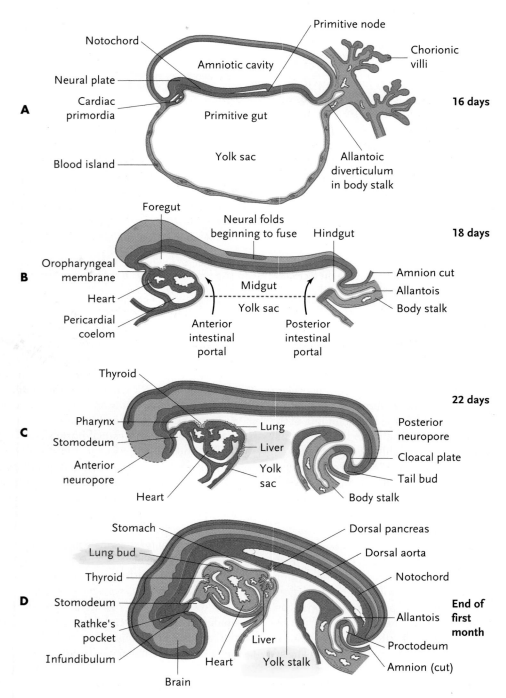

Figure 5-25 Sagittal sections through human embryos showing the early establishment of the digestive system. **A**, At 16 days. **B**, At 18 days. **C**, At 22 days. **D**, At the **end of the first month**. (After Patten. From Carlson BM: *Patten's foundations of embryology,* ed 6, New York, 1996, McGraw-Hill.)

rection while the paired cardiac tubes are moving toward one another in the ventral midline (see Figure 5-22).

In the region of the hindgut the expansion of the embryo's body is not as prominent as it is in the cranial end, but nevertheless a less exaggerated ventral folding also occurs in that region. Even as the earliest signs of the tail fold are taking shape, a tubular evagination of the hindgut extends into the mesoderm of the body stalk. This evagination is called the **allantois** (Figure 5-25, *B*). In most mammals and birds the allantois represents a major structural adaptation for the exchange of gases and the removal of urinary wastes. Because of the efficiency of the placenta, however, the allantois never becomes a prominent structure in the human embryo. Nevertheless, because of the blood vessels that become associated with it, it remains a vital part of the link between the embryo and the mother (see Chapter 6).

Caudal to the allantois is another ectodermal-endodermal bilayer called the **cloacal plate**, or **proctodeal membrane** (see Figure 5-25, *C*). This membrane, which ultimately breaks down, covers the cloaca, which in the early embryo represents a common outlet for both the digestive and the urogenital systems. The shallow depression outside the proctodeal membrane is called the **proctodeum**.

As the gut becomes increasingly tubular, a series of local inductive interactions between the epithelium of the digestive tract and the surrounding mesenchyme initiate the formation of most of the major digestive and endocrine glands (e.g., thyroid gland, salivary glands, pancreas), the respiratory system, and the liver. In the region of the stomodeum, an induction between forebrain and stomodeal ectoderm initiates the formation of the anterior pituitary gland. (Further development of these organs is discussed in Chapters 13 and 14.)

BASIC STRUCTURE OF THE 4-WEEK-OLD EMBRYO

Gross Appearance

By the end of the fourth week of pregnancy the embryo, which is still only about 4 mm long, has established the rudiments of most of the major organ systems except for the limbs (which are still absent) and the urogenital system (which has developed only the earliest traces of the embryonic kidneys). Externally, the embryo is C-shaped, with a prominent row of somites situated along either side of the neural tube (Figures 5-26 and 5-27). Except for the rudiments

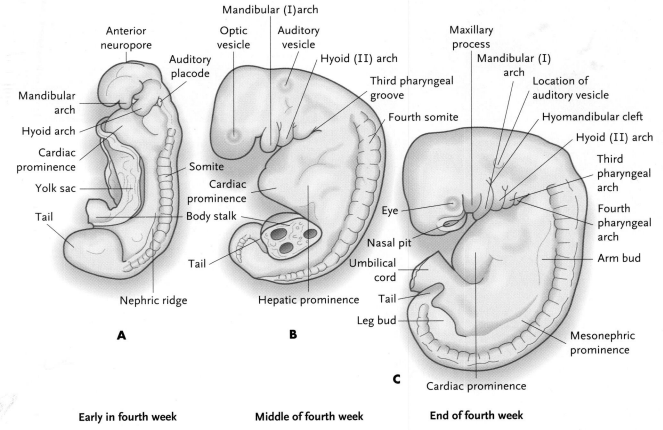

Early in fourth week   Middle of fourth week   End of fourth week

Figure 5-26 Gross development of human embryos during the period of early organogenesis. **A,** Early in the fourth week. **B,** Middle of the fourth week. **C,** End of the fourth week.

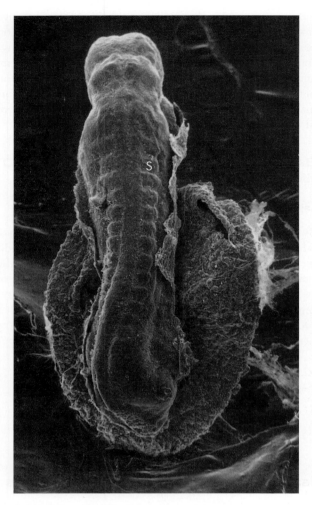

Figure 5-27 Scanning electron micrograph of a 3-mm human embryo approximately **26 days old**. *S,* Somite. (From Jirásek JE: *Atlas of human prenatal morphogenesis,* Amsterdam, 1983, Martinus Nijhoff.)

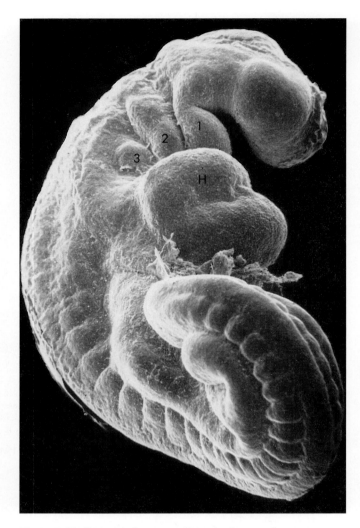

Figure 5-29 Scanning electron micrograph of a 4-mm human embryo **30 days old**. *1* to *3,* Pharyngeal arches; *H,* heart. (From Jirásek JE: *Atlas of human prenatal morphogenesis,* Amsterdam, 1983, Martinus Nijhoff.)

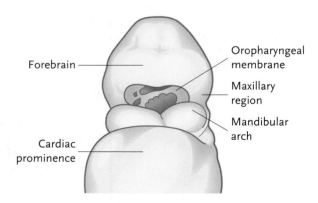

Figure 5-28 Face of a human embryo during the **fourth week** showing the breakdown of the oropharyngeal membrane.

of the eyes and ears and the oropharyngeal membrane, which is beginning to break down (Figure 5-28), the head is relatively featureless. In the cervical region, **pharyngeal arches** are prominent (Figures 5-26, *B* and *C,* and 5-29). The body stalk still occupies a significant part of the ventral body wall, and, cephalic to the body stalk, the heart and liver make prominent bulges in the contours of the ventral body wall. Posterior to the body stalk, the body tapers to a somewhat spiraled tail, which is prominent in embryos of this age.

Another prominent but little understood feature of embryos of this age is a ring of thickened ectoderm, called the **wolffian ridge,** that encircles the lateral aspect of the body (Figure 5-30). Its function is not well understood, but it spans the primordia of many structures (e.g., nose, eye, inner ear, pharyngeal arches, limbs) that require tissue interactions for their early development. What role the thickened ectoderm plays in early organogenesis remains to be determined.

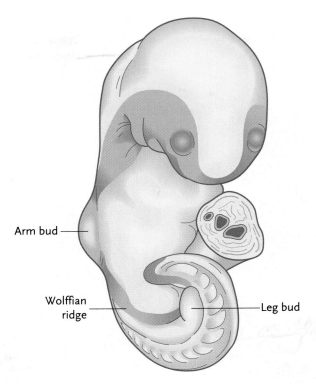

Arm bud

Wolffian ridge

Leg bud

Figure 5-30 Ventrolateral view of a 30-somite (4.2 mm) human embryo showing the thickened ectodermal ring *(blue)*. The portion of the ring between the upper and lower limb buds is the wolffian ridge. (Based on studies by O'Rahilly R, Gardner E: *Anat Embryol* 148:1-23, 1975.)

Circulatory System

At 4 weeks of age, the embryo has a functioning two-chambered heart and a blood vascular system that consists of three separate circulatory arcs (Figure 5-31). The first, the **intraembryonic circulatory arc,** is organized in a manner similar to that of a fish. A ventral aortic outflow tract from the heart splits into a series of aortic arches passing around the pharynx through the pharyngeal arches and then collecting into a cephalically paired dorsal aorta that distributes blood throughout the body. A system of cardinal veins collects the blood and returns it to the heart via a common inflow tract.

The second arc, commonly called the **vitelline** or **omphalomesenteric arc,** is principally an extraembryonic circulatory loop that supplies the yolk sac (see Figure 5-31). The third circulatory arc, also extraembryonic, consists of the vessels associated with the allantois. In the human, this third arc consists of the **umbilical vessels,** which course through the body stalk and spread in an elaborate network in the placenta and chorionic tissues. This set of vessels represents the real lifeline between the embryo and mother. Although the two extraembryonic circulatory loops do not persist as such after birth, the intraembryonic portions of these arcs are retained as vessels or ligaments in the adult body.

Derivatives of the Embryonic Germ Layers

By the end of the fourth week of development, primordia of most of the major structures and organs in the body have been laid down, many of them the result of local inductive interactions. Each of the embryonic germ layers contributes to the formation of many of these structures. Figure 5-32 summarizes the germ layer origins of most of the major structures in the embryonic body. This figure is designed to be a guide that will allow specific structures that are being studied to be viewed in the context of the whole body rather than something that should be memorized at this stage. Students have found that a table like this is useful for review at the end of an embryology course.

SUMMARY

- Evidence is increasing that the basic body plan of mammalian embryos is under the control of many of the same genes that have been identified to control morphogenesis in *Drosophila*. In this species the basic axes are fixed through the actions of maternal effect genes. Batteries of segmentation genes (gap, pair-rule, and segment-polarity genes) are then activated. Two clusters of homeotic genes next confer a specific morphogenetic character to each body segment. Because of their regulative nature, mam-

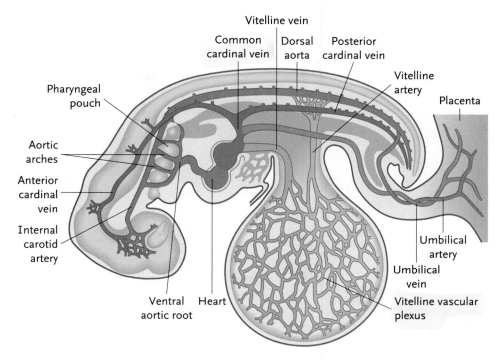

Figure 5-31 Basic circulatory arcs in the **4-week-old** human embryo.

malian embryos are not as rigidly controlled by genetic instructions as *Drosophila*.

- The homeobox, a highly conserved region of 183 base pairs, is found in multiple different genes in almost all animals. The homeobox protein is a transcription factor. Homeobox-containing genes are arranged along the chromosome in a specific order and are expressed along the craniocaudal axis of the embryo in the same order. Activation of homeobox genes may involve interactions with other morphogenetically active agents, such as retinoic acid and TGF-β.

- Many of the molecules that control development can be assigned to several broad groups. One group is the transcription factors, of which the products of homeobox-containing genes are just one of many types. A second category is signaling molecules, many of which are effectors of inductive interactions. Some of these are members of large families, such as the TGF-β and FGF families. A very important class of signaling molecules is the hedgehog proteins, which mediate the activities of many important organizing centers of the early embryo. Signaling molecules interact with responding cells by binding to specific surface or cytoplasmic receptors. These receptors represent the initial elements of complex signal transduction pathways, which translate the signal to an intracellular event that results in new patterns of gene expression in the responding cells.

- The response of dorsal ectodermal cells to primary induction is to thicken, forming a neural plate. Neurulation consists of lateral folding of the neural plate at hinge points to form a neural groove. Opposing sides of the thickened epithelium of the neural groove join to form a neural tube. The temporarily unclosed cranial and caudal ends of the neural tube are the anterior and posterior neuropores.

- Cranially, the neural tube subdivides into a primitive three-part brain consisting of the prosencephalon, mesencephalon, and rhombencephalon. The caudal part of the early brain also becomes subdivided into segments called *neuromeres*, of which the rhombomeres are most prominent. Specific homeobox genes are expressed in a regular order in the rhombomeres.

- As the neural tube closes, neural crest cells emigrate from the neural epithelium and spread through the body along well-defined paths. Secondary inductions acting on ectoderm in the cranial region result in the formation of several series of ectodermal placodes, which are the precursors of sense organs and sensory ganglia of cranial nerves.

- The embryonic mesoderm is subdivided into three craniocaudal columns: the paraxial, intermediate, and lateral plate mesoderm. Paraxial mesoderm is the precursor tissue to the paired somites and somitomeres. As the result of a complex series of inductive interactions involving a variety of signaling molecules, the epithelial somites become subdivided into sclerotomes (precursors of vertebral bodies) and dermomyotomes, which in turn form dermatomes (dermal precursors) and myotomes (precursors of axial muscles). In further subdivisions, precursor cells of limb muscles are found in the lateral halves of the somites, and precursor cells of axial muscles are found in the medial halves. The posterior half of one sclerotome joins with the anterior half of the next caudal somite to form a single vertebral body.

- Intermediate mesoderm forms the organs of the urogenital system. The lateral plate mesoderm splits to form somatic mesoderm (associated with ectoderm) and splanchnic mesoderm (associated with endoderm). The space between becomes the coelom. The limb bud arises from lateral plate mesoderm, and extraembryonic mesoderm forms the body stalk.

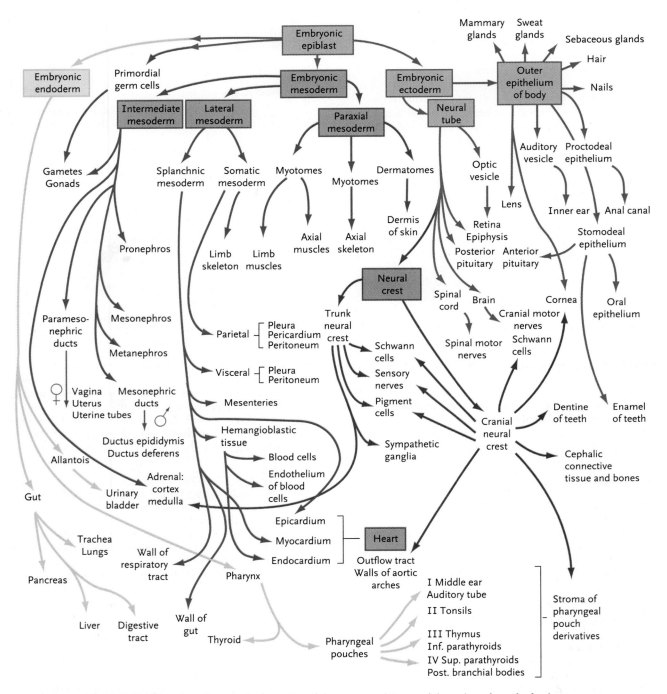

Figure 5-32 Flow chart showing the formation of the organs and tissues of the embryo from the fundamental germ layers. The arrows are color-coded according to the germ layer of origin of the structure (see Figure 4-1 for color code).

- Blood cells and blood vessels form initially from blood islands located in the mesodermal wall of the yolk sac. The heart, originating from a horseshoe-shaped region of splanchnic mesoderm anterior to the oropharyngeal membrane, forms two tubes on either side of the foregut. As the foregut takes shape, the two cardiac tubes come together to form a single tubular heart, which begins to beat around 22 days after fertilization.

- The embryonic endoderm initially consists of the roof of the yolk sac. As the embryo undergoes lateral folding, the endodermal gut forms cranial and caudal tubes (foregut and hindgut), but the middle region (midgut) remains open to the yolk sac ventrally. Regional specification of the gut begins with sonic hedgehog signals from the endoderm of the intestinal portals, which are translated to gradients of *Hox* gene expression in the neighboring mesoderm. As the tubular gut continues to take shape, the connection to the yolk sac becomes attenuated to form the yolk stalk. The future mouth (stomodeum) is separated from the foregut by an oropharyngeal membrane, and the hindgut is separated from the proctodeum by the cloacal plate. A ventral evagination from the hindgut is the allantois, which in many animals is an adaptation for removing urinary and respiratory wastes.

- In the 4-week-old embryo, the circulatory system includes a functioning two-chambered heart and a blood vascular system that consists of three circulatory arcs. In addition to the intraembryonic circulation, the extraembryonic vitelline circulatory arc, which supplies the yolk sac, and the umbilical circulation, which is associated with the allantois and supplies the placenta, are present.

REVIEW QUESTIONS

1. The sclerotome arises from cells that were located in the:
    A. Notochord
    B. Paraxial mesoderm
    C. Intermediate mesoderm
    D. Lateral mesoderm
    E. None of the above
2. The cardiogenic plate arises from:
    A. Embryonic endoderm
    B. Somatic mesoderm
    C. Splanchnic mesoderm
    D. Intermediate mesoderm
    E. Neural crest
3. An inductive stimulus from which structure stimulates the transformation of the epithelial sclerotome into secondary mesenchyme?
    A. Neural crest
    B. Somite
    C. Ectodermal placodes
    D. Embryonic endoderm
    E. Notochord
4. Which of these structures in the embryo is unsegmented?
    A. Somitomeres
    B. Neuromeres
    C. Notochord
    D. Somites
5. The intermediate mesoderm is the precursor of the:
    A. Urogenital system
    B. Heart
    C. Somites
    D. Body wall
    E. Vertebral bodies
6. What is a homeobox?
7. What forces are involved in the folding of the neural plate to form the neural tube?
8. What role do neuromeres play in the formation of the central nervous system?
9. From what structures do the cells that form skeletal muscles arise?
10. Where do the first blood cells of the embryo form?

REFERENCES

Alvarez IS, Schoenwolf GC: Expansion of surface epithelium provides the major extrinsic force for bending of the neural plate, *J Exp Zool* 261:340-348, 1992.

Amthor H and others: The expression and regulation of *follistatin* and a *follistatin-like* gene during avian somite compartmentalization and myogenesis, *Dev Biol* 178:343-362, 1996.

Bergquist H: Studies on the cerebral tube in vertebrates: the neuromeres, *Acta Zool* 33:117-187, 1952.

Brand-Saberi B and others: The formation of somite compartments in the avian embryo, *Int J Dev Biol* 40:411-420, 1996.

Christ B and others: Segmentation of the vertebrate body, *Anat Embryol* 197:1-8, 1998.

DeRobertis EM, Oliver G, Wright CVE: Homeobox genes and the vertebrate body plan, *Sci Am* 263(1):46-52, 1990.

Dietrich S, Schubert FR, Lumsden A: Control of dorsoventral pattern in the chick paraxial mesoderm, *Development* 124:3895-3908, 1997.

Duboule D, ed: *Guidebook to the homeobox genes*, Oxford, England, 1994, Oxford University Press.

Fishman MC, Chien KR: Fashioning the vertebrate heart: earliest embryonic decisions, *Development* 124:2099-2117, 1997.

French V and others: Mechanisms of segmentation, *Development* 104(suppl):1-254, 1980.

Gehring WJ: Homeotic genes, the homeobox, and the spatial organization of the embryo, *Harvey Lect* 81:153-172, 1987.

Graham A, Papalopulu N, Krumlauf R: The murine and *Drosophila* homeobox gene complexes have common features of organization and expression, *Cell* 57:367-378, 1989.

Hammerschmidt M, Brook A, McMahon AP: The world according to hedgehog, *Trends Genet* 13:14-21, 1997.

Jacobson AG: Somitomeres: mesodermal segments of the head and trunk. In Hanken J, Hall BK, eds: *The skull*, vol 1, *Development*, Chicago, 1993, University of Chicago Press.

Jacobson AG, Sater AK: Features of embryonic induction, *Development* 104:341-359, 1988.

Johnson RL, Tabin C: The long and short of hedgehog signaling, *Cell* 81:313-316, 1995.

Kingsley DM: The TGF-β superfamily: new members, new receptors, and new genetic tests of function in different organisms, *Genes Dev* 8:133-146, 1994.

Lassar AB, Munsterberg AE: The role of positive and negative signals in somite patterning, *Curr Opin Neurobiol* 6:57-63, 1996.

Lobe CG: Transcription factors and mammalian development, *Curr Topics Dev Biol* 27:351-382, 1992.

Lumsden A, Krumlauf R: Patterning the vertebrate neuraxis, *Science* 274:1109-1115, 1996.

Marcelle C, Stark MR, Bronner-Fraser M: Coordinate actions of BMPs, Wnts, Shh and Noggin mediate patterning of the dorsal somite, *Development* 124:3955-3963, 1997.

Mavillio F: Regulation of vertebrate homeobox-containing genes by morphogens, *Eur J Biochem* 212:273-288, 1993.

McGinnis W, Krumlauf R: Homeobox genes and axial patterning, *Cell* 68:283-302, 1992.

McMahon AP: The *Wnt* family of developmental regulators, *Trends Genet* 8:236-242, 1992.

Meier S: Development of the chick embryo mesoblast: formation of the embryonic axis and establishment of the embryonic pattern, *Dev Biol* 73:24-45, 1979.

Morris-Kay G: Retinoic acid and development, *Pathobiology* 60:264-270, 1992.

Müller F, O'Rahilly R: The timing and sequence of appearance of neuromeres and their derivatives in staged human embryos, *Acta Anat* 158:83-99, 1997.

Murtha MT, Leckman JF, Ruddle FH: Detection of homeobox genes in development and evolution, *Proc Natl Acad Sci USA* 88:10711-10715, 1991.

Nusse R, Varmus HE: *Wnt* genes, *Cell* 69:1073-1087, 1992.

O'Rahilly R, Müller F: The origin of the ectodermal ring in staged human embryos of the first 5 weeks, *Acta Anat* 122:145-157, 1985.

Ordahl CP, Le Douarin NM: Two myogenic lineages within the developing somite, *Development* 114:339-353, 1992.

Pourquie O and others: Lateral and axial signals involved in avian somite patterning: a role for BMP4, *Cell* 84:461-471, 1996.

Prior HM, Walter MA: Sox genes: architects of development, *Mol Med* 2:405-412, 1996.

Roberts DJ and others: Sonic hedgehog is an endodermal signal inducing *Bmp-4* and *Hox* genes during induction and regionalization of the chick hindgut, *Development* 121:3163-3174, 1995.

Rubenstein JLR and others: The embryonic vertebrate forebrain: the prosomeric model, *Science* 266:578-580, 1994.

Sasai Y, De Robertis EM: Ectodermal patterning in vertebrate embryos, *Dev Biol* 182:5-20, 1997.

Schoenwolf GC: Histological and ultrastructural studies of secondary neurulation in mouse embryos, *Am J Anat* 169:361-376, 1984.

Schoenwolf GC: Mechanisms of neurulation: traditional viewpoint and recent advances, *Development* 109:243-270, 1990.

Scott MP: Vertebrate homeobox nomenclature, *Cell* 71:551-553, 1992.

Smith JL, Schoenwolf GC: Neurulation: coming to closure, *Trends Neurol Sci* 20:510-517, 1997.

Sosic D and others: Regulation of *paraxis* expression and somite formation by ectoderm- and neural tube-derived signals, *Dev Biol* 185:229-243, 1997.

Tam PPL, Meier S, Jacobson AG: Differentiation of the metameric pattern in the embryonic axis of the mouse. II. Somitomeric organization of the presomitic mesoderm, *Differentiation* 21:109-122, 1982.

Tonegawa A and others: Mesodermal subdivision along the mediolateral axis in chicken controlled by different concentrations of BMP-4, *Development* 124:1975-1984, 1997.

Vaage S: The segmentation of the primitive neural tube in chick embryos (*Gallus domesticus*), *Adv Anat Embryol Cell Biol* 41(3):1-88, 1969.

van den Heuvel M, Ingham PW: "Smoothing" the path for hedgehogs, *Trends Cell Biol* 6:451-453, 1996.

Wehr R, Gruss P: Pax and vertebrate development, *Int J Dev Biol* 40:369-377, 1996.

Wilkie AOM and others: Functions of FGFs and their receptors, *Curr Biol* 5:500-507, 1995.

Williams BA, Ordahl CP: Emergence of determined myotome precursor cells in the somite, *Development* 124:4983-4997, 1997.

Wright CV and others: Interference with function of a homeobox gene in *Xenopus* embryos produces malformations of the anterior spinal cord, *Cell* 59:81-93, 1989.

Yamaguchi A: Regulation of differentiation pathway of skeletal mesenchymal cells in cell lines by TGF-β superfamily, *Semin Cell Biol* 6:165-173, 1995.

6

PLACENTA AND EXTRAEMBRYONIC MEMBRANES

One of the most characteristic features of human embryonic development is the intimate relationship between the embryo and mother. The fertilized egg brings little with it except genetic material. To survive and grow during intrauterine life, the embryo must maintain an essentially parasitic relationship with the body of the mother for acquiring oxygen and nutrients and eliminating wastes. It must also avoid being rejected like a foreign body by the immune system of its maternal host. These exacting requirements are met by the placenta and extraembryonic membranes that surround the embryo and serve as the interface between the embryo and mother.

The tissues that make up the fetal-maternal interface (**placenta** and **chorion**) are derivatives of the **trophoblast**, which separates from the inner cell mass and surrounds the cellular precursors of the embryo proper even as the cleaving zygote travels down the uterine tube on its way to implanting into the uterine wall (see Figure 3-17). Other extraembryonic tissues are derived from the inner cell mass. These include the **amnion** (an ectodermal derivative), which forms a protective fluid-filled capsule around the embryo; the **yolk sac** (an endodermal derivative), which in mammalian embryos no longer serves a primary nutritive function; the **allantois** (an endodermal derivative), which is associated with the removal of embryonic wastes; and the **extraembryonic mesoderm**, which forms the bulk of the umbilical cord, the connective tissue backing of the extraembryonic membranes, and the blood vessels that supply them.

EXTRAEMBRYONIC TISSUES

Amnion

The origin of the amniotic cavity within the ectoderm of the inner cell mass in the implanting embryo was described in Chapter 4 (see Figures 3-17 and 4-2). As the early embryo undergoes cephalocaudal and lateral folding, the amniotic membrane surrounds the body of the embryo like a fluid-filled balloon (Figure 6-1), allowing the embryo to be suspended in a liquid environment for the duration of pregnancy. The amniotic fluid serves as a buffer against mechanical injury to the fetus; in addition, it accommodates growth, allows normal fetal movements, and protects the fetus from adhesions.

The thin amniotic membrane consists of a single layer of extraembryonic ectodermal cells lined by a nonvascularized layer of extraembryonic mesoderm. Keeping pace with fetal growth, the amniotic cavity steadily expands until its fluid content reaches a maximum of nearly 1 L by weeks 33 to 34 of pregnancy (Figure 6-2).

In many respects, amniotic fluid can be viewed as a dilute transudate of maternal plasma, but the origins and exchange dynamics of amniotic fluid are complex and not completely understood. There appear to be two phases in amniotic fluid production. The first phase encompasses the first 20 weeks of pregnancy, during which the composition of amniotic fluid is quite similar to that of fetal fluids. During this period, the fetal skin is unkeratinized, and there is evidence that fluid and electrolytes are able to diffuse freely through the embryonic ectoderm of the skin. In addition, the amniotic membrane itself secretes fluid, and components of maternal serum pass through the amniotic membrane.

As pregnancy advances (especially after the week 20, when the fetal epidermis begins to keratinize), changes occur in the source of amniotic fluid. There is not complete agreement on the sources (and their relative contributions) of amniotic fluid in the second half of pregnancy. Nonetheless, there are increasing contributions from fetal urine, filtration from maternal blood vessels near the chorion laeve (which is closely apposed to the amniotic membrane at this stage), and possibly filtration from fetal vessels in the umbilical cord and chorionic plate.

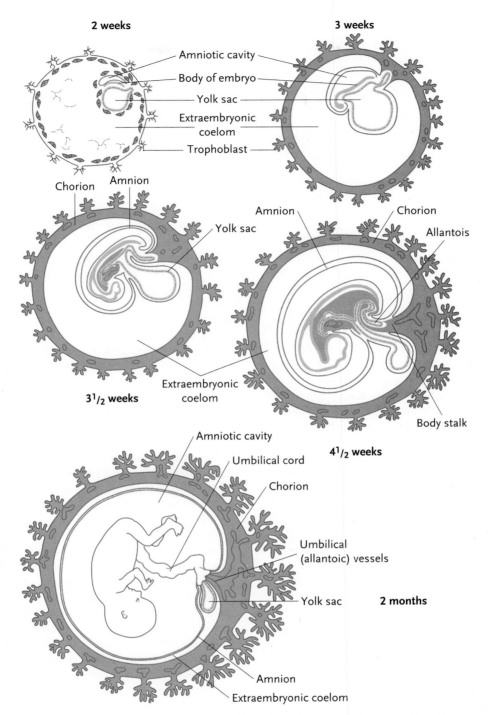

Figure 6-1 Human embryos showing the relationships of the chorion and other extraembryonic membranes. (Modified from Carlson BM: *Patten's foundations of embryology*, ed 6, New York, 1996, McGraw-Hill.)

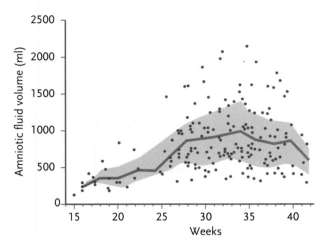

Figure 6-2 Volumes of amniotic fluid in women at various weeks of pregnancy. The lined and colored area represents the mean plus or minus standard deviation. Dots represent outlying values. (Data from Queenan JT and others: *Am J Obstet Gynecol* 114:34-38, 1972.)

In the third trimester of pregnancy, the amniotic fluid turns over completely every 3 hours, and at term, the fluid-exchange rate may approach 500 ml/hr. Although much of the amniotic fluid is exchanged across the amniotic membrane, fetal swallowing is an important mechanism in late pregnancy, with about 20 ml/hr of fluid being swallowed by the fetus. Swallowed amniotic fluid ultimately enters the fetal bloodstream after absorption through the gut wall. The ingested water can leave the fetal circulation through the placenta.

Clinical Correlation 6-1 discusses conditions related to the amount of amniotic fluid or substance concentrations in the fluid.

Yolk Sac

The yolk sac, which is lined by extraembryonic endoderm, is formed ventral to the bilayered embryo when the amnion appears dorsal to the embryonic disk (see Figure 4-2). In contrast to birds and reptiles, the yolk sac of mammals is small and devoid of yolk. Although vestigial in terms of its original function as a source of nutrition, the yolk sac remains vital to the embryo because of other functions that have become associated with it.

When it first appears, the yolk sac is in the form of a hemisphere bounded at the equatorial region by the dorsal wall of the primitive gut (see Figure 6-1). As the embryo grows and undergoes lateral folding and curvature along the craniocaudal axis, the connection between the yolk sac and forming gut becomes attenuated in the shape of a progressively narrowing stalk attached to a more spherical yolk sac proper at its distal end. In succeeding weeks the yolk stalk becomes very

long and attenuated as it is incorporated into the body of the umbilical cord. The yolk sac itself moves nearer the chorionic plate of the placenta (Figure 6-3).

The endoderm of the yolk sac is lined on the outside by well-vascularized extraembryonic mesoderm. Cells found in each of these layers contribute vital components to the body of the embryo. During the third week, **primordial germ cells,** which arise in the extraembryonic mesoderm near the base of the allantois, become recognizable in the lining of the yolk sac (see Figure 1-1). Soon these cells migrate into the wall of the gut and the dorsal mesentery as they make their way to the gonads, where they differentiate into oogonia or spermatogonia.

In the meantime, groups of extraembryonic mesodermal cells in the wall of the yolk sac become organized into **blood islands** (see Figure 5-24), and many of the cells differentiate into primitive blood cells. **Extraembryonic hematopoiesis** continues in the yolk sac until about the sixth week, when blood-forming activity becomes transferred to intraembryonic sites, especially the liver.

As the tubular gut forms, the attachment site of the yolk stalk becomes progressively less prominent, until by 6 weeks it has effectively lost contact with the gut. In a small percentage of adults, traces of the yolk duct persist as a fibrous cord or an outpouching of the small intestine known as a **Meckel's diverticulum** (see Figure 14-11, *A*). The yolk sac itself may persist throughout much of pregnancy, but it is not known to have a specific function in the fetal period. The proximal portions of the blood vessels of the yolk sac (the vitelline circulatory arc) persist as vessels that supply the midgut region.

Allantois

The allantois arises as an endodermally lined ventral outpocketing of the hindgut (see Figure 6-1). In the human embryo, it is just a vestige of the large, saclike structure that is used by the embryos of many mammals, birds, and reptiles as a major respiratory organ and repository for urinary wastes. Like the yolk sac, the allantois in the human retains only a secondary function, in this case respiration. However, in the human, this function is served by the blood vessels that differentiate from the mesodermal wall of the allantois. These vessels form the umbilical circulatory arc, consisting of the arteries and vein that supply the placenta (see Figure 5-31). (The postnatal fate of these vessels is discussed in Chapter 17.)

The allantois proper, which consists of little more than a cord of endodermal cells, is embedded in the umbilical cord. Later in development, the proximal part of the allantois (called the **urachus**) is continuous with the forming urinary bladder (see Figure 15-2). After birth, it becomes transformed into a dense fibrous cord (median umbilical ligament), which runs from the urinary bladder to the umbilical region (see Figure 17-18).

CLINICAL CORRELATION 6-1
Conditions Related to Amniotic Fluid

The normal amount of amniotic fluid at term is typically between 500 and 1000 ml. An excessive amount (over 2000 ml) is **hydramnios.** This condition is frequently associated with multiple pregnancies and **esophageal atresia** or **anencephaly** (a congenital anomaly characterized by gross defects of the head and often the inability to swallow [see Figure 7-4]). Such circumstantial evidence supports the important role of fetal swallowing in the overall balance of amniotic fluid exchange. Too little amniotic fluid (less than 500 ml) is **oligohydramnios.** This condition is often associated with bilateral **renal agenesis** (absence of kidneys) and points to the role of fetal urinary excretion in amniotic fluid dynamics. Oligohydramnios can also be a consequence of preterm rupture of the amniotic membrane, which occurs in about 10% of pregnancies.

There are many components, both fetal and maternal, in amniotic fluid; for example, over 200 proteins of both maternal and fetal origin have been detected in amniotic fluid. With the analytical tools available, much can be learned about the condition of the fetus by examining the composition of amniotic fluid. **Amniocentesis** involves removing a small amount of amniotic fluid by inserting a needle through the mother's abdomen and into the amniotic cavity. Because of the small amount of amniotic fluid in early embryos, amniocentesis is usually not performed until the thirteenth or fourteenth week of pregnancy. Amniotic fluid has bacteriostatic properties, which may account for the low incidence of infections after amniocentesis is performed.

Fetal cells present in the fluid can be cultured and examined for various chromosomal and metabolic defects. Recent techniques now permit the examination of chromosomes in the cells immediately obtained instead of having to wait up to 2 to 3 weeks for cultured amniotic cells to proliferate to the point of being suitable for genetic analysis. In addition to the detection of chromosomal defects (e.g., trisomies), it is possible to determine the sex of the fetus by direct chromosomal analysis. A high concentration of α-**fetoprotein** (a protein of the central nervous system) in amniotic fluid is a strong indicator of a neural tube defect. Fetal maturity can be assessed by determining the concentration of creatinine or the **lecithin/sphingomyelin ratio** (which is a reflection of the maturity of the lungs). The severity of **erythroblastosis fetalis** (Rh disease) can also be assessed by examination of amniotic fluid.

CHORION AND PLACENTA

Formation of the placental complex represents a cooperative effort between the extraembryonic tissues of the embryo and the endometrial tissues of the mother. (Early stages of implantation of the embryo and the decidual reaction of the uterine lining are described in Chapter 3.) After implantation is complete, the original trophoblast surrounding the embryo has undergone differentiation into two layers: the inner **cytotrophoblast** and the outer **syncytiotrophoblast** (see Figure 3-17, *D*). Lacunae in the rapidly expanding trophoblast have filled with maternal blood, and the connective tissue cells of the endometrium have undergone the decidual reaction (containing increased amounts of glycogen and lipids) in response to the trophoblastic invasion.

Formation of Chorionic Villi

In the early implanting embryo the trophoblastic tissues have no consistent gross morphological features; consequently, this is called the period of the **previllous embryo.** Late in the second week, defined cytotrophoblastic projections called **primary villi** begin to take shape (see Figure 4-2). Shortly thereafter, a mesenchymal core appears within an expanding villus, at which point it is properly called a **secondary villus** (Figure 6-4). Surrounding the mesenchymal core of the

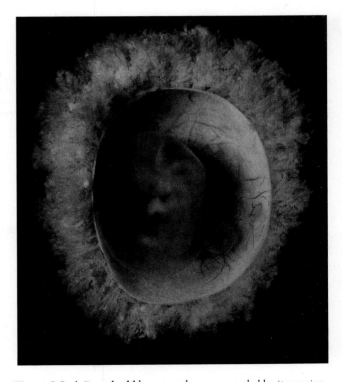

Figure 6-3 A 7-week-old human embryo surrounded by its amnion. The embryo was exposed by cutting open the chorion. The small sphere to the right of the embryo is the yolk sac. (Carnegie embryo No. 8537A, Chester Reather, Baltimore.)

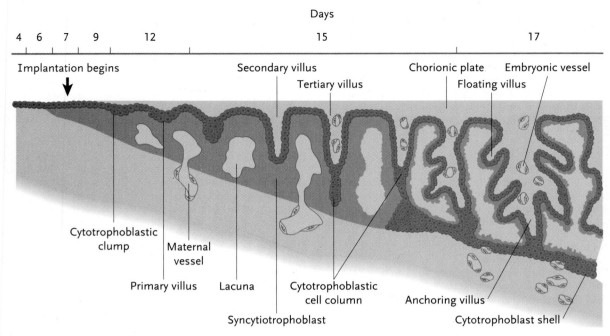

Days

4 6 7 9 12 15 17

Implantation begins   Secondary villus   Chorionic plate   Embryonic vessel

Tertiary villus   Floating villus

Cytotrophoblastic clump   Maternal vessel

Primary villus   Lacuna   Cytotrophoblastic cell column   Anchoring villus

Syncytiotrophoblast   Cytotrophoblast shell

Figure 6-4 Stages in the formation of a chorionic villus, starting with a cytotrophoblastic clump at the far left and progressing to an anchoring villus at right.

secondary villus is a complete layer of cytotrophoblastic cells, and outside of that is the syncytiotrophoblast. By definition, the secondary villus becomes a **tertiary villus** when blood vessels penetrate its mesenchymal core and newly formed branches. This occurs toward the end of the third week of pregnancy. Although individual villi undergo considerable branching, most of them retain the same basic structural plan throughout pregnancy.

The terminal portion of a villus remains trophoblastic, consisting of a solid mass of cytotrophoblast called a **cytotrophoblastic cell column** (see Figure 6-4) and a relatively thin covering of syncytiotrophoblast over that. The villus is bathed in maternal blood. A further development of the tip of the villus occurs when under the influence of the local hypoxic environment, the cytotrophoblastic cell column expands distally, penetrating the syncytiotrophoblastic layer (Figure 6-5). These cytotrophoblastic cells abut directly on maternal decidual cells and spread over them to form a complete cellular layer known as the **cytotrophoblastic shell**, which surrounds the embryo complex. The villi that give off the cytotrophoblastic extensions are known as **anchoring villi** (see Figure 6-4) because they represent the real attachment points between the embryo complex and the maternal tissues.

It is important to understand the overall relationships of the various embryonic and maternal tissues at this stage of development (see Figure 6-5). The embryo, attached by the **body stalk**, or **umbilical cord**, is effectively suspended in

the **chorionic cavity**. The chorionic cavity is bounded by the **chorionic plate**, which consists of extraembryonic mesoderm overlain with trophoblast. The chorionic villi extend outward from the chorionic plate, and their trophoblastic covering is continuous with that of the chorionic plate. The villi and the outer surface of the chorionic plate are bathed in a sea of continually exchanging maternal blood. Because of this, the human placenta is designated as the **hemochorial type.***

Although chorionic villi are structurally very complex, it is convenient to liken the basic structure of a villus complex to the root system of a plant. The anchoring villus is equivalent to the central tap root; by means of the cytotrophoblastic cell columns, it attaches the villus complex to the outer cytotrophoblastic shell. The unattached branches of the **floating villi** (see Figure 6-12) dangle freely in the maternal blood that fills the space between the chorionic plate and the outer cytotrophoblastic shell. All surfaces of the villi, chorionic plate, and cytotrophoblastic shell that are in contact with maternal blood are lined with a continuous layer of syncytiotrophoblast.

*Other mammals have various arrangements of tissue layers through which materials must pass to be exchanged between mother and fetus. For example, in an epitheliochorial placenta, which is found in pigs, the fetal component of the placenta (chorion) rests on the uterine epithelium instead of being directly bathed in maternal blood.

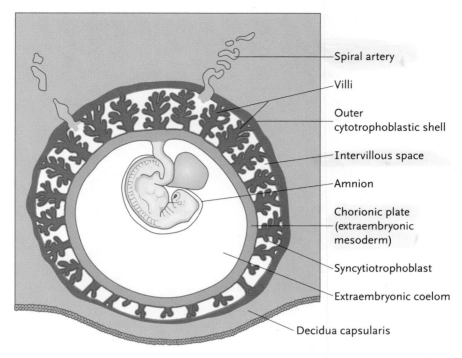

Spiral artery

Villi

Outer cytotrophoblastic shell

Intervillous space

Amnion

Chorionic plate (extraembryonic mesoderm)

Syncytiotrophoblast

Extraembryonic coelom

Decidua capsularis

Figure 6-5 Overall view of a **5-week-old** embryo plus membranes showing the relationships of the chorionic plate, villi, and outer cytotrophoblastic shell.

Maternal blood gains access to this syncytiotrophoblast-lined space through the open ends of the uterine spiral arteries, which pass through the cytotrophoblastic shell. The arteries were eroded by the invading trophoblast, but their lumens are invariably partially occupied by a plug of cytotrophoblastic cells, presumably an adaptation for controlling the flow of blood. For the first 12 weeks of embryonic life, the fluid that percolates through the intervillous spaces is a filtrate of maternal plasma and does not contain any blood cells. During this same period, the fetal erythrocytes contain embryonic hemoglobin, which is adapted to bind with oxygen under low tension. After 12 weeks, maternal erythrocytes appear in intervillous blood, and in an isoform transition the fetal erythrocytes begin to produce fetal hemoglobin, which requires a higher oxygen tension to bind oxygen efficiently. Having left the spiral arteries under relatively high pressure, the maternal blood freely percolates throughout the intervillous spaces and bathes the surfaces of the villi. The blood is then picked up by the open ends of uterine veins, which also penetrate the cytotrophoblastic shell (see Figure 6-10).

Gross Relations of Chorionic and Decidual Tissues

Within days after implantation of the embryo, the stromal cells of the endometrium undergo a striking transformation called the **decidual[†] reaction**. After the stromal cells swell as

the result of the accumulation of glycogen and lipid in their cytoplasm, they are known as **decidual cells** (Figure 6-6). The decidual reaction spreads throughout stromal cells in the superficial layers of the endometrium. The maternal decidua are given topographic names based on where they are located in relation to the embryo.

The decidual tissue that overlies the embryo and its chorionic vesicle is the **decidua capsularis,** whereas the decidua that lies between the chorionic vesicle and the uterine wall is the **decidua basalis** (see Figure 6-7). With continued growth of the embryo, the decidua basalis becomes incorporated into the maternal component of the definitive placenta. The remaining decidua, which consists of the decidualized endometrial tissue on the sides of the uterus not occupied by the embryo, is the **decidua parietalis**.

In human embryology the **chorion** is defined as the layer consisting of the trophoblast plus the underlying extraembryonic mesoderm (see Figure 6-1). The chorion forms a complete covering (**chorionic vesicle**) that surrounds the embryo, amnion, yolk sac, and body stalk. During the early period after implantation, primary and secondary villi project almost uniformly from the entire outer surface of the

[†]The term *deciduum* refers to tissues that are shed at birth, which include the extraembryonic tissues plus the superficial layers of the endometrial connective tissue and epithelium.

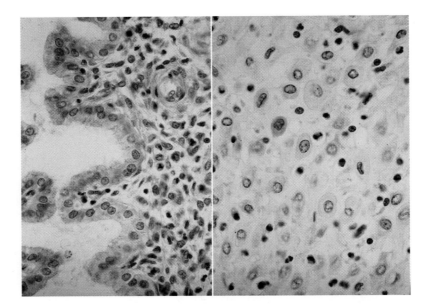

Figure 6-6 *Left*, Histological section through the endometrium during the late secretory stage of the endometrial cycle. A large uterine gland with an irregular epithelial border is on the left. On the right, note the stromal cells with compact nuclei and scanty cytoplasm. *Right*, Endometrial stroma, showing the decidual reaction. Note the expanded cytoplasm and less compact nuclei of the decidual cells. (Hematoxylin and eosin stain.) (Courtesy D. MacCallum, Ann Arbor, Mich.)

chorionic vesicle. The formation of tertiary villi, however, is asymmetrical, and the invasion of the cytotrophoblastic core of the primary villi by mesenchyme and embryonic blood vessels occurs preferentially in the primary villi located nearest the decidua basalis. As these villi continue to grow and branch, those located on the opposite side (the abembryonic pole) of the chorionic vesicle fail to keep up and eventually atrophy as the growing embryo complex bulges into the uterine cavity (Figure 6-7). The region that contains the flourishing chorionic villi and that ultimately becomes the placenta is the **chorion frondosum.** The remainder of the chorion, which ultimately becomes smooth, is the **chorion laeve** (Figure 6-8).

The overall growth of the chorionic vesicle (Figure 6-9), with its bulging into the uterine lumen, pushes the decidua capsularis progressively farther from the endometrial blood vessels. By the end of the first trimester, the decidua capsularis itself undergoes pronounced atrophy. Within the next month, portions of the atrophic decidua capsularis begin to disappear, leaving the chorion laeve in direct contact with the decidua parietalis on the opposite side of the uterus (see Figure 6-7). By mid-pregnancy, the chorion laeve has fused with the tissues of the decidua parietalis, thus effectively obliterating the original uterine cavity.

While the chorion laeve and decidua capsularis are undergoing progressive atrophy, the placenta takes shape in its definitive form and acts as the main site of exchange between the mother and embryo.

Formation and Structure of the Mature Placenta

As the distinction between the chorion frondosum and chorion laeve becomes more prominent, the limits of the placenta proper can be defined. The placenta consists of a fetal and a maternal component (Figure 6-10). The fetal component is that part of the chorionic vesicle represented by the chorion frondosum. It consists of the wall of the chorion, called the **chorionic plate,** and the chorionic villi that arise from that region. The maternal component is represented by the decidua basalis, but covering the decidua basalis is the fetally derived outer cytotrophoblastic shell. The intervillous space between the fetal and maternal components of the placenta is occupied by freely circulating maternal blood. In keeping with its principal function as an organ-mediating exchange between the fetal and maternal circulatory systems, the overall structure of the placenta is organized to provide a very large surface area (over 10 m^2) for that exchange.

Structure of the mature placenta

The mature placenta is disklike in shape, with a thickness of 3 cm and a diameter of about 20 cm (Table 6-1). A typical placenta weighs about 500 gm. The fetal side of the placenta is shiny because of the apposed amniotic membrane. From the fetal side, the attachment of the umbilical cord to the chorionic plate and the large placental branches of the umbilical arteries and vein radiating from it are evident.

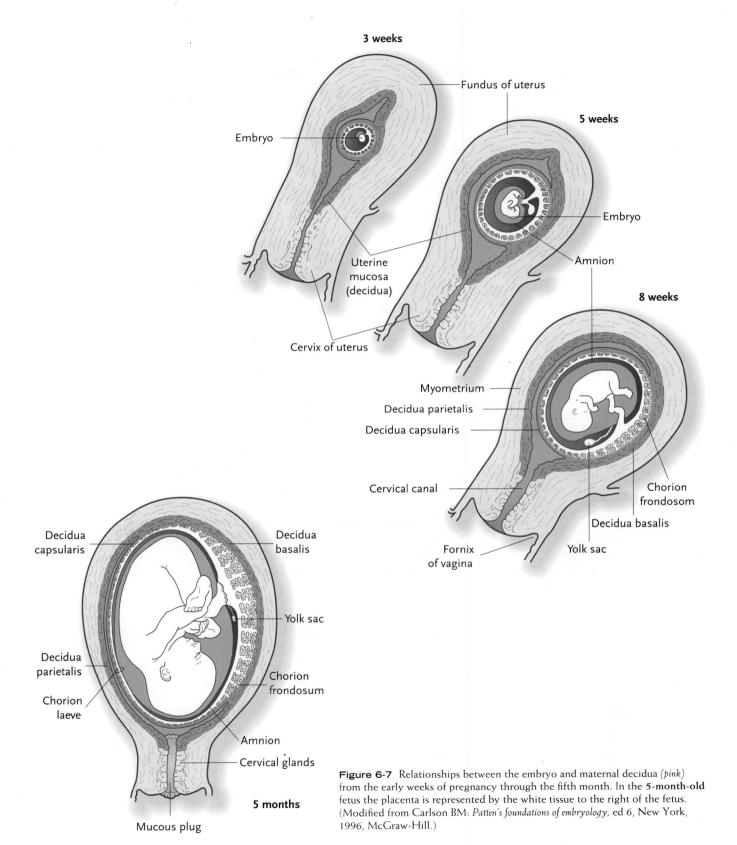

3 weeks

Embryo

Fundus of uterus

Uterine mucosa (decidua)

Cervix of uterus

5 weeks

Embryo

Amnion

8 weeks

Myometrium

Decidua parietalis

Decidua capsularis

Cervical canal

Fornix of vagina

Chorion frondosom

Decidua basalis

Yolk sac

Decidua capsularis

Decidua basalis

Yolk sac

Decidua parietalis

Chorion frondosum

Chorion laeve

Amnion

Cervical glands

5 months

Mucous plug

Figure 6-7 Relationships between the embryo and maternal decidua (*pink*) from the early weeks of pregnancy through the fifth month. In the **5-month-old** fetus the placenta is represented by the white tissue to the right of the fetus. (Modified from Carlson BM: *Patten's foundations of embryology*, ed 6, New York, 1996, McGraw-Hill.)

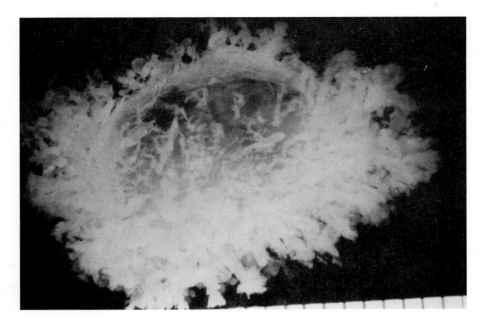

Figure 6-8 Early formation of the chorion laeve. The small bare area in this photograph of a human chorionic vesicle is a region where the chorionic villi have atrophied. This will enlarge in succeeding weeks. (From Gilbert-Barness E, ed: *Potter's pathology of the fetus and infant*, St Louis, 1997, Mosby.)

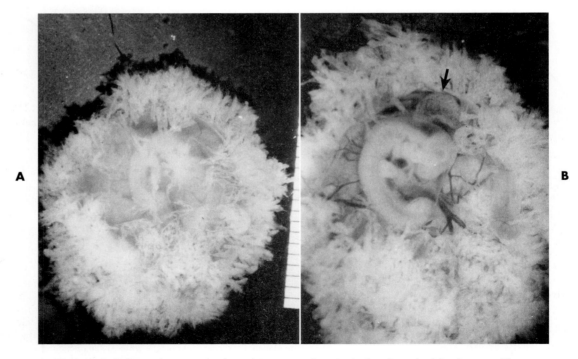

Figure 6-9 **A,** Intact chorionic vesicle containing an embryo in the **fourth week** of development. The outline of the embryo can be seen through the thinned chorion laeve region. **B,** Opened chorionic vesicle, showing the disposition of the embryo inside. The yolk sac is indicated by the arrow. (From Gilbert-Barness E, ed: *Potter's pathology of the fetus and infant*, St Louis, 1997, Mosby.)

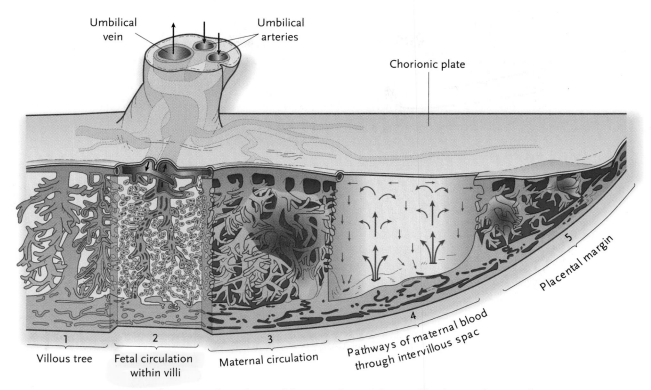

Umbilical vein
Umbilical arteries
Chorionic plate

1 Villous tree
2 Fetal circulation within villi
3 Maternal circulation
4 Pathways of maternal blood through intervillous spac
5 Placental margin

Figure 6-10 Structure and circulation of the mature human placenta. Blood enters the intervillous spaces from the open ends of the uterine spiral arteries. After bathing the villi, the blood (*blue*) is drained via endometrial veins. (From Bloom W, Fawcett DW: *Textbook of histology*, Philadelphia, 1986, WB Saunders.)

The maternal side of the placenta is dull and subdivided into as many as 35 lobes. The grooves between lobes are occupied by placental septa, which arise from the decidua basalis and extend toward the basal plate. Within a placental lobe are several cotyledons, each of which consists of a main stem villus and all its branches. The intervillous space in each lobe represents a nearly isolated compartment of the maternal circulation to the placenta.

Umbilical cord

The originally broad-based body stalk elongates and becomes relatively narrower as pregnancy progresses. The umbilical cord becomes the conduit for the umbilical vessels, which traverse its length between the fetus and the placenta (Figure 6-10). The umbilical vessels are embedded in a mucoid connective tissue that is often called **Wharton's jelly.**

The umbilical cord, which commonly attains a length of 50 to 60 cm by the end of pregnancy, is typically twisted many times. The twisting can be readily observed by gross exami-

nation of the umbilical blood vessels. In about 1% of full-term pregnancies, true knots occur in the umbilical cord. If they tighten as the result of fetal movements, they can cause anoxia and even death of the fetus.

Occasionally an umbilical cord contains two umbilical veins if the right umbilical vein does not undergo its normal degeneration (see Figure 16-11). Approximately 0.5% of mature umbilical cords contain only one umbilical artery. This condition is associated with a 15% to 20% incidence of associated cardiovascular defects in the fetus.

Placental circulation

Both the fetus and the mother contribute to the placental circulation (see Figure 6-10). The fetal circulation is contained in the system of umbilical and placental vessels. Fetal blood reaches the placenta through the two umbilical arteries, which ramify throughout the chorionic plate. Smaller branches from these arteries enter the chorionic villi and then break up into capillary networks in the terminal branches of the chorionic

TABLE 6-1   Developing Placenta

Age of embryo (weeks after fertilization)	Placental diameter (mm)	Placental weight (gm)	Placental thickness (mm)	Length of umbilical cord (mm)
6	—	6	—	—
10	—	26	—	—
14	70	65	12	180
18	95	115	15	300
22	120	185	18	350
26	145	250	20	400
30	170	315	22	450
34	195	390	24	490
38	220	470	25	520

Modified from Kaufmann P, Scheffen I. In Polin R, Fox W, eds: *Fetal and neonatal physiology*, vol 1, Philadelphia, 1992, WB Saunders, p 48.

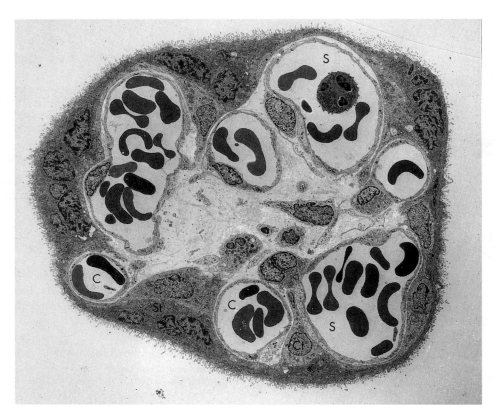

Figure 6-11 Low-power transmission electron micrograph through a typical terminal villus of a human placenta. *C,* Capillary; *Ct,* cytotrophoblast; *S,* sinusoid (dilated capillary); *St,* syncytiotrophoblast. (From Benirschke K, Kaufmann P: *Pathology of the human placenta,* ed 2, New York, 1990, Springer-Verlag.)

villi, where the exchange of materials with the maternal blood occurs (see Figure 6-14). From the villous capillary beds, the blood vessels consolidate into successively larger venous branches. These retrace their way through the chorionic plate into the large single umbilical vein and to the fetus.

In contrast to the fetal circulation, which is totally contained within blood vessels, the maternal blood supply to the placenta is a free-flowing lake that is not bounded by vessel walls. As a result of the trophoblast's invasive activities, roughly 80 to 100 spiral arteries of the endometrium open directly into the inter-

Embryo weight (gm)/ placental weight (gm)	Villous mass (gm)	Total villous surface area (cm^2)	Diffusion distance from maternal to fetal circulation (µm)	Mean trophoblastic thickness on villi (µm)
0.18	5	830	55.9	15.4
0.65	18	3020	—	—
0.92	28	5440	40.2	9.6
2.17	63	14,800	27.7	9.9
3.03	102	28,100	21.6	7.4
4.00	135	42,200	—	—
4.92	191	72,200	20.6	6.9
5.90	234	101,000	11.7	5.2
7.23	273	125,000	4.8	4.1

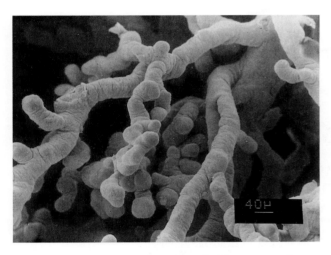

Figure 6-12 Scanning electron micrograph of long, intermediate, knoblike terminal (floating) villi from a normal placenta near the termination of pregnancy. (From Benirschke K, Kaufmann P: *Pathology of the human placenta*, ed 2, New York, 1990, Springer-Verlag.)

villous spaces and bathe the villi in about 150 ml of maternal blood, which is exchanged 3 to 4 times each minute.

The maternal blood enters the intervillous space under reduced pressure because of the cytotrophoblastic plugs that partially occlude the lumens of the spiral arteries. Nevertheless, the maternal blood pressure is sufficient to force the oxygenated maternal arterial blood to the bases of the villous trees at the chorionic plate (see Figure 6-10). The overall pressure of the maternal placental blood is about 10 mm Hg in the relaxed uterus. From the chorionic plate, the blood percolates over the terminal villi as it returns to venous outflow pathways located in the decidual (maternal) plate of the placenta. An adequate flow of maternal blood

to the placenta is vital to the growth and development of the fetus, and a reduced maternal blood supply to the placenta leads to a small fetus.

In the terminal (floating) villi, the fetal capillaries are located next to the trophoblastic surface to facilitate exchange between the fetal and maternal blood (Figure 6-11). The placental barrier of the mature placenta consists of the syncytiotrophoblast, its basal lamina, the basal lamina of the fetal capillary, and the capillary endothelium. Often the two basal laminae seem to be consolidated. In younger embryos a layer of cytotrophoblast is present in the placental barrier, but by 4 months the cytotrophoblastic layer begins to break up, and by 5 months, it is essentially gone. (Placental transfer is described on p. 118.)

Structure of a mature chorionic villus

Mature chorionic villi constitute a very complex mass of seemingly interwoven branches (Figure 6-12). The core of a villus consists of blood vessels and mesenchyme that is similar in composition to the mesenchyme of the umbilical cord (see Figure 6-11). Scattered among the mesenchymal cells are large **Hofbauer cells**, which function like fetal macrophages.

The villus core is covered by a continuous layer of syncytiotrophoblast, with minimum numbers of cytotrophoblastic cells beneath it. The surface of the syncytiotrophoblast is covered by immense numbers of microvilli (over 1 billion/cm^2 at term), which greatly increase the total surface area of the placenta (Figure 6-13). The size and density of the microvilli are not constant but change with increasing age of the placenta and differing environmental conditions. For example, under conditions of poor maternal nutrition or oxygen transport, the microvilli increase in prominence. Poor adaptation of the microvilli to adverse conditions can lead to newborns with low birth weight.

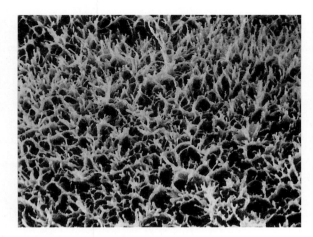

Figure 6-13 Scanning electron micrograph of the surface of the syncytiotrophoblast of a human placenta in the twelfth week of pregnancy. The numerous microvilli increase the absorptive surface of the placenta. (×9000.) (Courtesy S. Bergström, Uppsala, Sweden.)

The trophoblastic surface is not homogeneous but rather seems to be arranged into territories. Among the many functional components of the microvillous surface are (1) a wide variety of transport systems for substances ranging from ions to macromolecules, (2) hormone and growth factor receptors, (3) enzymes, and (4) numerous proteins with poorly understood functions. The placental surface is deficient or lacking in major histocompatibility antigens, the absence of which presumably plays a role in protecting against maternal immune rejection of the fetus and fetal membranes. In keeping with its active role in both synthesis and transport, the syncytiotrophoblast is well supplied with a high density and a wide variety of subcellular organelles.

Placental Physiology

Placental transfer

The transport of substances both ways between the placenta and the maternal blood that bathes it is facilitated by the great surface area of the placenta, which expands from 5 m² at 28 weeks to almost 11 m² at term. Approximately 5% to 10% of the human placental surface consists of scattered areas where the barrier between fetal and maternal blood is extremely thin, measuring only a few microns. These areas, sometimes called **epithelial plates**, appear to be morphological adaptations designed to facilitate the diffusion of substances between the fetal and maternal circulations (Figure 6-14).

The transfer of substances occurs both ways across the placenta. The bulk of the substances transferred from mother to fetus consists of oxygen and nutrients. The placenta represents the means for the final elimination of carbon dioxide and other fetal waste materials into the maternal circulation. Under some circumstances, other substances, some of them harmful, can

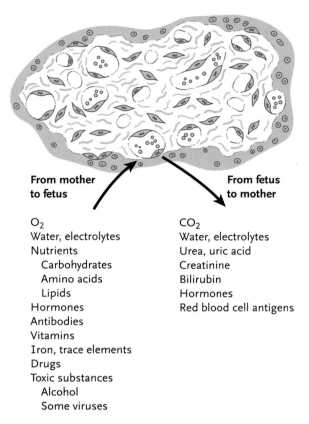

From mother to fetus	**From fetus to mother**
O_2	CO_2
Water, electrolytes	Water, electrolytes
Nutrients	Urea, uric acid
Carbohydrates	Creatinine
Amino acids	Bilirubin
Lipids	Hormones
Hormones	Red blood cell antigens
Antibodies	
Vitamins	
Iron, trace elements	
Drugs	
Toxic substances	
Alcohol	
Some viruses	

Figure 6-14 Exchange of substances across the placenta between the fetal and maternal circulation.

be transferred across the placenta. Clinical Correlation 6-2 describes abnormal placental transfer.

Gases, principally oxygen from the mother and carbon dioxide from the fetus, readily cross the placental barrier by diffusion. The amount of exchange is limited more by blood flow than by the efficiency of diffusion. The placenta is also permeable to carbon monoxide and many inhalational anesthetics. The latter can interfere with the transition of the newborn to independent function (e.g., breathing) if used during childbirth.

Like gases, water and electrolytes are readily transferred across the placenta. The rates of transfer are modified by colloid osmotic pressure in the case of water and the function of ion channels in the case of electrolytes. Fetal wastes (e.g., **urea, creatinine, bilirubin**) are rapidly transferred across the placenta from the fetal circulation to the maternal blood bathing the villi.

The placenta is highly permeable to certain nutrients such as **glucose**; on the other hand, it is considerably less permeable to **fructose** and several common disaccharides. Amino acids are transported across the placenta through the action of specific receptors. A certain degree of transfer of maternal free **fatty acids** occurs, but more must be learned about the mechanism of transfer. Vitamins, especially water-soluble ones, are transferred from the maternal to the fetal circulation.

Unfortunately, the placenta is permeable to substances that can be damaging to the embryo. Numerous maternally ingested drugs readily cross the placental barrier. Certain drugs can cause major birth defects if they reach the embryo during critical periods of morphogenesis. (Several classic examples of these are described in Chapter 7.) The placenta is highly permeable to alcohol, and excessive alcohol ingestion by the mother can produce **fetal alcohol syndrome** (see p. 136). The tragedy of newborns who are born addicted to heroin or crack cocaine is all too common in contemporary society.

In addition to drugs, certain infectious agents can penetrate the placental barrier and infect the fetus. Some (e.g., rubella virus) can cause birth defects if they infect the embryo at critical periods in development. Normally, bacteria cannot penetrate the placental barrier. Common viruses that can infect the fetus are rubella virus, cytomegalovirus, poliovirus, varicella virus, variola virus, human immunodeficiency virus, and coxsackieviruses. The spirochete *Treponema pallidum*, which causes syphilis, can cause devastating fetal infections. The protozoan parasite *Toxoplasma gondii* can cross the placental barrier and cause birth defects.

CELLULAR TRANSFER AND Rh INCOMPATIBILITY
Small quantities of fetal blood cells often escape into the maternal circulation, either through small defects in the placental vasculature or through hemorrhage at birth. If the fetal erythrocytes are positive for the Rh antigen and the mother is Rh negative, the presence of fetal erythrocytes in the maternal circulation can stimulate the formation of anti-Rh antibody by the immune system of the mother. The fetus in the first pregnancy is usually spared the effects of the maternal antibody (often because it has not formed in sufficient quantities), but in subsequent pregnancies, Rh-positive fetuses are attacked by the maternal anti-Rh antibodies, which make their way into the fetal bloodstream. This antibody causes hemolysis of the Rh-positive fetal erythrocytes, and the fetus develops **erythroblastosis fetalis**, sometimes known as **hemolytic disease**. In severe cases the bilirubin released from the lysed red blood cells causes jaundice and brain damage in addition to anemia. When recognized, this condition is treated by exchange transfusions of Rh-negative donor blood into either the fetus or the newborn. An indication of the severity of this condition can be gained by examining the amniotic fluid.

Steroid hormones cross the placental barrier from the maternal blood. Newborn males show evidence of the effects of exposure to maternal sex hormones. For example, the **prostatic utricle**, the vestigial rudiment of the uterine primordium (fused müllerian ducts [see Chapter 15]), is slightly enlarged in newborn males. Conversely, female fetuses exposed to testosterone or certain synthetic progestins (especially during the 1950s and 1960s before the effects were recognized) undergo masculinization of the external genitalia. Protein hormones are, in general, poorly transported across the placenta, although symptoms of maternal diabetes may be reduced during late pregnancy because of insulin produced by the fetus. Maternal thyroid hormone gains slow access to the fetus.

Some proteins are transferred very slowly through the placenta, mainly by means of pinocytosis (uptake by membrane-bound vesicles in the cells). Of considerable importance is the transfer of maternal antibodies, mainly of the immunoglobulin G class. Because of its immature immune system, the fetus produces only small amounts of antibodies. The transfer of antibodies from the mother provides a passive immunity of the newborn to certain common childhood diseases such as smallpox, diphtheria, and measles until the infant's immune system begins to function more efficiently.

Another maternal protein, **transferrin**, is important because, as its name implies, it carries iron to the fetus. The placental surface contains specific receptors for this protein. It appears that the iron is dissociated from its transferrin carrier at the placental surface and then is actively transported into the fetal tissues.

Placental Hormone Synthesis and Secretion

The placenta, specifically the syncytiotrophoblast, is an important endocrine organ during much of pregnancy. It produces both protein and steroid hormones.

The first protein hormone produced is **human chorionic gonadotropin (HCG)**, which is responsible for maintaining the corpus luteum and its production of progesterone and estrogens. With synthesis beginning even before implantation, the presence of this hormone in maternal urine is the basis for many of the common tests for pregnancy. The production of HCG peaks at approximately the eighth week of gestation and then gradually declines. By the end of the first trimester, the placenta produces enough progesterone and estrogens so that pregnancy can be maintained even if the corpus luteum is surgically removed. The placenta can independently synthesize progesterone from acetate or cholesterol precursors, but it does not contain the complete enzymatic apparatus for the synthesis of estrogens. For estrogen to be synthesized, the placenta must operate in concert with the fetal adrenal gland and possibly the liver; these structures possess the enzymes that the placenta lacks.

Another placental protein hormone is **chorionic somatomammotropin**, sometimes called **human placental lactogen**. Similar in structure to human growth hormone, it influences growth, lactation, and lipid and carbohydrate metabolism. The placenta also produces small amounts of **chorionic thyrotropin** and **chorionic corticotropin**. When they are secreted into the maternal bloodstream, some placental hormones stimulate changes in the metabolism and cardiovascular function of the mother. These changes ensure that appropriate types and amounts of fundamental nutrients and substrates reach the placenta for transport to the fetus.

A good example of a placental hormone that influences the mother is **human placental growth hormone**. This hormone, which differs by 13 amino acids from pituitary growth hormone, is produced by the syncytiotrophoblast. Placental growth hormone is not detectable in fetal serum, although it appears to influence growth of the placenta in a paracrine manner. This fetal hormone exerts a profound effect on the mother. During the first 15 to 20 weeks of pregnancy, maternal pituitary growth hormone is the main form present in the maternal circulation, but from 15 weeks to term, placental growth hormone gradually replaces maternal pituitary growth hormone to the extent that the maternally derived hormone becomes undetectable in the mother's serum. A major function of this hormone appears to be the regulation of maternal blood glucose levels so that the fetus is ensured of an adequate nutrient supply. Placental growth hormone secretion is stimulated by low maternal glucose levels. The increased hormone levels then stimulate gluconeogenesis in the maternal liver and other organs, thus increasing the supply of glucose available for fetal use.

In certain respects, the placenta duplicates the multilevel control system that regulates hormone production in the postnatal body. Cells of the cytotrophoblast produce a homologue of gonadotropin-releasing hormone (GnRH), as is normally done by the hypothalamus. GnRH then passes into the syncytiotrophoblast, where it, along with certain opiate peptides and their receptors (which have been identified in the syncytiotrophoblast), stimulates the release of HCG from the syncytiotrophoblast. The opiate peptides and their receptors are also involved in the release of chorionic somatomammotropin from the syncytiotrophoblast. Finally, HCG appears to be involved in regulating the synthesis and release of placental steroids from the syncytiotrophoblast.

In addition to hormones, the placenta also produces a wide variety of other proteins that have principally been identified immunologically. The functions of the dozens of placental proteins that have been discovered are still very poorly understood.

Placental Immunology

One of the major mysteries of pregnancy is why the fetus and placenta, which are immunologically distinct from the mother, are not recognized as foreign tissue and rejected by the mother's immune system. (Immune rejection of foreign tissues normally occurs by the activation of cytotoxic lymphocytes, but humoral immune responses are also possible.) Despite considerable research, the answer to this question is still unknown. Several broad explanations have been suggested to account for the unusual tolerance of the mother to the prolonged presence of the immunologically foreign embryo during pregnancy.

The first possibility is that the fetal tissues, especially those of the placenta, which constitute the direct interface between fetus and mother, do not present foreign antigens to the mother's immune system. To some extent this hypothesis is true, since neither the syncytiotrophoblast nor the nonvillous cytotrophoblast (**cytotrophoblastic shell**) expresses the two major classes of major histocompatibility antigens that trigger the immune response of the host in the rejection of typical foreign tissue grafts (e.g., a kidney transplant). However, these antigens are present on cells of the fetus and in stromal tissues of the placenta. The expression of minor histocompatibility antigens (e.g., the HY antigen in male fetuses [see Chapter 15]) follows a similar pattern. Nevertheless, other minor antigens are expressed on trophoblastic tissues. In addition, because of breaks in the placental barrier, fetal red and white blood cells are frequently found circulating in the maternal blood. These cells should be capable of sensitizing the mother's immune system.

A second major possibility is that the mother's immune system is somehow paralyzed during pregnancy so that it does not react to the fetal antigens to which it is exposed. Yet the mother is capable of mounting an immune response to infections or foreign tissue grafts. There still remains the possibility of a selective repression of the immune response to fetal antigens, although the Rh incompatibility response shows that this is not universally the case.

A third possibility is that local decidual barriers prevent either immune recognition of the fetus by the mother or the reaching of competent immune cells from the mother to the fetus. Again, there is evidence for a functioning decidual immune barrier, but in a significant number of cases that barrier is known to be breached through trauma or disease.

Currently, studies are being directed toward conditions such as recurrent spontaneous abortion with the hope of finding further clues to the complex immunological interrelationships between the fetus and mother. What is abundantly clear is that this is not a simple relationship. Nevertheless, the solution to this problem may yield information that might be applied to the problem of reducing the host rejection of tissue and organ transplants.

PLACENTA AFTER BIRTH

About 30 minutes after birth, the placenta, embryonic membranes, and remainder of the umbilical cord, along with much of the maternal decidua, are expelled from the uterus as the

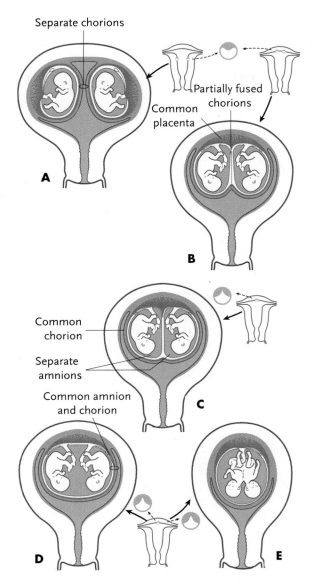

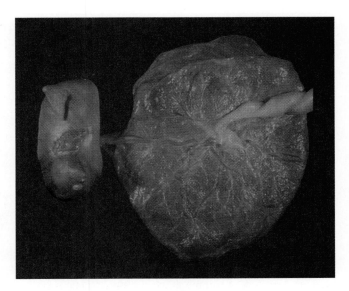

Figure 6-16 Fused twin placenta with an umbilical cord coming from its center and connecting to an anatomically normal fetus on the right. A shapeless acardiac monster is seen on the left. This condition is related to the siphoning of blood through a common circulation from the acardiac embryo to the other member of the pair. (Photograph #7702 from the Arey-Depeña Pediatric Pathology Photographic Collection, Human Development Anatony Center, National Museum of Health and Medicine, Armed Forces Institute of Pathology.)

Figure 6-15 Extraembryonic membranes in multiple pregnancies. A, Completely separate membranes in dizygotic or completely separated monozygotic twins. B, Common fused placenta, separate amnions, and partially fused chorions. C, Common placenta with separate or common fused vessels and separate amnions enclosed in a common chorion. D and E, Common placenta and amniotic cavity in separate or conjoined twins.

PLACENTA AND MEMBRANES IN MULTIPLE PREGNANCIES

Several different configurations of the placenta and extraembryonic membranes are possible in multiple pregnancies. Dizygotic twins or monozygotic twins resulting from complete separation of blastomeres very early in cleavage can have completely separate placentas and membranes if the two embryos implant in distant sites on the uterine wall (Figure 6-15, A). In contrast, if the implantation sites are closer together, the placentas and chorions (which were initially separate at implantation) can fuse, although the vascular systems of the two embryos remain separate (Figure 6-15, B).

When monozygotic twins form by splitting of the inner cell mass in the blastocyst, it is usual to have a common placenta and a common chorion, but inside the chorion the twin embryos each develop within separate amnions (Figure 6-15, C). In this case, there can be separate or fused vascular systems within the common placenta. When the vascular systems are fused, one twin may receive a greater proportion of the placental blood flow than the other. This may result in mild to severe stunting of growth of the embryo that receives the lesser amount of blood from the placenta. The twin from which the blood is siphoned is often highly misshapen and is commonly called an **acardiac monster** (Figure 6-16).

In conjoined twins and rarely in dizygotic twins with minimal separation of the inner cell mass, the embryos develop

afterbirth. The fetal surface of the placenta is smooth, shiny, and grayish because of the amnion that covers the fetal side of the chorionic plate. The maternal surface, on the other hand, is a dull red and may be punctuated with blood clots. The maternal surface of the placenta must be examined carefully because if a cotyledon is missing and is retained in the uterine wall, it could cause serious postpartum bleeding. Recognition of certain types of placental pathology can provide valuable clues to intrauterine factors that could affect the well-being of the newborn (see Clinical Correlation 6-3).

CLINICAL CORRELATION 6-3
Placental Pathological Conditions

Placental pathological conditions cover a wide spectrum, ranging from the abnormalities of implantation site to neoplasia to frank bacterial infections. Much can be learned about the past history and future prospects of a newborn by examining the placenta. This box deals only with those aspects of placental pathology that are relevant to developmental mechanisms.

ABNORMAL IMPLANTATION SITES
An abnormal implantation site within the uterine cavity is known as **placenta previa.** (Ectopic pregnancy is covered in Chapter 3.) When part of the placenta covers the cervical outlet of the uterine cavity, its presence is a mechanical obstacle in the birth canal. In addition, hemorrhage, which can be fatal to the fetus or even the mother, is a common consequence

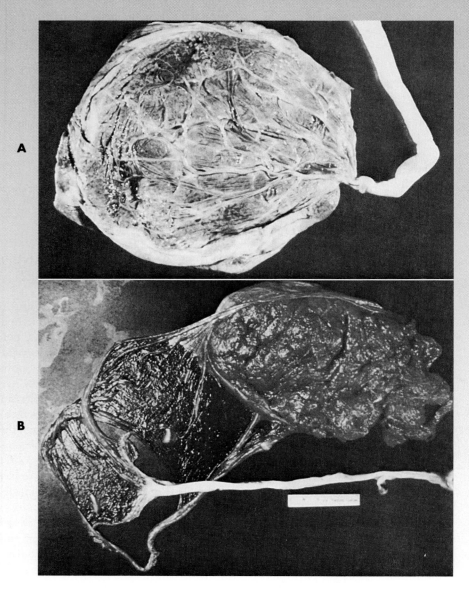

Figure 6-17 Variations in placental shape. **A,** Marginal insertion of the umbilical cord. **B,** Velamentous insertion of the umbilical cord. (From Nayeye RL: *Disorders of the placenta, fetus, and neonate,* St Louis, 1992, Mosby.)

CLINICAL CORRELATION 6-3
Placental Pathological Conditions—cont'd

of placenta previa as a result of the premature separation of part of the placenta from the uterus.

GROSS PLACENTAL ANOMALIES

Many variations in shape of the placenta have been described, but few appear to be of any functional significance. One involves marginal rather than central attachment of the umbilical cord (Figure 6-17, *A*).

If the umbilical cord attaches to the smooth membranes outside the boundaries of the placenta itself, the condition is known as a **velamentous insertion** of the umbilical cord (Figure 6-17, *B*).

The placenta itself can be subdivided into **accessory lobes** (Figure 6-17, *C*). It can also be completely divided into two parts, with smooth membrane between (Figure 6-17, *D*).

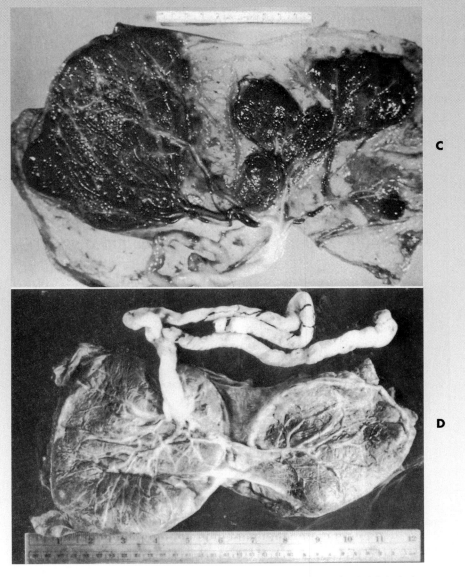

C

D

Figure 6-17, cont'd C, Placenta with accessory (succenturiate) lobes. D, Completely bilobed placenta.

Continued

CLINICAL CORRELATION 6-3
Placental Pathological Conditions—cont'd

HYDATIDIFORM MOLE

A **hydatidiform mole** is a noninvasive condition in which many of the chorionic villi are characterized by nodular swellings, giving them an appearance almost like bunches of grapes. Commonly, much of the villous surface of the placenta takes on this appearance; in addition, the embryo is either absent or not viable (Figure 6-18). The villi show no evidence of vascularization.

Genetic analysis has determined that hydatidiform moles represent the results of paternal imprinting where the female pronucleus of the egg does not participate in development (see Chapter 3). Instead, the chromosomal material is derived from two sperm that had penetrated the egg or by duplication of a single sperm pronucleus within the egg. The chromosomes of hydatidiform moles are paternally derived 46,XX, since the number of lethal genes in 46,YY embryos is not compatible with tissue survival.

CHORIOCARCINOMA

Choriocarcinomas are malignant tumors derived from embryonic cytotrophoblast and syncytiotrophoblast. These tumors are highly invasive into the maternal decidual tissues and blood vessels. Like hydatidiform moles, most choriocarcinomas contain only paternally derived chromosomes and are thus products of paternal imprinting.

BIOPSIES OF CHORIONIC VILLI

In recent years, biopsies of chorionic villi during the latter half of the second embryonic month have sometimes been performed instead of sampling of amniotic fluid. Performed with the assistance of ultrasonography, chorionic villus biopsies are obtained for the analysis of possible chromosomal disorders or the diagnosis of certain metabolic disorders.

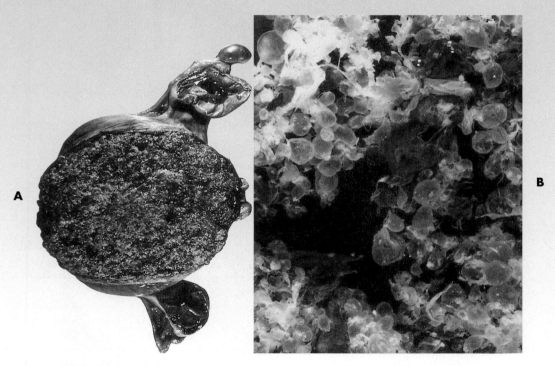

Figure 6-18 **A,** Distended uterus containing a hydatidiform mole. The ovaries (*top* and *bottom*) contain bilateral theca lutein cysts. **B,** View at greater magnification showing swollen villi. (**A** from Benirschke K, Kaufmann P: *Pathology of the human placenta,* ed 2, New York, 1990, Springer-Verlag. **B** courtesy K. Benirschke, San Diego.)

CLINICAL VIGNETTE

A 32-year-old woman's obstetrician notes that her weight gain during late pregnancy is excessive. At least part of her weight gain appears to be the result of a greater-than-normal volume of amniotic fluid. She lives in a remote rural area far from an imaging center. Amniocentesis is performed, and the laboratory report indicates the presence of a high level of α-fetoprotein in the amniotic fluid. The obstetrician is concerned that this pregnancy will not result in a normal single birth.

What condition does the doctor suspect and why?
A. Esophageal atresia
B. Renal agenesis
C. Triplets
D. Anencephaly
E. Placenta previa

within a single amnion and chorion and have a common placenta with a common blood supply (Figure 6-15, *D* and *E*). This and the previously described conditions can be readily determined by examination of the membranes of the afterbirth. At one time it was thought that it could be determined whether twins were monozygotic or dizygotic by simple examination of the membranes. Although in most cases the correct inference can be made, this method is by no means foolproof. Other methods ranging from simple observation of gender, eye color, and fingerprint patterns to determination of blood types or even deoxyribonucleic acid (DNA) fingerprinting should be used for a definitive determination. In the current age of organ and cell transplantation, it can be vital to know whether twins are monozygotic in the event that one develops a condition that can be treated by a transplant.

SUMMARY

- The extraembryonic membranes consist of the chorion (the combination of trophoblast plus underlying extraembryonic mesoderm), amnion, yolk sac, and allantois.
- The amnion, a thin ectodermal membrane lined with mesoderm, grows to enclose the embryo like a balloon. It is filled with a clear fluid, which is generated from many sources such as the fetal skin, the amnion itself, the fetal kidneys, and possibly the fetal vessels. At term the volume of amniotic fluid approaches 1 L. Amniotic fluid is removed by exchange across the amniotic membrane and by fetal swallowing.
- The yolk sac is a ventral endodermally lined structure that does not serve a nutritive function in mammalian embryos. Mesodermal blood islands in the wall of the yolk sac form the first blood cells and vessels. Primordial germ cells are recognizable in the wall of the yolk sac, but they originate in extraembryonic mesoderm at the base of the allantois.
- The allantois is a small, endodermally lined diverticulum off the ventral side of the hindgut. It does not serve a direct function of respiration or storage of wastes in humans. These functions are

carried out through the placenta and the umbilical vessels that arise in conjunction with the allantois.

- Chorionic villi form as outward projections from the trophoblast. Primary villi consist of projections of trophoblast alone. When a mesenchymal core forms within a villus, it is a secondary villus, and when the mesenchyme becomes vascularized, the villus is a tertiary villus. As villi mature, the cytotrophoblast in some villi grows through the syncytiotrophoblast as cytotrophoblastic cell columns and makes contact with the maternal endometrial tissue. Cytotrophoblast continues to grow around the blood-filled space surrounding the chorion to form a cytotrophoblastic shell, which is the direct interface between the fetal and maternal tissues. Villi that make direct contact with maternal tissues are anchoring villi; villi that do not make such contact are floating villi. Because chorionic villi float in a pool of maternal blood, the human placenta is designated as a hemochorial placenta.
- Stimulated by the implanting embryo, endometrial stromal cells undergo the decidual reaction. Maternal tissues that are lost at childbirth are, collectively, the decidua. The decidua basalis underlies the placenta; the decidua capsularis encircles the remainder of the chorion like a capsule; portions of the uterine wall not occupied by the fetal chorion are the decidua parietalis. As the fetal chorion matures, it becomes subdivided into a chorion laeve, in which the villi regress, and the chorion frondosum, which is the region of chorion nearest the basal tissues of the endometrium. The chorion frondosum ultimately develops into the placenta.
- The mature placenta consists of the wall of the chorion (the chorionic plate) and numerous villi protruding from it. The fetal surface of the placenta is smooth and shiny because of the apposed amniotic membrane. The maternal surface is dull and lobulated, with cotyledons of numerous placental villi and their branches. The umbilical cord (formerly the body stalk) enters the middle of the placenta. Blood from the fetus reaches the placenta via the umbilical arteries. These branch out into numerous small vessels, terminating into capillary loops in the ends of the placental villi. There, oxygen, nutrients, and wastes are exchanged between fetal and maternal blood, which bathes the villi. Fetal blood returns to the body of the mature fetus via a single umbilical vein. Maternal blood exiting open-ended spiral arteries of the endometrium bathes the placental villi.
- The transfer of substances from fetal to maternal blood must occur across the endothelium of the fetal capillaries, a basal lamina, and trophoblastic tissues before reaching the maternal blood. The transfer of substances is accomplished by both passive and active mechanisms. In addition to normal substances, alcohol, certain drugs, and some infectious agents can pass from the maternal blood into the fetal circulation and interfere with normal development. If a fetus is Rh positive and the mother is Rh negative, maternal anti-Rh antibodies from a previous pregnancy can pass to the fetus to cause erythroblastosis fetalis.
- The placenta produces a wide variety of hormones, many of which are normally synthesized in the hypothalamus and anterior pituitary gland. The first hormone released is HCG, which serves as the basis of many pregnancy tests. Other placental hormones are chorionic somatomammotropin (human placental lactogen), steroid hormones, and chorionic thyrotropin and corticotropin.
- The fetal and placental tissues are immunologically different from those of the mother, but the placenta and fetus are not im-

munologically rejected. The reason is still not clear, but some explanations involve reduced antigenicity of the trophoblastic tissues, paralysis of the mother's immune system during pregnancy, and local immunological barriers between the fetus and mother.

- The placenta is delivered about 30 minutes after the fetus as the afterbirth. Inspection of the placenta can reveal placental pathological conditions, missing cotyledons, or the arrangement of membranes in multiple pregnancies. The last finding can help to determine whether a multiple birth is monozygotic in origin. Placental pathological findings include abnormal gross shape, benign hydatidiform moles, and malignant choriocarcinomas.

REVIEW QUESTIONS

1. In the mature placenta, which fetal tissue directly interfaces with the maternal uterine connective tissue?
   A. Cytotrophoblast
   B. Syncytiotrophoblast
   C. Extraembryonic mesoderm
   D. Decidual cells
   E. None of the above
2. Which condition is related to paternal imprinting?
   A. Accessory placental lobes
   B. Placenta previa
   C. Oligohydramnios
   D. Single umbilical artery
   E. Hydatidiform mole
3. Blood vessels associated with which structure enter the fetal component of the placenta?
   A. Decidua basalis
   B. Allantois
   C. Amnion
   D. Yolk sac
   E. Decidua parietalis
4. What type of cells invades the maternal spiral arteries and reduces the flow of blood from their open ends?
   A. Hofbauer cells
   B. Syncytiotrophoblast
   C. Fetal erythrocytes
   D. Cytotrophoblast
   E. Amniotic epithelium
5. Which condition of the extraembryonic membranes can be found in uteri containing identical twins?
   A. Common placenta and amniotic membrane
   B. Common placenta and chorion, separate amnions
   C. Separate placentas and extraembryonic membranes
   D. Common placenta, partially fused chorions
   E. All of the above
6. A 28-year-old Rh-negative woman's second son is born severely jaundiced. What statement most likely characterizes her first child?
   A. Male
   B. Female
   C. Rh positive
   D. Rh negative
   E. Hydramnios
7. Why is the human placenta designated a hemochorial type of placenta?
8. Through what layers of a placental villus must a molecule of oxygen pass to go from the maternal blood into the embryonic circulation?
9. What embryonic hormone has served as the basis for many standard pregnancy tests and why?
10. Why must a pregnant woman be very careful of what she eats and drinks?

REFERENCES

Ahmed MS, Cemerikic B, Agbas A: Properties and functions of human placental opioid system, *Life Sci* 50:83-97, 1991.

Alsat E and others: Human placental growth hormone, *Am J Obstet Gynecol* 177:1526-1534, 1997.

Aplin JD: Implantation, trophoblast differentiation and haemochorial placentation: mechanistic evidence in vivo and in vitro, *J Cell Sci* 99:681-692, 1991.

Benirschke K, Kaufmann P: *Pathology of the human placenta*, ed 2, New York, 1990, Springer-Verlag.

Billingham RE, Beer AE: Reproductive immunology: past, present and future, *Prospect Biol Med* 27:259-275, 1984.

Bohn H, Dati F, Lueben G: Human trophoblast specific products other than hormones. In Loke YW, Whyte A, eds: *Biology of trophoblast*, Amsterdam, 1983, Elsevier Science, pp 317-352.

Bohn H, Winckler W, Grundmann U: Immunochemically detected placental proteins and their biological functions, *Arch Gynecol Obstet* 249:107-118, 1991.

Boyd JD, Hamilton WJ: *The human placenta*, Cambridge, England, 1970, Heffer & Sons.

Chamberlain GVP, Wilkinson AW, eds: *Placental transfer*, Tunbridge Wells, Kent, England, 1979, Pitman Medical.

Cullen TS: *Embryology, anatomy and diseases of the umbilicus, together with diseases of the urachus*, Philadelphia, 1916, WB Saunders.

Dallaire L, Potier M: Amniotic fluid. In Milunsky A, ed: *Genetic disorders and the fetus*, New York, 1986, Plenum, pp 53-97.

Dearden L, Ockleford CD: Structure of human trophoblast: correlation with function. In Loke YW, Whyte A, eds: *Biology of trophoblast*, Amsterdam, 1983, Elsevier Science, pp 69-110.

Demir R and others: Classification of human placental stem villi: review of structural and functional aspects, *Micros Res Techn* 38:29-41, 1997.

Enders AC: Trophoblast differentiation during the transition from trophoblastic plate to lacunar stage of implantation in the rhesus monkey and human, *Am J Anat* 186:85-98, 1989.

Faber JJ, Thornburg KL, eds: *Placental physiology*, New York, 1983, Raven.

Foidart J-M and others: The human placenta becomes haemochorial at the 13th week of pregnancy, *Int J Dev Biol* 36:451-453, 1992.

Garnica AD, Chan W-Y: The role of the placenta in fetal nutrition and growth, *J Am Coll Nutr* 15:206-222, 1996.

Genbacev O and others: Regulation of human placental development by oxygen tension, *Science* 277:1669-1672, 1997.

Kaufmann P: Basic morphology of the fetal and maternal circuits in the human placenta, *Contrib Gynecol Obstet* 13:5-17, 1985.

Kaufmann P, Burton G: Anatomy and genesis of the placenta. In Knobil E, Neill JD, eds: *The physiology of reproduction*, ed 2, New York, 1994, Raven, pp 441-484.

Knoll BJ: Gene expression in the human placental trophoblast: a model for developmental gene regulation, *Placenta* 13:311-327, 1992.

Lavrey JP, ed: *The human placenta: clinical perspectives*, Rockville, Md, 1987, Aspen.

Loke YW, King A: *Human implantation*, Cambridge, England, 1995, Cambridge University Press.

Morriss FJ, Boyd RDH, Mahendran D: Placental transport. In Knobil E, Neill JD, eds: *The physiology of reproduction*, ed 2, New York, 1994, Raven, pp 813-861.

Naeye RL: *Disorders of the placenta, fetus, and neonate*, St Louis, 1992, Mosby.

Ramsey EM: *The placenta: human and animal*, New York, 1982, Praeger.

Schneider H: Placental transport function, *Reprod Fertil Dev* 3:345-353, 1991.

Schneider H: The role of the placenta in nutrition of the human fetus, *Am J Obstet Gynecol* 164:967-973, 1991.

Schroeder J: Review article: transplacental passage of blood cells, *J Med Genet* 12:230-242, 1975.

Sibley CP, Boyd RDH: Mechanisms of transfer across the human placenta. In Polin R, Fox W, eds: *Fetal and neonatal physiology*, vol 1, Philadelphia, 1992, WB Saunders, pp 62-74.

Truman P, Ford HC: The brush border of the human term placenta, *Biochem Biophys Acta* 779:139-160, 1984.

DEVELOPMENTAL DISORDERS: CAUSES, MECHANISMS, AND PATTERNS

Congenital malformations have attracted attention since the dawn of human history. When seen in either humans or animals, malformations were often interpreted as omens of good or evil. Because of the great significance attached to congenital malformations, they were frequently represented in folk art, either as sculptures or paintings. As far back as the classical Greek period, people speculated that maternal impressions during pregnancy (e.g., being frightened by an animal) caused development to go awry. In other cultures, women who gave birth to malformed infants were assumed to have had dealings with the devil or other evil spirits.

Earlier representations of malformed infants were often remarkable in their anatomical accuracy, and it is often possible to diagnose specific conditions or syndromes from the ancient art (Figure 7-1, *A*). By the Middle Ages, however, representations of malformations were much more imaginative, with hybrids of humans and other animals often represented (Figure 7-1, *B*).

Among the first applications of scientific thought to the problem of congenital malformations were those of the sixteenth-century French surgeon, Ambrose Paré, who suggested a role for hereditary factors and mechanical influences such as intrauterine compression in the genesis of birth defects. Less than a century later, William Harvey, who is also credited with first describing the circulation of blood, elaborated the concept of developmental arrest and further refined thinking on mechanical causes of birth defects.

In the early nineteenth century, Etienne Geoffroy de St. Hilaire coined the term **teratology,** which literally means "the study of monsters," as a descriptor for the newly emerging study of congenital malformations. Late in the nineteenth century, the scientific study of teratology was put on a firm foundation with the publication of several encyclopedic treatises that exhaustively covered the anatomical aspects of the recognized congenital malformations.

After the flowering of experimental embryology and genetics in the early twentieth century, laboratory researchers began to produce specific recognizable congenital anomalies by means of defined experimental genetic or laboratory manipulations on laboratory animals. This led to the demystification of congenital anomalies and to a search for rational scientific explanations for birth defects. Nevertheless, old beliefs are very tenacious, and even today patients may adhere to traditional beliefs.

The first of two major milestones in human teratology occurred in 1941, when Gregg in Australia recognized that the **rubella** virus was a cause of a recognizable **syndrome** of abnormal development, consisting of defects in the eyes, ears, and heart. About 20 years later, the tragic story of **thalidomide** sensitized the medical community to the potential danger of certain drugs and other environmental **teratogens** (agents that produce birth defects) to the developing embryo.

Thalidomide is a very effective sedative that was widely used in West Germany, Australia, and other countries during the late 1950s. Soon, physicians began to see infants born with extremely rare birth defects. One example is **phocomelia** (which means "seal limb"), a condition in which the hands and feet seem to arise almost directly from the shoulder and hip (Figure 7-2). Another is **amelia,** in which a limb is entirely missing. Only after some careful epidemiological detective work involving the collection of individual case reports and sorting of the drugs taken by mothers during the early period of their pregnancies, was it possible to identify thalidomide as the certain cause. Thalidomide is still a drug of choice in the treatment of leprosy, and it is currently used in South America, where infants with thalidomide embryopathy continue to be born. With the intense investigations that followed the thalidomide disaster, modern teratology came of age. It is remarkable, however, that despite much effort, the causes for most congenital malformations are still unknown.

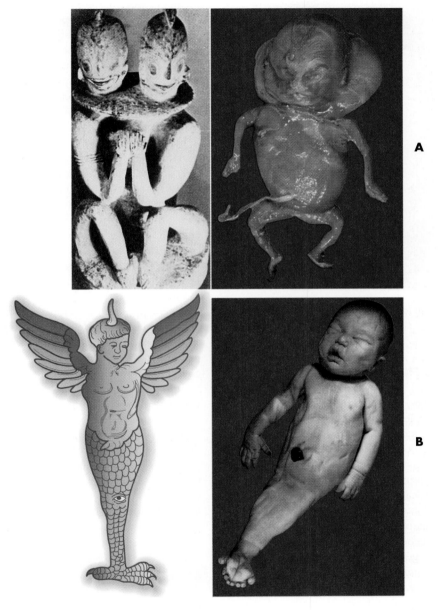

Figure 7-1 A, Chalk carving from New Ireland in the South Pacific showing dicephalic, dibrachic conjoined twins *(left)*. Note also the "collar" beneath the heads, which is a representation of the malformation cystic hygroma colli *(right)*. **B,** The bird-boy of Paré (about 1520) *(left)*. Stillborn fetus with sirenomelia (fused legs) *(right)*. Compare with the lower part of the bird-boy. (**A** *[left]* from Brodsky I: *Med J Aust* 1:417-420, 1943. **A** *[right]* and **B** *[right]* courtesy M. Barr, Ann Arbor, Mich.)

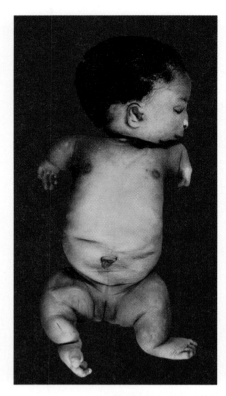

Figure 7-2 Phocomelia in all four limbs. This fetus had not been exposed to thalidomide. (Courtesy M. Barr, Ann Arbor, Mich.)

GENERAL PRINCIPLES

According to most studies, approximately 2% to 3% of all living newborns show at least one recognizable congenital malformation. This percentage is doubled when one considers anomalies diagnosed in children during the first few years after birth. With the decline in infant mortality caused by infectious diseases and nutritional problems, congenital malformations now rank high among the causes of infant mortality (currently over 20%), and an ever-increasing percentage (up to 30%) of infants admitted to neonatology or pediatric units come as a result of various forms of genetic diseases or congenital defects.

Congenital defects range from enzyme deficiencies caused by single nucleotide substitutions in the deoxyribonucleic acid molecule to very complex associations of gross anatomical abnormalities. Although medical embryology textbooks traditionally cover principally structural defects—congenital malformations—there is a continuum between purely biochemical abnormalities and those that are manifested as abnormal structures. This continuum includes defects that constitute abnormal structure, function, metabolism, and behavior.

According to contemporary theory, the genesis of congenital defects can be viewed as an interaction between the genetic endowment of the embryo and the environment in which it develops. The basic information is encoded in the genes, but as the genetic instructions unfold, the developing structures or organs are subjected to microenvironmental or macroenvironmental influences that either are compatible with or interfere with normal development. In the case of genetically based malformations or anomalies based on chromosomal aberrations, the defect is intrinsic and commonly expressed even in a normal environment. Purely environmental causes interfere with embryological processes in the face of a normal genotype. However, in other cases, environment and genetics interact. Penetrance (the degree of manifestation) of an abnormal gene or expression of one component of a genetically multifactorial cascade can sometimes be profoundly affected by environmental conditions.

One of the first clear-cut examples of the interactions between genetics and environment was provided in the 1950s by the experiments of Fraser on cleft palate formation in mice. In the presence of cortisone (the teratogen), 100% of the embryos of the A/J strain of mice developed cleft palate, whereas only about 20% of offspring of the C57BL strain were born with the anomaly. With crosses of the two strains, the incidence of cleft palate was approximately 40%. These results were ultimately shown to be related to strain-specific differences in the growth rate of the palatal shelves and to the width of the head at specific days of embryogenesis.

Several factors are associated with various types of congenital malformations. At present, they are understood more at the level of statistical associations than as points of interference with specific developmental controls, but they are important clues to why development can go wrong. Among the factors associated with increased incidences of congenital malformations are (1) parental age, (2) season of the year, (3) country of residence, (4) race, and (5) familial tendencies.

Well-known correlations exist between parental age and the incidence of certain malformations, a classic one being the increased incidence of **Down syndrome** (see Figure 7-9) in children born to women over 35 years of age. Other conditions are related to paternal age (Figure 7-3).

Some types of anomalies have a higher incidence among infants born at certain seasons of the year. For example, **anencephaly** (Figure 7-4) occurs more frequently in January. Recognizing that the primary factors leading to anencephaly occur during the first month of embryonic life, researchers must seek the potential environmental causes that are more prevalent in April. Anencephaly has been shown to be highly correlated with maternal **folic acid deficiency.** Its high incidence in pregnancies beginning in the early spring may relate to nutritional deficiencies of mothers during the late winter months. Folic acid supplementation in the diet of women of child-bearing age significantly reduces the incidence of neural tube defects, such as anencephaly.

The relationship between the country of residence and an increased incidence of specific malformations can be related to various factors, including racial tendencies, local environmental factors, and even governmental policies. A classic example of the last is the incidence of severely malformed infants as a result of exposure to thalidomide. These cases were concentrated in West Germany and Australia because the drug was commonly sold in these locations. Because thalidomide was

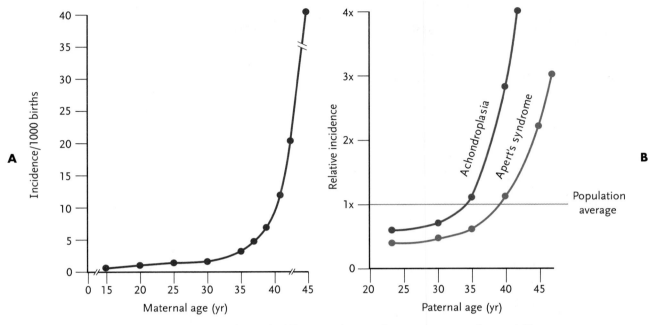

Figure 7-3 The increased incidence of (**A**) Down syndrome with increasing maternal age and (**B**) achondroplasia and Apert's syndrome with increasing paternal age. Apert's syndrome (acrocephalosyndactyly) is characterized by a towering skull and laterally fused digits.

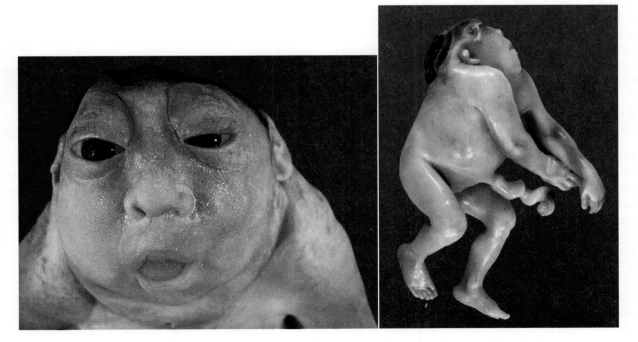

Figure 7-4 Frontal (*left*) and lateral (*right*) views of anencephaly. (Courtesy M. Barr, Ann Arbor, Mich.)

TABLE 7-1   Incidence of Neural Tube Defects

Site	Incidence*
India	0.6
Ireland	10
United States	1
Worldwide	2.6

*Per 1000 live births

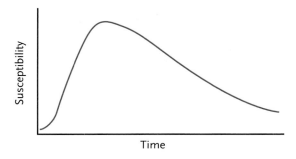

Figure 7-5 Generalized susceptibility curve to teratogenic influences by a single organ.

not approved by the Food and Drug Administration (FDA), the United States was spared from this epidemic of birth defects. Another classic example of the influence of country as a factor in the incidence of malformations is seen in neural tube defects (Table 7-1). The reason neural tube defects (especially anencephaly) are so common in Ireland has been the topic of much speculation. In light of the recognition of the importance of folic acid in the prevention of neural tube defects, it is possible that the high incidence of anencephaly in Ireland has resulted from poor nutrition in pregnant women during the winter.

Race is a factor in many congenital malformations and a variety of diseases. In humans as well as mice, there are racial differences in the incidence of cleft palate. The incidence of cleft palate among Caucasians is twice as high as it is among African Americans and twice as high among Orientals as among Caucasians.

A number of malformations, particularly those with a genetic basis, are found more frequently with certain families, especially if there is any degree of consanguinity in the marriages over the generations. A good example is the increased occurrence of extra digits among some families within the American Amish community.

Periods of Susceptibility to Abnormal Development

At certain critical periods during pregnancy, embryos are more susceptible to agents or factors causing abnormal development than at other times. The results of many investigations have allowed the following generalization: Insults to the embryo during the first 3 weeks of embryogenesis (the early period before organogenesis begins) are unlikely to result in defective development because they either kill the embryo or are compensated for by the powerful regulatory properties of the early embryo. The period of maximal susceptibility to abnormal development occurs between weeks 3 and 8, which is the period when most of the major organs and body regions are first being established. Major structural anomalies are unlikely to occur after the eighth week of pregnancy because by this point, most organs have become well established. Anomalies arising from the third to the ninth month of pregnancy tend to be functional (e.g., mental retardation) or involve disturbances in the

growth of already-formed body parts. Such a simplified view of susceptible periods does not, however, take into account the possibility that a teratogen or some other harmful influence might be applied at an early stage of development but not be expressed as a developmental disturbance until later during embryogenesis. On the other hand, certain other influences (e.g., intrauterine diseases, toxins), may result in the destruction of all or parts of structures that have already been formed.

Typically, a developing organ has a curve of susceptibility to teratogenic influences similar to that illustrated in Figure 7-5. Before the critical period, exposure to a known teratogen has little influence on development. During the first days of the critical period, the susceptibility, measured as incidence or severity of malformation, increases sharply and then declines over a much longer period.

Different organs have different periods of susceptibility during embryogenesis (Figure 7-6). Organs that form the earliest (e.g., heart) tend to be sensitive to the effects of teratogens earlier than those that form later (e.g., external genitalia). Some very complex organs, especially the brain and major sense organs, show prolonged periods of high susceptibility to the disruption of normal development.

Not all teratogenic influences act on the same developmental periods (Table 7-2). Some cause anomalies if the embryo is exposed to them early in development, but they are innocuous at later periods of pregnancy. Others affect only later developmental periods. A good example of the former is thalidomide, which has a very narrow and well-defined danger zone during the embryonic period (4 to 6 weeks). In contrast, tetracycline, which stains bony structures and teeth, exerts its effects after hard skeletal structures in the fetus have been formed.

Patterns of Abnormal Development

Although isolated structural or biochemical defects are not rare, it is common to find multiple abnormalities in the same individual. This can result from a number of reasons. One possibility is that a single teratogen acted on the primordia of several organs during susceptible periods of development. Another is that a genetic or chromosomal defect spanned genes

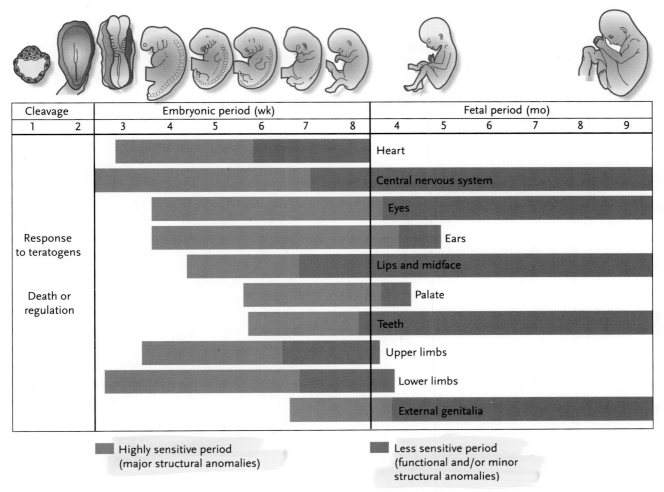

Figure 7-6 Periods and degrees of susceptibility of embryonic organs to teratogens. (Modified from Moore KL, Persaud TVN: *The developing human*, ed 5, Philadelphia, 1993, WB Saunders.)

TABLE 7-2   Developmental Times at Which Various Human Teratogens Exert Their Effects

Teratogens	Critical periods (gestational days)	Common malformations
Rubella virus	0-60	Cataract or heart malformations
	0-120+	Deafness
Thalidomide	21-40	Reduction defects of limbs
Adrogenic steroids	Earlier than 90	Clitoral hypertrophy and labial fusion
	Later than 90	Clitoral hypertrophy only
Coumadin anticoagulants	Earlier than 100	Nasal hypoplasia
	Later than 100	Possible mental retardation
Radioiodine therapy	Later than 65-70	Fetal thyroid deficiency
Tetracycline	Later than 120	Staining of dental enamel in primary teeth
	Later than 250	Staining of crowns of permanent teeth

Modified from Persaud TVN, Chudley AE, Skalko RG, eds: *Basic concepts in teratology*, New York, 1985, Liss.

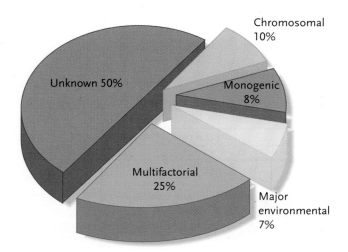

Figure 7-7 Major causes of congenital malformations. (Data from Persaud TVN, Chudley AE, Skalko RG, eds: *Basic concepts in teratology,* New York, 1985, Liss.)

affecting a variety of structures or that a single metabolic defect affected different developing structures in different ways.

CAUSES OF MALFORMATIONS

Despite considerable research over the past 50 years, the cause of at least 50% of human congenital malformations remains unknown (Figure 7-7). Of the other 50%, roughly 25% are genetically based (chromosomal defects or mutations based on mendelian genetics), and less than 10% are attributed to environmental factors or physical or chemical teratogens. Multifactorial causes account for the rest.

Genetic Factors

Genetically based malformations can be caused by abnormalities of chromosomal division or mutations of genes. Chromosomal abnormalities are usually classified as structural or numerical errors. These arise during cell division, especially meiosis. Numerical errors of chromosomes result in **aneuploidy**, defined as a total number of chromosomes other than the normal 46.

Abnormal chromosome numbers

Polyploidy. Polyploidy is the condition in which the chromosomal number is a higher multiple than 2 of the haploid number (23) of chromosomes. In the majority of cases, polyploid embryos abort spontaneously early in pregnancy. In fact, a high percentage of spontaneously aborted fetuses show major chromosomal abnormalities. Causes for polyploidy, especially triploidy, are likely to be either the fertilization of an egg by more than one sperm or the lack of separation of a polar body during meiosis.

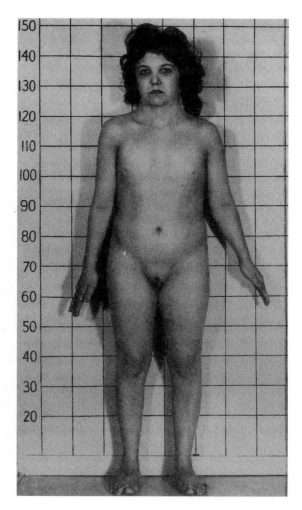

Figure 7-8 Woman with Turner's syndrome. Note the short stature, webbed neck, and infantile sexual characteristics. (From Connor J, Ferguson-Smith M: *Essential medical genetics,* ed 2, Oxford, England, 1987, Blackwell Scientific.)

Monosomy and Trisomy. Monosomy (the lack of one member of a chromosome pair) and **trisomy** (a triplet instead of the normal chromosome pair) are typically the result of nondisjunction during meiosis (see Figure 1-7). When this happens, one gamete shows monosomy and the other shows trisomy of the same chromosome.

In most cases, embryos with monosomy of the autosomes or sex chromosomes are not viable. However, some individuals with monosomy of the sex chromosomes (45, XO genotype) can survive (Figure 7-8). Such individuals, who are said to have **Turner's syndrome**, exhibit a female phenotype, but the gonads are sterile.

Three autosomal trisomies produce infants with characteristic associations of anomalies. The best known is **trisomy 21**, also called **Down syndrome**. Individuals with Down syndrome are typically mentally retarded and have a characteristic broad face with a flat nasal bridge, wide-set eyes, and prominent epicanthic folds. The hands are also broad, and

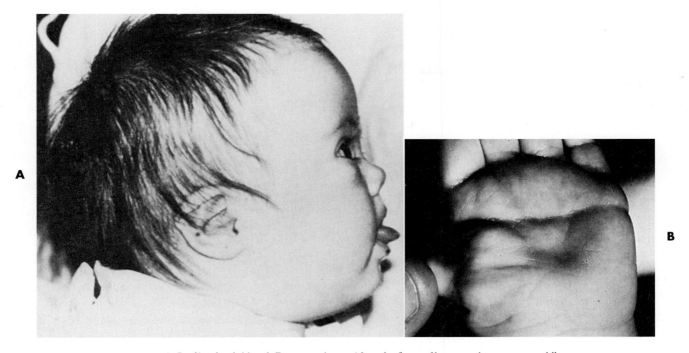

Figure 7-9 A, Profile of a child with Down syndrome. Note the flat profile, protruding tongue, saddle-shaped bridge of nose, and low-set ears. B, Hand of an infant with Down syndrome, showing the prominent simian crease that crosses the entire palm. (A from Garver K, Marchese S: *Genetic counseling for clinicians*, Chicago, 1986, Mosby. B from Fanaroff A, Martin RJ: *Neonatal-perinatal medicine*, ed 6, St Louis, 1997, Mosby.)

Figure 7-10 A, Front and lateral views of the head of a 34-week-old fetus with trisomy 13. This fetus shows pronounced cebocephaly with a keel-shaped head, a flattened nose, abnormal ears, and a reduction of forebrain and upper facial structures. B, Rocker-bottom feet from a fetus with trisomy 18. Note the prominent heels and somewhat convex profile of the soles of the feet. (A courtesy M. Barr, Ann Arbor, Mich. B from Nyberg D, Mahony B, Pretorious D: *Diagnostic ultrasound of fetal anomalies*, St Louis, 1990, Mosby.)

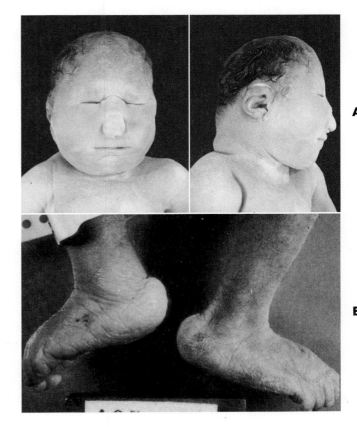

the palmar surface is marked by a characteristic transverse **simian crease** (Figure 7-9). Heart defects, especially atrial and ventricular septal defects, are common, with an incidence approaching 50%. Duodenal atresia and other intestinal anomalies are also seen in patients with Down syndrome. Individuals with Down syndrome are prone to the early appearance of Alzheimer disease and typically have a shortened life span.

Other trisomies of chromosomes 13 and 18 result in severely malformed fetuses, many of which do not survive to birth. Both **trisomy 13** and **trisomy 18** infants show severe mental retardation and other defects of the central nervous system. Cleft lip and cleft palate are common. Polydactyly is often seen in trisomy 13, and infants with both syndromes exhibit other anomalies of the extremities such as "**rocker bottom feet,**" meaning a rounding under and protrusion of the heels (Figure 7-10). Most infants born with trisomy 13 or 18 die within the first 1 or 2 months after birth.

TABLE 7-3 Variations in Numbers of Sex Chromosomes

Sex chromosome complement	Incidence	Phenotype	Clinical factors
XO	1:3000	Immature female	Turner syndrome: short stature, webbed neck, high and arched palate
XX		Female	Normal
XY		Male	Normal
XXY	1:1000	Male	Klinefelter syndrome: small testes, infertility, often tallness with long limbs
XYY	1:1000	Male	Tall, normal appearance; reputed difficulty with impulsive behavior
XXX	1:1000	Female	Normal appearance, mental retardation (up to one third of cases), fertility (in many cases)

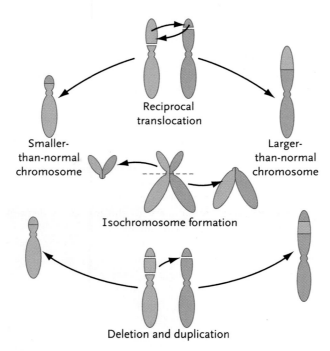

Figure 7-11 Different types of structural errors of chromosomes.

TABLE 7-4 Genetic Mutations Leading to Abnormal Development

Condition	Characteristics
AUTOSOMAL DOMINANT	
Achondroplasia	Dwarfism caused mainly by shortening of limbs
Aniridia	Absence of iris (usually not complete)
Crouzon syndrome (craniofacial dysostosis)	Premature closure of certain cranial sutures, leading to flat face and towering skull
Neurofibromatosis	Multiple neural crest–derived tumors on skin, abnormal pigment areas on skin
Polycystic kidney disease (adult onset, type III)	Numerous cysts in kidneys
AUTOSOMAL RECESSIVE	
Albinism	Absence of pigmentation
Polycystic kidney disease (perinatal type I)	Numerous cysts in kidneys
Congenital phocomelia syndrome	Limb deformities
X-LINKED RECESSIVE	
Hemophilia	Defective blood clotting
Hydrocephalus	Enlargement of cranium
Ichthyosis	Scaly skin
Testicular feminization syndrome	Female phenotype caused by inability to respond to testosterone

Abnormal numbers of the sex chromosomes are relatively common and can be detected by examination of the sex chromatin (X chromosome) or the fluorescence reactions of the Y chromosomes. Some of the various types of deletions and duplications of the sex chromosomes are summarized in Table 7-3.

Abnormal chromosome structure

Various abnormalities of chromosome structure can give rise to malformations in development. Some chromosomal abnormalities result from chromosome breakage induced by environmental factors such as radiation and certain chemical ter-

atogens. This type of structural error is usually unique to a given individual and is not transmitted to succeeding generations.

Other types of structural abnormalities of chromosomes are generated during meiosis and if present in the germ cells, can be inherited. Common types of errors in chromosome

TABLE 7-5   Infectious Diseases that Can Cause Birth Defects

Infectious agent	Disease	Congenital defects
VIRUSES		
Rubella virus	German measles	Cataracts, deafness, cardiovascular defects, fetal growth retardation
Cytomegalovirus	Cytomegalic inclusion disease	Microcephaly, microphthalmia, cerebral calcification, intrauterine growth retardation
SPIROCHETES		
Treponema pallidum (syphilis)	Syphilis	Dental anomalies, deafness, mental retardation, skin and bone lesions, meningitis
PROTOZOA		
Toxoplasma gondii	Toxoplasmosis	Microcephaly, hydrocephaly, cerebral calcification, microphthalmia, mental retardation, prematurity

structure are **reciprocal translocations, isochromosome formation,** and **deletions,** and **duplications** (Figure 7-11). One well-defined congenital malformation resulting from a deletion in the short arm of chromosome 5 is the **cri du chat syndrome.** Infants with this syndrome are severely retarded, have microcephaly, and make a cry that sounds like the mewing of a cat.

Genetic mutations

Many genetic mutations are expressed as morphological abnormalities. These can be dominant or recessive genes of either the autosomes or the sex chromosomes. For some of these conditions (e.g., hemophilia, Lesch-Nyhan syndrome, muscular dystrophy, cystic fibrosis), the molecular or biochemical lesion has been identified, but the manner in which these defects are translated into abnormal development is unclear. Many of these conditions are extensively discussed in textbooks of human genetics, and only representative examples are listed here (Table 7-4).

Environmental Factors

Various environmental factors are linked with birth defects. These range from chemical teratogens and hormones to maternal infections and nutritional factors. Although the list of suspected teratogenic factors is long, relatively few are unquestionably teratogenic in humans.

Maternal infections

After the recognition in 1941 that rubella was the cause of a spectrum of developmental anomalies, several other maternal diseases have been implicated as direct causes of birth defects. With infectious diseases, however, it is important to distinguish those that cause malformations by interfering with early stages in the development of organs and structures from those that interfere by destroying structures already formed. The same pathogenic organism can cause lesions by interference with embryonic processes or by destruction of differentiated tissues, depending on when the organism attacks the embryo.

Most infectious diseases that cause birth defects are viral, with **toxoplasmosis** (caused by the protozoan *Toxoplasma gondii*) and syphilis (caused by the spirochete *Treponema pallidum*) being notable exceptions. (A summary of the infectious diseases known to cause birth defects in humans is given in Table 7-5.)

The time of infection is very important in relation to the types of effects on the embryo. Rubella causes a high percentage of malformations during the first trimester, whereas cytomegalovirus infections usually kill the embryo during the first trimester. The agents of both syphilis and toxoplasmosis cross the placental barrier during the fetal period and to a large extent cause malformations by destroying existing tissues.

Chemical teratogens

Many substances are known to be teratogenic in animals or are associated with birth defects in humans, but for only a relatively small number is there convincing evidence that links the substance directly to congenital malformations in humans (Table 7-6). This makes testing drugs for teratogenicity difficult, since what can cause a high incidence of severe defects in animal fetuses (e.g., cortisone and cleft palate in mice) may not cause malformations in other species of animals or in humans. Conversely, the classic teratogen thalidomide is highly teratogenic in humans, rabbits, and some primates but not in commonly used laboratory rodents.

Folic Acid Antagonists.   At one time, folic acid antagonists, which are known to be highly embryolethal, were used in clinical trials as **abortifacients** (agents causing abortion).

TABLE 7-6   Chemical Teratogens in Humans

Agent	Effects
Alcohol	Growth and mental retardation, microcephaly, various malformations of face and trunk
Androgens	Masculinization of females, accelerated genital development in males
Anticoagulants (warfarin, dicumarol)	Skeletal abnormalities; broad hands with short fingers; nasal hypoplasia; anomalies of eye, neck, central nervous system
Antithyroid drugs (e.g., propyl-thiouracil, iodide)	Fetal goiter, hypothyroidism
Chemotherapeutic agents (methotrexate, aminopterin)	Variety of major anomalies throughout body
Diethylstilbestrol	Cervical and uterine abnormalities
Lithium	Heart anomalies
Organic mercury	Mental retardation, cerebral atrophy, spasticity, blindness
Phenytoin (Dilantin)	Mental retardation, poor growth, microcephaly, dysmorphic face, hypoplasia of digits and nails
Isotretinoin (Accutane)	Craniofacial defects, cleft palate, ear and eye deformities, nervous system defects
Streptomycin	Hearing loss, auditory nerve damage
Tetracycline	Hypoplasia and staining of tooth enamel, staining of bones
Thalidomide	Limb defects, ear defects, cardiovascular anormalies
Trimethadione and paramethadione	Cleft lip and palate, microcephaly, eye defects, cardiac defects, mental retardation
Valproic acid	Neural tube defects

Although three fourths of the pregnancies were terminated, almost a fourth of the embryos that survived to term were severely malformed. A classic example of an embryotoxic folic acid antagonist is **aminopterin**, which produces multiple severe anomalies such as anencephaly, growth retardation, cleft lip and palate, hydrocephaly, hypoplastic mandible, and low-set ears. These dramatic effects of folic acid antagonists underscore the importance of adequate amounts of folic acid in the diet to promote normal development.

Androgenic Hormones. The administration of androgenic hormones to pregnant women either to treat tumors or to prevent threatened abortion resulted in the birth of hundreds of female infants with varying degrees of masculinization of the external genitalia. The anomalies consisted of clitoral hypertrophy and often varying amounts of fusion of the genital folds to form a scrotumlike structure (Figure 7-12).

Anticonvulsants. Several commonly used anticonvulsants are known or strongly suspected to be teratogenic. Diphenylhydantoin produces a "fetal hydantoin syndrome" of anomalies, including growth anomalies, craniofacial defects, nail and digital hypoplasia, and mental retardation in up to a third of embryos exposed to hydantoin during pregnancy (Figure 7-13). Trimethadione also produces a syndrome of anomalies involving low-set ears, cleft lip and palate, and skeletal and cardiac anomalies.

Sedatives and Tranquilizers. Thalidomide is highly teratogenic when administered even as infrequently as once during a very narrow window of pregnancy, especially between days 25 and 50, when even a single dose of 100 mg can be sufficient to cause birth defects. This represents the period when the primordia of most major organ systems are being

established. The most characteristic lesions produced are gross malformations of the limbs, but the thalidomide syndrome also includes malformations of the cardiovascular system, absence of the ears, and assorted malformations of the urinary system, gastrointestinal system, and face. Despite years of intensive research, the mechanism by which thalidomide produces malformations is still unknown. Lithium carbonate, a commonly used agent for certain psychoses, is known to cause malformations of the heart and great vessels if administered early during pregnancy.

Antineoplastic Agents. Several antineoplastic agents are highly teratogenic, in large part because they are designed to kill or incapacitate rapidly dividing cells. Among these is aminopterin. Methotrexate and the combination of busulfan and 6-mercaptopurine cause severe anomalies of multiple organ systems. The use of these drugs during pregnancy is a difficult medical decision that must consider the lives of both the mother and the fetus.

Alcohol. Accumulated evidence now leaves little doubt that maternal consumption of alcohol during pregnancy can lead to a well-defined constellation of developmental abnormalities that includes poor postnatal growth rate, mental retardation, heart defects, and hypoplasia of facial structures (Figure 7-14). This is now popularly known as **fetal alcohol syndrome**. Ingestion of as little as 3 ounces of alcohol in a day during the first 4 weeks of pregnancy can lead to extremely severe malformations of the **holoprosencephaly** type (see p. 305). Exposure to alcohol later in pregnancy is less likely to cause major anatomical defects in the fetus, but because of the complex course of physiological maturation in the brain throughout pregnancy, more subtle behavioral defects can result.

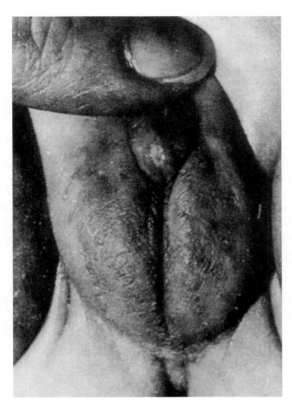

Figure 7-12 Ambiguous external genitalia in a newborn with pseudohermaphroditism. (From Reed GB, Claireaux AE, Bain AD: *Diseases of the fetus and newborn*, St Louis, 1989, Mosby.)

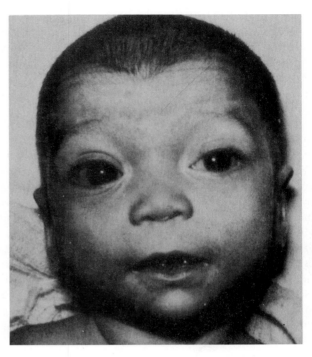

Figure 7-13 Face of an infant with fetal hydantoin syndrome. This infant has prominent eyes, hypertelorism (increased space between the eyes), micrognathia, and microcephaly. (From Wigglesworth JS, Singer DB: *Textbook of fetal and perinatal pathology*, 2 vols, Oxford, England, 1991, Blackwell Scientific.)

Retinoic Acid (Vitamin A). Derivatives of retinoic acid are used in the treatment of acne, but in recent years it has been established that retinoic acid acts as a potent teratogen when taken orally, especially during the period of organogenesis. Major defects produced by retinoic acid are neural tube anomalies, cleft palate, hypoplasia of lower facial structures, and heart and thymic defects. This pattern of gross abnormalities coincides very closely with a major site of retinoic acid action in the early embryo.

Retinoic acid acts through a complex sequence of cytoplasmic binding proteins and nuclear receptors, which ultimately affect the expression of certain *Hox* genes, especially those expressed in the anterior rhombomeres of the forming hindbrain. Excess retinoic acid causes an anterior shift of expression of key *Hox* genes (e.g., *Hoxb-1* [see Figure 10-10]), resulting in alterations of the more anterior rhombomeres and the neural crest cells that are derived from them. As discussed later (see Figure 11-8), neural crest cells emanating from rhombomeres are instrumental in patterning many structures of the face and neck and also contribute to the developing heart and thymus—hence the pattern of retinoic acid–induced defects previously outlined. In view of the increasing recognition that retinoic acid or its metabolites play an important role in pattern formation during early development, extreme caution when using vi-

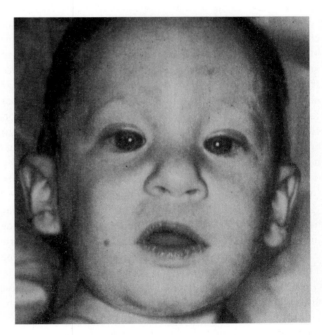

Figure 7-14 Face of an infant with fetal alcohol syndrome showing a long and thin upper lip, shortened and upwardly slanting palpebral fissures, epicanthic folds, and mild hirsutism. (From Wigglesworth JS, Singer DB: *Textbook of fetal and perinatal pathology*, 2 vols, Oxford, England, 1991, Blackwell Scientific.)

tamin A in doses above those needed for basic nutritional requirements is recommended.

Antibiotics. The use of two antibiotics during pregnancy is associated with birth defects. Streptomycin in high doses can cause inner ear deafness. Tetracycline given to the mother during late pregnancy crosses the placental barrier and seeks sites of active calcification in the teeth and bones of the fetus. Tetracycline deposits cause a yellowish discoloration of teeth and bones and in high doses, can interfere with enamel formation.

Other Drugs. A number of other drugs, such as the anticoagulant warfarin, are known to be teratogenic, and others are strongly suspected. However, firm proof of a drug's teratogenicity in humans is not easy to obtain. Several drugs, such as agent orange and some of the social drugs (e.g., LSD, marijuana), have often been claimed to cause birth defects, but the evidence to date is not entirely convincing. On the other hand, several studies have shown a variety of complications in pregnancy resulting from the use of cocaine, which can readily cross the placental barrier. In addition to structural malformations in organs such as the brain, cocaine use has been linked to intrauterine growth retardation, premature labor, and spontaneous abortion, as well as postnatal behavioral disturbances, such as attention deficit.

Physical factors

Ionizing Radiation. Ionizing radiation is a potent teratogen, and the response is both dependent on the dose and related to the stage at which the embryo is irradiated. In addition to numerous animal studies, there is direct human experience based on survivors of the Japanese atomic bomb blasts and pregnant women who were given large doses of radiation (up to several thousand rads) for therapeutic reasons. There is no evidence that doses of radiation at diagnostic levels (only a few millirads) pose a significant threat to the embryo. Nevertheless, because ionizing radiation can cause breaks in deoxyribonucleic acid and is also known to cause mutations, it is prudent for a woman who is pregnant to avoid exposure to radiation if possible, although the dose in a diagnostic x-ray examination is so small that the risk is minimal.

Although ionizing radiation can cause a variety of anomalies in embryos (e.g., cleft palate; microcephaly; malformations of the viscera, limbs, and skeleton), defects of the central nervous system are very prominent in irradiated embryos. The spectrum runs from spina bifida to mental retardation.

Other Physical Factors. A number of studies on the teratogenic effects of extremes of temperature and different concentrations of atmospheric gases have been conducted on experimental animals, but the evidence relating any of these factors to human malformations is still equivocal. One exception is the effect of excess concentrations of oxygen on prematurely born infants. When this was a common practice, **retrolental fibroplasia** developed in over 10% of premature infants weighing less than 3 pounds and in about 1% of those weighing between 3 and 5 pounds. When this was recognized, the practice of maintaining high concentrations of oxygen in incubators ceased, and this problem is now of only historical interest.

Maternal factors

A number of maternal factors have been implicated in the genesis of congenital malformations. **Maternal diabetes** is frequently associated with large birth weight and with stillbirths. Structural anomalies occur several times more frequently in infants of diabetic mothers than among the infants of mothers from the general population. Although there is a correlation between the duration and severity of the mother's disease and the effects on the fetus, the specific cause of interference with development has not been identified.

In general, maternal nutrition does not seem to be a major factor in the production of anomalies (folic acid being a notable exception), but if the mother is severely deficient in iodine, the newborn is likely to show the symptoms of cretinism (growth retardation, mental retardation, short and broad hands, short fingers, dry skin, and difficulty breathing).

There is now considerable evidence that **heavy smoking** by a pregnant woman leads to an increased risk of low birth weight and a low rate of growth after birth.

Mechanical factors

Although mechanical factors have been implicated in the genesis of congenital malformations for centuries, only in recent years has it been possible to relate specific malformations to mechanical causes. A number of the most common anomalies such as **clubfoot, congenital hip dislocations,** and even certain deformations of the skull can be attributed in large measure to abnormal intrauterine pressures imposed on the fetus. This can often be related to uterine malformations or a reduced amount of amniotic fluid (**oligohydramnios**).

Amniotic bands constricting digits or extremities of the fetus have been implicated as causes of intrauterine amputations (Figure 7-15). These bands form as the result of tears to the extraembryonic membranes during pregnancy.

DEVELOPMENTAL DISTURBANCES RESULTING IN MALFORMATIONS

Duplications and Reversal of Asymmetry

The classic example of a duplication is identical twinning. Under normal circumstances, both members of the twin pair are completely normal, but rarely the duplication is not complete and **conjoined twins** (sometimes referred to as *Siamese twins*) result (see Figures 3-13 and 3-14). Twins can be conjoined at almost any site and to any degree. With modern sur-

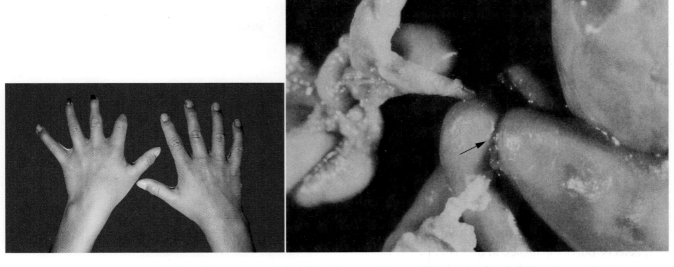

Figure 7-15 A, Digital amputations of the left hand presumably caused by amniotic bands. **B,** Amniotic bands involving the umbilical cord and limbs of a fetus. The arrow shows a constriction ring around the thigh. (**A** courtesy M. Barr, Ann Arbor, Mich. **B** from Wigglesworth JS, Singer DB: *Textbook of fetal and perinatal pathology,* 2 vols, Oxford, England, 1991, Blackwell Scientific.)

gical techniques, it is now possible to separate members of some conjoined pairs. A type of conjoined twinning is the condition of **parasitic twinning,** in which one member of the pair is relatively normal but the other is represented by a much smaller body, often consisting of just the torso and limbs, attached to an area such as the mouth or lower abdomen of the host twin (see Figure 3-15).

In a high number of conjoined twins, one member of the pair has reversed symmetry in relation to the other (see Figure 3-14). Over a century ago, the biologist Oscar Bateson compiled a large number of instances of reversals of symmetry in duplicated structures throughout the animal kingdom. His recognition of this phenomenon is now called **Bateson's rule.** (An example of this rule as it applies to a limb duplication is illustrated in Figure 9-9.)

In rare instances (approximately 1 in 10,000 births), an otherwise normal individual is found to have a partial or complete reversal of symmetry of the internal organs. The cause of this condition, called **situs inversus** (see Figure 3-16), has remained obscure, but recent research on the genetics and molecular basis of body asymmetry (see p. 69) promises to clarify this question in the near future.

Faulty Inductive Tissue Interactions

Absent or faulty induction early in development (e.g., induction of the central nervous system) is incompatible with life, but there are malformations consistent with disturbances in later inductions. Absence of the lens (**aphakia**) or a kidney (**renal agenesis**) could result from an absent or abnormal inductive interaction.

Absence of Normal Cell Death

Genetically or **epigenetically** (environmental influences imposed on the genetic background) controlled cell death is an important mechanism in sculpting a number of regions of the body. The absence of normal interdigital cell death has been implicated in **syndactyly** (webbed digits) (see Figure 9-13, *A*) and abnormal persistence of the tail (see Figure 8-20, *A*, for normal tail). The latter phenomenon has sometimes been considered an example of **atavism** (the persistence of phylogenetically primitive structures).

Failure of Tube Formation

The formation of a tube from an epithelial sheet is a fundamental developmental mechanism. A classic case of failure of tube formation is seen in the family of spina bifida anomalies, which are based on the incomplete fusion of the neural tube (see Figure 10-39). (Some of the possible mechanisms involved in normal formation of the neural tube are given in Chapter 10.)

Disturbances in Tissue Resorption

Some structures present in the early embryo must be resorbed for subsequent development to proceed normally. Good examples of this are the membranes that cover the future oral and anal openings. These membranes are composed of opposing sheets of ectoderm and endoderm, but if mesodermal cells become interposed between the two and this tissue becomes vascularized, breakdown typically fails to occur. **Anal atresia** is a common anomaly of this type (see Figure 14-15).

Failure of Migration

Migration is an important developmental phenomenon that occurs at the level of cells or entire organs. The neural crest is a classic example of massive migrations at the cellular level, and disturbances in migration can cause abnormalities in any of the structures for which the neural crest is a precursor (e.g., thymus, outflow tracts of the heart, adrenal medulla). At the organ level, the kidneys undertake a prominent migration into the abdominal cavity from their origin in the pelvic region, and the testes migrate from the abdominal cavity into the scrotum. **Pelvic kidneys** (see Figure 15-14) and undescended testes (**cryptorchidism**) are not rare.

Developmental Arrest

Early in the history of teratology, some malformations were recognized as the persistence of structures in a state that was normal at an earlier stage of development. Many of the patterns of **cleft lip** and **cleft palate** (see Figs. 13-17 and 13-18) are examples of developmental arrest, although it is incorrect to assume that development has been totally arrested since the sixth to eighth weeks of embryogenesis.

Another example of the persistence of an earlier stage in development is a **thyroglossal duct** (see Figure 13-29), in which persisting epithelial cells mark the path of the thyroid gland as it migrates from the base of the tongue to its normal position.

Destruction of Formed Structures

A number of teratogenic diseases or chemicals produce malformations by the destruction of structures already present. If the structure is in the early primordial stage, any tissues to which the primordium would normally give rise are missing or malformed. Interference with the blood supply of a structure can cause unusual patterns of malformations. For example, in the genesis of **phocomelia** (see Figure 7-2), damage to proximal blood vessels could destroy the primordia of the proximal limb segments, but the cells of the distal limb bud that gives rise to the hands or feet could be spared if the distal microvasculature of the limb bud remained intact.

Failure to Fuse or Merge

If two structures such as the palatal shelves fail to meet at the critical time, they are likely to remain separate. Similarly, the relative displacements of mesenchyme (**merging**) that are involved in the shaping of the lower jaw may not occur on schedule or in adequate amounts. This accounts for some malformations of the lower face.

Hypoplasia and Hyperplasia

The normal formation of most organs and complex structures requires a precise amount and distribution of cellular proliferation. If cellular proliferation in a forming organ is ab-

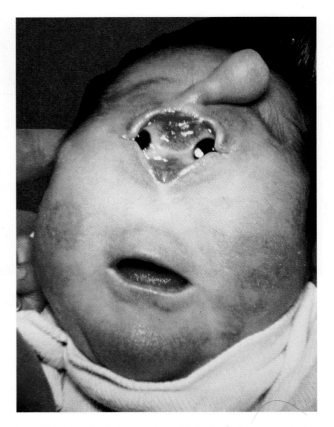

Figure 7-16 Cyclopia in a newborn. Note the fleshy proboscis above the partially fused eye. (Courtesy M. Barr, Ann Arbor, Mich.)

normal, the structure can become too small (**hypoplastic**) or too large (**hyperplastic**). Even relatively minor growth disturbances can cause severe problems in complex regions such as the face. Occasionally, **gigantism** of a structure such as a digit or whole limb occurs. The mechanism underlying this excessive growth remains obscure.

Receptor Defects

Some congenital malformations can be attributed to defects in specific receptor molecules. One of the earliest recognized is the **testicular feminization syndrome,** in which the lack of testosterone receptors results in the development of a typical female phenotype in a genetic male (see Figure 8-12).

Defective Fields

Proper morphogenesis of many regions of the body is under the control of poorly understood morphogenetic fields. These regions of the body are under the control of an overall developmental blueprint. Disturbances in the boundaries or overall controls of fields can sometimes give rise to massive anomalies. One example is the fusion of lower limb fields, which is probably associated with a larger defect in the field controlling the development of the caudal region of the body. This mermaidlike

Only a few decades ago, birth defects were diagnosed only after the fact, and sometimes it was years after birth before certain defects could be discovered and treated. Although this can still happen today, technological changes have permitted the earlier diagnosis and treatment of certain congenital malformations.

One of the first advances was the technology associated with karyotyping and sex chromosome analysis. Initially these techniques were applied after birth to diagnose conditions based on abnormalities in chromosome number or structure. After the development of amniocentesis (the removal of samples of amniotic fluid during early pregnancy), chromosomal analysis could be applied to cells in the amniotic fluid. This was particularly useful in the diagnosis of Down syndrome, but it also permitted the prenatal diagnosis of the gender of the infant. Biochemical analysis of amniotic fluid has permitted the diagnosis of

a number of inborn errors of metabolism and neural tube defects (the latter through the detection of **S-100 protein,** which leaks through the open neural tube into the amniotic fluid).

More recently, techniques have been developed for the direct sampling of tissue from the chorionic villi. The risk-to-benefit ratio of this technique is still being debated.

With the development of modern imaging techniques such as ultrasound, computed tomography, and magnetic resonance imaging, visualization of fetal morphological structures is now possible (see Figures 17-11 to 17-14). These images can now serve as a direct guide to surgeons, who are attempting to correct certain malformations by intrauterine surgery. Because surgical wounds in fetuses typically heal without scarring, there are distinct advantages to fetal corrective surgery (see Chapter 17).

anomaly is called **sirenomelia** (see Figure 7-1, *B*), an extreme example of what is called the **caudal regression syndrome.**

Effects Secondary to Other Developmental Disturbances

Because so much of normal development involves the tight interlocking of individual processes or building on completed structures, it is not surprising that a number of malformations are secondary manifestations of other disturbed embryonic processes. There are a number of examples in craniofacial development. Some cases of cleft palate have been attributed to a widening of the cranial base so that the palatal shelves, which may have been perfectly normal, are unable to make midline contact.

The single or widely separated tubular probosces that appear in certain major facial anomalies, such as **cyclopia** (Figure 7-16), are very difficult to explain unless it is understood that one of several primary defects, whether too much or too little tissue of the midface, prevented the two nasal primordia from joining in the midline. In the case of cyclopia, the primary defect is usually a deficiency of forebrain tissue, and the facial defects are secondary to that.

Germ Layer Defects

An understanding of normal development can explain the basis for a seemingly diverse set of anomalies. **Ectodermal dysplasias,** which are based on abnormalities in the ectodermal germ layer, can include malformations as diverse as thin hair, poorly formed teeth, short stature, dry and scaly skin, and hypoplastic nails. Other syndromes with diverse phenotypic abnormalities are related to defects of the neural crest (see Chapter 11).

CLINICAL VIGNETTE

A woman in her early forties who has chronic alcoholism, who smoked heavily, and who also occasionally used cocaine gave birth to an infant with severe anencephaly. She had previously given birth to a child who had a less severe form of spina bifida. Another child, although small in stature, seemed normal but had a behavioral problem in school.

What is a likely basis for such a history?

SUMMARY

- Developmental disorders have been recognized for centuries, but a direct connection between environmental teratogens and human birth defects was not demonstrated until 1941.
- Abnormal development is often the result of environmental influences imposed on genetic susceptibility. The factors involved in abnormal development include age, race, country, nutrition, and time of year. The study of abnormal development is teratology, and an agent that causes abnormal development is a teratogen.
- Genetic factors cause a significant number of birth defects. Abnormal chromosome numbers are associated with prenatal death and syndromes of abnormal structures. Common causes of abnormalities are monosomies and trisomies, which are often the result of nondisjunction during meiosis. Other malformations are based on abnormalities of chromosome structure. Certain malformations are based on genetic mutations.
- Among the environmental factors leading to defective development are maternal infections, chemical teratogens, physical factors such as ionizing radiation, maternal factors, and mechanical factors.

- A variety of disturbed developmental mechanisms may be involved in the production of a given congenital malformation. These include duplications, faulty inductive tissue interactions, absence of normal cell death, failure of tube formation, disturbances in tissue resorption, failure of migration, developmental arrest, destruction of an already formed structure, failure to fuse or merge, hypoplasia or hyperplasia, receptor defects, defective fields, effects secondary to other developmental disturbances, and germ cell layer defects.
- With technological developments, it is now possible to diagnose increasing numbers of birth defects in utero. Some of the diagnostic techniques are karyotyping and sex chromosome analysis on cells obtained from amniotic fluid, biochemical analysis of amniotic fluid, biochemical and molecular analysis of cells obtained from amniotic fluid or chorionic villus sampling, and imaging techniques, especially ultrasonography. There have been a few attempts to correct malformations by surgery in utero.

REVIEW QUESTIONS

1. Phocomelia is most likely to be seen after maternal exposure to which teratogenic agent during the first trimester of pregnancy?
   - A. Alcohol
   - B. Aminopterin
   - C. Androgens
   - D. Ionizing radiation
   - E. Thalidomide
2. Which of these anomalies can be attributed to a disturbance in tissue resorption?
   - A. Pelvic kidney
   - B. Cleft lip
   - C. Anal atresia
   - D. Renal agenesis
   - E. Amputated digit in utero
3. Which of the following is responsible for the largest percentage of congenital malformations?
   - A. Maternal infections
   - B. Chemical teratogens
   - C. Genetically based conditions
   - D. Ionizing radiations
   - E. Unknown factors
4. Folic acid deficiency is now felt to be a major cause of what class of malformations?
   - A. Trisomies
   - B. Neural tube defects
   - C. Ambiguous genitalia
   - D. Polyploidy
   - E. Duplications
5. Cleft palate is the result of a defect in what developmental mechanism?
   - A. Failure to fuse
   - B. Failure to merge
   - C. Faulty inductive tissue interaction
   - D. Disturbance in tissue resorption
   - E. Absence of normal cell death
6. An increased incidence of what condition is strongly associated with increasing maternal age?
   - A. Trisomy 18
   - B. Trisomy 21
   - C. Trisomy 13
   - D. Anencephaly
   - E. Ambiguous external genitalia

7. A woman who was in a car accident and suffered abdominal bruising during the fourth month of pregnancy gave birth to an infant with a cleft palate. She sued the driver of the other car for expenses associated with treatment of the birth defect, claiming that it was caused by the accident. You are asked to be a witness for the defense. What is your case?
8. A woman who took a new sedative during the second month of pregnancy felt somewhat nauseated after ingestion of the drug and stopped taking it after a couple of weeks. She gave birth to an infant who had a septal defect of the heart and sued the manufacturer of the drug, saying the defect was caused by the drug that made her nauseated. You are asked to be a witness for the manufacturer. What is your case?
9. What is a likely cause for a badly turned-in ankle in a newborn?
10. A 3-year-old child is much smaller than normal, has sparse hair, and has irregular teeth. What is a likely basis for this constellation of defects?

REFERENCES

Butterworth CE, Bendich, A: Folic acid and the prevention of birth defects, *Annu Rev Nutr* 16:73-97, 1996.

Buyse ML, ed: *Birth defects encyclopedia*, Dover, Mass, 1990, Centre for Birth Defects Information Services.

Catilla EE and others: Thalidomide, a current teratogen in South America, *Teratology* 54:273-277, 1996.

Coles CD: Prenatal alcohol exposure and human development. In Miller M, ed: *Development of the central nervous system: effects of alcohol and opiates*, New York, 1992, Wiley-Liss, pp 9-36.

Connor J, Ferguson-Smith N: *Essential medical genetics*, ed 2, Oxford, England, 1987, Blackwell Scientific.

Czeizel AE, Dudas I: Prevention of the first occurrence of neural-tube defects by periconceptional vitamin supplementation, *N Engl J Med* 327:1832-1835, 1992.

Erickson JD, ed: *Congenital malformations surveillance report*, *Teratology* 56:1-175, 1997.

Fanaroff A, Martin RJ: *Neonatal-perinatal medicine*, ed 6, St Louis, 1997, Mosby.

Frazer C: Of mice and children: reminiscences of a teratogeneticist, *Issues Rev Teratol* 5:1-75, 1990.

Ganapathy V, Leibach FH: Current topic: human placenta—a direct target for cocaine action, *Placenta* 15:785-795, 1994.

Hansen DK: The embryotoxicity of phenytoin: an update on possible mechanisms, *Proc Soc Exp Biol Med* 197:361-368, 1991.

Jones KL: *Smith's recognizable patterns of human malformation*, ed 4, Philadelphia, 1988, WB Saunders.

Kallen B, Mastroiacovo P, Robert E: Major congenital malformations in Down syndrome, *Am J Med Genet* 65:160-166, 1996.

Marshall H and others: Retinoids and *Hox* genes, *FASEB J* 10:969-978, 1996.

Miller MM: Effects of prenatal exposure to ethanol on cell proliferation and neuronal migration. In Miller M, ed: *Development of the central nervous system: effects of alcohol and opiates*, New York, 1992, Wiley-Liss, pp 47-69.

Miller RK and others: Periconceptional vitamin A use: how much is teratogenic? *Reprod Toxicol* 12:75-88, 1998.

Mills JL and others: Vitamin A and birth defects, *Am J Obstet Gynecol* 177:31-36, 1997.

Munger RG and others: Maternal alcohol use and risk of orofacial cleft birth defects, *Teratology* 54:27-33, 1996.

Naeye RL: *Disorders of the placenta, fetus, and neonate*, St Louis, 1992, Mosby.

Nishimura H, Okamoto N: *Sequential atlas of human congenital malformations*, Baltimore, 1976, University Park Press.

Nyberg D, Mahony B, Pretorious D: *Diagnostic ultrasound of fetal anomalies,* St Louis, 1990, Mosby.

Paré A: *On monsters and marvels,* Chicago, 1982, University of Chicago Press.

Pennington SN: Molecular changes associated with ethanol-induced growth suppression in the chick embryo, *Alcohol Clin Exp Res* 14:832-837, 1990.

Persaud TVN, Chudley AE, Skalko RG, eds: *Basic concepts in teratology,* New York, 1985, Liss.

Reed GB, Claireaux AE, Bain AD: *Diseases of the fetus and newborn,* St Louis, 1989, Mosby.

Saxén L, Rapola J: *Congenital defects,* New York, 1969, Holt, Rinehart & Winston.

Soprano DR, Soprano KJ: Retinoids as teratogens, *Annu Rev Nutr* 15:111-132, 1995.

Sulik KK, Alles AJ: *Teratogenicity of the retinoids.* In Saurat J-H, ed: *Retinoids: 10 years on,* Basel, Switzerland, 1991, Karger, pp 282-295.

Volpe JJ: Effect of cocaine use on the fetus, *N Engl J Med* 327:399-407, 1992.

Warkany J: *Congenital malformations,* St Louis, 1971, Mosby.

Wigglesworth JS, Singer DB: *Textbook of fetal and perinatal pathology,* 2 vols, Oxford, England, 1991, Blackwell Scientific.

Willis RA: *The borderland of embryology and pathology,* ed 2, London, 1962, Butterworths.

Wilson GN: Genomics of human dysmorphogenesis, *Am J Med Genet* 42:187-196, 1992.

Wilson JG, Fraser FC, eds: *Handbook of teratology,* vols 1-4, New York, 1977, Plenum.

Yen IH and others: The changing epidemiology of neural tube defects, *Am J Dis Control* 146:857-861, 1992.

II

DEVELOPMENT OF THE BODY SYSTEMS

8

INTEGUMENTARY, SKELETAL, AND MUSCULAR SYSTEMS

The construction of the tissues of the body involves developmental phenomena at two levels of organization. One is the level of individual cells, in which the cells that make up a tissue undergo increasing specialization through a process called **cytodifferentiation** (see discussion of restriction, determination, and differentiation, p. 70). At the next level of complexity, various cell types develop in concert to form specific tissues through a process called **histogenesis.** This chapter will cover the development of three important tissues of the body: skin, bone, and muscle. The histogenesis of each of these tissues exemplifies important aspects of development.

INTEGUMENTARY SYSTEM

The skin, consisting of the epidermis and dermis, is one of the largest structures in the body. The epidermis represents the interface between the body and its external environment, and its structure is well adapted for local functional requirements. Simple inspection of areas such as the scalp and palms shows that the structure of the integument varies from one part of the body to another. These local variations result from inductive interactions between the ectoderm and underlying mesenchyme. Abnormalities associated with the integumentary system are presented in Clinical Correlation 8-1, found near the end of this section.

Epidermis

Structural development

The outer layer of the skin begins as a single layer of ectodermal cells (Figure 8-1, A). As development progresses, the ectoderm becomes multilayered, and regional differences in structure become apparent.

The first stage in epidermal layering is the formation of a thin outer layer of flattened cells known as the **periderm** at the end of the first month of gestation (Figure 8-1, B). Cells of the periderm, which is present in the epidermis of all amniote embryos, appear to be involved in the exchange of water, sodium, and possibly glucose between the amniotic fluid and the epidermis.

By the third month the epidermis becomes a three-layered structure, with a mitotically active **basal** (or **germinative) layer,** an intermediate layer of cells (Figure 8-1, D) that represent the progeny of the dividing stem cells of the basal layer, and a superficial layer of peridermal cells bearing characteristic surface blebs (Figure 8-2). Peridermal cells contain large amounts of glycogen, but its function remains uncertain.

During the sixth month, the epidermis beneath the periderm undergoes differentiation into the definitive layers characteristic of the postnatal epidermis. Many of the peridermal cells undergo programmed cell death (**apoptosis**) and are sloughed into the amniotic fluid. The epidermis becomes a barrier between the fetus and the outside environment instead of a participant in exchanges between the two. The change in function of the fetal epidermis may have adaptive value, since it occurs at about the time when urinary wastes begin to accumulate in the amniotic fluid.

Immigrant cells in the epidermis

Despite its homogeneous histological appearance, the epidermis is really a cellular mosaic, with contributions from cells derived not only from surface ectoderm but also from other precursors, such as the neural crest or mesoderm. These cells play important specific roles in the function of the skin.

Early in the second month, **melanoblasts** derived from the neural crest migrate into the embryonic dermis; slightly later, they migrate into the epidermis. Although melanoblasts can be recognized early using stain with a monoclonal antibody (HMB-45, which reacts with a cytoplasmic antigen common

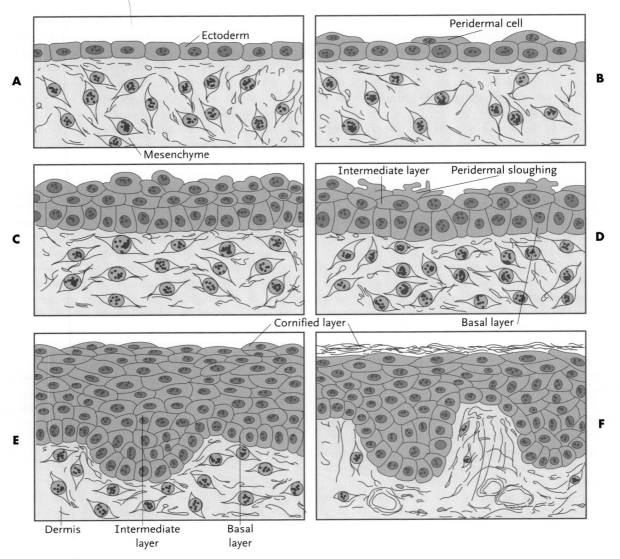

Figure 8-1 Stages in the histogenesis of human skin. **A**, At **1 month**. **B**, At **2 months**. **C**, At **2½ months**. **D**, At **4 months**. **E**, At **6 months**. **F**, After birth. (Modified from Carlson B: *Patten's foundations of embryology*, ed 6, New York, 1996, McGraw-Hill.)

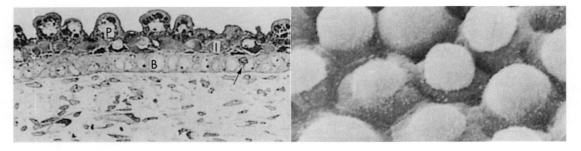

Figure 8-2 Light micrograph (*left*) and scanning electron micrograph (*right*) of the epidermis of a **10-week-old** human embryo. The prominent surface blebs seen in the scanning micrograph are represented by the irregular surface of the periderm (*P*) in the light micrograph. The arrow in the figure on the left points to a melanocyte in the basal layer (*B*) of the epidermis. I, Intermediate layer of epidermis. (From Sybert VP, Holbrook KA. In Reed G, Claireaux A, Bain A: *Diseases of the fetus and newborn*, St Louis, 1989, Mosby.)

to melanoblasts and **melanomas** [pigment cell tumors]), these cells do not begin to produce recognizable amounts of pigment until midpregnancy. This occurs earlier in heavily pigmented individuals than in those with light complexions. The differentiation of melanoblasts into mature **melanocytes** involves the formation of pigment granules called **melanosomes** from **premelanosomes.**

The number of pigment cells in the skin does not differ greatly among the various races, but the melanocytes of dark-skinned individuals contain more pigment granules per cell. **Albinism** is a genetic trait characterized by the lack of pigmentation, but albinos typically contain normal numbers of melanocytes in their skin. The melanocytes of albinos are generally unable to express pigmentation because they lack the enzyme **tyrosinase,** which is involved in the conversion of the amino acid tyrosine to **melanin.**

Late in the first trimester the epidermis is invaded by **Langerhans' cells,** which arise from precursors in the bone marrow. These cells are peripheral components of the immune system and are involved in the presentation of antigens; they cooperate with T lymphocytes (white blood cells involved in cellular immune responses) in the skin to initiate cell-mediated responses against foreign antigens. Although Langerhans' cells are not readily evident in ordinary histological preparations, they can be distinguished through antibodies directed toward cell-specific surface antigens or by histochemical demonstration of their high membrane-bound adenosinetriphosphatase activity. Langerhans' cells are present in low numbers (about 65 cells/mm^2 of epidermis) during the first two trimesters of pregnancy, but then their numbers increase several-fold to 2% to 6% of the total number of epidermal cells in the adult.

A third cell type in the epidermis, the **Merkel cell,** is of uncertain origin. Some evidence suggests that Merkel cells may differentiate from epidermal cell precursors, but experiments on birds involving the grafting of marked neural crest tissues indicate that precursors of Merkel cells migrate into the limb from the neural crest. These cells, which appear in palmar and plantar epidermis as early as 8 to 12 weeks of gestation, are associated with free nerve terminals. They function as slow-adapting mechanoreceptors in the skin, but cytochemical evidence suggests that they may also function as neuroendocrine cells at some stage.

Epidermal differentiation

Once the multilayered epidermis becomes established, a regular cellular organization and sequence of differentiation appears within it (Figure 8-3). **Stem cells*** of the basal layer

---

*Many types of tissues contain a population of **stem cells,** which have a high capacity for proliferation. Some of the daughter cells remain as stem cells, but other daughter cells become what in the epidermis are called **transit-amplifying cells.** These cells, which are located in the stratum basale and to some extent in the stratum spinosum, are capable of a few more mitotic divisions before permanently withdrawing from the cell cycle. The postmitotic cells are sometimes called **committed cells.** In the epidermis, these are the cells that undergo keratinization.

(stratum basale) divide and contribute daughter cells to the next layer, the **stratum spinosum.** The movement of epidermal cells away from the basal layer is preceded by a loss of adhesiveness to basal lamina components (e.g., fibronectin, laminin, and collagen types I and IV). These cellular properties can be explained by the loss of several **integrins** (membrane proteins that mediate the attachment of cells to extracellular matrix molecules). Cells of the stratum spinosum produce prominent bundles of **keratin** filaments, which converge on the patchlike desmosomes binding the cells to each other.

Keratohyalin granules, another marker of epidermal differentiation, begin to appear in the cytoplasm of the outer, postmitotic cells of the stratum spinosum and are prominent components of the stratum granulosum. Recent research has shown that keratohyalin granules are composed of two types of protein aggregates—one histidine rich and one sulfur rich—closely associated with bundles of keratin filaments. Because of their high content of keratin, epidermal cells are given the generic name **keratinocytes.** As the keratinocytes move into the stratum granulosum, their nuclei begin to show characteristic signs of terminal differentiation, such as a flattened appearance, dense masses of nuclear chromatin, and early signs of breaking up of the nuclear membrane. In these cells the bundles of keratin become more prominent, and the molecular weights of keratins that are synthesized are higher than in less mature keratinocytes.

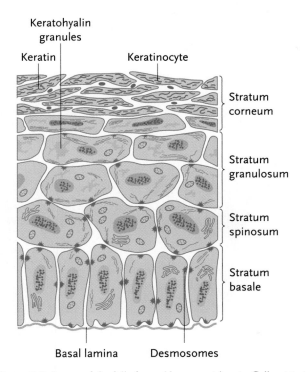

Figure 8-3 Layers of the fully formed human epidermis. Cells arising in the stratum basale undergo terminal differentiation into keratinocytes as they move toward the surface. (Modified from Carlson B: *Patten's foundations of embryology,* ed 6, New York, 1996, McGraw-Hill.)

As the cells move into the outer layer, the **stratum corneum**, they lose their nuclei and resemble very flattened bags densely packed with keratin filaments. The cells of this layer are interconnected by the histidine-rich protein **filaggrin**, which is derived from one of the granular components of keratohyalin. Depending on the region of the body surface, the cells of the stratum corneum accumulate to form approximately 15 to 20 layers of dead cells. In postnatal life, whether through friction or the degradation of the desmosomes and filaggrin, these cells are eventually shed (e.g., about 1300 cells/cm^2/hr in the human forearm) and commonly accumulate as house dust.

Biochemical work has correlated the expression of keratin proteins (members of a complex family of proteins) with specific stages of epidermal differentiation (Figure 8-4). Keratins of the family of intermediate cellular filaments are first expressed in cells of the two-layered epidermis during the second month

of pregnancy. Three of the keratins (40-, 45-, and 52-kDa) are characteristic of simple epithelia, and the other two (50- and 58-kDa) are typically seen in stratified epithelia. As the epidermis begins to stratify (at 9 to 12 weeks' gestation), the outer cells of the intermediate layer begin to express small amounts of 56.5- and 67-kDa keratins, which are characteristic of keratinized epidermis. In succeeding weeks the amounts of these two keratins increase greatly, whereas the prominence of the simple epithelial keratins (40-, 45-, and 52-kDa) declines during the late fetal period. The expression of filaggrin, the intercellular binding protein, is closely correlated with the later differentiation of the outer cornified layers of the fetal epidermis.

The proliferation of basal epidermal cells is under the control of a variety of growth factors. Some of these stimulate and others inhibit mitosis (Box 8-1). Keratinocytes commonly spend about 4 weeks in their passage from the basal

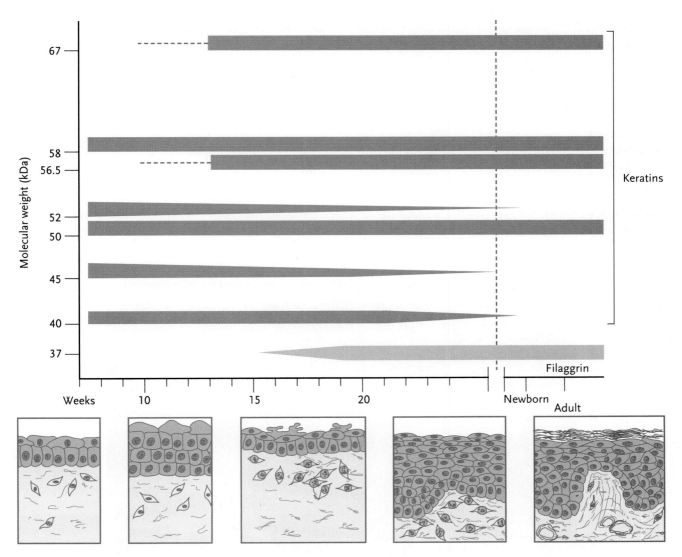

Figure 8-4 Expression of keratins and filaggrin during human fetal skin development. The lower figures show approximate stages in skin development at the times indicated. (Graph modified from Dale BA and others: *J Cell Biol* 101:1257-1269, 1985.)

layer of the epidermis to ultimate desquamation, but in some skin diseases, such as **psoriasis**, epidermal cell proliferation is poorly controlled, and keratinocytes may be shed within a week after their generation.

One of the prominent features of the skin, particularly the thick skin of the palms and soles, is the presence of epidermal ridges and creases. On the tips of the digits, the ridges form loops and whorls in fingerprint patterns that are unique to the individual. These patterns form the basis for the science of **dermatoglyphics**, in which the patterns constitute the foundation for genetic analysis or criminal investigation.

The formation of epidermal ridges is closely associated with the earlier appearance of **volar pads** on the ventral surfaces of the fingers and toes (Figure 8-5). Volar pads first form on the palms at about $6\frac{1}{2}$ weeks, and by $7\frac{1}{2}$ weeks, they have formed on the fingers. The volar pads begin to regress by about $10\frac{1}{2}$ weeks, but while they are present, they set the stage for the formation of the epidermal ridges, which occurs between 11 and 17 weeks. Similar events in the foot occur approximately a week later than those in the hand.

The pattern of the epidermal ridges is correlated with the morphology of the volar pads when the ridges first form. If a volar pad is high and round, the epidermal ridges form a whorl; if the pad is low, an arch results. A pad of intermediate height results in a loop configuration of the digital epidermal ridges. The timing of ridge formation also appears to influence the morphology: early formation of ridges is associated with whorls and late formation with arches. The primary basis for dermatoglyphic patterns is still not understood.

When the epidermal ridges first form, the tips of the digits are still smooth, and the fetal epidermis is covered with peridermal cells. Beneath the smooth surface, however, epidermal and dermal ridges begin to take shape (Figure 8-6). Late in the fifth month of pregnancy the epidermal ridges become recognizable features of the surface landscape.

Dermis

The dermis arises from mesodermal cells derived from the dermatome of the somites or other mesenchymal cells located just beneath the ectoderm. In the face and parts of the neck,

---

BOX 8-1   Peptide Factors that Affect Keratinocyte Proliferation

STIMULATORS

Epidermal growth factor
Transforming growth factor-α
Insulin
Insulin-like growth factors I and II
Fibroblast growth factor, acidic
Fibroblast growth factor, basic
Interleukin-1/ETAF

INHIBITORS

Transforming growth factor-β_1
Transforming growth factor-β_2
Interferon-α/β_1
Interferon-β_2
Interferon
Tumor necrosis factor

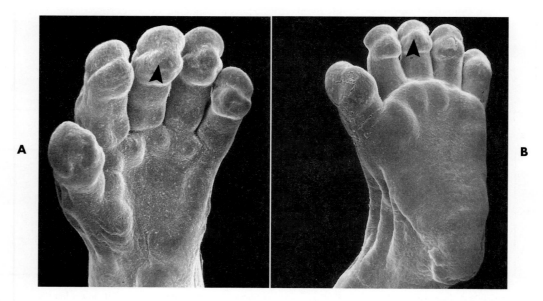

Figure 8-5 Scanning electron micrographs of the ventral surfaces of the hand (**A**) and the foot (**B**) of a human embryo at the **end of the second month**. Volar pads are prominent near the tips of the digits (*arrowheads*). (From Jirásek J: *Atlas of human prenatal morphogenesis*, Amsterdam, 1983, Martinus Nijhoff.)

dermal cells are descendants of the cranial neural crest ectoderm (see Figure 11-10).

The future dermis is initially represented by loosely aggregated mesenchymal cells that are highly interconnected by focal tight junctions on their cellular processes. These early dermal precursors secrete a watery intercellular matrix rich in glycogen and hyaluronic acid.

Early in the third month the developing dermis undergoes a transition from the highly cellular embryonic form to a state characterized by the differentiation of the mesenchymal cells into fibroblasts and the formation of increasing amounts of a fibrous intercellular matrix. The principal types of fibers are types I and III collagen and elastic fibers. The dermis becomes highly vascularized, with an early capillary network transformed into layers of larger vessels. Shortly after the eighth week, sensory nerves growing into the dermis and epidermis help complete reflex arcs, allowing the fetus to respond to pressure and stroking.

Dermal/epidermal interactions

The transformation of simple ectoderm into a multilayered epidermis depends on continuing inductive interactions with the underlying dermis. Dermal/epidermal interactions are also the basis for the formation of a wide variety of epidermal appendages and the appearance of regional variations in the structure of the epidermis.

For example, early in development the epidermis covering the palms and soles becomes significantly thicker than that elsewhere on the body. These regions also do not produce hairs, whereas hairs of some sort, whether coarse or extremely fine, form in regular patterns from the epidermis throughout most of the rest of the body.

Tissue recombination experiments on a variety of vertebrate species have shown that the underlying dermis determines the course of development of the epidermis and its

derivatives and that the ectoderm also influences the developmental course of the dermis. If the early ectodermal and mesenchymal components of the skin are enzymatically dissociated and grown separately, the ectodermal component remains simple ectoderm without differentiating into a multilayered epidermis with appropriate epidermal appendages. Similarly, isolated subectodermal mesenchyme retains its embryonic character without differentiating into dermis.

If ectoderm from one part of the body is combined with dermis from another area, the ectoderm differentiates into a regional pattern characteristic of underlying dermis rather than a pattern appropriate for the site of origin of the ectoderm (Figure 8-7). Cross-species recombination experiments have shown that even in distantly related animals, skin ectoderm and mesenchyme can respond to each other's inductive signals.

As in many other parts of the body, inductive interactions and subsequent morphogenesis of the skin and its appendages are mediated by the production and secretion of common signaling molecules. Specific regional morphogenesis of the skin and its appendages appears to be patterned through the actions of transcription factors, probably functioning in concert with the still poorly understood influences of retinoic acid, which exerts powerful effects on the skin.

Epidermal Appendages

As a result of inductive influences by the dermis, the epidermis produces a wide variety of appendages such as hair, nails, sweat and sebaceous glands, mammary glands, and even the enamel component of teeth. (The development of teeth is discussed in Chapter 13.)

Hair

Hairs are specialized epidermal derivatives that arise as the result of inductive stimuli from the dermis. There are many

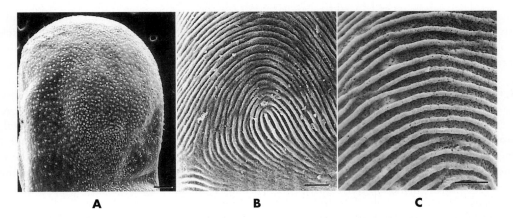

A   **B**   **C**

Figure 8-6 Scanning electron micrographs of human digital palmar skin in a **14-week-old** fetus. **A,** Low-power view of the palmar surface of a digit. **B,** Epidermal surface of the dermis of the fingertip showing the primary dermal ridges. **C,** Basal surface of the epidermis showing the epidermal ridges. *Bars,* 100 μm. (From Misumi Y, Akiyoshi T: *Am J Anat* 119:419, 1991.)

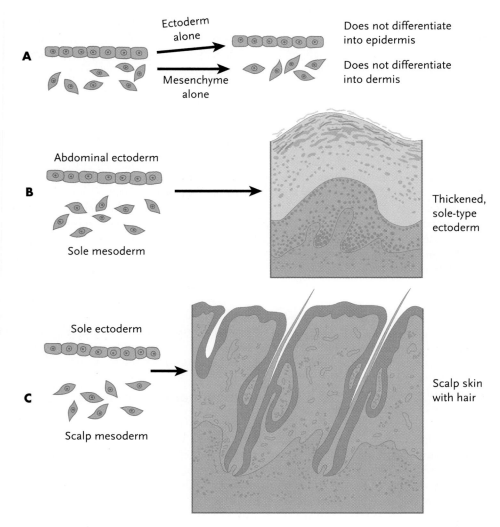

Figure 8-7 Recombination experiments illustrating the importance of tissue interactions in the differentiation of the skin. When separated (**A**), ectoderm and underlying mesenchyme do not differentiate. Recombinations (**B** and **C**) show that the dermis determines the nature of the ectodermal differentiation.

types of hairs, ranging from the coarse hairs of the eyelashes and eyebrows to the barely visible hairs on the abdomen and back. Regional differences in morphology and patterns of distribution are imposed on the epidermis by the underlying dermis.

Hair formation is first recognizable at about the twelfth week of pregnancy as regularly spaced epidermal downgrowths associated with small condensations of dermal cells called **dermal papillae** (Figure 8-8). Under the continuing influence of a dermal papilla, the epidermal downgrowth continues over the next few weeks and forms an early **hair peg**. In succeeding weeks the epidermal peg overgrows the dermal papilla, resulting in the shaping of an early **hair follicle**. At this stage the hair follicle still does not protrude beyond the outer surface of the epidermis, but in the portion of the follicle that penetrates deeply into the dermis, bulges in the epidermis (1) presage the formation of **sebaceous glands**, which

secrete an oily skin lubricant (**sebum**), and (2) are the attachment site for the tiny **arrector pili muscle**. The arrector pili is a mesodermally derived smooth muscle that lifts the hair to a near-vertical position in a cold environment. In many animals, this increases the insulation properties of the hair.

More is understood about the mechanisms underlying the formation of feathers than hairs. However, hairs are homologous with feathers, so it is highly likely that the fundamental mechanisms underlying feather formation will apply to hairs as well. The first step in the formation of an epidermal appendage, such as a hair or feather, is the action of mesenchymally produced growth factors, specifically bone morphogenetic proteins (BMPs) and fibroblast growth factors (FGFs), on the overlying ectoderm, causing the ectoderm to thicken into a **placode** for each hair that will form. The thickened ectodermal placodes then produce the signaling molecules—**FGF-2, sonic hedgehog**, and **BMP-2**—

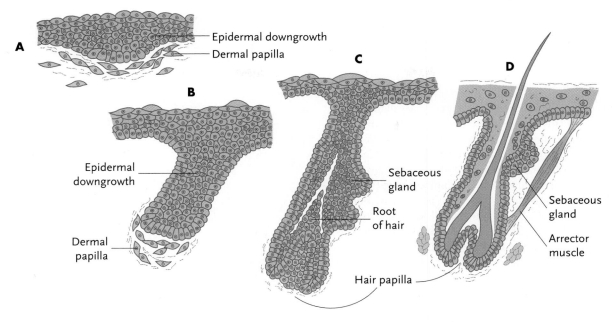

Figure 8-8 Differentiation of a human hair follicle. **A,** Hair primordium (**12 weeks**). **B,** Early hair peg (**15 to 16 weeks**). **C,** Bulbous hair follicle (**18 weeks**). **D,** Adult hair.

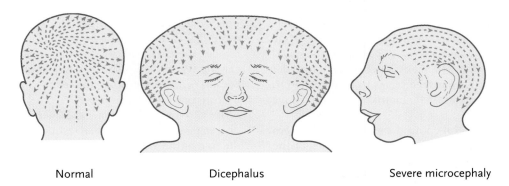

Normal   Dicephalus   Severe microcephaly

Figure 8-9 Patterns of whorls of hair in normal and abnormal fetuses.

which in turn cause the underlying mesenchyme to condense (dermal papilla). In a number of developing systems the class of homeobox-containing genes, **Msx,** is produced at times and places where cellular proliferation is prominent. This is the case in the formation of skin appendages, in which the production of Msx by the thickened ectoderm is associated with intense proliferation of both the ectoderm and the underlying dermis. Finally, the expression of various *Hox* genes appears important in determining the type of epidermal appendage that will form (e.g., eyebrow versus fine hair of cheek).

Erupted hairs are first seen on the eyebrows shortly after 16 weeks. Within a couple of weeks, they cover the scalp. The eruption of hairs follows a cephalocaudal gradient over the body. During the later stages of hair formation, the hair bulb becomes infiltrated with melanocytes, which provide color to the hair. Starting around the fifth month, the epi-

dermal cells of the hair shaft begin to undergo keratinization, forming firm granules of **trichohyalin,** which imparts hardness to the hair.

Products of the fetal sebaceous glands accumulate on the surface of the skin as **vernix caseosa.** This substance may serve as a protective coating for the epidermis, which is continually exposed to amniotic fluid. The first fetal hairs are very fine in texture and are close together. Known as **lanugo,** they are most prominent during the seventh and eighth months. Lanugo hairs are typically shed just before birth and are replaced by coarser definitive hairs, which arise from newly formed follicles.

The pattern of epidermal appendages such as hairs has been shown experimentally to relate to patterns generated in the dermis. Other studies have compared patterns of scalp hairs between normal embryos and those with cranial malformations (Figure 8-9) and have shown a correlation between whorls and the direction of hair growth and the tension on the epidermis at the time of formation of the hair follicles.

Mammary glands

As with many glandular structures, the mammary glands arise as epithelial (in this case, ectodermal) downgrowths into mesenchyme in response to inductive influences by the mesenchyme. The first morphological evidence of mammary gland development is the appearance of two bands of ectodermal thickenings called **milk lines** running along the ventrolateral body walls in embryos of both genders at about 6 weeks (Figure 8-10, A). The craniocaudal level and the extent along the milk lines at which mammary tissue develops vary among species. Comparing the location of mammary tissue in cows (caudal), humans (in the pectoral region), and dogs (along the length of the milk line) demonstrates the wide variation in location and number of mammary glands. In humans, supernumerary mammary tissue or nipples can be found anywhere along the length of the original milk lines (Figure 8-10, B).

Mammary ductal epithelial downgrowths (Figure 8-11) are associated with two types of mesoderm: fibroblastic and fatty. Experimental evidence suggests that inductive interactions with the fatty component of the connective tissue are responsible for the characteristic shaping of the mammary duct system. As with many developing glandular structures, the inductive message seems to be mediated to a great extent by the extracellular matrix of the connective tissue.

Although the mesoderm controls the branching pattern of the ductal epithelium, the functional properties of the mammary ducts are intrinsic to the epithelial component. An experiment in which mouse mammary ectoderm was combined with salivary gland mesenchyme illustrates this point. The mammary ducts developed a branching pattern characteristic of salivary gland epithelium, but despite this, the mammary duct cells produced one of the milk proteins, α-lactalbumin.

In keeping with their role as secondary sexual characteristics, mammary glands are extremely responsive to the hormonal environment. This has been shown by experiments conducted on mice. In contrast to the continued downgrowth of ductal epithelium in females, the mammary ducts in male mice respond to the presence of testosterone by undergoing a rapid involution. Female mammary ducts react similarly if they are exposed to testosterone. Further analysis has shown that the effect of testosterone is mediated through the mammary mesenchyme rather than acting directly on the ductal epithelium. Conversely, if male mammary ducts are allowed to develop in the absence of testosterone, they assume a female morphology.

The role of the mesoderm and **testosterone receptors** is well illustrated in experiments involving mice with a genetic

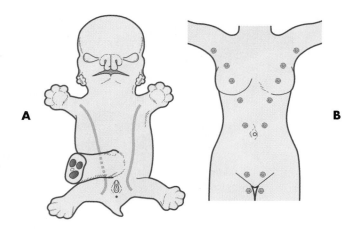

Figure 8-10 A, Milk lines (*blue*) in a generalized mammalian embryo. Mammary glands form along these lines. B, Common formation sites for supernumerary nipples or mammary glands along the course of the milk lines in the human.

mutant, **androgen insensitivity syndrome.** This is the counterpart of a human condition called the **testicular feminization syndrome,** in which genetic males lack testosterone receptors. Despite having high circulating levels of testosterone, these individuals develop female phenotypes, including typical female breast development (Figure 8-12, A), because without receptors, the tissue cannot respond to the testosterone.

In vitro recombination experiments on mice with androgen insensitivity have been instrumental in understanding the role of the mesoderm in mediating the effects of testosterone on mammary duct development (Figure 8-12, B). If mutant mammary ectoderm is combined with normal mesoderm in the presence of testosterone, the mammary ducts regress, but normal ectoderm combined with mutant mesoderm continues to form normal mammary ducts despite being exposed to high levels of testosterone. This shows that the genetic defect in testicular feminization is expressed in the mesoderm.

The postnatal development of female mammary gland tissue is also highly responsive to its hormonal environment. The simple mammary duct system that was laid down in the embryo remains in an infantile condition until it is exposed to the changing hormonal environment at the onset of puberty (Figure 8-13, A). Increasing levels of circulating estrogens and other, less prominent hormonal changes stimulate the proliferation of the mammary ducts and enlargement of the pad of fatty tissue that underlies it (Figure 8-13, B). The next major change in the complete cycle of mammary tissue development occurs during pregnancy, although minor cyclical changes in mammary tissue are detectable in each menstrual cycle. During pregnancy, increased amounts of progesterone, along with prolactin and placental lactogen, stimulate the development of secretory alveoli at the ends of

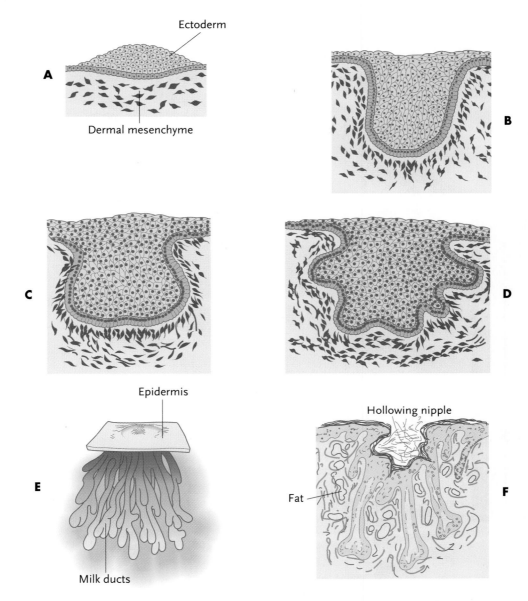

Figure 8-11 Stages in the embryonic development of the human mammary gland. A, Sixth week. B, Seventh week. C, Tenth week. D, Fourth month. E, Sixth month. F, Eighth month.

the branched ducts (Figure 8-13, C). With continuing development of the alveoli, the epithelial cells build up increased numbers of the cytoplasmic organelles, such as rough endoplasmic reticulum and the Golgi apparatus, that are involved in protein synthesis and secretion.

Lactation involves a number of reciprocal influences between the mammary glands and the brain. (These are summarized in Figure 8-13, D). Stimulated by prolactin secretion from the anterior pituitary, the alveolar cells synthesize milk proteins (**casein** and **α-lactalbumin**) and lipids. In a rapid response to the suckling stimulus, the ejection of milk is trig-

gered by the release of **oxytocin** by the posterior portion of the pituitary. Oxytocin causes the contraction of **myoepithelial cells,** which surround the alveoli. Suckling also causes an inhibition of the release of luteinizing hormone–releasing hormone by the hypothalamus, resulting in the inhibition of ovulation and a natural form of birth control.

With cessation of nursing, reduced prolactin secretion and the inhibitory effects of nonejected milk in the mammary alveoli result in the cessation of milk production. The mammary alveoli regress, and the duct system of the mammary gland returns to the nonpregnant state (Figure 8-13, E).

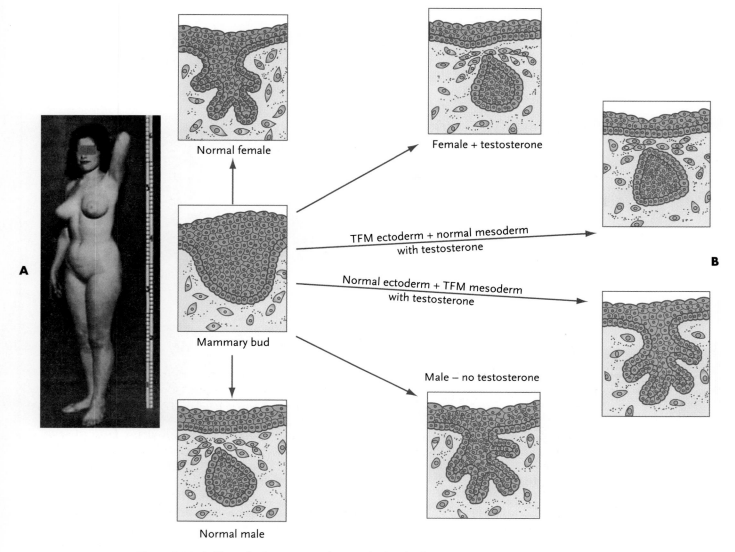

Figure 8-12 A, Testicular feminization, showing the female phenotype of an individual who had primary amenorrhea. Examination of the gonads after removal revealed immature testicular tubules. **B**, Roles of genetic specificity and testosterone in the development of mouse mammary gland tissue. With normal female mammary tissue *(top center)*, the addition of testosterone causes prospective duct tissue to detach and regress as in normal male development. Conversely, in the absence of testosterone, male ductal primordia *(bottom center)* assume a female configuration. In the testicular feminization mutant *(TFM)*, if normal mammary ectoderm is cultured with TFM mammary mesoderm in the presence of testosterone, mammary duct epithelium continues to develop *(lower right)*. If normal male mammary mesoderm is combined with TFM ectoderm in the presence of testosterone, the normal male pattern of separation and regression of mammary duct epithelium occurs *(upper right)*, showing that the genetic defect is expressed in TFM mesoderm. (**A** from Morris JM, Mahesh VB: *Am J Obstet Gynecol* 87:731, 1963. **B** based on studies by Kratochwil K: *J Embryol Exp Morphol* 25:141-153, 1971.)

Normal female

Female + testosterone

TFM ectoderm + normal mesoderm with testosterone

Mammary bud

Normal ectoderm + TFM mesoderm with testosterone

Male – no testosterone

Normal male

A

B

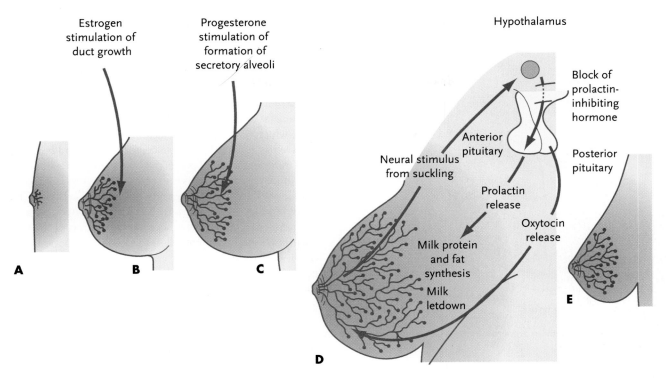

Figure 8-13 Development of the mammary ducts and hormonal control of mammary gland development and function. **A,** Newborn. **B,** Young adult. **C,** Adult. **D,** Lactating adult. **E,** Adult after lactation.

CLINICAL CORRELATION 8-1
Abnormalities of Skin Development

Several types of anomalies affect the integumentary system. **Ectodermal dysplasia** is a germ layer defect that can affect a number of ectodermal derivatives depending on the type and severity of the condition. In addition to abnormalities of the epidermis itself, this syndrome can include the absence or abnormalities of hairs and teeth and short stature (caused by anterior pituitary gland maldevelopment).

A number of relatively rare conditions are included among the genetically transmitted disorders of keratinization. **Ichthyosis** is characterized by scaling and cracking of a hyperkeratinized epidermis. Disorders of sweat glands are commonly associated with this condition. A more severe autosomal recessive disorder is a **harlequin fetus,** in which epidermal platelike structures form, with deep cracks between the structures, because the skin cannot expand to accommodate the increasing bulk of the fetus. Infants with this condition typically do not survive longer than a few weeks.

Angiomas of the skin (birthmarks) are vascular malformations characterized by localized red or purplish spots ranging in size from tiny dots to formations many inches in diameter. Angiomas consist of abnormally prominent plexuses of blood vessels in the dermis, and they may be raised above the level of the skin or a mucous membrane.

SKELETON

Skeletal tissue is present in almost all regions of the body, and the individual skeletal elements are quite diverse in morphology and tissue architecture. However, despite this diversity, there are some fundamental embryological commonalities.

All skeletal tissue arises from cells with a mesenchymal morphology, but the origins of the mesenchyme vary in different regions of the body. In the trunk the mesenchyme that gives rise to the segmented **axial skeleton** (i.e., vertebral column, ribs, sternum) originates from the sclerotomal portion of the mesodermal somites, whereas the appendicular skeleton (the bones of the limbs and their respective girdles) is derived from the mesenchyme of the lateral plate mesoderm.

The origins of the head skeleton are more complex. Some cranial bones (e.g., those making up the roof and much of the base of the skull) are mesodermal in origin, but the facial bones and some of the bones covering the brain arise from mesenchyme derived from the ectodermal neural crest.

The deep skeletal elements of the body typically first appear as cartilaginous models of the bones that will ultimately be formed (Figure 8-14). At specific periods during embryogenesis, the cartilage is replaced by true bone through the process of **endochondral ossification**. In contrast, the superficial bones of the face and skull form by the direct ossification of mesenchymal cells without an intermediate cartilaginous stage (**intramembranous bone formation**). Microscopic details of both intramembranous and

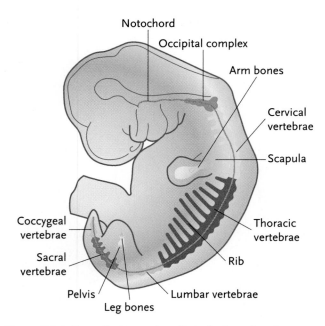

Figure 8-14 Precartilaginous primordia in the 9-mm long human embryo.

endochondral bone formation are presented in the standard histology texts and are not repeated here.

A common element of many mesenchymal cell precursors of skeletal elements is their migration or relative displacement from their site of origin to the area where the bone will ultimately form. The displacement can be relatively minor, such as the aggregation of cells from the sclerotome of the receding somite around the notochord to form the body (**centrum**) of a vertebra, or it can involve extensive migrations of cranial neural crest cells to their final destinations as membrane bones of the face.

To differentiate into defined skeletal elements, the mesenchymal precursor cells must often interact with elements of their immediate environment—typically epithelia with associated basal laminae—or components of the neighboring extracellular matrix. Details of the interactions vary among regions of the body. In the limb, for example, a continuous interaction between the **apical ectodermal ridge** (see Chapter 9) and the underlying limb bud mesoderm is involved in the specification of the limb skeleton. An inductive interaction between the sclerotome and notochord or neural tube initiates skeletogenesis of the vertebral column. In the head, preskeletal cells of the neural crest may receive information at levels ranging from the neural tube itself to sites along their path of migration to the region of their final destination. Inductive interactions between regions of the brain and the overlying mesenchyme stimulate formation of the membrane bones of the cranial vault.

Regardless of the sources and types of environmental information that are used by the skeletal precursor cells, after they arrive at their final destinations, these cells typically un-

dergo a local condensation before overt signs of differentiation occur. The condensation phase of bone formation is typically accompanied by the up-regulation of N-CAM, which is one of the molecules that mediates adhesion of the bone-forming cells and promotes the establishment of a prebone condensation.

Skeletal tissues differentiate from pluripotent mesenchymal cells, which have the ability to differentiate into fibrous connective tissue, fat cells, muscle cells, cartilage, and bone. Specific transcription factors are known to direct the differentiation of mesenchymal cells into both adipocytes (fat cells) and muscle cells (see p. 174). Recently a transcription factor, **Cbfa1** (**core binding factor a1**), which is a gene related to the pair rule genes of *Drosophila*, has been shown to control the differentiation of mesenchymal cells into **osteoblasts** (bone-forming cells), but the formation of cartilage is independent of this gene. Mice bearing homozygous mutants of *Cbfa1* form the cartilaginous models of endochondral bones, but these bones never ossify; instead they undergo some calcification but remain as calcified cartilage. Intramembranous bones of the head and face do not form in these mice. **Bone morphogenetic proteins (BMPs)**, especially BMP-2, BMP-4, and BMP-7, are involved in embryonic bone formation. BMPs operate at several stages in the formation of bone, but some evidence suggests that an early function is to stimulate the expression of Cbfa1. The morphogenesis of individual skeletal elements is often under complex sets of controls, ranging from pattens of *Hox* gene expression in the somite stage embryogenesis to inductive interactions between epithelia and mesenchymal precursor cells to mechanical influences that can act at any time from the early stages of morphogenesis to late postnatal life.

Axial Skeleton

Vertebral column and ribs

The earliest stages in establishing the axial skeleton were introduced in Chapter 5. Formation of the axial skeleton, however, is more complex than the simple subdivision of the paraxial mesoderm into somites and the medial displacement of sclerotomal cells to form primordia of the vertebrae. Each vertebra has a complex and unique morphology specified by controls operating at several levels and during several developmental periods.

According to the traditional view of vertebral development (see Figure 5-19), the sclerotomes split into cranial and caudal halves, and the densely packed caudal half of one sclerotome joins with the loosely packed cranial half of the next to form the centrum of a vertebra. Recent morphological research suggests that vertebral development is more complex than this model, as indicated by the scheme illustrated in Figure 8-15.

The vertebral column is divided into several general areas (see Figure 8-14): (1) an **occipital region**, which is incorporated into the bony structure of the base of the skull; (2) a

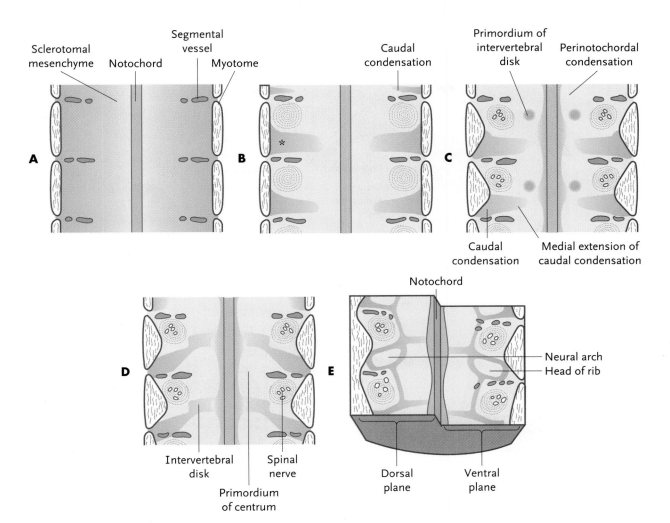

Figure 8-15 Frontal sections through the developing vertebral column. A, Early stage, showing sclerotomal mesenchyme with a lesser density of cells around the notochord than laterally. The segmental vessels mark the division between adjacent somites. B, Lateral sclerotomal mesenchyme shows a band of greater density (*asterisk*) in the caudal half. The density of cells around the notochord is still low. C, Transverse band of densely packed cells in the cranial portion of the sclerotome represents the primordium of the intervertebral disk. Although a thin layer of densely packed cells surrounds the notochord, the bulk of the primordium of the centrum of the vertebra is a triangular mass of loosely packed cells. The condensed primordium of the neural arch and transverse process extends diagonally from just caudal to the intervertebral disk to the caudal edge of the lateral border of the sclerotome. D, All components described in C are better defined. The centrum arises from mesenchyme extending continuously from the caudal half of one somite to the cranial half of the next. (Note the position of the intersegmental vessels.) The spinal nerves pass through the cranial half of the sclerotome. E, Left side shows a dorsal level through the developing vertebrae, with the neural arch visible. The right side shows a more ventral plane, with the head of the rib articulating with the centrum below the level of the neural arch and transverse process.(Based on studies by Verbout AJ: *Adv Anat Embryol Cell Biol* 90:1-122, 1985.)

cervical region, which includes the highly specialized **atlas** and **axis** that link the vertebral column to the skull; (3) the **thoracic region**, from which the true ribs arise; (4) the **lumbar region**; (5) a **sacral region**, in which the vertebrae are fused into a single **sacrum**; and (6) a **caudal region**, which represents the tail in most mammals and the rudimentary **coccyx** in humans. A typical vertebra arises from the fusion of several cartilaginous primordia. The centrum, which is derived

from the ventromedial sclerotomal portions of the paired somites (see Figure 5-18), surrounds the notochord and serves as a bony floor for the spinal cord (Figure 8-16). The **neural arches**, arising from lateral sclerotomal cells, fuse on either side with the centrum and along with other neural arches, form a protective roof over the spinal cord. Incomplete closure of the bony roof results in a common anomaly called **spina bifida occulta** (see Figure 10-40). The **costal process**

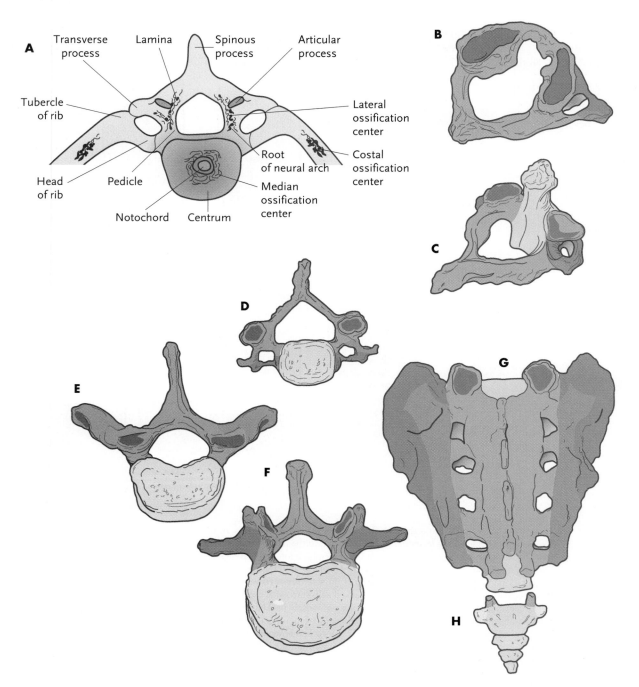

Figure 8-16 **A**, Structure of a thoracic vertebra. **B** to **H**, Specific types of vertebrae, with homologous structures shown in the same color. **B**, Atlas with axis shown in its normal position beneath. **C**, Axis. **D**, Cervical vertebra. **E**, Thoracic vertebra. **F**, Lumbar vertebra. **G**, Sacrum. **H**, Coccyx.

forms the true ribs at the level of the thoracic vertebrae. At other levels along the vertebral column the costal processes become incorporated into the vertebrae proper.

Development of an individual vertebra begins with a sonic hedgehog–mediated (shh-mediated) induction by the notochord on the early somite to form the sclerotome. Under the continuing influence of shh, the ventromedial portion of the somite will ultimately form the centrum of the vertebra. Formation of the dorsal part of the vertebra (the neural arch) is guided by a different set of developmental controls. An initial induction from the roof plate of the neural tube results in the expression of Pax-9 and the homeobox-containing gene *Msx-2*, which guides cells of the lateral sclerotome to form the neural arch.

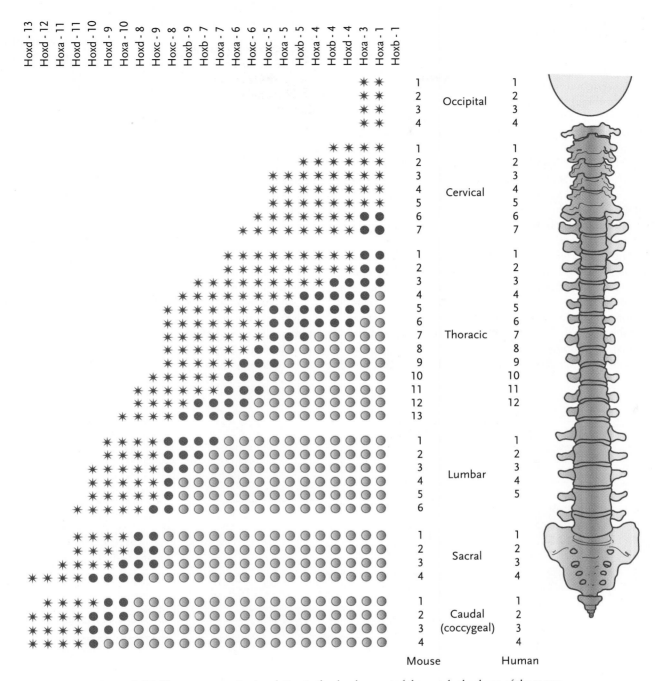

Figure 8-17 *Hox* gene expression in relation to the development of the vertebral column of the mouse. Note that the vertebral column of the mouse (*left*) has one more thoracic and one more lumbar vertebra than does the vertebral column of the human. Green asterisks indicate levels at which there is definite expression of the *Hox* gene indicated at the top of the column. Purple circles represent the caudal border where expression fades out. (Based on studies by Kessel M, Balling R, Gruss P: *Cell* 61:301-308, 1990.)

The fundamental regional characteristics of the vertebrae are specified by the actions of discrete combinations of homeobox-containing genes (Figure 8-17). Expression of the *Hox* genes begins with the first appearance of the presomitic mesoderm and for most genes persists until chondrification begins in the primordia of the vertebrae. Formation of the normal segmental pattern along the craniocaudal axis of the vertebral column may be ensured by the fact that most vertebrae are specified by a unique combination of *Hox* genes. For example, in the mouse the atlas (C-1) is characterized by the expression of *Hoxa-1, Hoxa-3, Hoxb-1,* and *Hoxd-4.* The axis (C-2) is specified by these four genes plus *Hoxa-4* and *Hoxb-4.* **Retinoic acid** (vitamin A) can cause cranial or caudal level shifts in the overall segmental organization of the vertebrae if applied at specific developmental periods. For example, if administered early, retinoic acid results in a cranial level shift (the last cervical vertebra is transformed into the first thoracic vertebra), and later administration causes a caudal level shift (thoracic vertebrae extend into the levels of the first two lumbar vertebrae). Such shifts in level are called **homeotic transformations** and are representative of the broad family of homeotic mutants described in Chapter 5. In about 5% of humans, there are minor variations in the number or proportions of vertebrae. The **Klippel-Feil syndrome**, sometimes called **brevicollis**, is characterized by a short neck with a reduced number of cervical vertebrae, a low hairline, and other assorted anomalies. These variations in vertebral organization are likely related to imbalances of the expression of key homeobox-containing gene products.

Among the vertebrae, the axis and atlas have an unusual morphology and distinctive origin (Figure 8-18). The centrum of the atlas is deficient, but the area of the centrum is penetrated by the protruding **odontoid process** of the axis. The odontoid process consists of three fused centra that are presumably equivalent: (1) a half-segment from the centrum of a transitional bone (the **proatlas**) not found in humans, (2) the centrum that should have belonged to the atlas, and

(3) the normal centrum of the axis. This arrangement permits a greater rotation of the head about the cervical spine. When the ubiquitously expressed *Hoxa-7* transgene was introduced into the germline of mice, the cranial part of the vertebral column was posteriorized. The base of the occipital bone was transformed into an occipital vertebra (the proatlas), and the atlas was combined with its centrum, resulting in an axis that did not possess an odontoid process.

The ribs arise from zones of condensed mesenchymal cells lateral to the centrum (see Figure 8-16). By the time ossification in the vertebrae begins, the ribs separate from the vertebrae. **Accessory ribs**, especially in the upper lumbar and lower cervical levels, are common, but estimates of the incidence vary widely from one series to the next. Somewhat less than 1% may be a realistic estimate. These and other common rib anomalies (**forked** or **fused ribs**) are typically asymptomatic and are usually detected on x-ray examination. They are probably the result of misexpression of specific *Hox* genes.

The **sternum** arises as a pair of cartilaginous bands that converge at the ventral midline as the ventral body wall consolidates (Figure 8-19). After the primordial sternal bands come together, they reveal their true segmental nature by secondarily subdividing into craniocaudal elements. Such sec-

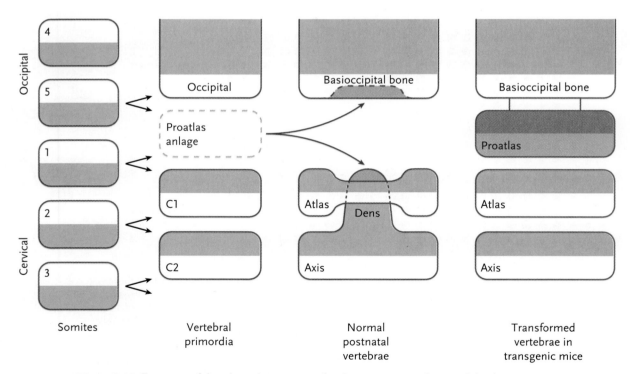

Figure 8-18 Formation of the atlas and axis in normal and transgenic mice. In normal development, cells from a proatlas anlage contribute to the formation of the basioccipital bone and the dens of the axis. The normal atlas forms an anterior arch (only a transient structure in other vertebrae) instead of a centrum. The cells that would normally form the centrum at the level of the atlas instead fuse with the axis to form the dens of the axis. In mice containing the *Hoxa-7* (A7) transgene, a proatlas forms, and the atlas and axis have the form of typical vertebrae (*right column*). (Based on studies by Kessel M, Balling R, Gruss P: *Cell* 61:301-308, 1990.)

ondary segmentation follows an early morphological and molecular course that closely parallels the formation of synovial joints (see p. 198). Many of these ultimately fuse as they ossify to form a common unpaired body of the sternum. Several common anomalies of the sternum (e.g., **split xiphoid process**) are readily understood from its embryological development. Malformations of the xiphoid process are seen in mice mutant for both *Hoxc-4* and *Hoxa-5*, and mice mutant for *Hoxb-4* have split sternums.

The **clavicle** is sometimes considered to be part of the appendicular skeleton because it connects the sternum to the shoulder. The clavicle is one of the first bones in the body to become ossified, with ossification well advanced by the eighth week. Recent studies of mice heterozygous for the *Cbfa1* gene have shed light not only on the nature of the clavicle but also on a poorly understood human syndrome. Such heterozygotes exhibit hypoplasia of the clavicle, delayed ossification of membrane bones (e.g., of the skull), and open anterior and posterior fontanelles in the skull. **Cleidocranial dysplasia** in humans exhibits all of these conditions, as well as supernumerary teeth. Without clavicles, affected individuals can approximate their shoulders in the anterior midline. The findings in this mutant suggest that the clavicle is a purely membranous bone and may

be a unique class of bone, being neither truly axial or appendicular in the usual sense.

Another late development is the disappearance of the notochord from the bodies of the vertebrae. Between the vertebrae the notochord expands into the condensed mesenchymal primordia of the intervertebral disks. In the adult the notochord persists as the **nucleus pulposus,** which constitutes the soft core of the disk. The bulk of the **intervertebral disk** consists of layers of fibrocartilage that differentiate from sclerotomally derived mesodermal cells. *Pax-1* is expressed continuously during the development of intervertebral disks. In a mouse mutant, *undulated, Pax-1* expression is deficient, and fusion of the vertebral bodies results. It appears that *Pax-1* expression and the subsequent formation of the intervertebral disks are important mechanisms in maintaining the individual segmental character of the vertebral column.

The caudal end of the axial skeleton is represented by a well-defined, tail-like appendage during much of the second month (Figure 8-20, *A*). During the third month, the tail normally regresses, largely through cell death and differential growth, to persist as the coccyx, but rarely a well-developed tail persists in newborns.

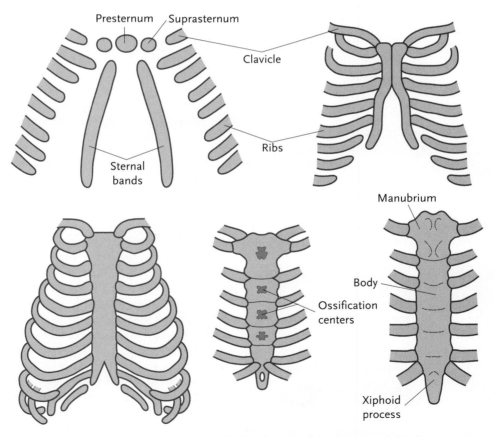

Figure 8-19 Successive stages in the development of the sternum and clavicle.

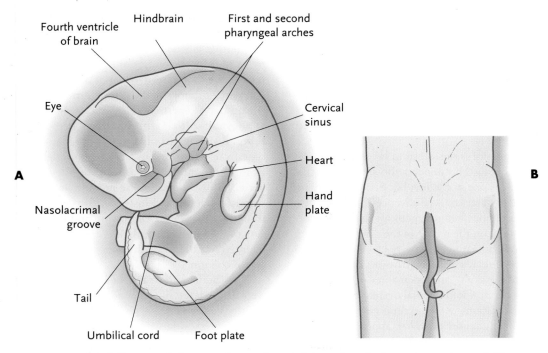

Figure 8-20 A, Drawing of a human embryo at the end of the **sixth week,** showing a prominent tail. Normally the tail regresses. **B,** Drawing of a persisting tail (9 inches long) in a **12-year-old boy.** (**B** modified from Patten BM: *Human embryology,* ed 3, New York, 1968, McGraw-Hill.)

Skull

The skull is a composite structure consisting of two major subdivisions: the **neurocranium,** which surrounds the brain, and the **viscerocranium,** which surrounds the oral cavity, pharynx, and upper respiratory passages. Each of these subdivisions in turn consists of two components, one in which the individual bones are first represented by cartilaginous models and are subsequently replaced by bone through endochondral ossification and another in which bone arises directly through the ossification of mesenchyme.

The phylogenetic and ontogenetic foundation of the skull is represented by the **chondrocranium,** which is the cartilaginous base of the neurocranium (Figure 8-21, *A*). The fundamental pattern of the chondrocranium has been remarkably preserved in the course of phylogeny. It is initially represented by several sets of paired cartilages. One group (parachordals, hypophyseal cartilages, and trabeculae cranii) is closely related to midline structures. Caudal to the parachordal cartilages are four **occipital sclerotomes.** Along with the parachordal cartilages the occipital sclerotomes, which are homologous with precursors of the vertebrae, fuse to form the base of the occipital bone. More laterally, the chondrocranium is represented by pairs of cartilage that are associated with epithelial primordia of the sense organs (olfactory organ, eyes, and auditory organ).

The individual primordial elements of the chondrocranium undergo several patterns of growth and fusion to form the structurally complex bones of the basicranium (the occipital, sphenoid, and temporal bones as well as much of the deep bony support of the nasal cavity) (Figure 8-21, *B*). In addition, some of these bones (e.g., the occipital and temporal bones) incorporate membranous components during their development, so in their final form, they are truly composite structures (Figure 8-21, *D*). Other components of the neurocranium, such as the parietal and frontal bones, are purely membranous bones (Box 8-2).

Virtually all the bones of the neurocranium arise as the result of an inductive influence of an epithelial structure on the neighboring mesenchyme. These interactions are typically mediated by growth factors and the extracellular matrix. Immunocytochemical studies have shown the transient appearance of **type II collagen** (the principal collagenous component of cartilage) at the sites and times during which the interactions leading to the formation of the chondrocranium take place. In addition to type II collagen, a **cartilage-specific pro-**

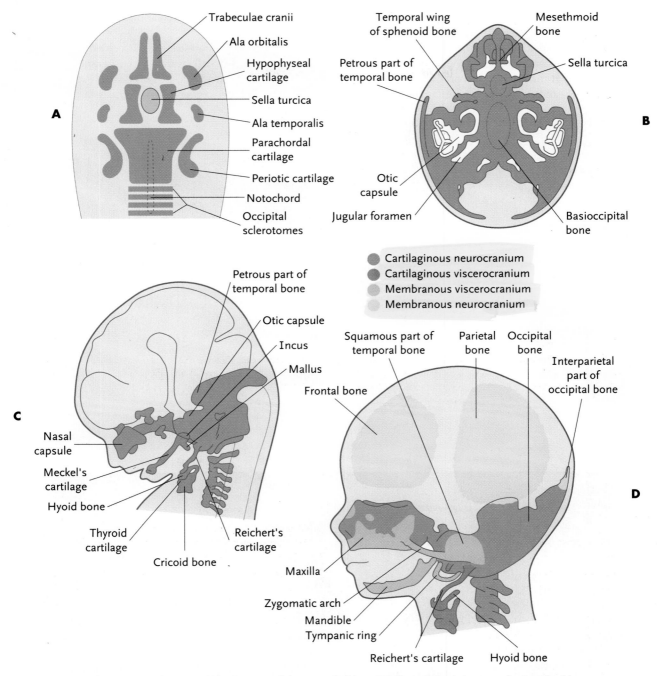

Figure 8-21 Origins and development of the major skull bones. **A,** Basic skeletal elements of a **6-week-old** embryo viewed from above. **B,** Chondrocranium of an **8-week-old** embryo viewed from above. **C,** Lateral view of the embryo illustrated in **B**. **D,** Skull of a **3-month-old** embryo. (Modified from Carlson B: *Patten's foundations of embryology*, ed 6, New York, 1996, McGraw-Hill.)

teoglycan also accumulates in areas of induction of chondrocranial elements. There is increasing evidence that epithelial elements in the head not only induce the skeleton but also control its morphogenesis. This contrasts with morphogenetic control of the appendicular skeleton, which is determined by the mesoderm rather than the ectoderm of the limb bud.

Elements of the membranous neurocranium (the paired parietal and frontal bones and the interparietal part of the occipital bone) arise as flat, platelike aggregations of bony spicules (trabeculae) from mesenchyme that has been induced by specific parts of the developing brain. These bones remain separate structures during fetal development, and even at birth, they are separated by connective tissue sutures. Intersections between sutures where more than two bones meet are occupied by broader areas of connective tissue called **fontanelles**. The most prominent fontanelles are the **anterior fontanelle**, located at the intersection of the two frontal and two parietal bones, and the **posterior fontanelle**, located at

the intersection of the parietal bones and the single occipital bone (Figure 8-22).

Like the neurocranium, the viscerocranium consists of two divisions: a **cartilaginous viscerocranium** and a **membranous viscerocranium**. In contrast to the neurocranium, the bones of the viscerocranium originate largely from neural

---

BOX 8-2 Embryological Origins of Bones of the Cranium

NEUROCRANIUM

Chondrocranium
  Occipital
  Sphenoid
  Ethmoid
  Petrous and mastoid part of temporal
Membranous neurocranium
  Interparietal part of occipital
  Parietal
  Frontal
  Squamous part of temporal

VISCEROCRANIUM

Pharyngeal Arch I

Cartilaginous viscerocranium
  Meckel's cartilage
    Malleus
    Incus

Membranous viscerocranium
  Maxillary process (superficial)
    Squamous part of temporal
    Zygomatic
    Maxillary
    Premaxillary
    Nasal?
    Lacrimal?
  Maxillary process (deep)
    Palatine
    Vomer
    Pterygoid laminae
  Mandibular process
    Mandible
    Tympanic ring

Pharyngeal Arch II

Cartilaginous viscerocranium
  Reichert's cartilage
    Stapes
    Styloid process

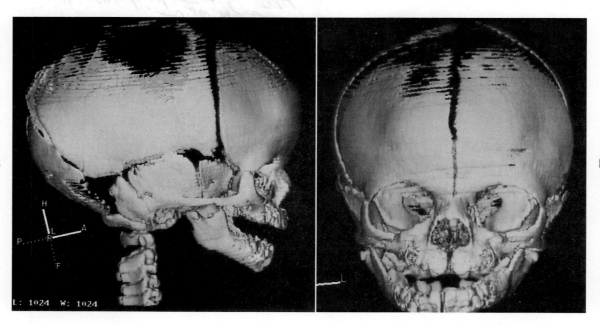

Figure 8-22 High-resolution computed tomographic scans of the skull of a **34½-week-old** fetus. **A**, Lateral view. **B**, Frontal view. The midline fissure in the forehead area is the metopic suture, which normally becomes obliterated after birth. The irregular black area above that is the anterior fontanelle, one of the "soft spots" in a newborn's head. In these images the skeletal anatomy was reconstructed by two-dimensional algorithms followed by three-dimensional reconstructions. (Courtesy R.A. Levy, H. Maher, and A.R. Burdi, Ann Arbor, Mich.)

crest–derived mesenchyme. Phylogenetically, the viscerocranium is related to the skeleton of the **branchial arches** (gill arches). Each branchial arch (more commonly called a *pharyngeal arch* in humans) is supported by a cartilaginous rod, which gives rise to a number of definitive skeletal elements characteristic of that arch (see Box 8-2). (Details of the organization and derivatives of the noncranial pharyngeal arch cartilages are discussed in Chapter 13 [see Figure 13-22].)

The membranous viscerocranium consists of a series of bones associated with the upper and lower jaws and the region of the ear (see Figure 8-21, *D*). These arise in association with the first arch cartilage (**Meckel's cartilage**) and take over some of the functions originally subserved by Meckel's cartilage, as well as a number of new ones, such as sound transmission in the middle ear. Clinical Correlation 8-2 discusses conditions resulting from skull deformities.

CLINICAL CORRELATION 8-2
Conditions Resulting from Skull Deformities

A number of conditions are recognizable by gross deformities of the skull. Although many of these are true congenital malformations, others fall into the class of deformities that can be attributed to mechanical stress during intrauterine life or childbirth. Some malformations of the skull are secondary to disturbances in development of the brain. In this category are conditions such as **acrania** and **anencephaly** (see Figure 7-4), which are associated with severe malformations of the brain; **microcephaly** (see Figure 8-9), in which the size of the cranial vault accommodates to a very small brain; and **hydrocephaly** (see Figure 10-36), a greatly enlarged cranial vault that represents the response of the skeleton of the head to an excessive buildup of cerebrospinal fluid.

One family of cranial malformations called **craniosynostosis** results from premature closure of certain sutures between major membrane bones of the neurocranium. Craniosynostosis is a feature of over 100 human genetic syndromes and is seen in 1 in 3000 live births. One type, the Boston variant, is a dominant gain of function mutant of the homeobox-containing gene *Msx-2* expressed in both the mesenchymal tissue of the early sutures and the underlying neural tissue. Exactly how this mutation is translated into premature suture closure in not known. Premature closure of the **sagittal suture** between the two parietal bones produces a long, keel-shaped skull referred to as **scaphocephaly** (Figure 8-23).

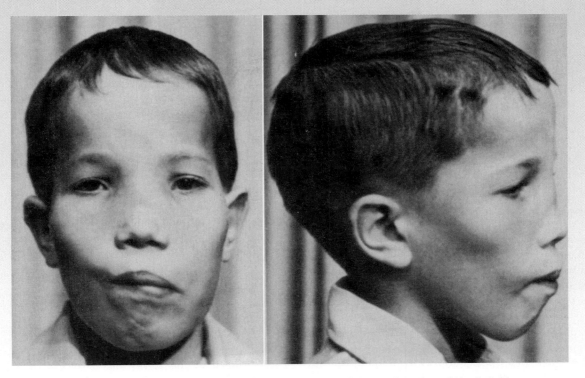

Figure 8-23 Frontal and lateral views of a boy with a narrow and elongated scaphocephalic skull. Note the high forehead and flat bridge of the nose. This patient had an associated facial palsy and mixed deafness. (From Goodman R, Gorlin R: *Atlas of the face in genetic disorders*, St Louis, 1977, Mosby.)

Continued

Oxycephaly, or turret skull, is the result of premature fusion of the **coronal suture,** which is located between the frontal and parietal bones. A dominant genetic condition, **Crouzon's syndrome,** has a gross appearance quite similar to that of oxycephaly, but the malformation of the cranial vault is typically accompanied by malformations of the face, teeth, and ears and occasional malformations in other parts of the body (Figure 8-24).

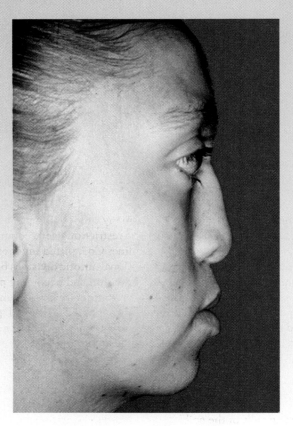

Figure 8-24 Lateral view of the flattened face of an individual with Crouzon's syndrome. (Courtesy A.R. Burdi, Ann Arbor, Mich.)

Appendicular Skeleton

The **appendicular skeleton** consists of the bones of the limbs and limb girdles. There are fundamental differences in organization and developmental control between the axial and appendicular skeleton. The axial skeleton forms a protective casing around soft internal tissues (e.g., brain, spinal cord, pharynx), and the mesenchyme forming the bones is induced by the organs that the bones surround. In contrast, the bones of the appendicular skeleton form a central supporting core of the limbs. Although interaction with an epithelium (the apical ectodermal ridge of the limb bud [see Chapter 9]) is required for the formation of skeletal elements in the limb, morphogenetic control of the limb is inherent in the mesoderm, with the epithelium playing only a stimulatory role.

All components of the appendicular skeleton begin as cartilaginous models, which convert to true bone by endochondral ossification later during embryogenesis. (Details of the formation of the appendicular skeleton are given in Chapter 9.)

MUSCULAR SYSTEM

Three types of musculature—skeletal, cardiac, and smooth—are formed during embryonic development. Virtually all skeletal musculature is derived from the paraxial mesoderm, specifically the somites or somitomeres (see Figure 5-16). Splanchnic mesoderm gives rise to the musculature of the heart (cardiac muscle) and the smooth musculature of the gut

TABLE 8-1 Embryologic Origins of the Major Classes of Muscle

Embryologic origin	Derived muscle	Innervation
Somitomeres 1 through 3 and prechordal plate	Most extrinsic eye muscles	Cranial nerves III and IV
Somitomere 4	Jaw-closing muscles	Cranial nerve V (mandibular branch)
Somitomere 5	Lateral rectus of eye	Cranial nerve VI
Somitomere 6	Jaw-opening and other second-arch muscles	Cranial nerve VII
Somitomere 7	Third-arch branchial muscles	Cranial nerve IX
Somites 1 and 2	Intrinsic laryngeal muscles and pharyngeal muscles	Cranial nerve X
Occipital somites (1 through 7)	Muscles of tongue, larynx, and neck	Cranial nerves XI and XII, cranial cervical nerves
Trunk somites	Trunk muscles, diaphragm, and limb muscles	Spinal nerves
Splanchnic mesoderm	Cardiac muscles	Autonomic
Splanchnic mesoderm	Smooth muscles of gut and respiratory tract	Autonomic
Local mesenchyme	Other smooth muscle: vascular, arrector pili muscles	Autonomic

From Carlson BM: *Patten's foundations of embryology,* ed 6, New York, 1996, McGraw-Hill.

and respiratory tracts (Table 8-1). Other smooth muscle, such as that of the blood vessels and the arrector pili muscles, is derived from local mesoderm.

The development of muscle can be studied at several different levels, ranging from the determination and differentiation of individual muscle cells, to the histogenesis of muscle tissue, and finally to the formation (morphogenesis) of entire muscles. Skeletal muscle will be used as an example to illustrate how development occurs and is controlled at these different levels of organization.

Skeletal Muscle

There is increasing evidence that certain cells of the epiblast are determined to become myogenic cells even before the somites are completely formed, but it is convenient to begin with the emergence of muscle precursor cells in the somites. For many decades the origin of the skeletal musculature was in question, with the somites and lateral plate mesoderm being likely candidates. This issue was finally resolved by tracing studies involving cellular markers (Box 8-3), and it is now known that virtually all of the skeletal muscle originates in somites or somitomeres. Early steps in the determination of myogenic cells in somites are summarized in Figure 5-18.

Determination and differentiation of skeletal muscle

The mature skeletal muscle fiber is a complex multinucleated cell that is specialized for contraction. Precursors of most muscle lineages (**myogenic cells**) have been traced to the myotome of the somite (see Figure 5-17). Although these cells look like the mesenchymal cells that can give rise to

many other cell types in the embryo, they have undergone a restriction event committing them to the muscle-forming line. Committed myogenic cells pass through several additional mitotic divisions before completing a terminal mitotic division and becoming **postmitotic myoblasts.**

Proliferating myogenic cells are kept in the cell cycle through the action of growth factors, such as **fibroblast growth factor (FGF)** and **transforming growth factor-β**. In the myotome of the somite, myogenic regulatory factors (see later section) are expressed in the muscle-forming regions. MyoD, one of these factors, removes the mesenchymal cells from the cell cycle by preventing their entry into the S phase and also stimulates their differentiation by turning on muscle-specific genes. Other growth factors, such as **insulin-like growth factor**, are also involved in promoting muscle differentiation.

Postmitotic myoblasts begin to transcribe the messenger ribonucleic acids (mRNAs) for the major contractile proteins **actin** and **myosin**, but the major event in the life cycle of a postmitotic myoblast is its fusion with other similar cells into a multinucleated **myotube** (Figure 8-26). The fusion of myoblasts is a precise process involving their lining up and adhering by Ca^{++}-mediated recognition mechanisms and the ultimate union of their plasma membranes.

Myotubes are intensively involved in mRNA and protein synthesis. In addition to forming actin and myosin, they synthesize a wide variety of other proteins, including the regulatory proteins of muscle contraction—**troponin** and **tropomyosin**. These proteins assemble into myofibrils, which are precisely arranged aggregates of functional contractile units called **sarcomeres**. As the myotubes fill with myofibrils, their nuclei, which had been arranged in regular central chains, migrate to the periphery of the myotube. At this stage

BOX 8-3   Tracing Studies Involving Cellular Markers

The origins of many tissues in embryos have been identified by grafting tissues from quail embryos into homologous sites in chick embryos. The nuclei of quail cells contain a distinctive mass of dense chromatin and also react with a species-specific monoclonal antibody, enabling researchers to distinguish quail from chick cells with great reliability (Figure 8-25).

If a putative precursor tissue is grafted from a quail into a chick embryo, the grafted quail tissue becomes well integrated into the chick host, and if cells migrate out of the graft, their pathway of migration into the host embryo can be clearly traced. Experiments involving this approach have been particularly useful in studies of muscle and the neural crest.

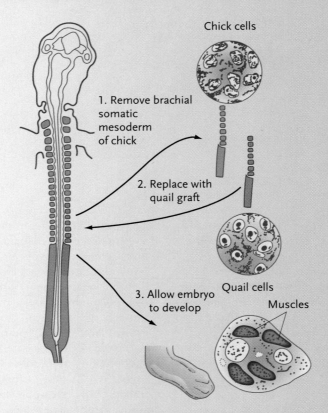

Figure 8-25 Principle of quail/chick grafting for the tracing of cells. *1* and *2*, Quail tissues are transplanted in place of the equivalent tissues removed from the chick embryo. The prominent nuclear chromatin mass in quail cells provides a permanent marker that can be used to trace the fate of the cells of the graft of quail tissue. *3*, When quail somites are grafted into a chick embryo at the appropriate level, the muscles of the limb are derived from quail and not chick cells.

the myotube is considered to have differentiated into a **muscle fiber**, the final stage in the differentiation of the skeletal muscle cell.

The development of a muscle fiber is not complete, however, with the peripheral migration of the nuclei of the myotube. The nuclei (**myonuclei**) of a multinucleated muscle fiber are no longer able to proliferate, but the muscle fiber must continue to grow in proportion to the rapid growth of the fetus and then the infant. Muscle fiber growth is accomplished by means of a population of myogenic cells, called

satellite cells, which take up positions between the muscle fiber and the basal lamina in which each muscle fiber encases itself (see Figure 8-26). Operating under a poorly understood control mechanism, satellite cells divide slowly during the growth of an individual. Some of the daughter cells fuse with the muscle fiber so that the muscle fiber contains an adequate number of nuclei to direct the continuing synthesis of contractile proteins required by the muscle fiber. After muscle fiber damage, satellite cells proliferate and fuse to form regenerating muscle fibers.

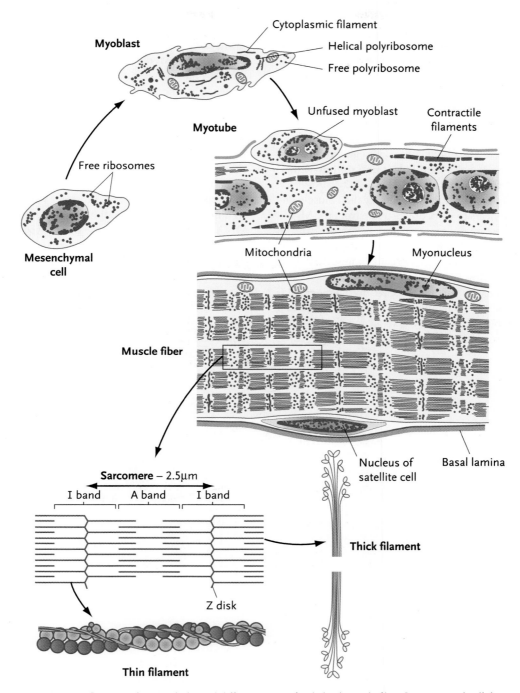

Figure 8-26 Stages in the morphological differentiation of a skeletal muscle fiber. Important subcellular elements in a muscle fiber are also shown.

A typical muscle is not composed of homogeneous muscle fibers. Instead, usually several types of muscle fibers are distinguished by their contractile properties and morphology and by their possession of different isoforms of the contractile proteins. For the purposes of this text, muscle fibers are considered to be either fast or slow.

Muscle Transcription Factors. Myogenesis begins with a restriction event that channels a population of mesenchymal cells into a lineage of committed myogenic cells. The molecular basis for this commitment is the action of members of families of **myogenic regulatory factors** that acting as master genetic regulators, turn on muscle-specific genes in the pre-muscle mesenchymal cells.

The first-discovered family of myogenic regulatory factors is a group of four basic helix-loop-helix transcription factors, sometimes called the **MyoD family** (Figure 8-27). Another, more recently discovered regulatory factor, called **muscle enhancer factor-2**, appears to work downstream from the MyoD family, but all of these myogenic regulatory factors are capable of converting nonmuscle cells (e.g., fibroblasts, adipocytes, chondrocytes, retinal pigment cells) to cells expressing the full range of muscle proteins.

As with many helix-loop-helix proteins, myogenic regulatory proteins of the MyoD family form dimers and bind to a specific deoxyribonucleic acid (DNA) sequence (CANNTG), called the **E box**, in the enhancer region of muscle-specific genes. The myogenic specificity of these proteins is encoded in the basic region (see Figure 8-27).

The regulatory activities of MyoD and other members of that family are themselves regulated by other regulatory proteins, which can modify their activities (Figure 8-28). For example, many cells contain a **transcriptional activator** designated E12. When a molecule of E12 forms a **heterodimer** with a molecule of MyoD, the complex binds more tightly to the muscle-enhancer region of DNA than does a pure MyoD dimer. This increases the efficiency of transcription of the muscle genes. On the other hand, a **transcriptional inhibitor** called **Id** (inhibitor of DNA binding) can form a heterodimer with a molecule of MyoD. Id contains a loop-helix-loop region but no basic region, which is the DNA-binding part of the molecule. The Id molecule has a greater binding affinity for a MyoD molecule than another molecule of MyoD and can thus displace one of the units of a MyoD dimer, resulting in more Id-MyoD heterodimers. These bind very poorly to DNA and often fail to activate muscle specific genes.

During muscle development, the myogenic regulatory factors of the MyoD family are expressed in a regular sequence (Figure 8-29). In mice the events leading to muscle formation begin in the somite, where both **Pax-3** and **myf-5**, working through apparently separate pathways, activate **MyoD**, causing certain cells of the dermomyotome to become committed to forming muscle. With increased levels of

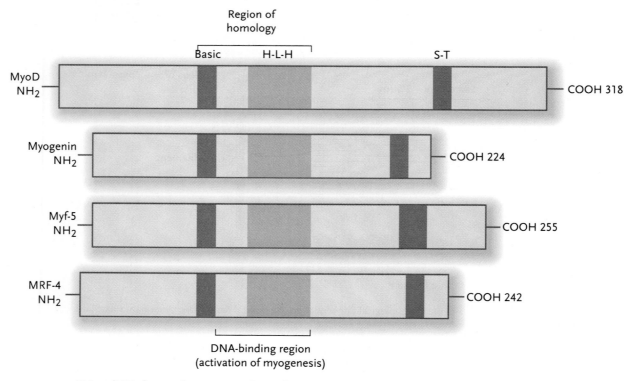

Figure 8-27 Structural comparison of several myogenic regulatory factors. *H-L-H,* Homologous helix-loop-helix regions; *S-T,* homologous serine/threonine-rich region.

MyoD, the mononuclear cells withdraw from the mitotic cycle and begin to fuse into myotubes. At this stage **myogenin** is expressed. Finally, in maturing myotubes, **MRF-4** is expressed. Interestingly, in knockout mice, the absence of a single myogenic regulatory factor (e.g., myf-5, MyoD) alone does not prevent the formation of skeletal muscle (although there may be other minor observable defects), but when myf-5 and MyoD are knocked out simultaneously, muscle fails to form. Another very instructive double knockout of Pax-3 and myf-5 produces mice that are totally lacking in muscles of the trunk and limbs, but the head musculature remains intact. This shows that in the very earliest stages of determination, different regulatory pathways are followed by muscle-forming cells of the head and trunk.

Because each of the regulators, activators, and inhibitors is itself a protein, their formation is subject to similar positive and negative controls. The complex examples of the regulation of the first steps in myogenesis give some idea of the multiple levels of the control of gene expression and the stages of cytodifferentiation in mammals. Although the molecular aspects of myogenesis are better understood than the stages underlying the differentiation of most cell types, it is unrealistic to think that similar sets of interlinked regulatory mechanisms do not operate in the differentiation of most cell types.

Histogenesis of muscle

Muscle as a tissue consists not only of muscle fibers but also of connective tissue, blood vessels, and nerves. Even the muscle fibers themselves are not homogeneous but can be separated into functionally and biochemically different types.

As muscles first form, the myoblasts are intermingled with future connective tissue mesenchyme. The role of the connective tissue in the morphogenesis of a muscle is discussed in the next section. Capillary sprouts grow into the forming muscle for nourishment, and motor nerve fibers enter shortly after the first myoblasts begin forming myotubes.

At one time, it was thought that all myoblasts were essentially identical and that their different characteristics (e.g., fast or slow) were imposed on them by their motor innerva-

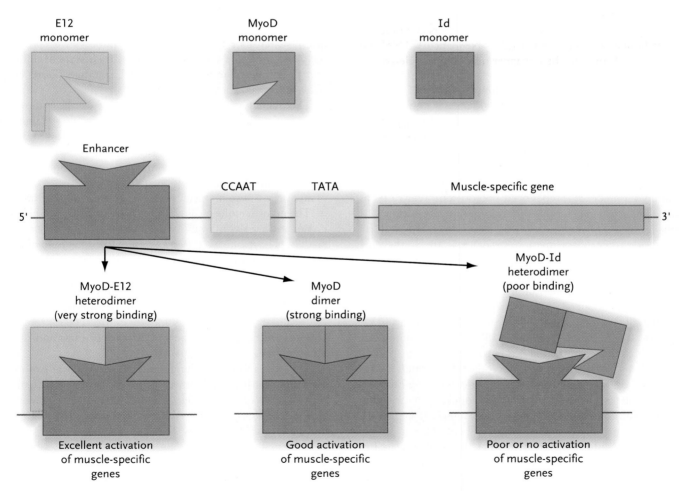

Figure 8-28 MyoD regulation of early myogenesis, showing interactions between MyoD and a transcriptional activator *(E12)* and a transcriptional inhibitor *(Id)*.

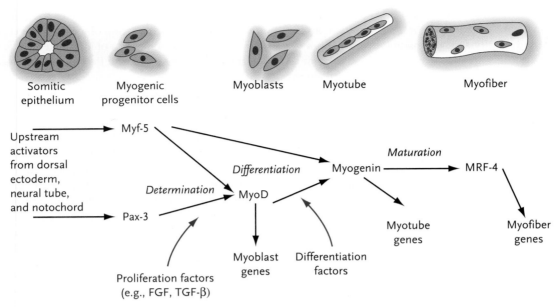

Figure 8-29 Schematic representation of early myogenesis, showing the sequence of expression of myogenic regulatory factors and other influences on the myogenic process.

tion. Recent research, however, has shown that in birds and several species of mammals, there are distinct populations of fast and slow muscle cells as early as the myoblast stage, well before nerve fibers reach the developing muscles.

Not only are there fast and slow myoblasts, but there are also early and late cellular isoforms of myoblasts, which have different requirements for serum factors and nerve interactions in their differentiation. When the earliest myoblasts fuse into myotubes, they give rise to **primary myotubes,** which form the initial basis for an embryonic muscle. The differentiation of primary myotubes occurs before motor nerve axons have entered the newly forming muscle. Subsequently, smaller **secondary myotubes** arising from late myoblasts form alongside the primary myotubes (Figure 8-30). By the time secondary myotubes form, early motor axons are present in the muscles, and there is evidence that the presence of nerves is required for the formation of secondary myotubes. A primary muscle fiber and its associated secondary muscle fibers are initially contained within a common basal lamina and are electrically coupled. These muscle fibers actively synthesize a wide variety of contractile proteins.

Early in their life history, embryonic muscle fibers are innervated by motor neurons. Although it has long been assumed that fast and slow motoneurons impose their own functional characteristics on the developing muscle fibers, it now appears that they may select muscle fibers of a compatible type through information contained on their cell surfaces. Initially, a motor nerve may terminate on both fast and slow muscle fibers, but ultimately, inappropriate connections are broken, so fast nerve fibers innervate only fast muscle fibers, and slow nerves innervate only slow muscle fibers. If the cur-

rent research data hold, nerve fibers will be viewed principally as helping muscle fibers maintain their state of differentiation rather than determining the qualitative differences between fast and slow muscle fibers.

The phenotypes of muscle fibers depend on the nature of the specific proteins that make up their contractile apparatus. There are qualitative differences between fast and slow muscle fibers in many of the contractile proteins, and within each type of muscle fiber, there is a succession of isoforms of major proteins during embryonic development. (The isoform transitions of **myosin** in a developing muscle fiber are used as an example.)

The myosin molecule is complex, consisting of two heavy chains and a series of four light chains (Figure 8-31). Mature fast fibers have one LC1, two LC2, and one LC3 light chain subunits; slow muscle myosin contains two LC1 and two LC2 light chain subunits. In addition, there are fast and slow forms (MHCf and MHCs) of the **myosin heavy chain** subunits. The myosin molecules possess adenosinetriphosphatase activity, and differences in this activity partly account for differences in the speed of contraction between fast and slow muscle fibers.

The myosin molecule undergoes a succession of isoform transitions during development. From the fetal period to maturity a series of three developmental isoforms of the myosin heavy chain (embryonic [MHCemb], neonatal [MHCneo], and adult fast [MHCf]) pass through a fast muscle fiber. (Developmental changes in the light and heavy chain subunits are summarized in Figure 8-31.) Other contractile proteins of muscle fibers (e.g., actin, troponin) pass through similar isoform transitions. After injury to muscle in the adult the regenerating muscle fibers undergo sets of cellular and molec-

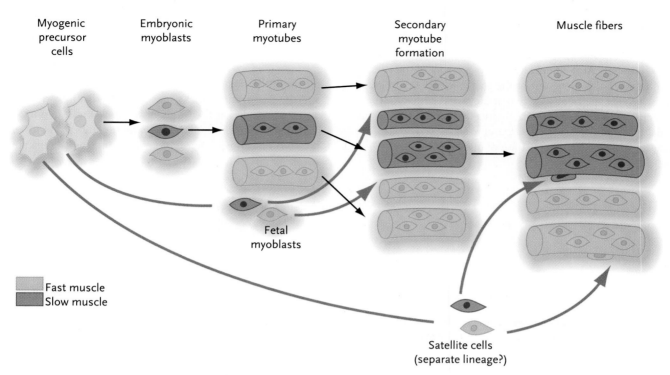

Figure 8-30 Stages in the formation of primary and secondary muscle fibers. A family of embryonic myoblasts contributes to the formation of the primary myotubes, and fetal myoblasts contribute to secondary myotubes. Doubts remain about the origin of satellite cells.

Myosin molecule

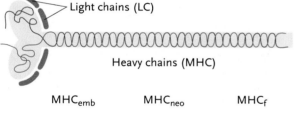

MHC_{emb}	MHC_{neo}	MHC_f
$LC1_{emb}$ $LC1_f$	$LC1_f$	$LC1_f$
$LC2_f$	$LC2_f$	$LC2_f$
	$LC3_f$	$LC3_f$
Fetal muscle	Neonatal muscle	Adult fast muscle

Figure 8-31 Changes in myosin subunits during the development of a fast muscle fiber. A schematic representation of the myosin molecule is also shown.

ular isoform transitions that closely recapitulate those occurring in normal ontogenesis.

The phenotype of muscle fibers is not irreversibly fixed. Even postnatal muscle fibers possess a remarkable degree of plasticity. They respond to exercise by undergoing hypertrophy or becoming more resistant to fatigue. On the other hand, they adapt to inactivity or denervation by becoming atrophic. All these changes are accompanied by various changes in gene expression. Many other types of cells can also modify their phenotypes in response to changes in the environment, but the molecular changes are not always as striking as those seen in muscle fibers.

Morphogenesis of muscle

At a higher level of organization, muscle development involves the formation of anatomically identifiable muscles. The overall form of a muscle is determined principally by its connective tissue framework rather than the myoblasts themselves. Experiments have shown that myogenic cells from somites are essentially interchangeable. For example, myogenic cells from somites that would normally form muscles of the trunk can participate in the formation of normal leg muscles. In contrast, the cells of the connective tissue component of the muscles appear to be imprinted with the morphogenetic blueprint.

Muscles of the Trunk and Limbs. Quail/chick grafting experiments have clearly shown that the major groups of skeletal muscles in the trunk and limbs arise from myogenic precursors located in the somites. In the thorax the intrinsic muscles of the back are derived from cells in the myotomes, whereas ventrolateral muscles (e.g., intercostal muscles) arise from epithelially organized ventral buds of the somites (Figure 8-32). In the limb regions, myogenic cells migrate from the epithelium of the ventrolateral dermomyotome quite early during development. More cranial myogenic cells originating in similar regions of the somites migrate into the developing tongue. At the lumbar levels, precursors of the abdominal muscles also move out of the epithelium of ventrolateral somitic buds. It is highly likely that the **prune-belly syndrome,** which is characterized by the absence of the abdominal musculature (Figure 8-33), will be found to be caused by a molecular deficiency in this population of myogenic cells.

Recent experiments have shown different cellular behavior in areas of the myotomes adjacent to limb and nonlimb regions. In thoracic segments, cells of the dermatome surround the lateral edges of the myotome. This is followed by an increase in the number of myotubes formed in the myotome and the penetration of the muscle primordia into the body wall. In contrast, at the levels of the limb buds, dermatome cells die before surrounding the early myotubes that form in the myotome. These myotubes neither increase significantly

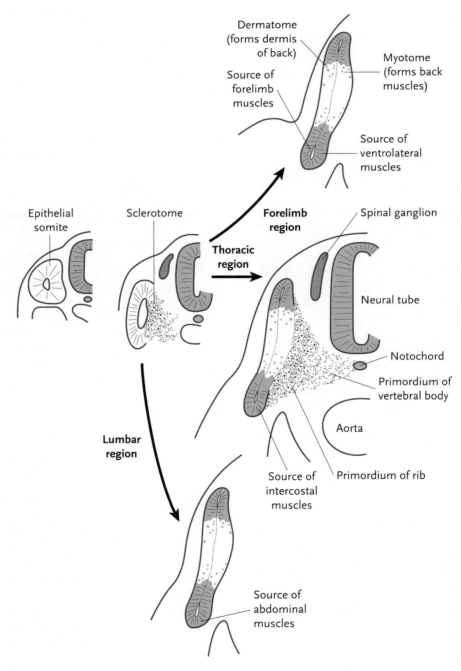

Figure 8-32 Origin of the trunk muscles from the somites in the forelimb, thoracic, and lumbar regions. (Modified from Theiler K: *Adv Anat Embryol Cell Biol* 112:1-99, 1988.)

in number nor move out from the myotomes to form separate muscle primordia.

Several experiments suggest that influences of the body regions surrounding the somites play a role in the early steps of the release and morphogenesis of myogenic precursor cells from the somites. If a chick limb bud is removed, the dermatome cells do not die; rather, they surround the myotomes, allowing an increase in the number of myotubes that form in the myotomes. In contrast, when a limb bud is grafted onto a thoracic level, cells of the dermatome die, and the underlying muscle primordia fail to mature. In another experimental approach, if somites or pieces of paraxial mesoderm are grafted in a rotated position with the medial edge facing laterally, myogenic cells migrate from the new lateral edge, indicating again that activities of cells within the somites respond to local environmental influences.

After their origin from the somites, the muscle primordia of the trunk and abdomen become organized into well-defined groups and layers (Figure 8-34). (Morphogenesis of the limb

muscles is discussed in Chapter 9.) The results of a number of experiments have demonstrated fundamental differences in cellular properties between the cellular precursors of limb muscles and axial muscles. These are summarized in Table 8-2.

Muscles of the Head and Cervical Region. The skeletal muscle of the head and neck is mesodermal in origin. Quail/chick grafting experiments have shown that the paraxial mesoderm, specifically the somitomeres, constitutes the main source of the cranial musculature, although some question still remains about the origin of the extraocular muscles. There is evidence that at least some of the cells that make up the extraocular muscles arise from the prechordal plate of the early embryo. There is increasing evidence that in some aspects, myogenesis in the head differs significantly from that in the trunk. Different controls at the level of myogenic determination between the head and the trunk have already

TABLE 8-2   Differences Between Cellular Precursors of Axial and Limb Muscles

Axial muscles	Limb muscles
Are located in medial half of somite	Are located in lateral half of somite
Differentiate largely in situ	Migrate into limb buds before differentiating
Differentiate initially as mononucleate myocytes	Differentiate initially as multinucleate myocytes
Myogenic determination factors (Myf-5, MyoD) are expressed at or before the onset of myotome formation	Expression of myogenic determination genes is delayed until limb muscle masses begin to coalesce
Differentiation seems strongly influenced by neural tube and notochord	Migration and differentiation are little influenced by axial structures

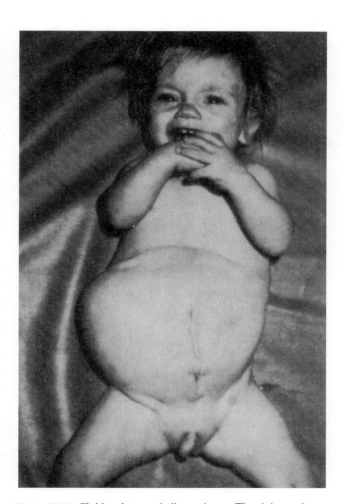

Figure 8-33 Child with prune-belly syndrome. The abdominal musculature is absent or very hypoplastic. Urinary defects commonly accompany this defect. Note the characteristic dimples on the knees. (From Wigglesworth J, Singer D: *Textbook of fetal and perinatal pathology,* Oxford, England, 1991, Blackwell Scientific.)

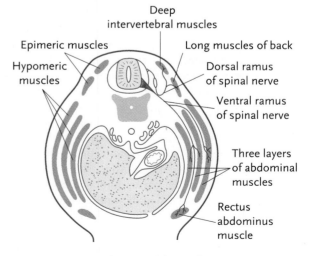

Figure 8-34 Groups and layers of trunk muscles.

been discussed. Also, a number of the craniofacial muscles have different phenotypic properties from trunk muscles (e.g., myosin isoforms and possibly elements of neuromuscular control of phenotype).

As with muscles in the trunk, muscles in the head and neck arise by the movement of myogenic cells away from the paraxial mesoderm through mesenchyme (either neural crest derived or mesodermal) on their way to their final destination. As in the trunk, the morphogenesis of muscles in the cranial region appears to be determined by information inherent in the connective tissues that ensheathe the muscles. There is no early level specificity in the paraxial myogenic cells. This has been determined by grafting somites or somitomeres from one craniocaudal level to another. In these cases, the myogenic cells that leave the grafted structures form muscles normal for the region into which they migrate rather than muscles appropriate for the level of origin of the grafted somites.

Despite evidence that suggests the interchangeability of embryonic somites in muscle formation, other experimental data show the existence of well-defined positional properties of skeletal muscles (e.g., their ability to make connections with nerves from different axial levels and certain aspects of gene expression). These findings indicate a strong imprinting on the muscle fibers according to a pronounced rostrocaudal gradient. The time at which this form of axial specificity is imposed on the developing muscle fibers is not known.

Certain muscles of the head, in particular those of the tongue, arise from the occipital somites in the manner of trunk muscles and undergo extensive migrations into the enlarging head. Their more caudal level of origin is evidenced by the innervation by the **hypoglossal nerve** (twelfth cranial nerve), which, according to some comparative anatomists, is a series of highly modified spinal nerves. Despite their final location in the head, these muscles are subjected to the same early molecular regulation of myogenesis as trunk muscles.

Anomalies of skeletal muscles

Variations and anomalies of skeletal muscles are common. Some, such as the absence of portions of the pectoralis major muscle, are associated with malformations of other structures. Further discussion of anomalies of specific muscles requires a level of anatomical knowledge beyond that assumed for this text.

Muscular dystrophy is a family of genetic diseases characterized by the repeated degeneration and regeneration of various groups of muscles during postnatal life. In Duchenne muscular dystrophy, which occurs in young boys, a membrane-associated protein called **dystrophin** is lacking from the muscle fibers. Although the exact function of dystrophin is still uncertain, its absence appears to make the muscle fibers more susceptible to damage when physically stressed.

Cardiac Muscle

Although a striated muscle, cardiac muscle differs from skeletal muscles in many aspects of embryonic development. Derived from the splanchnic mesoderm of the early embryo, cardiac muscle cells arise from cells present in the myocardium. Differences between the differentiation of cardiac and skeletal muscle appear early, since MyoD and other common master regulators of skeletal muscle differentiation are not expressed in early cardiac muscle development. Nevertheless, early cardiac and skeletal muscle cells express isoforms of molecules that are characteristic of mature cells of the other type. For example, both cardiac and skeletal muscle cells in the embryo express high levels of cardiac α-actin; however, after birth, expression of this molecule declines in skeletal muscle but remains high in cardiac muscle. Interestingly, in cardiac hypertrophy, mature cardiac muscle cells begin to express large amounts of skeletal α-actin mRNA.

Even early cardiac myoblasts contain relatively large numbers of myofibrils in their cytoplasm, and they are capable of undergoing pronounced contractions. In the embryo the mononucleated cardiac myocytes face a difficult problem: the cells of the developing heart must continue to contract while the heart is increasing in mass. This functional requirement necessitates that cardiac myocytes undergo mitosis even though their cytoplasm contains many bundles of contractile filaments (Figure 8-35). Cells of the body often lose their ability to divide when their cytoplasm contains structures characteristic of the differentiated state. Cardiac myocytes deal with this problem by partially disassembling their contractile filaments during mitosis. In contrast to skeletal muscle, cardiac myocytes do not undergo fusion but rather remain as individual cells, although they may become binucleated. Cardiac myocytes keep in close structural and functional contact through **intercalated disks,** which join adjacent cells to one another.

Later in development a network of cardiac muscle cells undergoes an alternative pathway of differentiation characterized by increased size, a reduction in the concentration of myofibrils, and a greatly increased concentration of glycogen in the cytoplasm. These cells form the **conducting system,** parts of which are called **Purkinje fibers.** Purkinje fibers also express a different profile of contractile protein isoforms from either atrial or ventricular myocytes.

Smooth Muscle

As with cardiac muscle, much of the smooth muscle in the body arises from splanchnic mesoderm. Exceptions are the ciliary muscle and sphincter pupillae muscles of the eye, which are derived from neural crest ectoderm, and much of the vascular smooth muscle, which frequently arises from the local mesoderm. Very little is known about the morphology and mechanisms underlying the differentiation of smooth muscle cells.

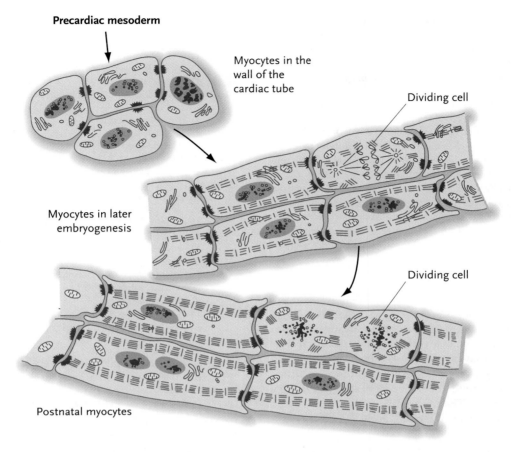

Precardiac mesoderm

Myocytes in the wall of the cardiac tube

Dividing cell

Myocytes in later embryogenesis

Dividing cell

Postnatal myocytes

Figure 8-35 Stages in the histogenesis of cardiac muscle. During mitosis, the contractile filaments undergo a partial disassembly. (Modified from Rumyantsev P: *Cardiomyocytes in processes of reproduction, differentiation and regeneration [in Russian]*, Leningrad, 1982, Nauka.)

SUMMARY

- The epidermis starts as a single layer of ectoderm, to which a single superficial layer of peridermal cells is added. As other layers are added, three cell types migrate from other sources: (1) melanoblasts (pigment cells) from the neural crest, (2) Langerhans' cells (immune cells) from precursors in the bone marrow, and (3) Merkel cells (mechanoreceptors), probably from the neural crest.

- In the multilayered epidermis, unspecialized cells from the stratum basale differentiate as they move through the various layers toward the surface of the epidermis. The cells produce increasing amounts of intracellular keratins and filaggrin; the latter is involved in the interconnections of the keratinocytes, the final differentiated form of the epidermal cell.

- The dermis arises from mesodermal cells derived from the dermatome of the somites. Dermal/epidermal interactions underlie the formation of epidermal appendages such as hairs. In mammary glands, hormonal influences are important in the development of the duct system after the ductal epithelium is induced.

- Skeletal tissue arises from the mesenchyme of either mesodermal or neural crest origin. There are two major subdivisions of the skeleton: the axial skeleton of the trunk and the appendicular skeleton of the limbs.

- The fundamental organization of the cranial components of the vertebral column is closely associated with expression of the

CLINICAL VIGNETTE

A pediatrician noticed that a new patient, a 1½-year-old boy, had a shorter-than-normal neck and hair that went farther down the neck than usual. A family history produced no evidence of other similarly affected relatives. X-ray examination revealed that the boy's neck contained only six cervical vertebrae. The pediatrician then asked if the mother could remember taking or being exposed to certain compounds during early pregnancy.

1. Which of the following did the doctor suspect as possibly being related to the boy's condition?
   A. Folic acid
   B. Retinoic acid
   C. Cocaine
   D. Thalidomide
   E. Alcohol
2. A disturbance in what class of molecules was suspected to underlie this condition?
   A. *Hox* genes
   B. *Pax* genes
   C. Myogenic regulatory factors
   D. FGF
   E. Hedgehog proteins

homeobox-containing genes. Superimposed on this is the induction of many components of the axial skeleton by underlying ectodermal (usually neural) structures. Individual vertebrae are composite structures consisting of components derived from two adjoining somites.

- The skull consists of two subdivisions: the neurocranium, which surrounds the brain, and the viscerocranium, which surrounds the oral cavity. The base of the neurocranium (chondrocranium) is initially represented by several sets of paired cartilage. These later become transformed into bone. Most bones surrounding the brain are formed by intramembranous bone, which differentiates directly from mesenchyme. The viscerocranium is also derived from cartilaginous and membranous components.

- Skeletal muscle fibers undergo a sequence of differentiation from mononuclear myoblasts. First, they fuse to form multinucleated myotubes, and then they mature into skeletal muscle fibers. Mononucleated reserve cells (satellite cells) can proliferate and fuse to growing or mechanically stressed muscle fibers.

- Pax-3 and myf-5 (a member of the MyoD transcription factor family) stimulate myogenic progenitor cells of the trunk to form myoblasts. Other regulatory factors can activate (e.g., E12) or inhibit (e.g., Id) the activities of muscle regulatory factors. Early myogenic cells are kept in the cell cycle by growth factors such as FGF and transforming growth factor-β. Myoblasts are characterized by the expression of MyoD, and growth factors such as insulin-like growth factor promote their fusion and differentiation into myotubes, which express myogenin.

- The first multinucleated muscle fibers to form are primary myotubes. Secondary myotubes form around them. Innervation by motor nerve fibers is necessary for the full differentiation of muscle fibers. During the differentiative process, several sets of isoforms of myosin subunits and other contractile proteins appear in sequence in the muscle fibers.

- Skeletal muscles of the limbs and trunk arise from cellular precursors in the somites. The cranial musculature arises from the somitomeres. Dorsal and ventral muscles of the trunk arise from precursors located in different regions of the somites. The limb musculature also arises from cells in the ventrolateral regions of the somites. These cells migrate into the limb buds.

- Cardiac muscle arises from splanchnic mesoderm. Cardiomyocytes differ from skeletal muscle cells in that they can divide mitotically after they are highly differentiated and contain contractile filaments.

REVIEW QUESTIONS

1. Satellite cells of muscle are activated under which of these conditions?
   - A. Normal muscle fiber growth
   - B. Muscle fiber regeneration
   - C. Muscle fiber hypertrophy
   - D. All of the above
   - E. None of the above
2. Which cellular component of the epidermis is a peripheral outpost of the immune system and functions to present antigens to other immune cells?
   - A. Merkel cells
   - B. Keratinocytes
   - C. Basal cells
   - D. Melanocytes
   - E. Langerhans' cells
3. Which structure is mesodermal in origin?
   - A. Hair shaft
   - B. Mammary duct
   - C. Sebaceous gland
   - D. Arrector pili muscle
   - E. None of the above
4. Craniosynostosis is caused by an abnormal developmental course of the:
   - A. Foramen magnum
   - B. Cranial sutures
   - C. Basicranium
   - D. Jaws
   - E. None of the above
5. Which myogenic regulatory factor is expressed latest in the development of a muscle fiber?
   - A. Myogenin
   - B. MyoD
   - C. MRF-4
   - D. myf-5
   - E. Pax-3
6. In the let-down of milk during lactation, the myoepithelial cells contract in response to:
   - A. Progesterone
   - B. Oxytocin
   - C. Estrogens
   - D. Lactalbumin
   - E. Casein
7. What component of the developing skin determines the nature of the hairs that form or the thickness of the epidermis in the fetus?
8. A male has two bilaterally symmetrical brownish spots about 8 mm in diameter located on the skin about 3 inches below each nipple. What is one explanation for them?
9. Why is cranial bone typically not found over an area where part of the brain is missing?
10. How was it determined that the limb musculature arises from the somites?

REFERENCES

Skin

Adams JC, Watt FM: Changes in keratinocyte adhesion during terminal differentiation: reduction in fibronectin binding precedes $\alpha_5 \beta_1$ integrin loss from the cell surface, *Cell* 63:425-435, 1990.

Babler WJ: Embryologic development of epidermal ridges and their configurations, *Birth Defects* 27:95-112, 1991.

Chuong C-M and others: Early events during avian skin appendage regeneration: dependence on epithelial-mesenchymal interaction and order of molecular reappearance, *J Invest Dermatol* 107:639-646, 1996.

Cummins H: The topographic history of the volar pads (walking pads; Tastballen) in the human embryo, *Carnegie Contr Embryol* 113:103-126, 1929.

Duernberger H, Kratochwil K: Specificity of time interaction and origin of mesenchymal cells in the androgen response of the embryonic mammary gland, *Cell* 19:465-471, 1980.

Goldsmith LA, ed: *Physiology, biochemistry, and molecular biology of the skin*, ed 2, New York, 1991, Oxford University.

Halata Z, Grim M, Christ B: Origin of spinal cord meninges, sheaths of peripheral nerves, and cutaneous receptors, including Merkel cells, *Anat Embryol* 182:529-537, 1990.

Holbrook KA: Structure and function of the developing human skin. In Goldsmith LA, ed: *Physiology, biochemistry, and molecular biology of the skin*, ed 2, New York, 1991, Oxford University Press, pp 63-110.

Imagawa W and others: Control of mammary gland development. In Knobil E, Neill JD, eds: *The physiology of reproduction*, ed 2, New York, 1994, Raven, pp 1033-1063.

Jones PH, Harper S, Watt FM: Stem cell patterning and fate in human epidermis, *Cell* 80:83-93, 1995.

Kimura S: Embryologic development of flexion creases, *Birth Defects* 27:113-129, 1991.

Krey AK and others: Morphogenesis and malformations of the skin, NICHD/NIADDK research workshop, *J Invest Dermatol* 88:464-473, 1987.

Millar S: The role of patterning genes in epidermal differentiation. In Cowin P, Klymkowsky MW, eds: *Cytoskeletal-membrane interactions and signal transduction*, Austin, Texas, 1997, Landes Bioscience, pp 87-102.

Polakowska RR and others: Apoptosis in human skin development: morphogenesis, periderm, and stem cells, *Dev Dynam* 199:176-188, 1994.

Sakakura T, Sakagami Y, Nishizuka Y: Dual origin of mesenchymal tissues participating in mouse mammary gland morphogenesis, *Dev Biol* 91:202-207, 1982.

Saxod R: Ontogeny of the cutaneous sensory organs, *Microscop Res Tech* 34:313-333, 1996.

Sengel P: *Morphogenesis of skin*, Cambridge, Mass, 1976, Cambridge University Press.

Skeleton

Balling R and others: Development of the skeletal system, *Ciba Found Symp* 165:132-143, 1992.

Bosma JF, ed: *Symposium on development of the basicranium*, DHEW Pub No (NIH) 76-989, Washington, DC, 1976, US Government Printing Office.

Hall BK: Divide, accumulate, differentiate: cell condensation in skeletal development revisited, *Int J Devel Biol* 39:881-893, 1995.

Hall BK: The evolution of connective and skeletal tissues. In Hinchliffe JR, Hurle JM, Summerbell D, eds: *Developmental patterning of the vertebrate limb*, New York, 1991, Plenum, pp 303-311.

Hanken J, Hall BK, eds: *The skull*, vol 1, *Development*, Chicago, 1993, University of Chicago Press.

Horan GSB and others: Mutations in paralogous *Hox* genes result in overlapping homeotic transformations of the axial skeleton: evidence for unique and redundant function, *Dev Biol* 169:359-372, 1995.

Kessel M: Molecular coding of axial positions by *Hox* genes, *Semin Dev Biol* 2:367-373, 1991.

Kessel M: Respecification of vertebral identities by retinoic acid, *Development* 115:487-501, 1992.

Kessel M, Balling R, Gruss P: Variations of cervical vertebrae after expression of a *Hox-1.1* transgene in mice, *Cell* 61:301-308, 1990.

Liu YH and others: Premature suture closure and ectopic cranial bone in mice expressing msx2 transgenes in the development skull, *Proc Natl Acad Sci USA* 92: 6137-6141,1995.

Monsoro-Burq A-H and others: Heterogeneity in the development of the vertebra, *Proc Natl Acad Sci USA* 91:10435-10439, 1994.

Rodan GA, Harada S-I: The missing bone, *Cell* 89:677-680, 1997.

Schierhorn H: Ueber die Persistenz der embryonalen Schwanzknospe beim Menschen, *Anat Anz* 127:307-337, 1970.

Sensenig EC: The early development of the human vertebral column, *Carnegie Contr Embryol* 33:21-42, 1949.

Theiler K: Vertebral malformations, *Adv Anat Embryol Cell Biol* 112:1-99, 1988.

Verbout AJ: The development of the vertebral column, *Adv Anat Embryol Cell Biol* 90:1-122, 1985.

Vortkamp A and others: Regulation of rate of cartilage differentiation by Indian hedgehog and PTH-related protein, *Science* 273:613-622, 1996.

Muscle

Arnold H-H, Braun T: Targeted inactivation of myogenic factor genes reveals their role during mouse myogenesis: a review, *Int J Dev Biol* 40:345-363, 1996.

Christ B: Entwicklung und Biologie des Bewegungsapparates. In Staubesand J, ed: *Benninghoff Makroskopische und mikroskopische Anatomie des Menschen*, Munich, 1985, Urban & Schwarzenberg, pp 167-180.

Christ B, Cihák R, eds: *Development and regeneration of skeletal muscles*, Basel, Switzerland, 1986, Karger.

Christ B, Jacob M, Jacob HJ: On the origin and development of the ventrolateral abdominal muscles in the avian embryo: an experimental and ultrastructural study, *Anat Embryol* 166:87-102, 1983.

Christ B and others: The somite-muscle relationship in the avian embryo. In Hinchliffe JR, Hurle JM, Summerbell D, eds: *Developmental patterning of the vertebrate limb*, New York, 1991, Plenum, pp 265-271.

Hans-Henning A, Braun T: Targeted inactivation of myogenic factor genes reveals their role during mouse myogenesis: a review, *Int J Dev Biol* 40:345-363, 1996.

Kieny M and others: Origin and development of avian skeletal musculature, *Reprod Nutr Dev* 28(3B):673-686, 1988.

Ludolph DC, Konieczny SF: Transcription factor families: muscling in on the myogenic program, *FASEB J* 9:1595-1604, 1995.

Maroto M and others: Ectopic Pax-3 activates MyoD and myf-5 expression in embryonic mesoderm and neural tissue, *Cell* 89:139-148, 1997.

Noden DM: The embryonic origins of avian cephalic and cervical muscles and associated connective tissues, *Am J Anat* 168:257-276, 1983.

Olson EN: Signal transduction pathways that regulate skeletal muscle gene expression, *Mol Endocrinol* 7:1369-1378, 1993.

Olson EN, Rosenthal N: Homeobox genes and muscle patterning, *Cell* 79:9-12, 1994.

Ott M-O and others: Early expression of the myogenic regulatory gene, *myf-5*, in precursor cells of skeletal muscle in the mouse embryo, *Development* 111:1097-1107, 1991.

Rong PM and others: The neural tube/notochord complex is necessary for vertebral but not limb and body wall striated muscle differentiation, *Development* 115:657-672, 1992.

Rumyantsev PP: *Cardiomyocytes in processes of reproduction, differentiation and regeneration (in Russian)*, Leningrad, 1982, Nauka.

Sanes JR, Donoghue MJ, Merlie JP: Positional differences among adult skeletal muscle fibers. In Kelly AM, Blau HM, eds: *Neuromuscular development and disease*, New York, 1992, Raven, pp 195-209.

Sasson D: Myogenic regulatory factors: dissecting their role and regulation during vertebrate embryogenesis, *Dev Biol* 156:11-23, 1993.

Sassoon D and others: Expression of two myogenic regulatory factors myogenin and MyoD1 during mouse embryogenesis, *Nature* 341:303-307, 1989.

Tajabkhsh S and others: Redefining the genetic hierarchies controlling skeletal myogenesis, *Cell* 89:127-138, 1997.

9

LIMB DEVELOPMENT

Limbs are remarkable structures that are designed almost solely for mechanical functions: motion and force. These functions are achieved through the coordinated development of various tissue components. No single tissue in the limb takes shape without reference to the other tissues with which it is associated. The limb as a whole develops according to a master blueprint that reveals itself sequentially with each successive stage in limb formation. Many of the factors that control limb development cannot be seen by examining morphology alone, but rather must be demonstrated by experimental means or through the localization of molecules. Despite remarkable recent progress in understanding the molecular basis of the tissue interactions that control limb development, many fundamental questions remain poorly understood. Important among these are what initiates the development of a limb, what determines the individual identity of the digits, and how a developing extremity turns out to be an arm or a leg. Limb anomalies are common and highly visible. Many of these are now understood to be reflections of disturbances in specific cellular or molecular interactions that are fundamental to limb development. These are discussed in Clinical Correlation 9-1 at the end of the chapter.

INITIATION OF LIMB DEVELOPMENT

Limb formation begins relatively late in embryonic development with the activation of a group of mesenchymal cells in the **somatic mesoderm** of the **lateral plate** (Figure 9-1). The initial stimulus for limb development remains poorly understood. There is evidence that localized secretion of **fibroblast growth factor-8 (FGF-8)** is an important component of the initial stimulus, but the tissue origin of the stimulus for limb formation remains in doubt. That stimulus in turn may depend on the local action of **retinoic acid**. If the local synthesis and action of retinoic acid are inhibited, limb formation fails to occur. If a small bead containing FGF-8 is implanted into flank mesoderm, an extra limb will develop at that site. Despite these advances in knowledge, we are still far from understanding how limb formation is activated and why limbs form where they do.

The mesodermal limb primordia form at discrete locations beneath a broad band of thickened ectoderm that encircles the ventrolateral aspect of the embryo (see Figure 5-30). In the earliest stages of limb development the limb mesoderm is the prime mover. It influences the overlying ectoderm to be a functional part of an interacting mesodermal-ectodermal primordium that has sufficient developmental information to form a limb even if isolated from the rest of the body (a so-called **self-differentiating system**).

The primacy of the early limb mesoderm was demonstrated long ago by transplantation experiments on amphibian embryos. If early limb mesoderm is removed, a limb fails to form. However, if the same mesoderm is transplanted to the flank of an embryo, a supernumerary limb grows at that site. In contrast, if the ectoderm overlying the normal limb

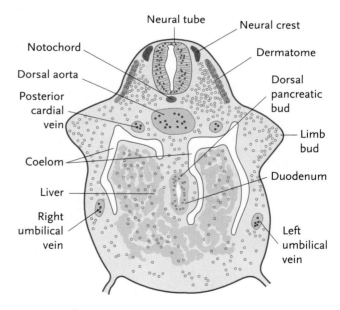

Figure 9-1 Cross section through the trunk at an early stage of limb bud development, showing the position of the limb bud in relation to that of the somite (dermatome) and other major structures. The limb bud is an outgrowth of the body wall (lateral plate mesoderm).

mesoderm is removed, new ectoderm heals the defect, and a limb forms. If the original ectoderm that was removed is grafted to the flank, no limb forms. These experiments show that in *early* limb development, mesoderm is the primary bearer of the limb blueprint and ectoderm is only secondarily co-opted into the system.

In rare instances, individuals are born without one or sometimes all limbs (**amelia**) (Figure 9-2). In some cases this probably reflects a disturbance in the production of the normal signaling molecules for initiating limb development or the cellular receptors for these molecules.

REGULATIVE PROPERTIES AND AXIAL DETERMINATION

The early limb primordium is a highly regulative system, with properties very similar to those described for the cleaving embryo (see p. 44). These properties can be summarized with the following experiments (Figure 9-3):

1. If part of a limb primordium is removed, the remainder reorganizes to form a complete limb.

2. If a limb primordium is split into two halves and these are prevented from fusing, each half gives rise to a complete limb (the twinning phenomenon).

3. If two equivalent halves of a limb primordium are juxtaposed, one complete limb forms.

4. If two equivalent limb disks are superimposed, they reorganize to form a single limb (see section on tetraparental embryos, p. 45).

5. In some species, disaggregated limb mesoderm can reorganize and form a complete limb.

The organization of the limb is commonly related to three linear axes based on the cartesian coordinate system. The anteroposterior* axis runs from the first (anterior) to the fifth (posterior) digit. The back of the hand or foot is dorsal, and

*Because of different conventions in the use of axial terms, some human embryologists would take exception to the axial terminology presented here. Specifically, according to strict human terminology, *anterior* means "ventral," and *posterior* means "dorsal." However, the axial terminology used in this chapter (*anterior* means "cranial," and *posterior* means "caudal") is so uniformly used in the experimental and comparative embryological literature that the student referring to the original literature in the field of limb development would find it very confusing to use human axial terminology.

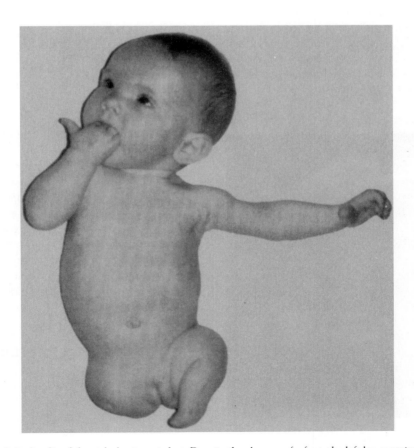

Figure 9-2 Amelia of the right leg in an infant. Despite the absence of a foot, the left leg contains an upper and a lower leg segment. (From Connor JM, Ferguson-Smith MA: *Essential medical genetics,* ed 3, Oxford, England, 1991, Blackwell Scientific.)

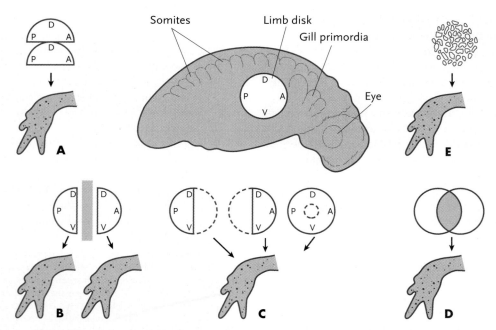

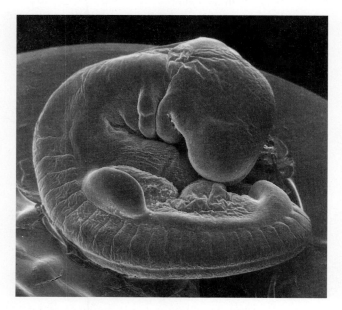

Figure 9-3 Experiments demonstrating regulative properties of limb disks in amphibian embryos. **A,** Combining two identical halves of limb disks results in a single limb. **B,** Separation of two halves of a limb disk by a barrier results in each half forming a normal limb of the same polarity. **C,** After various types of tissue removal, the remaining limb tissue regulates to form a normal limb. **D,** Combining two disks results in the formation of a single normal limb. **E,** Mechanical disruption of a limb disk is followed by reorganization of the pieces and the formation of a normal limb. *A,* Anterior; *D,* dorsal; *P,* posterior; *V,* ventral. (Based on studies by Harrison RG: *J Exp Zool* 32:1-136, 1921; and Swett FH: *Q Rev Biol* 12:322-339, 1937.)

Figure 9-4 Scanning electron micrograph of a **34-day-old** human embryo (5 mm), with 34 pairs of somites. Toward the lower left, the right arm bud protrudes from the body. (From Jirásek JE: *Atlas of human prenatal morphogenesis,* Amsterdam, 1983, Martinus Nijhoff.)

the palm or sole is ventral. The proximodistal axis extends from the base of the limb to the tips of the digits.

Experiments involving the transplantation and rotation of limb primordia in lower vertebrates have shown that these axes are fixed in a sequential order: anteroposterior to dorsoventral to proximodistal. Before all three axes are specified, a left limb primordium can be converted into a normal right limb simply by rotating it with respect to the normal body axes. These axes are important as reference points in several aspects of limb morphogenesis. Evidence indicates a similar sequence of axial specifications in certain other primordia, such as those of the retina and inner ear.

OUTGROWTH OF THE LIMB BUD

Shortly after its initial establishment, the limb primordium begins to bulge from the body wall (late in the first month for the human upper extremity [Figure 9-4]). At this stage the limb bud consists of a mass of similar-looking mesodermal cells covered by a layer of ectoderm. Despite its apparently simple structure, the limb bud contains enough intrinsic information to guide its development, since if a mammalian limb

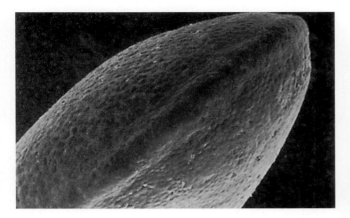

Figure 9-5 Scanning electron micrograph of the flattened limb bud of a human embryo showing the prominent apical ectodermal ridge traversing the apical border. (From Kelley RO, Fallon JF: *Dev Biol* 51:241-256, 1976.)

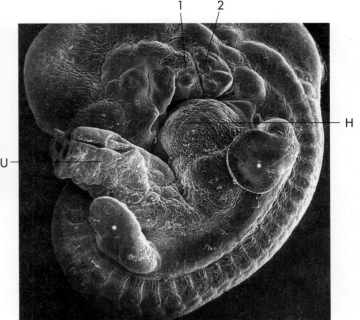

Figure 9-6 Scanning electron micrograph of a **40-day-old** human embryo (10 mm). The arm and leg buds (*asterisks*) are in the flattened paddle stage. *H,* Heart; *U,* umbilical cord; *1, 2,* pharyngeal arches 1 and 2. (From Jirásek JE: *Atlas of human prenatal morphogenesis,* Amsterdam, 1983, Martinus Nijhoff.)

bud is transplanted to another region of the body or is cultured in vitro, a recognizable limb forms.

A distinctive feature is the presence of a ridge of thickened ectoderm (**apical ectodermal ridge**) located along the anteroposterior plane of the apex of the limb bud (Figure 9-5). During much of the time when the apical ectodermal ridge is present, the hand- and foot-forming regions of the developing limb bud are paddle shaped, with the apical ridge situated along the rim of the paddle (Figure 9-6). Experiments have shown that the apical ectodermal ridge interacts with the underlying limb bud mesoderm to promote outgrowth of the developing limb. Other aspects of limb development such as morphogenesis (the development of form) are guided by information contained in the mesoderm.

This section outlines many of the ways in which the limb bud mesoderm and ectoderm interact to control limb development. Recognition of these developmental mechanisms is important in understanding the genesis of a number of limb malformations.

Apical Ectodermal Ridge

The human apical ectodermal ridge is a multilayered epithelial structure (Figure 9-7) characterized by the presence of numerous gap junctions through which the cells are interconnected. A basal lamina is interposed between the apical ridge and the underlying mesodermal cells.

Although the apical ectodermal ridge has been recognized morphologically for many years, its role in limb development was not understood until it was subjected to experimental analysis. Removal of the apical ridge results in an arrest of limb development, leading to distal truncation of the limb (Figure 9-8). In the *limbless* mutant in chickens, early limb development is normal; later the apical ectodermal ridge disappears, and further wing development ceases. If mutant ectoderm is placed over normal wing bud

mesoderm, limb development is truncated, whereas combining mutant mesoderm with normal ectoderm results in more normal limb development, suggesting that the ectoderm is defective in this mutant. Studies involving the *limbless* mutant have shown that the normal apical ectodermal ridge forms at the junction of the dorsal and ventral ectoderm and that in the absence of the juxtaposition of ectoderm with dorsal and ventral properties (e.g., the *limbless* mutant), an apical ectodermal ridge cannot be maintained. Conversely, the presence of an additional apical ectodermal ridge on a limb bud, whether experimentally transplanted or through genetic mutation (e.g., diplopodia), results in the formation of a supernumerary limb (Figure 9-9).

Recent studies have shown that the outgrowth-promoting signal produced by the apical ectodermal ridge is FGF. In the earliest stages of limb formation, the lateral ectoderm begins to produce FGF-8 as it thickens to form an apical ectodermal ridge. As the limb bud begins to grow out, the apical ridge also produces FGF-2 throughout its entire length and FGF-4 in its posterior half (see Figure 9-15). If the apical ectodermal ridge is removed, outgrowth of limb bud mesoderm can be supported by the local application of either FGF-2 or FGF-4. Other studies have shown that in mutants characterized by deficient or absent outgrowth of the limb, the mutant ectoderm fails to produce FGF. The effects of the FGF produced by the apical ectoderm on the underlying mesoderm are discussed later in this chapter.

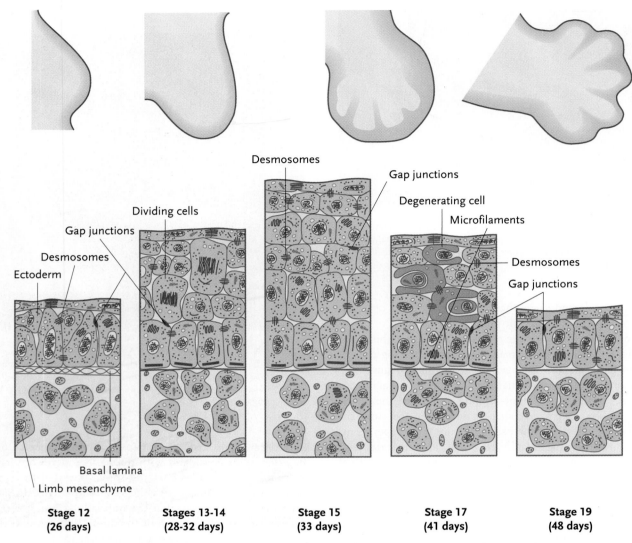

Figure 9-7 Changes in structure during the buildup and regression of the human apical ectodermal ridge. Beneath the early ridge, the basal lamina is double layered with cross-links. At later stages, it is a single-layered structure. (Modified from Kelley RO, Fallon JF: *Dev Biol* 51:241-256, 1976.)

Mesoderm of the Early Limb Bud

Structure and composition

The mesoderm of the early limb bud consists of homogeneous mesenchymal cells supplied by a well-developed vascular network. The mesenchymal cells are embedded in a matrix consisting of a loose meshwork of collagen fibers and ground substance, with hyaluronic acid and glycoproteins being prominent constituents of the latter. There are no nerves in the early limb bud.

It is not possible to distinguish different cell types within the early limb bud mesenchyme by their morphology alone. Nevertheless, mesenchymal cells from several sources are present (Figure 9-10). Initially the limb bud mesenchyme con-

sists exclusively of cells derived from the lateral plate mesoderm. These cells give rise to the skeleton, connective tissue, and some blood vessels. Mesenchymal cells derived from the somites migrate into the limb bud as precursors of muscle cells. Another population of migrating cells is that from the neural crest, which ultimately form the Schwann cells of the nerves and pigment cells (**melanocytes**).

Mesodermal-ectodermal interactions and the role of mesoderm in limb morphogenesis

Limb development occurs as the result of continuous interactions between the mesodermal and ectodermal components of the limb bud. The ectoderm stimulates outgrowth of

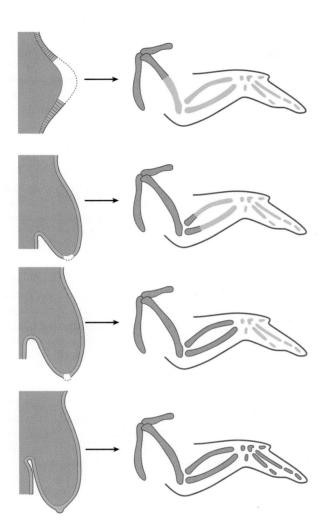

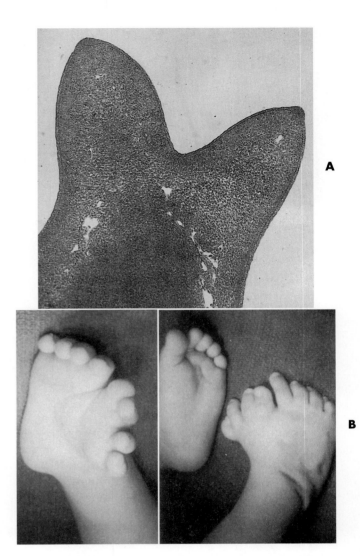

Figure 9-8 *Top three,* Effect of removing the apical ectodermal ridge at successively later stages on the development of the avian wing bud. The more mature the wing bud, the more skeletal elements form after apical ridge removal. Missing structures are shown in light gray. *Bottom,* Normal development of an untouched wing bud. (Based on Saunders JW: *J Exp Zool* 108:363-403, 1948.)

Figure 9-9 A, Duplicated wing bud in a chick with eudiplopodia. Under the influence of a secondary apical ectodermal ridge, a supernumerary limb bud forms. B, Diplopodia in the human. Dorsal and ventral views of the right foot, where duplication has occurred along the anteroposterior axis. (**A** from Goetinck P: *Dev Biol* 10:71-79, 1964. **B** courtesy D. Hootinck, Buffalo, NY.)

the limb bud by promoting mitosis and preventing differentiation of the distal mesodermal cells of the limb bud. Although the apical ridge promotes outgrowth, its own existence is reciprocally controlled by the mesoderm. If an apical ridge from an old limb bud is transplanted onto the mesoderm of a young wing bud, the limb grows normally until morphogenesis is complete. However, if old limb bud mesoderm is covered by young apical ectoderm, limb development ceases at a time appropriate for the age of the mesoderm and not that of the ectoderm.

Similar reciprocal transplantation experiments have been used to demonstrate that the overall shape of the limb is determined by the mesoderm and not the ectoderm. This is most dramatically represented by experiments done on birds be-

cause of the great differences in morphology between the extremities. For example, if leg bud mesoderm in the chick embryo is covered with wing bud ectoderm, a normal leg covered with scales develops. In a somewhat more complex example, if chick leg bud ectoderm is placed over duck wing bud mesoderm, a duck wing covered with chicken feathers forms. Such experiments, which have sometimes involved mosaics of avian and mammalian limb bud components, show that the overall morphology of the limb is determined by the mesodermal component and not the ectoderm. In addition, the regional characteristics of the ectodermal appendages (e.g., scalp hair versus body hair in the case of mammals) is also dictated by the mesoderm. Cross-species grafting experiments, however, show that the nature of the ectodermal

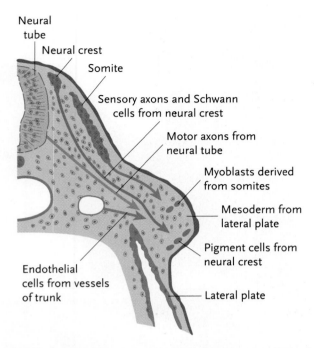

Neural tube
Neural crest
Somite
Sensory axons and Schwann cells from neural crest
Motor axons from neural tube
Myoblasts derived from somites
Mesoderm from lateral plate
Pigment cells from neural crest
Lateral plate
Endothelial cells from vessels of trunk

Figure 9-10 The different types of cells that enter the limb bud.

appendages formed (e.g., hair versus feathers) is appropriate for the species from which the ectoderm was derived.

Polydactyly is a condition characterized by supernumerary digits and exists as a mutant in birds. Reciprocal transplantation experiments between mesoderm and ectoderm have shown that the defect is inherent in the mesoderm and not the ectoderm. Polydactyly in humans (Figure 9-11) is typically inherited as a genetic recessive trait and is commonly found in populations such as certain American Amish communities, where the total genetic pool is relatively restricted.

Cell death and the development of digits

Although it may seem paradoxical, genetically programmed **cell death (apoptosis)** is important in the development of a number of structures in the body. In the forelimb, it is prominently manifested in the future axillary region, between the radius and ulna, and in the interdigital spaces (Figure 9-12). Experiments on avian embryos have shown that to a certain stage, mesodermal cells scheduled to die could be spared by transplanting them to areas in which cell death did not normally occur. However, after a certain time, a "death clock" was set (an example of determination), and the cells could no longer be rescued.

As limb development proceeds, changes become apparent in the apical ectodermal ridge. Instead of remaining continuous around the entire apex of the limb, the ridge begins to break up, leaving intact segments of thickened ridge epithelium covering the digital rays. Between the digits, the ridge re-

gresses (see Figure 9-12, A). As the digital primordia continue to grow outward, cell death sculpts the interdigital spaces (see Figure 9-12, C). A number of developmentally important molecules, including **bone morphogenetic protein-2 (BMP-2)**, **BMP-4, BMP-7, Msx-1**, and a retinoic acid receptor, are expressed in the interdigital mesodermal cells. The exact mechanism of interdigital cell death remains to be elucidated, but some elements of the process are beginning to be understood. The thinning of the apical ectodermal ridge over the interdigital areas appears to reduce the amount of FGF transmitted to the interdigital mesenchyme and serves as an early step in the apoptotic process. If FGF-2 or FGF-4 is supplied to interdigital mesenchyme, cell death is inhibited. Some investigators have proposed that the BMPs, especially BMP-4, are also part of the signal leading to cell death, not only in the interdigital region but also in other areas of the body.

If interdigital cell death does not occur, a soft tissue web connects the digits on either side. This is the basis for the normal development of webbed feet on ducks and the abnormal formation of **syndactyly** (Figure 9-13, A) in humans. BMP is not found in the interdigital mesoderm in developing duck feet, although it is found in other regions of cell death in the duck limb.

All human digits contain three phalangeal segments except for the first digits (thumb and great toe), which consist of only two segments. Some investigators have attributed the development of diphalangeal first digits to the actions of a small zone of cell death that is thought to occur at the tip of the first digital primordium. On rare occasions an individual is born with a triphalangeal thumb (Figure 9-13, B), which could be related to the absence of normally occurring cell death at the tip of the primordium of the thumb.

Zone of polarizing activity and morphogenetic signaling

During the course of experiments investigating morphogenetic cell death, researchers grafted mesodermal cells from the posterior base of the avian wing bud into the anterior margin. This manipulation resulted in the formation of a supernumerary wing, which was a mirror image of the normal wing (Figure 9-14). Much subsequent experimentation has shown that this posterior region, called the **zone of polarizing activity (ZPA)**, acts as a signaling center and determines the organization of the limb along its anteroposterior axis. The signal itself has been shown to be **sonic hedgehog**, a molecule that mediates various tissue interactions in the embryo (see Table 5-3). As seen in the next section, sonic hedgehog not only organizes tissues along the anteroposterior axis but also maintains the structure and function of the apical ectodermal ridge. In the absence of the ZPA or sonic hedgehog, the apical ridge regresses.

Cross-species grafting experiments have demonstrated that mammalian (including human) limb buds also contain a functional ZPA. A transplanted ZPA acts on the apical ecto-

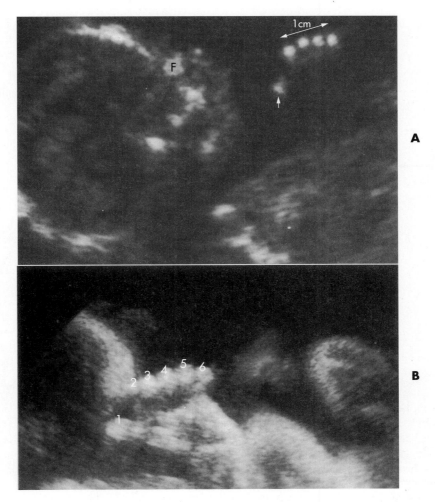

Figure 9-11   Ultrasound images of normal (A) and polydactylous (six digits) (B) hands of human fetuses **16** and **31 weeks old.** In both cases the digits are imaged in cross section. *Arrow,* Thumb; *F,* face; *1,* thumb; *2 to 6,* fingers on polydactylous hand. (A from Bowerman R: *Atlas of normal fetal ultrasonographic anatomy,* St Louis, 1992, Mosby. B from Nyberg D and others: *Diagnostic ultrasound of fetal anomalies,* St Louis, 1990, Mosby.)

dermal ridge, eliciting a growth response from the mesenchymal cells just beneath the part of the ridge adjacent to the transplanted ZPA. As few as 50 cells from the ZPA can stimulate supernumerary limb formation. Other structures, such as pieces of Hensen's node, notochord, and even feather germs, are able to stimulate the formation of supernumerary limbs if grafted into the anterior margin of the limb. Since these experiments were conducted, all of the implanted tissues have been shown to be sources of sonic hedgehog.

Model of Morphogenetic Control of the Developing Limb

A virtual explosion of information on gene expression during a period of 3 or 4 years, superimposed on a firm base of experimental embryological findings, permits the construction of a tentative model of morphogenetic control of limb development. Limb development appears to be initiated by the release of signaling molecules (possibly FGF-8) from localized regions of the trunk. The net result of this inductive signal is the expression of FGF-8 in the ectoderm covering the future limb mesoderm and its ultimate localization to only the region that will form the apical ectodermal ridge.

During this early period, before there is any detectable outgrowth of the limb, important developmental events also fix the dorsoventral axis of the limb field. Initially the mesoderm contains dorsoventral patterning information, but this is soon transferred to the ectoderm. The dorsal ectoderm then develops a morphogenetic signaling center, characterized by the expression of Wnt-7a (Table 9-1). Wnt-7a induces the expression of a homeobox-containing gene, *Lmx1,* in the dorsal

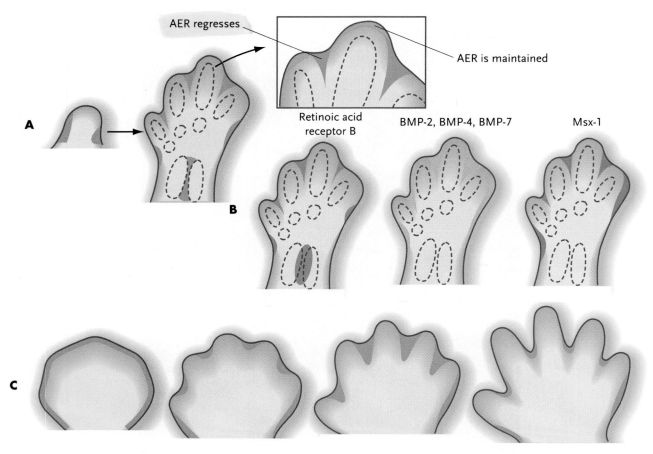

Figure 9-12 Cell death in development of the hand and digits. **A,** Cell death in the chick limb bud. **B,** Gene expression in zones of cell death of the chick embryo. **C,** Cell death in the developing human hand. *AER,* Apical ectodermal ridge; *BMP,* bone morphogenetic protein.

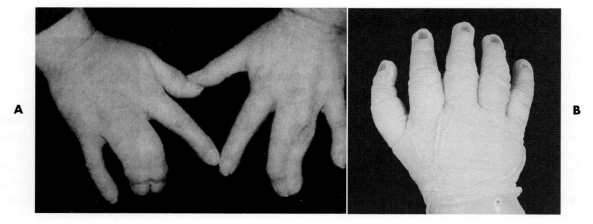

Figure 9-13 **A,** Syndactyly in the human. **B,** Triphalangeal thumb in a human fetus. (**A** from Connor J, Ferguson-Smith M: *Essential medical genetics,* ed 2, Oxford, England, 1987, Blackwell Medical. **B** courtesy M. Barr, Ann Arbor, Mich.)

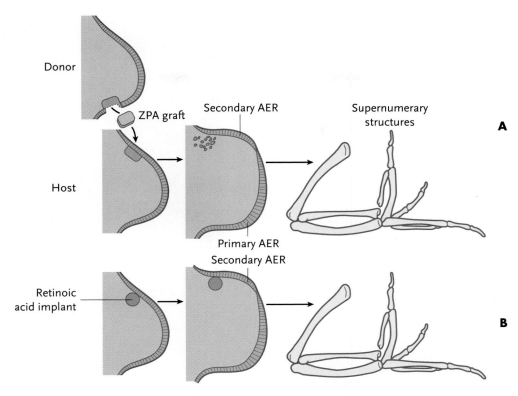

Figure 9-14 **A,** Grafting of the zone of polarizing activity *(ZPA)* into the anterior border of the avian limb bud results in the formation of a secondary apical ectodermal ridge and a supernumerary limb. **B,** Implantation of a bead soaked in retinoic acid into the anterior border of the limb bud also stimulates the formation of a supernumerary limb. *AER,* Apical epidermal ridge.

TABLE 9-1   Axial Control in the Developing Limb

Axis	Signaling center	Molecular signal
Proximodistal	Apical ectodermal ridge	FGF-2, FGF-4, FGF-8
Anteroposterior	ZPA	Sonic hedgehog
Dorsoventral	Dorsal ectoderm	Wnt-7a (dorsal)
	Ventral ectoderm	En-1 (ventral)

mesoderm beneath it, and at roughly the same time the ventral ectoderm begins to express En-1 (Figure 9-15, *A*). This combination of molecular events instructs the mesoderm of the future limb bud to become dorsal under the influence of Wnt-7a or ventral under the influence of En-1. En-1 appears to inhibit the expression of Wnt-7a in the ventral tissues.

In a manner still poorly understood, the ectoderm at the boundary between the dorsal and ventral limb ectoderm thickens to form the apical ectodermal ridge. Early dorsal ectoderm expresses a gene called **radical fringe**. The apical ectodermal ridge forms at the boundary between cells that do and do not express radical fringe. As it does with Wnt-7a, En-1

inhibits the expression of radical fringe in ventral tissues. The cells of the early apical ectodermal ridge express a variety of genes, such as FGF-2, FGF-4, FGF-8, BMP-2, BMP-4, and Msx-2. The events that have occurred to this point are considered to belong to the **initiation phase** of limb development.

The initiation phase of limb development is followed by the **outgrowth phase**. This phase begins with the secretion of FGF by the apical ectodermal ridge and its influence on the underlying mesoderm (Figure 9-15, *B*). The FGF produced by the ridge has two principal effects. Interacting with Wnt-7a produced by the dorsal ectoderm, FGF-8 from the apical ectodermal ridge stimulates the expression of **sonic hedgehog** in the

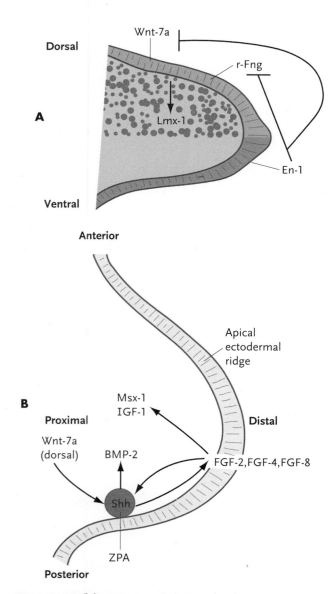

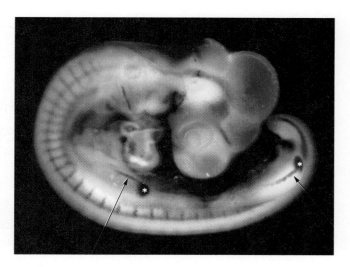

Figure 9-16 Whole-mount preparation (double in situ hybridization) of a chick embryo showing the expression of FGF-4 in the apical ectodermal ridge *(arrows)* and somites. In addition to the bases of the limb buds (dark spots indicated by *asterisks*), sonic hedgehog is expressed in the notochord, floor plate, gut, some branchial arches, midbrain, and forebrain. (Courtesy A. López-Martínez and J.F. Fallon, Madison, Wis.)

Figure 9-15 Schematic representations of molecular control of limb development. **A,** Molecular control of the dorsoventral axis. En-1 inhibits both Wnt-7a and r-Fng. **B,** Molecular control along the anteroposterior and proximodistal axes. *r-Fng,* Radical fringe; *ZPA,* zone of polarizing activity.

posterior mesoderm (the ZPA) (Figure 9-16). In turn, under the influence of sonic hedgehog, FGF-4 begins to be expressed in the posterior half of the apical ectodermal ridge. Once the production of FGF-4 is induced, FGF-4 and sonic hedgehog form a positive feedback loop, and each stimulates the formation of the other. FGF secreted by the apical ectodermal ridge, working through **insulin-like growth factor-1,** also stimulates the proliferation of mesodermal cells throughout the entire limb bud.

Simultaneous with the establishment of the ZPA, an orderly sequence of expression of the homeobox-containing genes **Hoxd-9** to **Hoxd-13** (Figure 9-17, *A* and *B*), as well as

certain of the **Hoxa** genes, occurs in the early limb bud. What stimulates the expression of the *Hox* genes is not presently known. Evidence in some vertebrates suggests that the *Hoxa* genes are mostly involved in patterning along the proximodistal axis and that the *Hoxd* genes are also involved in patterning along the anteroposterior axis. Studies on mice have shown limb defects corresponding to zones of *Hoxa* and *Hoxd* expression (Figure 9-18). Mutations of Hoxa-13 and Hoxd-13 cause characteristic patterns of **polysyndactyly** as well as reduction defects of the digits resulting from shortness of the phalanges (Figure 9-19).

The establishment of the ZPA and its secretion of the sonic hedgehog protein set up a signaling center that organizes limb development along the anteroposterior axis. Sonic hedgehog induces the expression of BMP-2 in the posterior mesoderm. In addition, it acts reciprocally on the apical ectodermal ridge. In the absence of sonic hedgehog activity, the apical ridge fails to be maintained.

The apical ectodermal ridge acts as the organizing center for the proximodistal axis of the limb by stimulating the proliferation of the mesodermal cells. Just beneath the apical ectodermal ridge is a region of distal mesoderm that is several hundred microns thick; this region has been called the **progress zone** (Figure 9-20). Cells in the progress zone divide actively and are not morphogenetically determined. As the limb bud grows out, however, mesodermal cells that are far enough proximal to escape the influence of the apical ectodermal ridge become fixed in their ultimate morphogenetic fate so that cells leaving the progress zone early ultimately form proximal skeletal elements (e.g., humerus, femur) and cells leaving later form elements of the forearm or hand in the

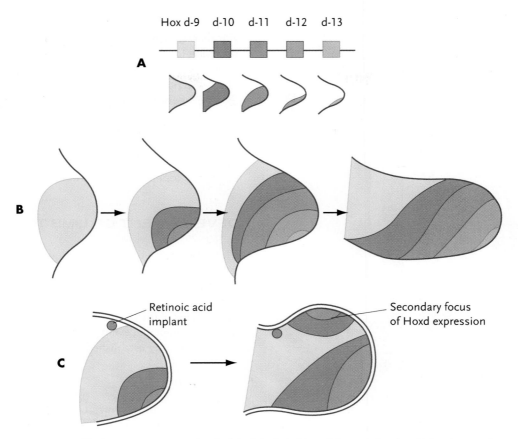

Figure 9-17 *Hoxd* gene expression in the chick limb bud. **A,** Map of this gene family and distribution of individual gene products. **B,** Development of the aggregate pattern of *Hoxd* gene expression over time in the normal limb bud. **C,** The development of a secondary focus of *Hoxd* gene expression in the area of supernumerary limb formation caused by an implant of retinoic acid. (Based on Tabin CJ: *Development* 116:289-296, 1992.)

upper limb. Cells in the progress zone are characterized by their expression of the *Msx-1* gene, and as they leave the progress zone, expression of this gene ceases. There is something about the environment of the progress zone that stimulates *Msx-1* expression because if mesodermal cells that have left the progress zone (and consequently cease production of *Msx-1*) are transplanted back into the progress zone, they reexpress that molecule (see Figure 9-20, *B*). In addition, the positional values (see later section) of the transplanted cells are reset so that they can now form more distal structures than they would have done had they not been transplanted.

A major unanswered question in limb development is what causes an arm to become an arm and a leg to become a leg. It is quite clear that the development of upper and lower extremities involves many common mechanisms, but the question of what determines the difference in form between arms and legs is far from answered. Molecular embryologists are just

beginning to identify certain types of homeobox-containing genes that are differentially expressed between arms and legs, but a coherent explanation for the difference still eludes them.

Many of the newer molecular data fit into an older model of **positional information**. According to this concept, cells of a developing structure, such as limb mesoderm, are exposed to environmental signals. In some manner, these cells are able to receive and interpret the signals and then differentiate according to this information. A specific example relating to limb development involves the influence of the ZPA on the developing limb. According to the classic theory, the ZPA produces a diffusible **morphogen** (a molecule capable of influencing morphogenesis). As the morphogen diffuses through the mesoderm, its concentration decreases with time and distance, setting up a concentration gradient. The cells along the anteroposterior axis of the limb bud can sense the different concentrations of the morphogen (presumably sonic

Hoxa, Hoxd

9   10   11   12   13

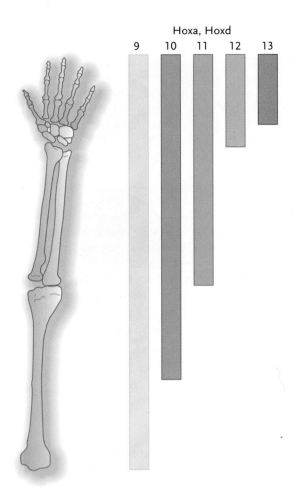

Figure 9-18 Levels of *Hox* gene expression in relation to skeletal components of the limb. Molecular data from the mouse are superimposed on the human limb skeleton.

hedgehog protein or a molecule induced by sonic hedgehog) and then differentiate accordingly (Figure 9-21, *A*). An explanation for the formation of a supernumerary limb when a piece of posterior mesoderm (or retinoic acid) is transplanted to the anterior margin of the limb bud (see Figure 9-14, *A*) is that the anterior mesodermal cells are now exposed to a high concentration of the morphogen and are tricked into thinking that they should develop into posterior structures. A second apical ectodermal ridge is induced over the graft, and a duplicate array of *Hoxd* gene expression appears (Figure 9-17, *C*) before the formation of a mirror image supernumerary limb.

DEVELOPMENT OF LIMB TISSUES

The morphogenetic events previously described take place largely during the early stages of limb development when the limb bud consists of a homogeneous-appearing mass of mesodermal cells covered by ectoderm. The differentiation and histogenesis of the specific tissue components of the limb are later developmental events that build on the morphogenetic blueprint already established.

Skeleton

The skeleton is the first major tissue of the limb to show signs of overt differentiation. Its gross morphology, whether normal or abnormal, closely reflects the major pattern-forming events that shape the limb as a whole. Formation of the skeleton can be first seen as a condensation of mesenchymal cells in the central core of the proximal part of the limb bud. Even before undergoing condensation, these cells are determined to form cartilage, and if they are transplanted

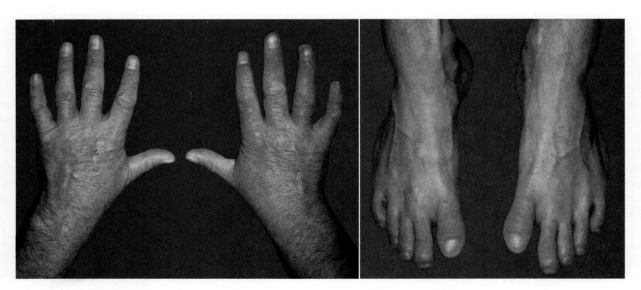

Figure 9-19 Hands and feet of a person with a mutation of the *Hoxa-13* gene. Both thumbs and great toes are more proximally situated than normal. In addition, some phalanges are shortened, and the nails are hypoplastic. (Courtesy J.W. Innis, Ann Arbor, Mich.)

to other sites or into culture, they differentiate only into cartilage. However, other mesenchymal cells that would normally form connective tissue retain the capacity to differentiate into cartilage if they are transplanted into the central region of the limb bud.

The ectoderm of the limb bud exerts an inhibitory effect on cartilage differentiation, so cartilage does not form in the region just beneath the ectoderm. In vitro studies suggest that the inhibition is mediated by a diffusible material secreted by the ectoderm. Whether this is the same mechanism that maintains the integrity of the progress zone remains to be determined.

The condensed cells comprising the precartilaginous aggregates express both BMP-2 and BMP-4. As skeletal development continues, their expression becomes progressively restricted to the cells that will become the perichondrium or periosteum surrounding the bones. BMP-3 transcripts are first seen in cartilage, rather than precartilage, but this growth factor also becomes ultimately located in the perichondrium. The translocation of expression of these BMP molecules to the perichondrium reflects their continuing role in the earliest phases of differentiation of skeletal tissues.

In contrast, another BMP (BMP-6) is expressed only in areas of maturing (hypertrophying) cartilage within the limb bones. **Indian hedgehog,** a molecule related to sonic hedgehog, is also expressed in the same regions of hypertrophying cartilage (which is also marked by the presence of type X collagen), and this signaling molecule may actually induce the expression of BMP-6.

Differentiation of the cartilaginous skeleton occurs in a proximodistal sequence, and in mammals the postaxial structures of the distal limb segments differentiate before the preaxial structures. For example, the sequence of formation of the digits is from the fifth to the first (Figure 9-22). The postaxial skeleton of the arm is considered to be the ulna, digits 4 and 5, and the corresponding carpal elements. The

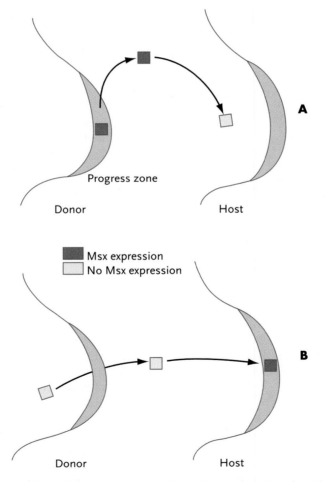

Figure 9-20 Msx-1 expression and the progress zone. **A,** If Msx-1–expressing tissue from the progress zone is transplanted into more proximal regions of the limb bud, it soon stops expressing that molecule. **B,** If proximal mesenchyme that has already stopped expressing Msx-1 is transplanted back into the progress zone, it reexpresses the molecule.

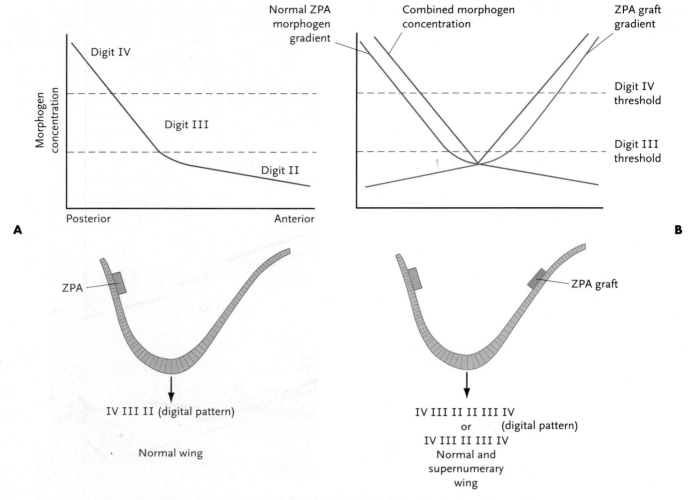

Figure 9-21 A, Diminishing concentration gradient of the hypothetical morphogen released from the ZPA. The lowest concentration (*below the lower dashed line*) is compatible with the formation of digit II; the highest concentration (*above the upper dashed line*) is compatible with the formation of digit IV. B, Explanation of the formation of duplicate limb structures after a ZPA graft. The additive level of the two morphogen gradients from the normal and grafted ZPAs determines the types of digits that form.

radius, digits 1 through 3, and the corresponding carpal bones constitute the preaxial skeleton. Such terminology is often used to classify certain limb defects called **hemimelias**, in which many or all of the preaxial or postaxial components of the limb are missing (Figure 9-23).

One of the characteristic features in differentiation of the limb skeleton is the formation of joints. Joint formation occurs by the transverse splitting of precartilaginous rods rather than by the apposition of two separate skeletal elements. The morphology of joint formation has been well described, but the molecular underpinnings of joint formation are just beginning to be understood. Joint formation is first apparent when transverse strips of highly condensed cells cross a precartilaginous rod (Figure 9-24). At this stage, **growth/differ-**

entiation factor-5 (Gdf-5), a member of the BMP family, is expressed in the zone of cell density. Condensation is followed by cell death and matrix changes in the region of the future joint. Then the skeletal elements on either side of the joint form articular cartilage, and a fluid-filled gap forms between them. Additional condensations of mesenchymal cells form the joint capsule, ligaments, and tendons. During later development, muscular activity is required to maintain the integrity of the joint, but early joint development is completely independent of muscular activity. A well-known mutant, called **brachypodism**, involves a shortening of the limb and the lack of development of certain joints, specifically those between the proximal and middle phalanges. In this mutant, Gdf-5 expression is also absent in these joint regions.

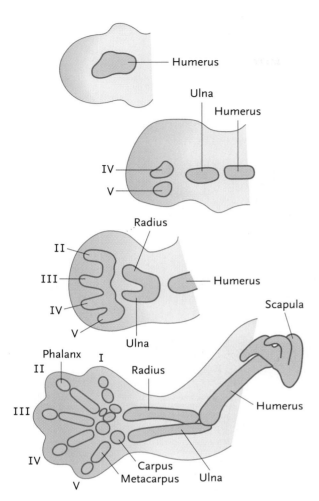

Figure 9-22 Formation of the skeleton in the mammalian forelimb.

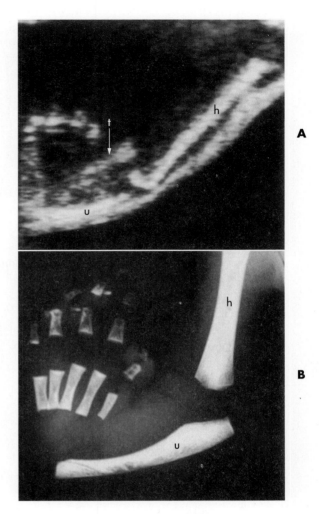

Figure 9-23 Radial hemimelia (absent radius) in a **27-week-old** fetus. **A,** Ultrasound image showing a thumb (*arrow*) but no radius. **B,** Postnatal x-ray image confirming the absent radius. *u,* Ulna; *h,* humerus. (From Nyberg D and others: *Diagnostic ultrasound of fetal anomalies,* St Louis, 1990, Mosby.)

Musculature

The musculature of the limb is derived from myogenic cells that migrate into the very early limb bud from the ventral part of the dermomyotome of the somite. These cells are stimulated to leave the somite and migrate toward the limb through the stimulus of **scatter factor (hepatic growth factor),** which is produced by the proximal cells of the limb-forming area. Before migrating, the premuscle cells in the somite express **c-met,** which is a specific receptor for scatter factor. The premyogenic cells, which are morphologically indistinguishable from the other mesenchymal cells but which express Pax-3, spread throughout the limb bud. In the splotch mutant, which is characterized by the absence of Pax-3 expression, muscle cells do not populate the limb bud. The migrating premuscle cells keep pace with the elongation of the limb bud, although cells expressing characteristic muscle molecules (e.g., MyoD) are not seen in the progress zone. Some experimental evidence suggests that premyogenic cells are not present in the progress zone; other ex-

periments have shown that the environment of the progress zone suppresses the expression of MyoD and other muscle-specific molecules, possibly through the mitosis-promoting influence of the FGFs in that area.

Shortly after the condensations of the skeletal elements take shape, the myogenic cells themselves begin to coalesce into two common muscle masses: one the precursor of the flexor muscles and the other giving rise to the extensor muscles. The next stage in muscle formation is the splitting of the **common muscle masses** into anatomically recognizable precursors of the definitive muscles of the limb. Little is known about the mechanisms that guide the splitting of the common muscle masses. The fusion of myoblasts into early myotubes begins to occur during these early stages of muscle development.

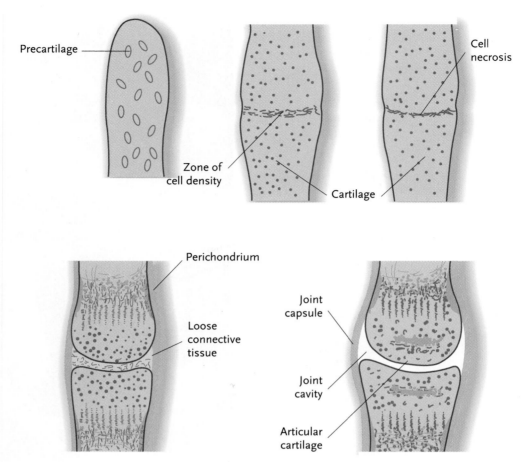

Figure 9-24 Sequence of the formation of the joints in the limbs.

Considerable evidence suggests that myogenic precursor cells do not possess intrinsic information guiding their morphogenesis. Rather, it appears that the myogenic cells follow the lead of connective tissue cells, which are the bearers and effectors of the morphogenetic information required to form anatomically correct muscles. In experiments in which the somites normally associated with a limb bud are removed and replaced by somites from elsewhere along the body axis, myogenic cells are morphogenetically neutral. Muscle morphogenesis is typically normal even though the muscle fiber precursors are derived from abnormal sources.

Through the removal of somites, the use of x-radiation, and the analysis of certain mutants such as *wingless*, it has been shown that the tendons and connective tissue components of a muscle are derived from the limb bud mesoderm, whereas the muscle fibers themselves are somite derived. In situations in which myogenic cells are prevented from entering the limb bud, morphologically appropriate tendons still form, but these tendons are not attached to "muscles." In the same limbs, other connective tissue cells form a model of the muscle, even though it does not contain muscle fibers.

Depending on the specific muscle, the migration, fusion, or displacement of muscle primordia may be involved in the genesis of the final form of the muscle. In one case, genetically programmed cell death, apoptosis, is responsible for the disappearance of an entire muscle layer (the **contrahentes muscle**) in the flexor side of the human hand. The myogenic cells differentiate to the myotube stage; they then accumulate with glycogen and soon degenerate. The contrahentes muscle layer is preserved in most of the great apes. The reason it degenerates in the human hand at such a late stage in its differentiation is not understood.

Although limb muscles assume their definitive form in the very early embryo, they must undergo considerable growth in both length and cross-sectional area to keep up with the overall growth of the embryo. This is accomplished by the division of the satellite cells (see Chapter 8) and the fusion of their progeny with the muscle fibers. The added satellite cell nuclei increase the potential of the muscle fiber to produce structural and contractile proteins, which increase the cross-sectional area of each muscle fiber. Accompanying this addition to the nuclear complement of the muscle fibers is

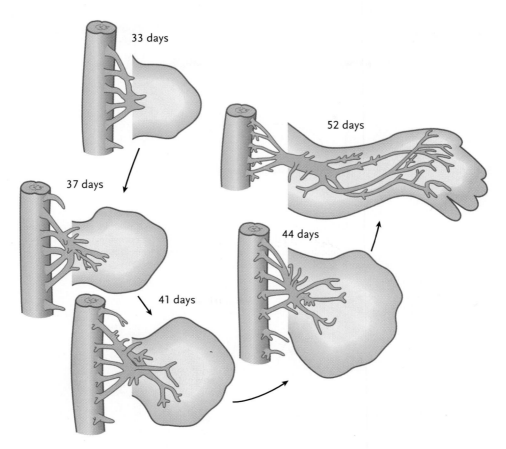

33 days

37 days

41 days

44 days

52 days

Figure 9-25 Development of the nerve pattern of the human upper extremity. (Based on Shinohara H and others: *Acta Anat* 138:265-269, 1990.)

their lengthening by the addition of more sarcomeres, usually at the ends of the muscle fibers. The formation of new muscle fibers typically ceases at or shortly after birth. Although the muscles are capable of contracting in the early fetal period, their physiological properties continue to mature until after birth.

Innervation

Motor axons originating in the spinal cord enter the limb bud at an early stage of development (during the fifth week) and begin to grow into the dorsal and ventral muscle masses before the latter have split up into primordia of individual muscles (Figure 9-25). Tracing studies have shown a high degree of order in the projection of motor neurons into the limb. Neurons located in medial positions in the spinal cord send axons to the ventral muscle mass, whereas those located more laterally in the spinal cord supply the dorsal muscle mass. Similarly, a correlation exists between the craniocaudal position of neurons in the cord with the anteroposterior pattern of innervation of limb muscles within the common muscle masses.

For example, the rostralmost neurons innervate the most anterior muscle primordia.

Local cues at the base of the limb bud seem to guide the entering pathways of nerve fibers into the limb bud. If a segment of the spinal cord opposite the area of limb bud outgrowth is reversed in the craniocaudal direction, the motor neurons change the direction of their outgrowth and enter the limb bud in their normal positions (Figure 9-26). If larger segments of spinal cord are reversed and the neurons are at considerable distances from the level of the limb bud, their axons do not find their way to their normal locations in the limb bud. The muscles themselves apparently do not provide specific target cues to the ingrowing axons, since if muscle primordia are prevented from forming, the main patterns of innervation in the limb are still normal.

Sensory axons enter the limb bud after the motor axons and use them for guidance. Similarly, neural crest cell precursors of Schwann cells lag slightly behind the outgrowth of motor axons into the limb bud. Cells of the neural crest surround both motor and sensory nerve fibers to form the coverings of the nerves in the limbs. By the time digits have

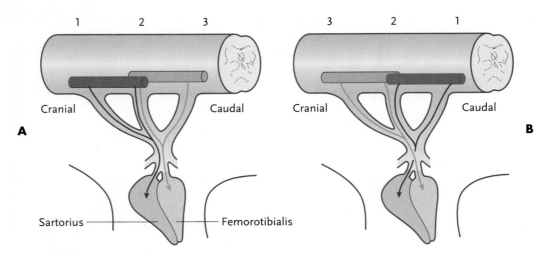

Cranial   Caudal   Cranial   Caudal

A   **B**

Sartorius   Femorotibialis

Figure 9-26 Pathways taken by axons from specific pools of motoneurons in the spinal cord to limb muscles in the hindlimb of the chick embryo. **A,** Normal limb. **B,** After reversal of three segments of the embryonic spinal cord, axons originating from the spinal cord pass through abnormal pathways to innervate the muscles that they were originally destined to innervate. (Modified from Brown M and others: *Essentials of neural development,* Cambridge, Mass, 1990, Cambridge University Press.)

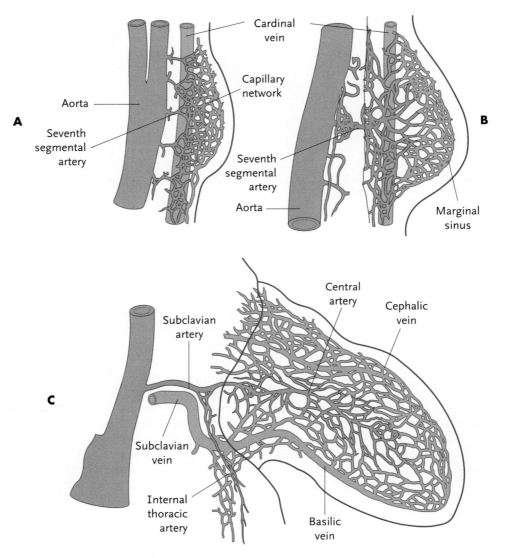

Figure 9-27 Early stages in the development of the vascular pattern in the mammalian limb bud. **A,** Equivalent of a **4-week-old** human embryo. **B,** Equivalent of **5-week-old** human embryo. **C,** Equivalent of a **6-week-old** human embryo.

formed in developing limbs, the basic elements of the gross pattern of innervation in the adult limb have been established.

Vasculature

The earliest vasculature of the limb bud is derived from endothelial cells arising from several segmental branches of the aorta and the cardinal veins and to some extent from **angioblasts** (endothelial cell precursors) endogenous to the limb bud mesoderm. Initially, the limb vasculature consists of a fine capillary network, but soon, some channels are preferentially enlarged, resulting in a large central artery that supplies blood to the limb bud (Figure 9-27). From the central artery, the blood is distributed to the periphery via a mesh of capillaries and then collects into a **marginal sinus**, which is located beneath the apical ectodermal ridge. Blood in the marginal sinus drains into peripheral venous channels, which carry it away from the limb bud.

Even in the earliest limb bud there is a peripheral avascular zone of mesoderm within about 100 μm of the ectoderm of the limb bud (Figure 9-28, A). The avascular region persists until the digits have begun to form. Angioblasts are present in the avascular zone, but they are isolated from the functional capillaries. Experimental studies have clearly shown that the proximity of ectoderm is inhibitory to vasculogenesis in the limb bud mesoderm. If the ectoderm is removed, vascular channels form to the surface of the limb bud mesoderm, and if a piece of ectoderm is placed into the deep limb mesoderm, an avascular zone forms around it (Figure 9-28, B). Degradation products of hyaluronic acid, which is secreted by the ectoderm, appear to be the inhibitory agents.

Just before the skeleton begins to form, avascular zones appear in the areas where the cartilaginous models of the bones will take shape. Neither the stimuli for the disappearance of the blood vessels nor the fate of the endothelial cells that were present in these regions is understood at this time.

The pattern of the vascular channels changes constantly as the limb develops, mainly by the outgrowth of sprouts from existing channels, the regression of original channels, and the coalescence of the sprouts to form new ones. Such a mechanism accounts for the distal progression of the marginal sinus. With the establishment of the digital rays, the apical portion of the marginal sinus breaks up, but the proximal channels of the marginal sinus persist into adulthood as the **basilic** and **cephalic veins** of the arm (see Figure 9-27, C).

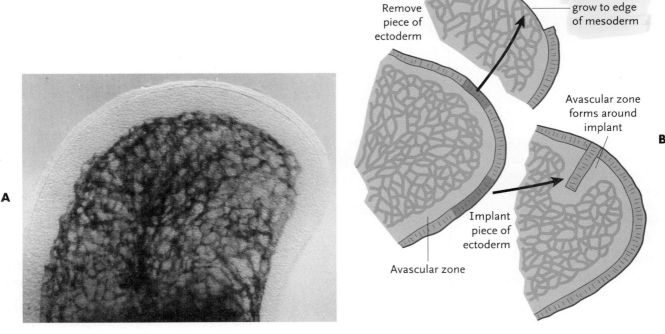

Figure 9-28 A, Photomicrograph of a quail wing bud with ink-injected blood vessels. **B**, Experiments illustrating the inhibitory effect of limb ectoderm on vascularization of the subjacent mesoderm. *Left*, Normal limb bud with an avascular zone beneath the ectoderm. *Upper right*, After removal of a piece of ectoderm, capillaries grow to the edge of the mesoderm in the region of removal. *Lower right*, A zone of avascularity appears around a piece of implanted ectoderm. (**A** courtesy R. Feinberg. Based on Feinberg RN, Noden DM: *Anat Rec* 231:136-144, 1991.)

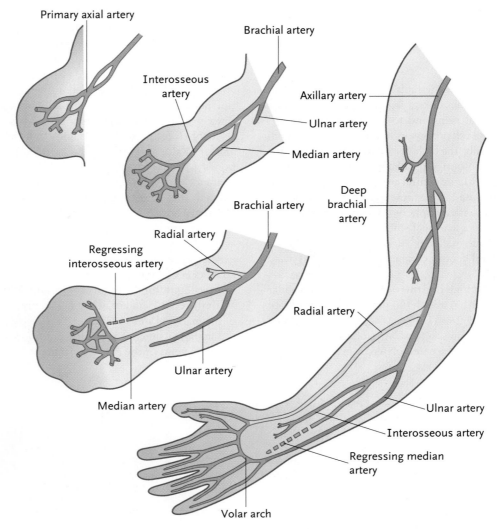

Figure 9-29 Formation of arteries in the human arm.

Similar major changes take place in the arterial channels that course through the developing limb (Figure 9-29). Branches arising from the primary axial artery ultimately take ascendancy, especially in the forearm, leaving the original primary axial artery a relatively minor vessel (the **interosseous artery**) in the forearm.

SUMMARY

- Limbs arise from the lateral plate mesoderm and the overlying ectoderm under the influence of an inductor (possibly FGF-8 from the intermediate mesoderm). The early limb bud is a highly regulative system that can compensate for a variety of surgical disturbances and still form a normal limb. The axes of the limb are fixed in an anteroposterior, dorsoventral, and proximodistal sequence.
- The early limb bud mesoderm stimulates the overlying ectoderm to form an apical ectodermal ridge that stimulates the outgrowth of the limb through proliferation of the underlying mesodermal

cells. FGF-2 and FGF-4 are secreted by the apical ridge and can induce outgrowth in the absence of the ridge. The overall morphogenesis of the limb is determined by properties of the mesoderm, whereas the ectoderm acts in a more permissive sense.
- Cell death is an important mechanism in normal limb development. Regions of programmed cell death include the axillary region and the interdigital spaces. In the absence of interdigital cell death, syndactyly results.
- A ZPA located in the posterior mesoderm acts as a biological signaler and plays an important role in the anteroposterior organization of the limb by releasing sonic hedgehog. Wnt-7a, which is released by dorsal ectoderm, is the organizer of dorsoventrality in the limb bud. According to the concept of positional information, cells in the developing limb are exposed to positional cues (such as the signal from the ZPA) that allow them to determine their relative position within the limb bud. The cells then process this information and differentiate accordingly. Proximodistal control of morphogenesis may reside in the progress zone, a narrow band of mesoderm beneath the apical ectodermal ridge.

CLINICAL CORRELATION 9-1
Limb Anomalies

Because they are so obvious, limb anomalies are frequently described in the literature. For many, however, the etiology remains unknown, especially when individual cases are considered. Some human anomalies parallel those that can be produced by specific experimental manipulations. Many other limb malformations cannot be attributed to disturbances of specific mechanisms.

A number of limb anomalies have been attributed to vascular anomalies, but it is not always easy to know whether the vascular abnormalities preceded or accompanied the overall defective development in the limb. One of the persisting explanations for the proximal reduction defect in **phocomelia** (see Figure 7-2), in which the distal limb structures are well formed, is secondary damage to the blood vessels in the proximal part of the limb bud after the pattern for distal hand or foot structures has been established. This would then cause regression of proximal limb structures.

Some of the most commonly encountered limb defects can be attributed to mechanical causes. **In-trauterine amputations** by amniotic bands, presumably caused by tears in the amnion, can result in the loss of parts of digits or even hands or feet (see Figure 7-15). Other deformities, such as **clubfoot (talipes equinovarus)** and some cases of congenital dislocations, have been attributed to persistent mechanical pressures of the uterine wall on the fetus, particularly in cases of **oligohydramnios** (see Chapter 6).

Other limb anomalies are familial and have a genetic basis as either dominant or recessive traits. Although some of the anomalies such as amelia and polydactyly are known to exist as mutants in laboratory animals, the developmental defect underlying the genesis of a given human defect may not be the same as the one in the animal model; several defective mechanisms can give rise to the same phenotype.

A very rare limb deformity is **macromelia** (or **macrodactyly**), in which a limb or a digit is considerably enlarged over normal. Such abnormalities are sometimes associated with neurofibromatosis, and the neural crest may be involved in this defect.

- Retinoic acid exerts a profound effect on limb morphogenesis and can cause the formation of a supernumerary limb if applied to the anterior border of the limb bud, but its exact role in limb development remains obscure. Expression of a variety of homeobox-containing genes follows well-defined patterns in the normally developing limb. Some patterns of gene expression are profoundly altered in limbs treated with retinoic acid.

- The skeleton of the limb arises from lateral plate mesoderm. The ectoderm of the limb bud inhibits cartilage formation in the mesoderm cells immediately beneath it. This could explain the reason the skeleton of the vertebrate limb forms in a central position.

- Limb muscles arise from cells derived from somitic mesoderm. These cells express Pax-3 during their migration into the limb bud. Myogenic cells first form dorsal and ventral common muscle masses, which later split into primordia of individual muscles. Morphogenetic control of muscles resides in the associated connective tissue rather than in the muscle cells themselves. Later stages in muscle development may involve cell death, the fusion of muscle primordia, and the displacement of muscle primordia to other areas.

- Nerves grow into the developing limb bud and become associated with the common muscle masses as they split into individual muscles. Local cues are important in guiding growing axons into the developing limb.

- The vasculature of the limb bud arises from cells budding off the aorta and cardinal veins as well as from endogenous mesodermal cells. The early vascular pattern consists of a central artery, which drains into a peripheral marginal sinus and then into peripheral venous channels. Blood vessels do not form beneath the ectoderm or in the central cartilage-forming regions.

- Limb anomalies can form as the result of genetic mutations, drug effects, disturbed tissue interactions, and purely mechanical effects.

CLINICAL VIGNETTE

After a normal pregnancy and labor, a 32-year-old woman gave birth to a 7-lb boy who had a duplication of his right foot along the anteroposterior axis. To the left of a single big toe (hallux) were four additional toes arranged in a mirror-symmetrical fashion so that the pattern of digits in that foot was 543212345, with 1 being the common hallux. Two older siblings were normal.

How can you explain this malformation on the basis of developmental mechanisms learned in this chapter?

REVIEW QUESTIONS

1. Which of the following molecules plays an important role in the determination of the dorsoventral axis of the developing limb?
    A. Msx-1
    B. Wnt-7a
    C. Hoxd-13
    D. Pax-1
    E. FGF-8
2. What molecule is associated with myogenic cells migrating into the limb bud from the somites?
    A. Shh
    B. BMP-7
    C. FGF-4
    D. Pax-3
    E. En-1

3. What is the principal function of the apical ectodermal ridge?
   A. Stimulating outgrowth of the limb bud
   B. Setting up the anteroposterior axis of the limb bud
   C. Determining the specific characteristics of the ectodermal appendages of the limb
   D. Determining the pattern of neural ingrowth into the limb
   E. Attracting the subcutaneous plexus of capillaries in the limb bud
4. In the developing limb the sonic hedgehog (Shh) gene product is produced in the:
   A. Progress zone
   B. Region of interdigital cell death
   C. ZPA
   D. Apical ectodermal ridge
   E. Common muscle mass
5. The connective tissue of the limb arises from the:
   A. Paraxial mesoderm
   B. Neural crest
   C. Intermediate mesoderm
   D. Somitic mesoderm
   E. Lateral mesoderm
6. The formation of clubfoot (talipes equinovarus) is associated with:
   A. A misplaced ZPA
   B. Defective cellular migration from somites
   C. Thalidomide
   D. Oligohydramnios
   E. A neural crest defect
7. A baby whose mother underwent chorionic villus sampling during pregnancy was born with the tips of two digits missing. What is a possible cause?
8. A woman who underwent amniocentesis during pregnancy gave birth to a child with a duplicated thumb. What is a possible cause?
9. If the somites close to a limb-forming region are experimentally removed, the limbs form without muscles. Why?
10. A child is born with webbed fingers (syndactyly). What is the reason for this anomaly?

REFERENCES

Brand-Saberi B and others: Scatter factor/hepatocyte growth factor (SF/HGF) induces emigration of myogenic cells at interlimb level in vivo, *Dev Biol* 179:303-308, 1996.

Brook WJ, Diaz-Benjumea FJ, Cohen SM: Organizing spatial pattern in limb development, *Annu Rev Cell Dev Biol* 12:161-180, 1996.

Christ B, Jacob HJ, Jacob M: Experimental analysis of the origin of the wing musculature in avian embryos, *Anat Embryol* 150:171-186, 1977.

Cihák R: Ontogenesis of the skeleton and intrinsic muscles of the human hand and foot, *Adv Anat Embryol Cell Biol* 46:1-194, 1972.

Coelho CND and others: Altered expression of the chicken homeobox-containing genes GHox-7 and GHox-8 in the limb buds of *limbless* mutant chick embryos, *Development* 113:1487-1493, 1991.

Cohn MJ and others: Fibroblast growth factors induce additional limb development from the flank in chick embryos, *Cell* 80:739-746, 1995.

Dealy CN, Kosher RA: IGF-1, insulin and FGFs induce outgrowth of the limb buds of amelic mutant chick embryos, *Development* 122:1323-1330, 1996.

Dylevsky I: Connective tissue of the hand and foot, *Acta Univ Carol [Med Mongr]* 127:1-195, 1988.

Dylevsky I: Growth of the human embryonic hand, *Acta Univ Carol [Med Monogr]* 114:1-139, 1986.

Fallon JF and others: FGF-2: apical ectodermal ridge growth signal for chick limb development, *Science* 264:104-107, 1994.

Feinberg RN: Vascular development in the embryonic limb bud. In Feinberg RN, Sherer GK, Auerbach R, eds: *The development of the vascular system,* Basel, Switzerland, 1991, Karger, pp 136-148.

Feinberg RN, Noden DM: Experimental analysis of blood vessel development in the avian wing bud, *Anat Rec* 231:136-144, 1991.

Fernandez-Teran M and others: Limb initiation and development is normal in the absence of the mesonephros, *Dev Biol* 189:246-255, 1997.

Ganan Y and others: Role of TGFβs and BMPs as signals controlling the position of the digits and the areas of interdigital cell death in the developing chick autopod, *Development* 122:2349-2357, 1996.

Grieshammer U and others: The chick limbless mutation causes abnormalities in limb bud dorsal-ventral patterning: implications for the mechanism of apical ridge formation, *Development* 122:3851-3861, 1996.

Grim M, Wachtler F: Muscle morphogenesis in the absence of myogenic cells, *Anat Embryol* 183:67-70, 1991.

Harrison RG: On relations of symmetry in transplanted limbs, *J Exp Zool* 32:1-136, 1921.

Herault Y, Duboule D: Le contrôle génétique du développement des membres, *Ann Genet* 39:222-232, 1996.

Heymann S and others: Regulation and function of SF/HGF during migration of limb muscle precursor cells in chicken, *Dev Biol* 180:566-578, 1996.

Hinchliffe JR, Johnson DR: *The development of the vertebrate limb,* Oxford, England, 1980, Clarendon.

Izpisua-Belmonte J-C, Duboule D: Homeobox genes and pattern formation in the vertebrate limb, *Dev Biol* 152:26-36, 1992.

Izpisua-Belmonte J-C and others: Expression of the homeobox Hox-4 genes and the specification of position in chick wing development, *Nature* 350:585-589, 1991.

Johnson RL, Tabin CJ: Molecular models for vertebrate limb development, *Cell* 90:979-990, 1997.

Kelley RO, Fallon JF: Ultrastructural analysis of the apical ectodermal ridge during morphogenesis. I. The human forelimb with special reference to gap junctions, *Dev Biol* 51:241-256, 1976.

Laufer E and others: Expression of radical fringe in limb-bud ectoderm regulates apical ectodermal ridge formation, *Nature* 386:366-373, 1997.

Logan C and others: The role of engrailed in establishing the dorsoventral axis of the chick limb, *Development* 124:2317-2324, 1997.

Maini PK, Solursh M: Cellular mechanisms of pattern formation in the developing limb, *Int Rev Cytol* 129:91-133, 1991.

Marigo A and others: Conservation in hedgehog signaling: induction of a chicken patched homolog by sonic hedgehog in the developing limb, *Development* 122:1225-1233, 1996.

Michaud JL, Lapointe F, Le Douarin NM: The dorsoventral polarity of the presumptive limb is determined by signals produced by the somites and by the lateral somatopleure, *Development* 124:1453-1463, 1997.

Mrázková O: Blood vessel ontogeny in upper extremity of man as related to developing muscles, *Acta Univ Carol [Med Monogr]* 115:1-114, 1986.

Muragaki Y and others: Altered growth and branching patterns in synpolydactyly caused by mutations in Hoxd 13, *Science* 272:548-551, 1996.

Nelson CE and others: Analysis of Hox gene expression in the chick limb bud, *Development* 122:1449-1466, 1996.

Niswander L and others: Function of FGF-4 in limb development, *Mol Reprod Dev* 39:83-89, 1994.

Riddle RD and others: Sonic hedgehog mediates the polarizing activity of the ZPA, *Cell* 75:1401-1416, 1993.

Rijli FM, Chambon P: Genetic interactions of Hox genes in limb development: learning from compound mutants, *Curr Opin Genet Dev* 7:481-487, 1997.

Robert B and others: The apical ectodermal ridge regulates Hox-7 and Hox-8 gene expression in developing limb buds, *Genes Dev* 5:2363-2374, 1991.

Robert E, Harris J, Kallen BAJ: The epidemiology of preaxial limb formations, *Reprod Toxicol* 11:653-662, 1997.

Ros MA, Sefton M, Nieto MA: *Slug*, a zinc finger gene previously implicated in the early patterning of the mesoderm and the neural crest, is also involved in chick limb development, *Development* 124:1821-1829, 1997.

Ros MA and others: Apical ridge dependent and independent mesodermal domains of and *GHox-8* expression in chick limb buds, *Development* 116:811-818, 1992.

Ros MA and others: The limb field mesoderm determines initial limb bud anteroposterior asymmetry and budding independent of sonic hedgehog or apical ectodermal gene expressions, *Development* 122:2319-2330, 1996.

Rubin L, Saunders JW: Ectodermal-mesodermal interactions in the growth of limb buds in the chick embryo: constancy and temporary limits of the ectodermal induction, *Dev Biol* 28:94-112, 1972.

Sassoon D: *Hox* genes: a role for tissue development, *Am J Respir Cell Mol Biol* 7:1-2, 1992.

Saunders JW: The proximodistal sequence of origin on the parts of the chick wing and the role of the ectoderm, *J Exp Zool* 108:363-403, 1948.

Saunders JW, Gasseling MT: Ectodermal-mesenchymal interactions in the origin of limb symmetry. In Fleischmajer R, Billingham RE, eds: *Epithelial-mesenchymal interactions*, Baltimore, 1968, Williams & Wilkins, pp 78-97.

Saunders JW, Gasseling MT, Saunders LC: Cellular death in morphogenesis of the avian wing, *Dev Biol* 5:147-178, 1962.

Seichert V: Significance of the differential growth, relative tissue shifts and the vascular bed in limb development, *Acta Univ Carol [Med Monogr]* 125:1-162, 1988.

Shinohara H and others: Development of innervation patterns in the upper limb of staged human embryos, *Acta Anat* 138:265-269, 1990.

Stephens TD: The wolffian ridge: history of a misconception, *Isis* 73:254-259, 1982.

Storm EE, Kingsley DM: Joint patterning defects caused by single and double mutations in members of the bone morphogenetic protein (BMP) family, *Development* 122:3969-3979, 1996.

Stratford T, Horton C, Maden M: Retinoic acid is required for the initiation of outgrowth in the chick limb bud, *Curr Biol* 6:1124-1133, 1996.

Stratford TH, Kostakopoulou K, Maden M: Hoxb-8 has a role in establishing early anterior-posterior polarity in chick forelimb but not hindlimb, *Development* 124:4225-4234, 1997.

Summerbell D, Lewis JW, Wolpert L: Positional information in chick limb morphogenesis, *Nature* 244:492-496, 1973.

Swett FH: Determination of limb-axes, *Q Rev Biol* 12:322-339, 1937.

Tabin CJ: The initiation of the limb bud: growth factors, *Hox* genes, and retinoids, *Cell* 80:671-674, 1995.

Tabin CJ: Why we have (only) five fingers per hand: *Hox* genes and the evolution of paired limbs, *Development* 116:289-296, 1992.

Tanaka M and others: Induction of additional limb at the dorsal-ventral boundary of a chick embryo, *Dev Biol* 182:191-203, 1997.

Tickle C, Eichele G: Vertebrate limb development, *Annu Rev Cell Biol* 10:121-152, 1994.

Uhthoff HK: *The embryology of the human locomotor system*, Berlin, 1990, Springer-Verlag.

Wolpert L: Positional information revisited, *Development* 107(suppl):3-12, 1989.

Yang Y, Niswander L: Interaction between the signalling molecules Wnt-7a and shh during vertebrate limb development: dorsal signals regulate anteroposterior patterning, *Cell* 80:939-947, 1995.

Zwilling E: Limb morphogenesis, *Adv Morphogen* 1:301-330, 1961.

10

NERVOUS SYSTEM

Many fundamental developmental processes are involved in the formation of the nervous system. Some of these dominate certain stages of embryogenesis; others occur only at limited times and in restricted locations. The major processes follow:

1. **Induction**, including both primary induction of the nervous system by the underlying notochord and secondary inductions driven by neural tissues themselves
2. **Proliferation**, first as a response of the neuroectodermal cells to primary induction and later to build up critical numbers of cells for virtually all aspects of morphogenesis of the nervous system
3. **Pattern formation**, in which cells respond to genetic or environmental cues in forming the fundamental subdivisions of the nervous system
4. **Intercellular communication** and the adhesion of like cells
5. **Cell migration**, of which there are a variety of distinct patterns in the nervous system
6. **Cellular differentiation** of both neurons and glial cells
7. Formation of specific connections or **synapses** between cells
8. **Stabilization** or **elimination** of specific interneuronal connections, sometimes associated with massive episodes of cell death of unconnected neurons
9. Progressive **development of integrated patterns** of neuronal function, which results in coordinated reflex movements

ESTABLISHMENT OF THE NERVOUS SYSTEM

As described in Chapter 4, primary induction of the nervous system results in the formation of a thickened ectodermal **neural plate** overlying the notochord. Molecular studies conducted mainly on amphibians have shed new light on mechanisms of neural induction. Much of the dorsal ectoderm in gastrulating embryos produces the signaling protein, **bone morphogenetic protein-4 (BMP-4)**, which appears to inhibit the dorsal ectoderm from forming neural tissue. Instead of sending positive inductive signals to the overlying ectoderm, neural inductors, **noggin** and **chordin** (and follistatin in amphibians), block the inhibitory influence of BMP-4, thus allowing the dorsal ectoderm to form neural tissue (the neural plate [see Figure 4-10]). Under the influence of noggin and chordin alone, the induced neural plate develops forebrain characteristics, whereas neural ectoderm induced in the presence of **fibroblast growth factor-8 (FGF-8)** forms caudal neural plate (spinal cord). Neural ectoderm induced in the presence of both noggin and FGF-8 develops midbrain and hindbrain characteristics. Shortly after neural induction, the neural plate begins to fold into the **neural tube** (see Figure 5-11).

During these earliest stages in the establishment of the nervous system, a striking change occurs in the distribution of **cell adhesion molecules (CAMs)** on the surfaces of the ectodermal cells. CAMs protrude from the plasma membrane. Cells of a similar type typically adhere by means of Ca^{++} ions, which bind CAMs of one cell to those of the other (see Figure 4-15). In chick embryos, cells of the early epiblast express both **N-CAM** and **L-CAM** (E-cadherin) before primary induction takes place. As the neural plate takes shape after the primary inductive event, the profound changes that have occurred in the ectoderm are reflected not only in the shapes of the cells but also in their expression of CAMs. Neuroepithelial cells lose their L-CAM and express only N-CAM, whereas the noninduced ectodermal cells lose N-CAM but retain L-CAM.

The neural tube, which is the structural manifestation of the earliest stages in establishing the nervous system, is a prominent structure. In the human, it dominates the cephalic end of the embryo (see Figure 5-10). This chapter describes the way the neural tube develops into the major morphological and functional components of the nervous system.

EARLY SHAPING OF THE NERVOUS SYSTEM

Closure of the neural tube first occurs in the region where the earliest somites appear; closure spreads both cranially and caudally (see Figure 5-10). The unfused regions of the neural tube are known as the **cranial** and **caudal neuropores**. Even before the closure of the neuropores (24 days' gestation for the cranial neuropore and 26 days' gestation for the caudal neuropore), some fundamental subdivisions in the early nervous system can be distinguished. The future spinal cord and brain are recognizable, and within the brain the forebrain (**prosencephalon**), midbrain (**mesencephalon**), and hindbrain (**rhombencephalon**) are distinguishable (Figure 10-1, *A*).

A prominent force in shaping the early nervous system is the overall bending of the cephalic end of the embryo into a C-shape. Associated with this bending is the appearance at the end of the third week of a prominent **cephalic flexure** of the brain at the level of the mesencephalon (see Figure 10-1, *A*). Soon the brain almost doubles back on itself at the cephalic flexure. At the beginning of the fifth week a **cervical flexure** appears at the boundary between the hindbrain and the spinal cord.

By the fifth week the original three-part brain has become further subdivided into five parts (Figures 10-1, *B*, and 10-2). The prosencephalon gives rise to the **telencephalon** (endbrain), with prominent lateral outpocketings that ultimately form the cerebral hemispheres, and a more caudal **diencephalon**. The diencephalon is readily recognizable because of the prominent lateral **optic vesicles** that extend from its lateral walls. The mesencephalon, which is sharply bent by the cephalic flexure, remains undivided and tubular in its overall structure. The roof of the rhombencephalon becomes very thin, and there are early indications of the subdivision

of the rhombencephalon into a **metencephalon** and a more caudal **myelencephalon**. These five subdivisions of the early brain represent a fundamental organization that persists through adulthood. Many further structural and functional components give added layers of complexity to the brain over the next several weeks of embryonic life.

HISTOGENESIS WITHIN THE CENTRAL NERVOUS SYSTEM

Proliferation Within the Neural Tube

Shortly after induction, the thickening neural plate and early neural tube organize into a pseudostratified epithelium (Figure 10-3). In this type of epithelium the nuclei appear to be located in several separate layers within the elongated neuroepithelial cells. The nuclei undertake extensive shifts of position within the cytoplasm of the neuroepithelial cells.

The neuroepithelial cells are characterized by a high degree of mitotic activity, and the position of the nuclei within the neural tube and their stage in the mitotic cycle are closely correlated (Figure 10-4). The synthesis of deoxyribonucleic acid (DNA) occurs in nuclei located near the **external limiting membrane** (the basal lamina surrounding the neural tube). As these nuclei prepare to go into mitosis, they migrate within the cytoplasm toward the lumen of the neural tube, where they undergo mitotic division. Nuclei of the resulting two daughter cells migrate up the cytoplasm toward the external limiting membrane. At this point they have two options: (1) to undergo DNA

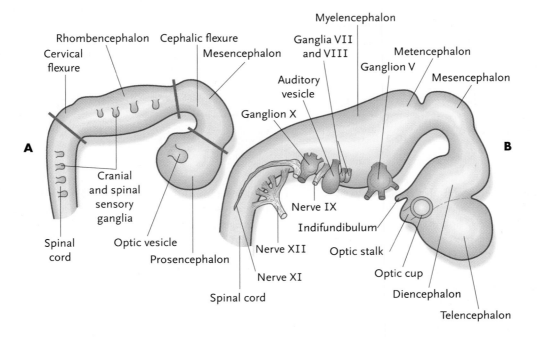

Figure 10-1 Basic anatomy of the three-part (**A**) and five-part (**B**) human brain.

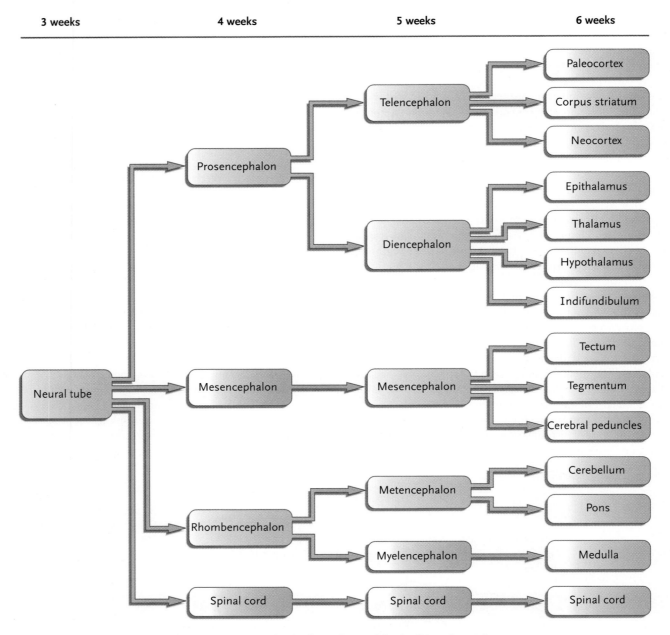

Figure 10-2 Increasing levels of complexity of the developing human brain.

synthesis again and feed back into the mitotic cycle or (2) to leave the mitotic cycle permanently and ultimately take up positions beneath the external limiting membrane as **neuroblasts.** The neuroblasts, cellular precursors of neurons, begin to produce cell processes that ultimately become axons and dendrites.

Cell Lineages in Histogenesis of the Central Nervous System

The origins of most cells found in the mature central nervous system can be traced to **multipotential stem cells** within the early neuroepithelium (Figure 10-5). These cells undergo nu-

merous mitotic divisions before maturing into **bipotential progenitor cells,** which give rise to either neuronal or glial progenitor cells. This developmental bifurcation is accompanied by a change in gene expression. Multipotential stem cells express an intermediate filament protein called **nestin.** Nestin is down-regulated as descendants of bipolar progenitor cells separate into neuronal progenitor cells, which express **neurofilament protein,** and glial progenitor cells, which express **glial fibrillary acidic protein.**

The **neuronal progenitor cells** give rise to a series of neuroblasts. The earliest **bipolar neuroblasts** possess two slender cytoplasmic processes that contact both the external limiting

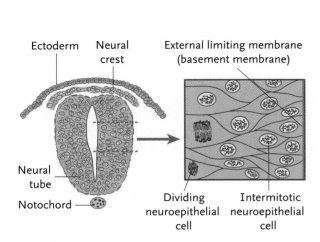

Figure 10-3 *Left,* Cross section through the early neural tube. *Right,* Higher magnification of a segment of the wall of the neural tube.

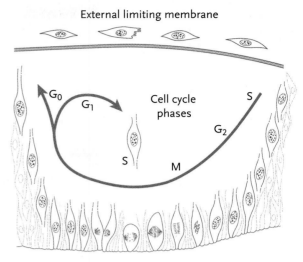

Figure 10-4 Mitotic events in the early neural tube. In pseudostratified cells of the early neural tube, nuclei that synthesize DNA (S phase) are located near the external limiting membrane. Nuclei then move toward the inner margin of the neural tube, where mitosis occurs. The nuclei of daughter cells then move outward toward the external limiting membrane, where cells containing them either undergo another round of DNA synthesis or differentiate into neuroblasts (G_0).

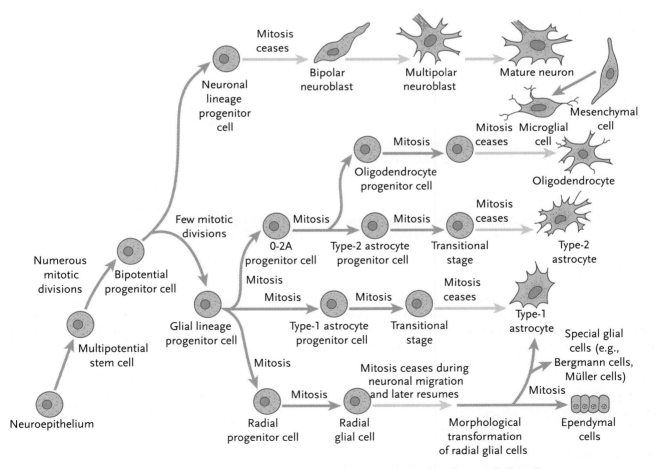

Figure 10-5 Cell lineages in the developing central nervous system. (Based on Cameron R, Rakić P: *Glia* 4:124-127, 1991.)

membrane and the central luminal border of the neural tube. By retracting the inner process, a bipolar neuroblast loses contact with the inner luminal border in the process of becoming a **unipolar neuroblast**. The unipolar neuroblasts accumulate large masses of rough endoplasmic reticulum (**Nissl substance**) in their cytoplasm and then begin to send out several cytoplasmic processes. At this point, they are known as **multipolar neuroblasts**. Their principal developmental activities are to send out axonal and dendritic processes and to make connections with other neurons or end organs.

The other major lineage stemming from the bipotential progenitor cells is the glial line. **Glial progenitor cells** continue to undergo mitosis, and their progeny split into several lines. One, the **O-2A progenitor cell** (see Figure 10-5), is a precursor to two lines of glial cells that ultimately form the **oligodendrocytes** and **type-2 astrocytes**. Another glial lineage gives rise to **type-1 astrocytes**. The origins of oligodendrocytes has long been a matter for debate, but recent studies have shown that human oligodendrocytes arise from progenitor cells located in the ventral ventricular zone (see Figure 10-6) alongside the floor plate. From there, they spread throughout the brain and spinal cord and ultimately form the myelin coverings around neuronal processes in the white matter. The formation of oligodendrocyte precursors depends on an inductive signal from the notochord (possibly sonic hedgehog). If notochord is transplanted alongside dorsal neural tube, oligodendrocyte precursors differentiate there, showing that cells with the potential to form oligodendrocytes reside in that area, but normally do not develop because of the lack of an adequate inductive signal.

The third glial lineage has a more complex history. Radial progenitor cells give rise to **radial glial cells**, which act as guide wires in the brain for the migration of young neurons (see Figure 10-21). When the neurons are migrating along the radial glial cells during midpregnancy, they inhibit the proliferation of the radial glial cells. After neuronal cell migration, the radial glial cells, now free from the inhibitory influence of the neurons, reenter the mitotic cycle. Their progeny can transform into a number of cell types. Some can seemingly cross lineage lines and differentiate into type-1 astrocytes (see Figure 10-5). Other progeny differentiate into various specialized glial cell types or even into **ependymal cells**. According to some authors, the remaining neuroepithelial cells represent another source of ependymal cells.

Not all cells of the central nervous system originate in the neuroepithelium. **Microglial cells**, which serve a phagocytic function after damage to the brain, are mesodermally derived immigrant cells. Microglia are not found in the developing brain until it is penetrated by blood vessels.

Fundamental Cross-Sectional Organization of the Developing Neural Tube

The developing spinal cord is a useful prototype for studying the overall structural and functional features of the central nervous system because it preserves its fundamental organization through much of development. With the beginning of cellular differentiation in the neural tube, the neuroepithelium thickens and appears layered. The layer of cells closest to the lumen (**central canal**) of the neural tube remains epithelial and is called the **ventricular zone** (the **ependymal zone** in older literature). This zone, which still contains mitotic cells, ultimately becomes the **ependyma,** a columnar epithelium that lines the ventricular system and central canal of the central nervous system (Figure 10-6). Farther from the ventricular zone is the **intermediate** (formerly called **mantle**) **zone,** which contains the cell bodies of the differentiating postmitotic neuroblasts. As the neuroblasts continue to produce axonal and dendritic processes, the processes form a peripheral **marginal zone** that contains neuronal processes but not neuronal cell bodies.

As the spinal cord matures, the ventricular zone becomes the gray matter, in which the cell bodies of the neurons are located. The marginal zone is called the *white matter* because of the color imparted by the numerous tracts of myelinated nerve fibers in that layer (see Figure 10-6). During development, the proliferating progenitor cell populations in the ventricular zone become exhausted, and the remaining cells differentiate into the epithelium of the ependymal layer.

Once the basic layers in the spinal cord are established, a number of important topographical features can be recognized in cross sections of the cord. A **sulcus limitans** within

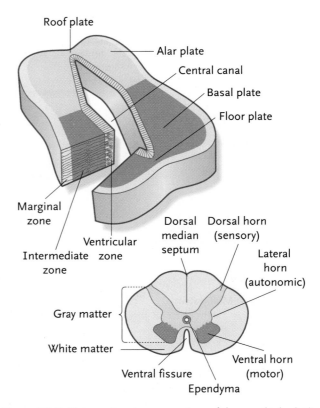

Figure 10-6 Major regions in cross sections of the neural tube (*top*) and spinal cord (*bottom*).

the central canal divides the cord into a dorsal **alar plate** and a ventral **basal plate** on each side of the central canal. The right and left alar plates are connected dorsally over the central canal by a thin **roof plate**, and the two basal plates are connected ventrally by a **floor plate**.

The basal plate represents the motor component of the spinal cord. Axons arising from neurons located in the **ventral horn** of the gray matter exit the spinal cord as **ventral motor roots** of the spinal nerves (see Figure 10-13). The gray matter of the alar plate, called the **dorsal horn**, is associated with sensory functions. Sensory axons from the spinal ganglia (neural crest derivatives) enter the spinal cord as dorsal roots and synapse with neurons in the dorsal horn. A small projection of gray matter between the dorsal and ventral horns at spinal levels T1 to L2 contains cell bodies of autonomic neurons. This projection is called the **lateral horn** or sometimes the **intermediolateral gray column** (see Figure 10-6).

The floor plate is far more than an anatomical connection between the right and left basal plates. Cells of the future floor plate are the first to differentiate in the neural plate after primary induction of the nervous system. Experimental work has demonstrated a specific inductive influence of the notochord on the neuroepithelial cells that overly it. If an extra notochord is grafted along the lateral surface of the neural tube, the neuroepithelial cells closest to it acquire the properties of floor plate cells (Figure 10-7). Conversely, if a segment of normal notochord is removed, the neuroepithelial cells overlying it do not acquire the properties of floor plate cells.

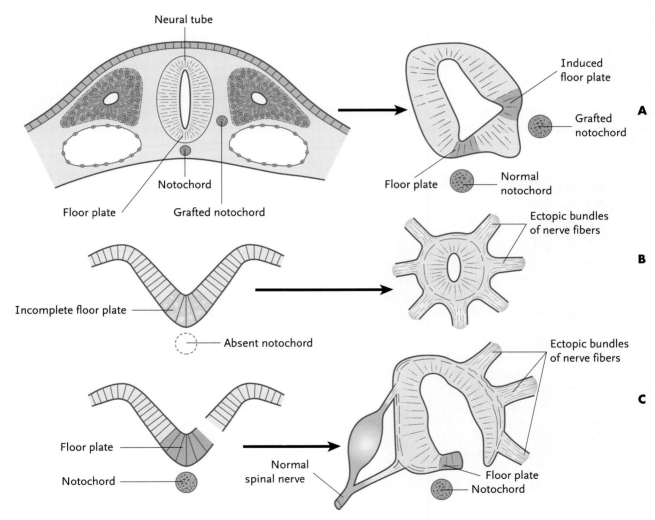

Figure 10-7 Experiments illustrating the influence of the notochord on development of the floor plate and exit sites of nerves from the spinal cord. **A,** Grafting an extra notochord near the neural tube induces a secondary floor plate. **B,** In the absence of a notochord, a very incomplete floor plate forms, and nerve fibers exit from multiple sites around the spinal cord. **C,** Slitting the neural plate on one side of the floor plate removes the wall of the neural tube from the influence of the notochord, allowing the disorganized exit of nerve fibers from that part of the spinal cord. (Modified from Hirano S, Fuse S, Sohal GS: *Science* 251:310-313, 1991.)

Through its action on the floor plate, the notochord also exerts a profound effect on the organization of the dorsal and ventral roots that enter and leave the spinal cord. If the notochord is absent, the neural tube closes, but recognizable dorsal and ventral roots are absent. Numerous ectopic nerve fibers appear in their place (Figure 10-8). If the future floor plate is split, the side of the neural tube on which the notochord is located develops normal dorsal and ventral roots, whereas the side lacking these structures gives off ectopic nerves (see Figure 10-7, C).

Recent studies have provided a molecular basis for cross-sectional pattern formation within the early neural plate and neural tube (Figure 10-9). In the early neural plate the homeobox-containing transcription factors, Pax-3, Pax-7, Msx-1, and Msx-2, are expressed throughout the neural plate. Even before the neural plate has folded over to become the neural tube, the notochord, which is adherent to the midline neural plate at this stage, releases **sonic hedgehog**. Local hedgehog signaling stimulates the neural plate cells directly above the notochord to transform into **floor plate**. One of the first stages of this transformation is the repression of Pax-3 and Pax-7 expression, which allows the neuroectodermal cells near the midline of the neural plate to adopt a ventral fate (i.e., floor plate, basal plate). Cells of the floor plate itself then become sites of production of sonic hedgehog. Sonic hedgehog pro-

duced by both the notochord and the floor plate then diffuses laterally through the neural plate and induces cells on either side of the floor plate to become **motor neurons**.

In addition to inducing motor neurons, the floor plate plays other roles in the developing nervous system. A number of groups of neuronal processes cross from one side of the central nervous system to the other through the floor plate as **commissural axons**. These axons, leading from neuronal cell bodies located in the dorsal half of the neural tube, are attracted to the floor plate by specific molecules produced in that region, (e.g., **netrin 1**). In mutant animals lacking netrin 1, commissural axons are disorganized and do not cross to the other side through the floor plate. Not only does the floor plate attract certain types of axons, but it also repels others. A specific example is the trochlear nerve (cranial nerve IV), whose axons do not cross to the other side from their cell bodies of origin because of some yet undefined repellent molecules present in the floor plate.

Development of the cross-sectional organization of the neural tube involves not only a ventralizing influence from the notochord but also an opposing dorsalizing influence from the epidermal ectoderm adjacent to the developing neural tube. In the lateral regions of the neural plate (future dorsal region of the neural tube), BMP-4 and BMP-7, expressed by nonneural ectoderm at the ectodermal-lateral neural plate junction, exert a dorsalizing inductive effect on the neuroectodermal cells by elevating levels of Pax-3, Pax-7, Msx-1, and Msx-2. This results in the formation of the roof plate and the alar plate. In addition, the same inductive influence stimulates the expression of a transcription factor, **slug**, in future neural crest cells before they have left the neural tube. After closure of the neural tube, the BMP influence induces the formation of sensory interneurons in the dorsal half (alar plate) of the spinal cord.

CRANIOCAUDAL PATTERN FORMATION AND SEGMENTATION

Through neural induction, the early central nervous system becomes organized into broad regions that will develop cranial, middle, and caudal characteristics (see p. 66). This is soon followed by the appearance of the morphological subdivisions outlined in Figure 10-2. At an even finer level, segments called **rhombomeres** appear in the region of the hindbrain (see Figure 5-12), and a less distinct series of subdivisions called **prosomeres** appears in the forebrain.

Patterning in the Hindbrain and Spinal Cord Regions

The rhombomeres, which were introduced in Chapter 5, are the morphological reflection of a highly segmentally ordered pattern of expression of a variety of developmentally prominent genes (Figure 10-10). **Krox-20** and the **Hox** genes ap-

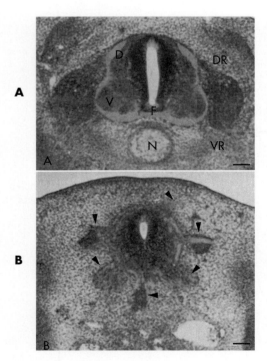

Figure 10-8 **A,** Photomicrograph of a normal embryonic quail spinal cord. **B,** In an experiment in which the notochord was absent, the spinal cord is disorganized and has multiple exit sites of nerve fibers (see Figure 12-7, *B*). Arrowheads indicate ectopic spinal nerves. *D,* Dorsal; *V,* ventral; *DR,* dorsal root; *VR,* ventral root; *N,* notochord; *F,* floor plate. (From Hirano S, Fuse S, Sohol GS: *Science* 251:310-313, 1991.)

pear to be particularly important in determining the segmental nature of the hindbrain. If *Krox*-20 is knocked out in mice, rhombomeres 3 and 5 fail to form. *Krox*-20 acts upstream of the *Hox* genes and exerts local regulatory control over them. *Krox*-20 also acts upstream from genes for receptors that restrict cell intermingling between odd- and even-numbered rhombomeres. In a manner still poorly understood, retinoic acid appears to exert an even broader control of *Hox* gene expression. As is the case in segmentation of the vertebrae (see pp. 161-162), excess retinoic acid causes an anterior shift in *Hox* gene expression and a corresponding posterior shift in

rhombomeres so that a given rhombomere is transformed into the next most posterior one. By the same token a deficiency in retinoic acid results in the formation of a small hindbrain without posterior rhombomeres.

The correspondence between the rhombomeres of the developing hindbrain and other structures of the cranial and pharyngeal arch region is remarkable (see Chapter 13). The cranial nerves, which have a highly ordered pattern by which they supply structures derived from the pharyngeal arches and other structures in the head, have an equally highly ordered origin with respect to the rhombomeres (Figure 10-11).

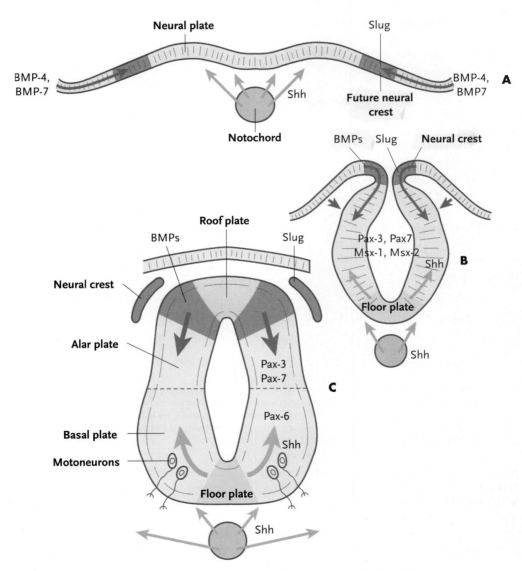

Figure 10-9 Dorsal and ventral signaling in the early central nervous system. **A,** Signals from sonic hedgehog *(Shh)* *(orange arrows)* in the notochord induce the floor plate. **B,** In the dorsal part of the future neural tube, BMP-4 and BMP-7 *(green arrows)* from the ectoderm adjacent to the neural tube induces slug in the future neural crest and maintains Pax-3 and Pax-7 expression dorsally. Ventrally, sonic hedgehog, now produced by the floor plate, induces motoneurons. **C,** Sonic hedgehog, produced by the floor plate, suppresses the expression of dorsal *Pax* genes *(Pax-3* and *Pax-7)* in the ventral half of the neural tube.

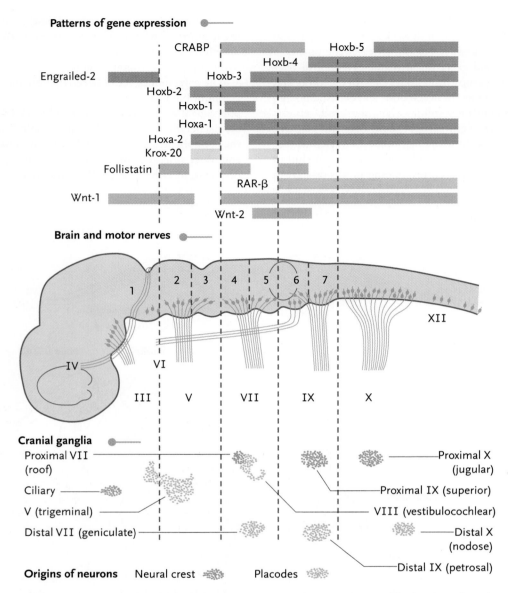

Figure 10-10 Patterns of *Hox* and other gene expression in relation to anatomical landmarks in the early mammalian embryo. The bars refer to craniocaudal levels of expression of a given gene product. Cranial sensory nerves derived from the neural crest and placodal precursors are laid out in proper register. *CRABP*, Cytoplasmic retinoic acid–binding protein; *RAR*, retinoic acid receptor. (Modified from Noden DM: *J Craniofac Genet Dev Biol* 11:192-213, 1991.)

For example, cranial nerve V innervates structures derived from the first pharyngeal arch. Cranial nerves VII and IX innervate the second and third arch structures, respectively. In embryos of birds, the species studied most extensively, cell bodies of the motor components of cranial nerves V, VII, and IX are initially found exclusively in rhombomeres 2, 4, and 6. Dye injection studies have shown that the progeny of a single neuroblast remain within the rhombomere containing the injected cell, suggesting that rhombomeres have the properties of cellular compartments. Axons contributing to a cranial nerve extend laterally within the rhombomere and converge on a common exit site in the craniocaudal midpoint of the

rhombomere. At a slightly later stage in development, motor neurons originating in the next more posterior rhombomere (3, 5, 7) extend axons laterally. However, before the axons reach the margin of the rhombomere, they cross into rhombomeres 2, 4, or 6 and converge on the motor axon exit site in the even-numbered rhombomere. Comparative studies indicate species differences in the relationship between rhombomeres and origins of the cranial nerves. Relationships between neuromeres and cranial nerves are outlined in Table 10-1.

The cell bodies (within the central nervous system the collection of cell bodies of a single cranial nerve is called a **nucleus**) of the cranial nerves that innervate the pharyngeal

NERVOUS SYSTEM   **217**

TABLE 10-1 Relationship Among Neuromeres, Pharyngeal Arches, Cranial Nerves, and the Neural Crest

Primary neuromeres	Secondary neuromeres	Exits of cranial nerves			Neural crest	Pharyngeal arches
		SSA	SVE	GSE		
P	T	I				
	D1	II				
	D2					
M	M1			III	} Mesencephalic	
	M2					
	Isthmus			IV		
Rh A	r 1				Trigeminal	} 1
	r 2		V			
	r 3				Otic	} 2
Rh B	r 4	VIII	VII			
	r 5				Glossopharyngeal	} 3
Rh C	r 6		IX	VI	Vagal	} 4-6
	r 7		X, XI			
Rh D	r 8			XII	Hypoglossal	

Adapted from Müller F, O'Rahilly R: *Acta Anat* 158:83-99, 1997.
SSA, Special somatic afferent; *SVE*, special visceral efferent; *GSE*, general somatic efferent; *P*, prosencephalon; *T*, telencephalon; *D*, diencephalon; *M*, mesencephalon; *Rh*, rhombencephalon; *r*, rhombomere.

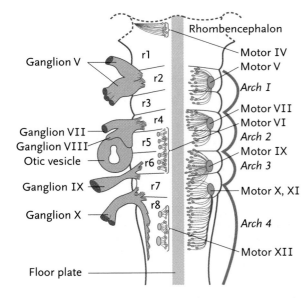

Figure 10-11 Origin of cranial nerves in relation to rhombomeres (*r*) in the developing brain. (Based on Lumsden A, Keynes R: *Nature* 337:424-428, 1989.)

arches arise in register along the craniocaudal axis. The motor nuclei of other cranial nerves that innervate somatic structures (e.g., extraocular muscles or the tongue) arise in a different craniocaudal column along the hindbrain and do not occupy contiguous rhombomeres (see Figure 10-11).

Direct and indirect evidence indicates that properties of the walls of the rhombomeres prevent axons from straying

into inappropriate neighboring rhombomeres. One cellular property, which is also characteristic of regions of somites that restrict the movement of neural crest cells, is the ability of cells of the wall of the rhombomere to bind specific lectins. In apparent contradiction to the compartmentalization just described, processes growing from sensory neuroblasts and from nerves of a tract called the *medial longitudinal fasciculus* are free to cross rhombomeric boundaries. Blood vessels first enter the hindbrain in the region of the floor plate soon after the emergence of the motor axons and spread within the interrhombomeric junctions. The way the vascular branches recognize the boundaries of the rhombomeres is not known.

In contrast to the hindbrain, the pattern of nerves emanating from the spinal cord does not appear to be determined by craniocaudal compartmentalization within the cord. Rather, the segmented character of the spinal nerves is dictated by the somitic mesoderm along the neural tube. Outgrowing motor neurons from the spinal cord and migrating neural crest cells can easily penetrate the anterior mesoderm of the somite, but they appear to be repulsed by the posterior half of the somite. This results in a regular pattern of spinal nerve outgrowth, with one bilateral pair of spinal nerves per body segment. Rotating the early neural tube about its craniocaudal axis does not result in an abnormal pattern of spinal nerves. This further strengthens the viewpoint that the pattern of spinal nerves is not generated within the neural tube itself. Despite many studies on molecular differences between anterior and posterior somitic mesoderm, the exact molecular basis for the repulsion or attraction of spinal nerves by specific regions of the somites remains unknown.

Patterning in the Midbrain Region

One of the fundamental patterning mechanisms in the midbrain region is a molecular signaling center located at the border between the mesencephalon and metencephalon (see Figure 5-13). The principal signaling molecule appears to be **FGF-8**, which is expressed in a narrow ring at the anterior border of the first rhombomere, a subdivision of the metencephalon. Acting with **Wnt-1**, FGF-8 induces the expression of the engrailed genes, **En-1** and **En-2**, which are expressed in decreasing concentrations at increasing distances from the FGF-8 signaling center (see Figure 5-13). This signaling center induces and polarizes the dorsal midbrain region and the cerebellum. Grafts of the signaling center, called the *isthmic region,* or beads releasing FGF-8 alone into more cranial regions of the forebrain of the avian embryo induce a second tectum (dorsal mesencephalon or colliculi in mammals). Similarly, isthmic grafts into regions of the hindbrain can induce supernumerary cerebellar structures.

One byproduct of the recent molecular studies is the realization that in some species, at least, the boundary between the future midbrain and hindbrain does not correspond to the anatomical constriction between the mesencephalon and rhombencephalon. Instead, it is located cranial to that constriction in a plane marked by the posterior limit of expression of the homeobox-containing gene, **Otx-2**.

Patterning in the Forebrain Region

Although some investigators have subdivided the early forebrain into segments called **prosomeres** (Figure 10-12), very

little definitive information exists concerning the control of patterning in the forebrain. Studies with marked cells indicate that in contrast with the rhombomeres, cells can migrate through the boundaries of the prosomeres. Especially in the region of the future telencephalon, there does not seem to be major compartmentalization. A narrow band of **sonic hedgehog** expression at the border between the future dorsal and ventral thalamus has been suggested to be a forebrain signaling center, but more research is necessary to verify that hypothesis. Although the embryonic forebrain is not underlain by notochord and does not possess a floor plate, sonic hedgehog is nevertheless expressed in a craniocaudal strip along the ventral telencephalon and diencephalon. As is the case in the early spinal cord, sonic hedgehog induces ventral motor neurons in these forebrain regions.

PERIPHERAL NERVOUS SYSTEM

Structural Organization of a Peripheral Nerve

The formation of a peripheral nerve begins with the outgrowth of axons from motor neuroblasts located in the basal plate (the future ventral horn of the gray matter) of the spinal cord (Figure 10-13). Near the dorsal part of the spinal cord, thin processes also begin to grow from neural crest–derived neuroblasts that have aggregated to form the spinal ganglia. **Dendrites,** which conduct impulses toward the nerve cell body, grow from the sensory neurons toward the periphery. **Axons,** which conduct impulses away from the cell body, penetrate the dorsolateral aspect of the spinal cord and terminate in the dorsal horn (the gray matter of the alar plate). Within the gray matter, short interneurons connect the terminations of the sensory axons to the motor neurons. These three con-

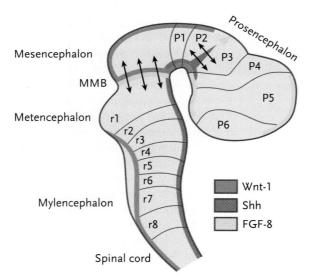

Figure 10-12 Generalized brain of a vertebrate embryo showing segmentation in the hindbrain (rhombomeres [*r*]) and forebrain (prosomeres [*P*]) and the distribution of major signaling molecules. The midbrain/hindbrain signaling region is indicated by the arrows just rostral to the first rhombomere. The arrows between the second and third prosomeres represent a hypothetical signaling region in the forebrain. *MMB,* Mesencephalic-metencephalic border. (Adapted from Bally-Cuif L, Wassef M: *Curr Opin Genet Dev* 5:450-458, 1995.)

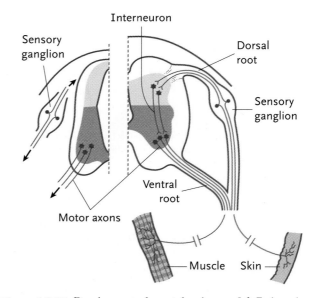

Figure 10-13 Development of a peripheral nerve. *Left,* Early embryo. *Right,* Fetus.

nected neurons (motor, sensory, and interneuron) constitute a simple **reflex arc** through which a sensory stimulus can be translated into a simple motor response. Autonomic nerve fibers are also associated with typical spinal nerves.

Within a peripheral nerve the neuronal processes can be myelinated or unmyelinated. At the cellular level, **myelin** is a multilayered spiral sheath consisting largely of phospholipid material that is formed by individual **Schwann cells** (neural crest derivatives) wrapping themselves many times around a nerve process like a jelly roll (Figure 10-14). This wrapping serves as a form of insulation that determines to a great extent the character of the electrical impulse (action potential) traveling along the neuronal process. **Unmyelinated nerve fibers** are also embedded in the cytoplasm of Schwann cells, but they lack the characteristic spiral profiles of myelinated processes (see Figure 10-14).

The Schwann cells that surround myelinated and unmyelinated axons are different not only in their morphology but also, not surprisingly, in their patterns of gene expression. Through the actions of a family of growth factor–like proteins (**neuregulins**), the axon associated with a Schwann cell precursor promotes the differentiation of the Schwann cell and helps determine whether it will produce myelin or form

a nonmyelinating Schwann cell. Schwann cell precursors that are not associated with axons do not receive neuregulin support and undergo programmed cell death, a mechanism that preserves an appropriate ratio of Schwann cells to axons.

Within the central nervous system the color of the white matter is the result of its high content of myelinated nerve fibers, whereas the gray matter contains unmyelinated fibers. Schwann cells are not present in the central nervous system; instead, myelination is accomplished by oligodendrocytes. Although one Schwann cell in a myelinated peripheral nerve fiber can wrap itself around only one axon or dendrite, a single oligodendroglial cell can myelinate several nerve fibers in the central nervous system.

Patterns and Mechanisms of Neurite Outgrowth

The outgrowth of **neurites** (axons or dendrites) involves many factors both intrinsic and extrinsic to the neurite. Although similar in many respects, the outgrowth of axons and dendrites differs in fundamental ways.

An actively elongating neurite is capped by a **growth cone** (Figure 10-15). Growth cones are characterized by an ex-

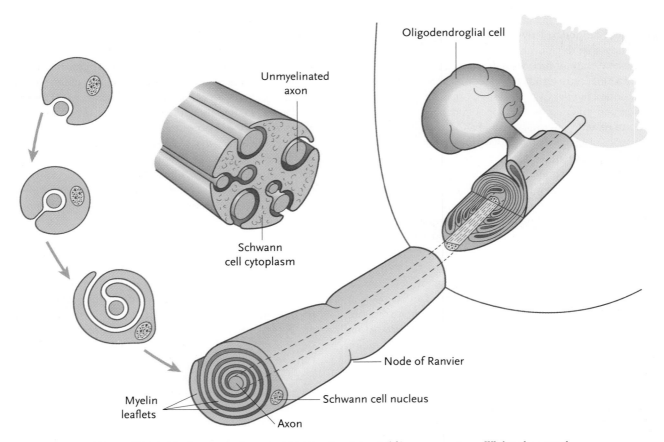

Figure 10-14 Myelination in the central (*right*) and peripheral (*left*) nervous systems. Within the central nervous system, myelin is formed by oligodendroglial cells. In the peripheral nervous system, Schwann cells wrap around individual axons. The inset shows a segment through a region of unmyelinated nerve fibers embedded in the cytoplasm of a single Schwann cell.

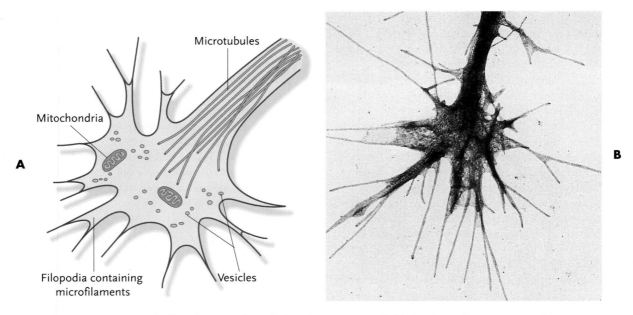

Figure 10-15 **A,** Growth cone at the end of an elongating axon. **B,** High-voltage electron micrograph of a growth cone in culture. (**A** from Landis S: *Annu Rev Physiol* 45:567-580, 1983. **B** courtesy K. Tosney, Ann Arbor, Mich.)

panded region of cytoplasm with numerous spikelike projections called **filopodia.** In vitro and in vivo studies of living nerves show that the morphology of an active growth cone is in a constant state of flux, with filopodia regularly extending and retracting as if testing the local environment. Growth cones contain numerous cytoplasmic organelles, but much of the form and function of the filopodia depends on the large quantities of **actin** microfilaments that fill these processes. In the presence of agents that disrupt actin filaments, the filopodia retract and the growth cones cease to function normally.

Whether growth cones progress forward, remain static, or change directions depends in large measure on their interactions with the local environment. If the environment is favorable, a filopodium remains extended and adheres to the substrate around it, whereas other filopodia on the same growth cone retract. Depending on the location of the adhering filopodia, the growth cone may lead the neurite to which it is attached straight ahead or change its direction of outgrowth. This outgrowth appears to be guided by four broad types of environmental influences: **chemoattraction, contact attraction, chemorepulsion,** and **contact repulsion.** It now appears that outgrowing nerve processes find themselves in different environments every couple hundred microns and that some environments give them signals to continue extending forward, whereas other environments may act as "stop" signals or "turn" signals.

Growth cones can respond to concentration gradients of diffusible substances (e.g., nerve growth factor) or to weak local electrical fields. A major family of chemoattractant molecules is called the **netrins.** The repulsive counterparts to

the netrins are members of a family of secreted proteins called **semaphorins.**

Growth cones can also respond to fixed physical or chemical cues from the microenvironment immediately surrounding them. For example, the caudal half of the somite repulses the ingrowth of motor axons and of neural crest cells into that area. Repulsion is manifested by the collapse of the growth cone and the retraction of the filopodia. On the other hand, extracellular matrix glycoproteins such as **fibronectin** and especially **laminin** strongly promote the adhesion and outgrowth of neurites. Integral membrane proteins (**integrins**) on the neurites bind specifically to arginine-glycine-asparagine sequences on the glycoproteins and promote adhesion to the substrate containing these molecules.

Other molecules, such as **N-cadherin, N-CAM,** and **L1,** are involved in intercellular adhesion at various stages of cell migration or neurite elongation. N-cadherin, which uses Ca^{++} as an ionic agent to bind two like molecules together, is heavily involved in the intercellular binding of cells in neuroepithelia. It also plays a role in the adhesion of parallel outgrowing neurites. In a peripheral nerve, one **pioneering axon** typically precedes the others in growing toward its target. Other axons then follow, forming **fascicles** (bundles) of axons. Fasciculation is facilitated by intercellular adhesion proteins such as L1, which help bind parallel nerve fibers. If antibodies to the L1 protein are administered to an area of neurite outgrowth, fasciculation is disrupted. N-CAM is present on the surfaces of most embryonic nerve processes and muscle fibers and is involved in the initiation of neuromuscular contacts. Antibodies to N-CAM interfere with the development of neu-

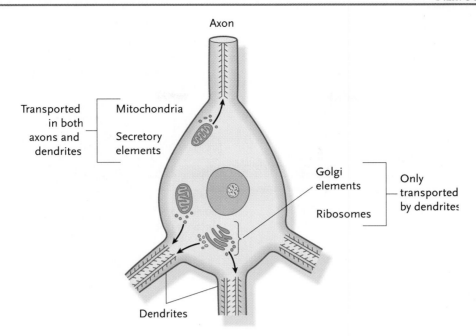

Axon

Transported in both axons and dendrites

Mitochondria

Secretory elements

Golgi elements

Ribosomes

Only transported by dendrites

Dendrites

Figure 10-16 Polarity in a developing neuron. In the axon, microtubules have only one polarity, but in dendrites, microtubules with opposite polarities are present.

romuscular junctions in embryos. Outgrowing neurites interact with many other molecules, the full extent of which is just becoming apparent.

Although the growth cone can be thought of as the director of neurite outgrowth, other factors are important for the elongation of axons. Essential to the growth and maintenance of axons and dendrites is **axonal transport**. In this intracellular process, materials produced in the cell body of the neuron are carried to the ends of these neurites, which can be several feet long in humans.

The cytoskeletal backbone of an axon is an ordered array of microtubules and neurofilaments. **Microtubules** are long, tubular polymers composed of **tubulin** subunits. As an axon extends from its cell body, tubulin subunits are transported down the axon and polymerize onto the distal end of the microtubule. The assembly of **neurofilaments** is organized in a similar polarized manner. The site of these cytoskeletal additions is close to the base of the growth cone, meaning that the axon elongates by being added to distally rather than being pushed out by an addition to its proximal end near the neuronal cell body. A characteristic accompaniment of axonal growth is the production of large amounts of **growth-associated proteins (GAPs)**. Particularly prominent among these is **GAP-43**, which serves as a substrate for protein kinase C and is concentrated in the growth cone.

Outgrowing axons and dendrites differ in several important ways. In contrast to axons, dendrites contain microtubules with polarity running in both directions (Figure 10-16). Another prominent difference is the absence of GAP-43 protein in growing dendrites. One of the first signs of polarity

of a developing neuron is the concentration of GAP-43 in the outgrowing axon and its disappearance from the dendritic processes.

Neurite/Target Relations During Development of a Peripheral Nerve

Developing neurites continue to elongate until they have contacted an appropriate end organ. In the case of motor neurons, that end organ is a developing muscle fiber. Dendrites of sensory neurons relate to a number of types of targets. The end of the neurite must first recognize its appropriate target, and then it must make a functional connection with it.

In the case of motor neurons, evidence that very specific cues guide individual nerves and axons to their muscle targets is increasing. Tracing and transplantation studies have shown that outgrowing motor nerves to limbs supply the limb muscles in a well-defined order and that after minor positional dislocations, they will seek out the correct muscles (see Figure 9-26). Recent evidence suggests that even at the level of neurons, "fast" axons are attracted to the precursors of fast muscle fibers and "slow" axons to those of slow muscle fibers. There are many similar examples of target specificity in dendrites in the peripheral nervous system and of both dendrites and axons in the central nervous system.

When a motor axon and a muscle fiber meet, a complex series of changes in both the nerve and muscle fibers marks the formation of a functional **synapse**, in this case called a **neuromuscular junction** (Figure 10-17). The early changes consist of (1) the cessation of outgrowth of the axon, (2) the prepa-

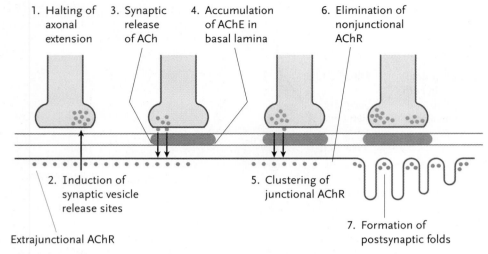

1. Halting of axonal extension
3. Synaptic release of ACh
4. Accumulation of AChE in basal lamina
6. Elimination of nonjunctional AChR
2. Induction of synaptic vesicle release sites
5. Clustering of junctional AChR
Extrajunctional AChR
7. Formation of postsynaptic folds

Figure 10-17 *Major steps in the formation of a neuromuscular junction. ACh, Acetylcholine; AChE, acetylcholinesterase; AChR, acetylcholine receptors.*

ration of the nerve terminal for the ultimate release of appropriate neurotransmitter molecules, and (3) modifications of the muscle fibers at the site of nerve contact so that the neural stimulus can be received and translated into a contractile stimulus. Both neural and muscular components of the neuromuscular junction are involved in stabilizing the morphological and functional properties of this highly specialized synapse.

One of the first signs of specialization at an incipient neuromuscular junction is the formation of synaptic vesicles, which is caused by an influence of the muscle fiber. These vesicles store and ultimately release the neurotransmitter substance **acetylcholine** from the nerve terminal (see Figure 10-17). Before the developing muscle fiber is contacted by the motor neuron, **acetylcholine receptors** (nonjunctional type) are scattered throughout the length of the muscle fiber. After initial nerve contact, myonuclei in the vicinity of the neuromuscular junction produce junction-specific acetylcholine receptors that reside on nerve-induced postjunctional folds of the muscle fiber membrane, and the scattered nonjunctional receptors disappear. Between the nerve terminal and the postsynaptic apparatus of the muscle fiber lies a basal lamina containing molecules that stabilize the acetylcholine receptors at the neuromuscular junction and also **acetylcholinesterase**, an enzyme produced by the muscle fiber.

Factors Controlling Numbers and Kinds of Connections Between Neurites and End Organs in the Peripheral Nervous System

At many stages in the formation of a peripheral nerve, interactions between the outgrowing neurites and the target structure influence the numbers and quality of either the nerve fibers or the targets. The existence of such mechanisms was

demonstrated in the early 1900s by transplanting limb buds onto flank regions. The motor nerves and sensory ganglia that supplied the grafted limbs were substantially larger than the contralateral spinal nerves, which innervated only structures of the body wall. Examination of the spinal cord at the level of the transplant revealed larger ventral horns of gray matter containing more motor neurons than normal for levels of the spinal cord that supply only flank regions.

Additional experiments of this type cast light on normal anatomical relations, which show relatively larger volumes of gray matter and larger nerves at levels from which the normal limbs are innervated. Deletion experiments, in which a limb bud is removed before neural outgrowth, or the congenital absence of limbs results in deficient numbers of peripheral neurons and reduced volumes of gray matter in the affected regions.

Neuronal **cell death (apoptosis)** plays an important role in normal neural development. For example, when a muscle is first innervated, far more than the normal adult number of neurons supply it. At a critical time in development, massive numbers of neurons die. There seem to be a number of reasons for this seemingly paradoxical phenomenon, including the following:

1. Some axons fail to reach their normal target, and cell death is a way of eliminating them.
2. Cell death could be a way of reducing the size of the neuronal pool to something appropriate to the size of the target.
3. Similarly, cell death could compensate for a presynaptic input that is too small to accommodate the neurons in question.
4. Neuronal cell death may also be a means of eliminating connection errors between the neurons and their specific end organs.

All of these reasons for neuronal cell death may be part of a general biological strategy that reduces superfluous initial connections to ensure that enough correct connections have been made. The other developmental strategy, which seems to be much less used, is to control the outgrowth and connection of neurites with their appropriate end organs so tightly that there is little room for error from the beginning. Because of the overall nature of mammalian development, such tight developmental controls would rob the embryo of the overall flexibility it needs to compensate for genetically or environmentally induced variations in other aspects of development.

The mechanisms by which innervated target structures prevent the death of the neurons that supply them are only beginning to be understood. A popular hypothesis is that the target cells release chemical **trophic factors** that neurites take up, usually by binding to specific receptors. The trophic factor then sustains the growth of the neurite. The classic example of a trophic factor is **nerve growth factor,** which supports the outgrowth and prevents the death of sensory neurons. Several other well-characterized molecules are also candidates for trophic factors.

AUTONOMIC NERVOUS SYSTEM

The autonomic nervous system is the component of the peripheral nervous system that subserves many of the involuntary functions of the body, such as glandular activity and motility within the digestive system, heart rate, vascular tone, and sweat gland activity. It is divided into two major divisions, the sympathetic and parasympathetic nervous systems. Components of the **sympathetic nervous system** arise from the thoracolumbar levels (T1 to L2) of the spinal cord, whereas the **parasympathetic nervous system** has a widely separated dual origin from the cranial and sacral regions. Both components of the autonomic nervous system consist of two tiers of neurons: **preganglionic** and **postganglionic.** Postganglionic neurons are derivatives of the neural crest (see Chapter 11).

Sympathetic Nervous System

Preganglionic neurons of the sympathetic nervous system arise from the **intermediate horn** (visceroefferent column) of the gray matter in the spinal cord. At levels from T1 to L2, their myelinated axons grow from the cord through the ventral roots, paralleling the motor axons that supply the skeletal musculature (Figure 10-18). Shortly after the dorsal and ventral roots of the spinal nerve join, the preganglionic sympathetic axons, which are derived from the neuroepithelium of the neural tube, leave the spinal nerve via a **white communicating ramus.** They soon enter one of a series of **sympathetic ganglia** to synapse with neural crest–derived postganglionic neurons.

The sympathetic ganglia, the bulk of which are organized as two chains running ventrolateral to the vertebral bodies, are laid down by neural crest cells that migrate from the closing neural tube along a special pathway (see Figure 11-4). Once the **migrating sympathetic neuroblasts** have reached the site at which the **sympathetic chain ganglia** form, they spread both cranially and caudally until the extent of the chains approximates that seen in the adult. Some of the sympathetic neuroblasts migrate farther ventrally than the level of the chain ganglia to form a variety of other **collateral ganglia** (e.g., **celiac** and **mesenteric ganglia**), which occupy somewhat variable positions within the body cavity. The **adrenal medulla** can be broadly viewed as a highly modified sympathetic ganglion.

The outgrowing preganglionic sympathetic neurons either terminate within the chain ganglia or pass through on their way to more distant sympathetic ganglia to form synapses with the cell bodies of the second-order postganglionic sympathetic neuroblasts (see Figure 10-18). Axons of some postganglionic neuroblasts, which are unmyelinated, leave the chain ganglia as a parallel group and reenter the nearest spinal nerve through the **gray communicating ramus.** Once in the spinal nerve, these axons continue to grow until they reach appropriate peripheral targets, such as sweat glands, arrector pili muscles, and walls of blood vessels. Axons of other postganglionic sympathetic neurons leave their respective ganglia as tangled **plexuses** of nerve fibers and grow toward other visceral targets.

Parasympathetic Nervous System

Although also organized on a preganglionic and postganglionic basis, the parasympathetic nervous system has a distribution quite different from that of the sympathetic system. Like those of the sympathetic nervous system, preganglionic parasympathetic neurons originate in the visceroefferent column of the central nervous system. However, the levels of origin of these neuroblasts are in the midbrain and hindbrain (specifically associated with cranial nerves III, VII, IX, and X) and in the second to fourth sacral segments of the developing spinal cord. Axons from these preganglionic neuroblasts grow long distances before they meet the neural crest–derived postganglionic neurons. These are typically embedded in scattered small ganglia or plexuses in the walls of the organs that they innervate.

The neural crest precursors of the postganglionic neurons often undertake extensive migrations (e.g., from the hindbrain to final locations in the walls of the intestines). The migratory properties of the neural crest precursors of parasympathetic neurons are impressive, but this population of cells also undergoes a tremendous expansion until the final number of enteric neurons approximates the number of neurons in the spinal cord. Evidence is increasing that factors in the gut wall stimulate the mitosis of the neural crest cells migrating there. A striking demonstration of the stimulatory powers of the gut is the ability of pieces of gut wall transplanted along the neural

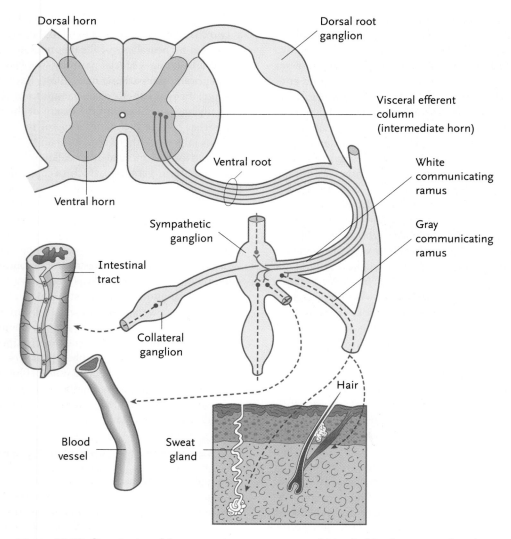

Figure 10-18 Organization of the autonomic nervous system at the level of the thoracic spinal cord. First-order sympathetic neurons are indicated by solid blue lines; second-order sympathetic neurons are indicated by dashed green lines.

tube to cause a great expansion of the region of the neural tube closest to the graft (Figure 10-19).

Differentiation of Autonomic Neurons

At least two major steps are involved in the differentiation of autonomic neurons. The first is the determination of certain migrating neural crest cells to differentiate into autonomic neurons instead of the other possible neural crest derivatives.

At early stages the neural crest cells have the option of becoming components of either the sympathetic or parasympathetic system. This was demonstrated by level-shift transplantations of neural crest cells in birds. For example, when the cephalic neural crest, which would normally form parasympathetic neurons, was transplanted to the level of somites 18 to 24, the transplanted cells migrated and settled into the adrenal medulla as **chromaffin cells**, which are part

of the sympathetic nervous system. Conversely, trunk neural crest cells transplanted into the region of the head often migrated into the lining of the gut and differentiated into postganglionic parasympathetic neurons.

A second major step in the differentiation of autonomic neurons involves the choice of the neurotransmitter that the neuron will use. Typically, parasympathetic postganglionic neurons are **cholinergic** (i.e., they use acetylcholine as a transmitter), whereas sympathetic neurons are **adrenergic** (noradrenergic) and use norepinephrine as a transmitter.

As they arrive at their final destinations, autonomic neurons are noradrenergic. They then enter a phase during which they select the neurotransmitter substance that will characterize their mature state. Considerable experimental evidence suggests that the choice of transmitter proceeds independently of other concurrent events, such as axonal elongation and the innervation of specific target organs.

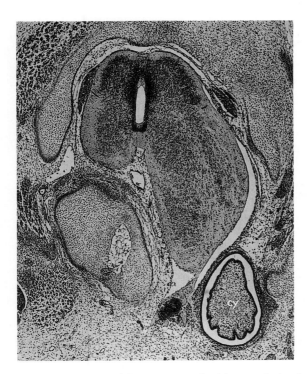

Figure 10-19 Influence of the gut on growth of the neural tube. A graft of quail duodenum was placed between the neural tube and somites of a chick embryo host. The spinal cord on the side near the graft of gut has greatly enlarged, causing secondary distortion of the musculoskeletal structures near it. *cy,* Cyst of donor endoderm. (From Rothman TP and others: *Dev Biol* 124:331-346, 1987.)

At surprisingly late stages in their development, autonomic neurons still retain flexibility in their choice of neurotransmitter. For example, sympathetic neurons in newborn rats are normally adrenergic, and if grown in standard in vitro culture conditions, they produce large amounts of norepinephrine and negligible amounts of acetylcholine. If the same neurons are cultured in a medium that has been conditioned by the presence of cardiac muscle cells, they undergo a functional conversion and instead produce large amounts of acetylcholine (Figure 10-20).

An example of a natural transition of the neurotransmitter phenotype from noradrenergic to cholinergic occurs in the sympathetic innervation of sweat glands in the rat. Neurotransmitter transitions depend on target-derived cues. One such cue is **cholinergic differentiation factor,** a glycosylated basic 45-kDa protein. This molecule, which is present in cardiomyocyte-conditioned medium, is one of a number of chemical environmental factors that can exert a strong influence on late phases of differentiation of autonomic neurons.

Congenital Aganglionic Megacolon (Hirschsprung's Disease)

If a newborn exhibits symptoms of complete constipation in the absence of any demonstrable physical obstruction, the cause is usually an absence of parasympathetic ganglia from the lower (sigmoid) colon and rectum. This condition, commonly called **aganglionic megacolon** or **Hirschsprung's disease,** is normally attributed to the absence of colonization of the wall of the lower colon by neural crest–derived parasympathetic neuronal precursors, presumably of sacral origin because of their distribution. In rare cases, greater parts of the colon lack ganglia.

LATER STRUCTURAL CHANGES IN THE CENTRAL NERVOUS SYSTEM*

Histogenesis Within the Central Nervous System

A major difference between the brain and spinal cord is the organization of the gray and white matter. In the spinal cord the gray matter is centrally located, with white matter surrounding it (see Figure 10-6). In many parts of the brain, this arrangement is reversed, with a large core of white matter and layers of gray matter situated superficial to this core.

One of the fundamental processes in histogenesis within the brain is cell migration. From their sites of origin close to the ventricles in the brain, neuroblasts migrate toward the periphery following set patterns. These patterns often result in a multilayering of the gray substance of the brain tissue. Key players in the migratory phenomenon are radial glial cells, which extend radially toward the periphery long processes from cell bodies located close to the ventricular lumen (Figure 10-21). Young postmitotic neurons, which are typically simple bipolar cells, wrap themselves around the radial glial cells and use them as guides on their migrations from their sites of origin to the periphery.

In areas of brain cortex characterized by multiple layers of gray matter, the large neurons populating the innermost layer migrate first. The remainder of the layers of gray matter are formed by smaller neurons migrating through the first layer and other previously formed layers to set up a new layer of gray matter at the periphery. With this pattern of histogenesis, the outermost layer of neurons is the one formed last, and the innermost is the layer formed first. In a mouse mutant called **weaver,** specific behavioral defects are related to abnormal function of the cerebellum. The morphological basis for this mutant is an abnormality of the radial glial cells in the cerebellum and a consequent abnormal migration of the cells that normally form the granular layer of the cerebellar cortex. Another mutant, called **reeler,** is characterized by abnormal behavior and the absence of normal cortical layering. Recently a protein, called **reelin,** has been shown to be missing in the reeler mutant. Its exact cellular function has not yet been determined, but

---

*The later changes in the central nervous system are so extensive that an exhaustive treatment of even one aspect, such as morphology, is well beyond the scope of this book. This section instead stresses fundamental aspects of the organization of the central nervous system and summarizes the major changes in the organization of the brain and spinal cord.

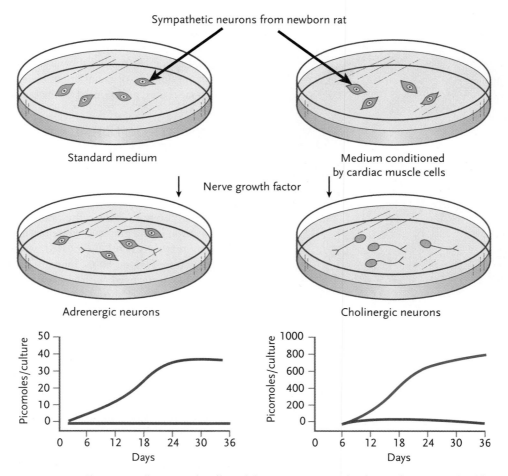

Figure 10-20 Experiment illustrating the effect of the environment on the choice of transmitter by differentiating sympathetic neurons. In standard medium, they become adrenergic; in medium conditioned by cardiac muscles, they become cholinergic. Levels of norepinephrine are in red; levels of acetylcholine are in blue. (Based on Patterson PH and others: *Sci Am* 239[1]:50-59, 1978.)

it may serve as a stop signal for radial neuronal migration or as an insertional signal for migrating neurons.

Increasing evidence indicates that the seemingly featureless cerebral cortex is a matrix of discrete **columnar radial units** that consist of radial glial cells and the neuroblasts that migrate along them. There may be as many as 200 million radial units in the human cerebral cortex. The radial units begin as proliferative units, with most cortical neurons generated between days 40 and 125. As with many aspects of neural differentiation, the number of radial units seems to be sensitive to their own neural input. For example, in cases of **congenital anophthalmia** (the absence of eyes), neural input from visual pathways to the area of the occipital cortex associated with vision is reduced. This results in both gross and microscopic abnormalities of the visual cortex, principally related to a reduced number of radial units in that region.

Spinal Cord

In the spinal cord, inputs from many peripheral sensory nerves are distributed as local reflex arcs or are channeled to the brain through tracts of axons. Also, motor messages originating in the brain are distributed to appropriate peripheral locations via motor tracts and ventral (motor) roots of individual spinal nerves. Although several aspects of spinal cord organization were discussed earlier in this chapter, some are briefly reviewed because of their value in understanding basic brain organization.

The early spinal cord is divided into alar and basal plate regions, which are precursors for the sensory and motor regions of the cord (see Figure 10-6). The mature cord has a similar organization, but these regions are further subdivided into somatic and visceral components. Within the brain, still another layer of input and output is added with "special" components. These are summarized in Box 10-1.

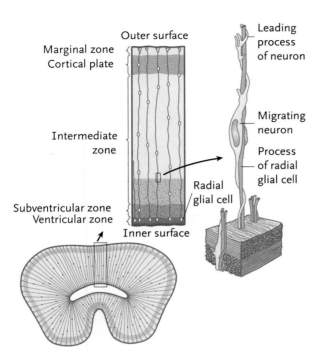

Figure 10-21 Radial glial cells and their association with peripherally migrating neurons during the development of the brain. (Based on Rakić P: *Birth Defects Orig Article Series* II[7]:95-129, 1975.)

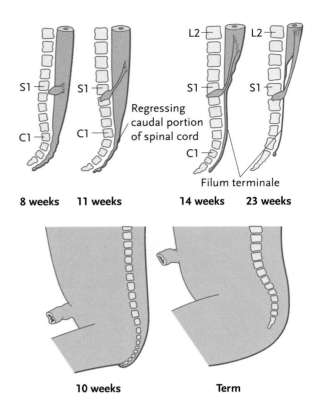

Figure 10-22 *Top,* Changes in the level of the end of the spinal cord in relation to bony landmarks in the vertebral column during fetal development. *Bottom,* Development of the curvature of the spine.

BOX 10-1   Functional Regions in the Spinal Cord and Brain

ALAR PLATE (AFFERENT OR SENSORY)

General somatic afferent: sensory input from the skin, joints, and muscles

Special visceral afferent: sensory input from the taste buds and pharynx

General visceral afferent: sensory input from the viscera and heart

BASAL PLATE (EFFERENT: MOTOR OR AUTONOMIC)

General visceral efferent: autonomic (two-neuron) links from the intermediate horn to the viscera

Special visceral efferent: motor nerves to striated muscles of the pharyngeal arches

General somatic efferent: motor nerves to the striated muscles other than those of the pharyngeal arches

---

A gross change of the spinal cord that is of clinical significance is the relative shortening of the cord in relation to the vertebral column (Figure 10-22). In the first trimester the spinal cord extends the entire length of the body, and the spinal nerves pass through the intervertebral spaces directly opposite their site of origin. In later months, growth of the posterior part of the body outstrips that of both the vertebral column and the spinal cord, but growth of the cord lags significantly behind that of the vertebral column. This disparity is barely apparent in the cranial and thoracic regions, but at birth the spinal cord terminates at the level of L3. By adulthood, the cord terminates at the L2.

The consequence of this growth disparity is the considerable elongation of the lumbar and sacral dorsal and ventral spinal nerve roots to accommodate the increased distance between their point of origin and the appropriate intervertebral space. This gives them the collective appearance of a horse's tail (hence their name, **cauda equina**). A thin, filament-like **filum terminale** extending from the end of the spinal cord proper to the base of the vertebral column marks the original excursion of the spinal cord. This arrangement is convenient for the clinician because the space below the termination of the cord is a safe place from which to withdraw cerebrospinal fluid for analysis.

Myelencephalon

The **myelencephalon,** the most caudal subdivision of the rhombencephalon (see Figure 10-2), develops into the **medulla oblongata** of the adult brain (Figures 10-1, *B,* and 10-23). It is in many respects a transitional structure between the brain and spinal cord, and the parallels between its functional organization and that of the spinal cord are readily ap-

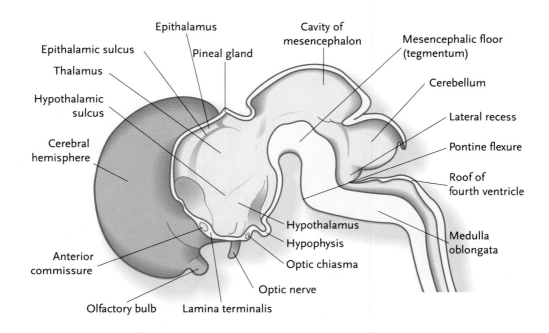

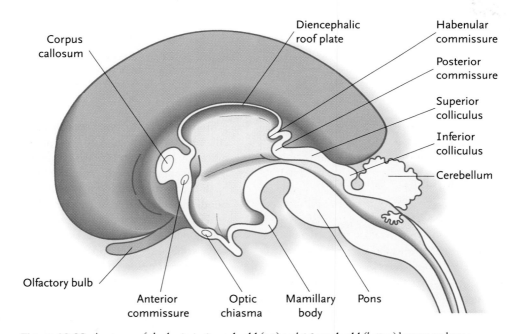

Figure 10-23 Anatomy of the brain in **9-week-old** (*top*) and **16-week-old** (*bottom*) human embryos.

parent (Figure 10-24). Much of the medulla serves as a conduit for tracts that link the brain with input and output nodes in the spinal cord, but it also contains centers for the regulation of vital functions such as the heart beat and respiration.

The fundamental arrangement of alar and basal plates with an intervening sulcus limitans is retained almost unchanged in the myelencephalon. The major topographical change from the spinal cord is a pronounced expansion of the roof plate to form the characteristic thin roof overlying the ex-

panded central canal, which in the myelencephalon is called the **fourth ventricle** (see Figure 10-35). (Details of the ventricles and the coverings of the brain and spinal cord are presented later in this chapter.)

Special visceral **afferent** (leading toward the brain) and **efferent** (leading from the brain) columns of nuclei (aggregations of neuronal cell bodies in the brain) appear in the myelencephalon to accommodate structures derived from the pharyngeal arches.

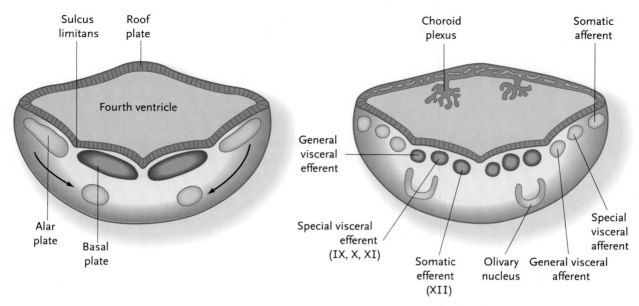

Figure 10-24 Cross sections through the developing myelencephalon at early (*left*) and later (*right*) stages of embryonic development. Motor tracts (from the basal plate) are shown in green; sensory tracts (from the alar plate) are orange. (Modified from Sadler T: *Langman's medical embryology*, ed 6, 1990, Williams & Wilkins.)

Metencephalon

The **metencephalon**, the more cranial subdivision of the hindbrain, consists of two main parts: the **pons**, which is directly continuous with the medulla, and the **cerebellum**, a phylogenetically newer and ontogenetically later-appearing component of the brain (see Figure 10-23). The formation of these structures depends on the functioning of engrailed-1 in the early midbrain/hindbrain region.

As its name implies, the pons serves as a bridge that carries tracts of nerve fibers between higher brain centers and the spinal cord. Its fundamental organization remains like that of the myelencephalon, with three sets of afferent and efferent nuclei (Figure 10-25). In addition to these, other special pontine nuclei, which originated from alar plate–derived neuroblasts, are present in the ventral white matter. The caudal part of the pons also has an expanded roof plate similar to that of the myelencephalon.

The cerebellum is both structurally and functionally complex, but phylogenetically, it arose as a specialization of the vestibular system and was involved with balance. Other functions, such as the orchestration of general coordination and involvement in auditory and visual reflexes, were later superimposed.

The future site of the cerebellum is first represented by the **rhombic lips** of the 5- to 6-week-old embryo (Figure 10-26). The rhombic lips are located at the cranial edge of the thinned roof of the fourth ventricle, and they project partly into the ventricle. Until the end of the third month the expansion of the rhombic lips is mainly inward, but thereafter the rapid

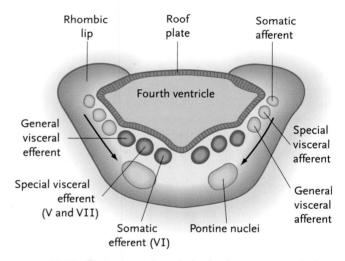

Figure 10-25 Cross section through the developing metencephalon. Motor tracts are green; sensory tracts are orange. (Modified from Sadler T: *Langman's medical embryology*, ed 6, 1990, Williams & Wilkins.)

growth in volume of the cerebellum is directed outward (Figure 10-27).

As the volume of the developing cerebellum expands, the two lateral rhombic lips join in the midline, giving the early cerebellar primordium a dumbbell appearance. The cerebellum then enters a period of rapid development and external expansion. Internally, the cerebellum undergoes a complex process of histogenesis. (Generally, the processes underlying

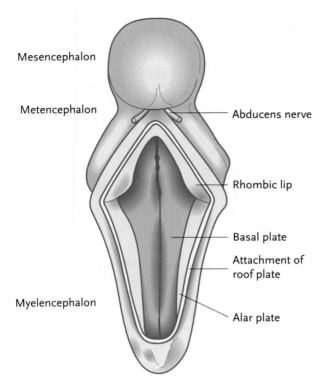

Figure 10-26 Dorsal view of the midbrain and hindbrain of a 5-week-old embryo. The roof of the fourth ventricle has been opened.

Labels in figure: Mesencephalon, Metencephalon, Myelencephalon, Abducens nerve, Rhombic lip, Basal plate, Attachment of roof plate, Alar plate

the cellular organization of the cerebellum can be appreciated by reviewing the section on histogenesis of the cerebral cortex [see Figure 10-21].) Histogenesis of the cerebellum continues until well after birth. Many fibers emanating from the vast number of neurons generated in the cerebellum leave the cerebellum through a pair of massive **superior cerebellar peduncles**, which grow into the mesencephalon.

Mesencephalon

The **mesencephalon, or midbrain,** is structurally a relatively simple part of the brain in which the fundamental relationships between the basal and alar plates are essentially preserved (Figure 10-28). In the region of the alar plates, neuroblasts migrate toward the roof (**tectum**), forming two prominent pairs of bulges collectively called the **corpora quadrigemina**. The caudal pair, called the **inferior colliculi,** are relatively simple in structure and are functionally part of the auditory system. The **superior colliculi** take on a more complex layered architecture through the migration patterns of the neuroblasts that give rise to it. The superior colliculi are an integral part of the visual system, and they serve as an important synaptic relay station between the optic nerve and the visual areas of the cerebral (occipital) cortex. Connections between the superior and inferior colliculi help coordinate visual and auditory reflexes.

The primitive mesencephalic basal plates develop into the structurally less well-defined region called the **tegmentum**. In the tegmentum are located the somatic efferent nuclei of cranial nerves III and IV, which supply most of the extrinsic muscles of the eye. A small visceroefferent nucleus, the **Edinger-Westphal nucleus,** is responsible for innervation of the pupillary sphincter muscle of the eye. Two pairs of prominent nuclei of gray matter, the **nucleus ruber** (red nucleus) and **substantia nigra,** are still of uncertain origin.

The third major region of the mesencephalon is represented by prominent ventrolateral bulges of white matter called the **cerebral peduncles**. A number of the major descending fiber tracts pass through these structures on their way from the cerebral hemispheres to the spinal cord.

Diencephalon

Cranial to the mesencephalon, the organization of the developing brain becomes so highly modified that it is difficult to relate later morphology to the fundamental alar plate/basal plate plan. In fact, it is widely believed that the forebrain structures (diencephalon and telencephalon) are highly modified derivatives of the alar plates and roof plate without significant representation by basal plates.

Development of the early diencephalon is characterized by the appearance of two pairs of prominent swellings on the lateral walls of the **third ventricle**. These swellings line the greatly expanded central canal in this region (see Figure 10-23). The largest pair of masses represents the developing **thalamus,** in which neural tracts from higher brain centers synapse with those of other regions of the brain and brainstem. Among the many thalamic nuclei are those that receive input from the auditory and visual systems and transmit them to the appropriate regions of the cerebral cortex. In later development the thalamic swellings may thicken to the point where they meet and fuse in the midline across the third ventricle. This connection is called the **massa intermedia**.

Ventral to the thalamus, the swellings of the **incipient hypothalamus** are separated from the thalamus by the **hypothalamic sulcus**. As mentioned earlier, the hypothalamus receives input from many areas of the central nervous system. It also acts as a master regulatory center, controlling many basic homeostatic functions such as sleep, temperature control, hunger, fluid and electrolyte balance, emotions, and rhythms of glandular secretion (e.g., of the pituitary). A number of its functions are neurosecretory; therefore the hypothalamus serves as a major interface between the neural integration of sensory information and the humoral environment of the body.

In early embryos (specifically, those around 7 to 8 weeks' gestational age), a pair of less prominent bulges dorsal to the thalamus mark the emergence of the **epithalamus** (see Figure 10-23), a relatively poorly developed set of nuclei

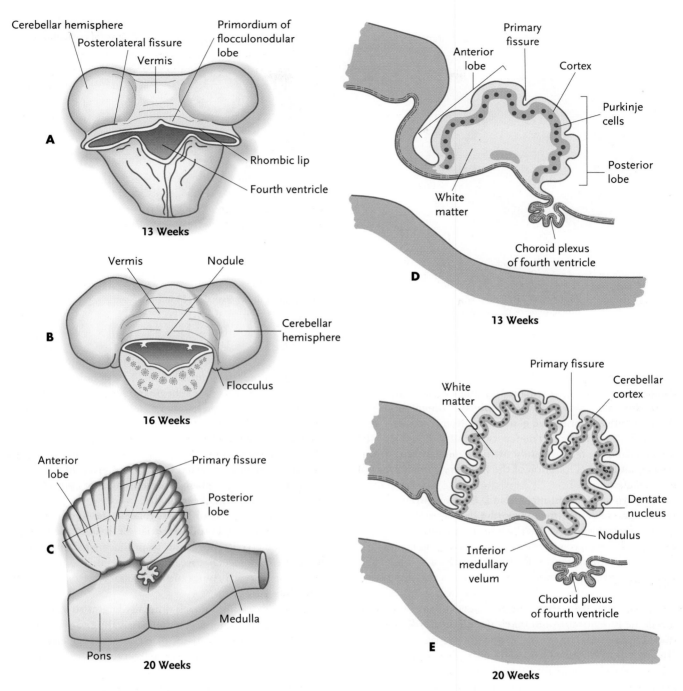

Figure 10-27 Development of the cerebellum. A and B, Dorsal views. C, Lateral view. D and E, Sagittal sections.

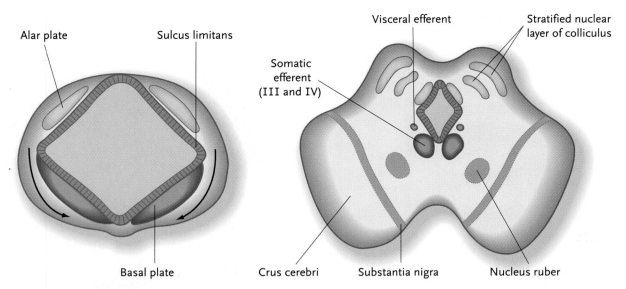

Figure 10-28 Cross sections through the early and later developing mesencephalon. Motor tracts are green; sensory tracts are orange. (Modified from Sadler T: *Langman's medical embryology*, ed 6, 1990, Williams & Wilkins.)

relating to masticatory and swallowing functions. The most caudal part of the diencephalic roof plate forms a small diverticulum that becomes the **epiphysis (pineal body)**, a phylogenetically primitive gland that often serves as a light receptor. Under the influence of light/dark cycles, the pineal gland secretes (mainly at night) **melatonin,** a hormone that inhibits function of the pituitary-gonadal axis of hormonal control.

The **hypophysis** (pituitary gland) develops from two initially separate ectodermal primordia that secondarily unite. One of the primordia, called the **infundibular process,** forms as a ventral downgrowth from the floor of the diencephalon. The other primordium is **Rathke's pouch,** a midline outpocketing from the stomodeal ectoderm that extends toward the floor of the diencephalon as early as the fourth week. An inductive event from the overlying diencephalon first stimulates the formation of a **Rathke's pouch primordium** in the dorsal stomodeal ectoderm. Through the action of **Rpx** (Rathke's pouch homeobox-containing gene) and the Lim-type homeobox-containing genes **Lhx-3** and **Lhx-4,** Rathke's pouch primordium forms the definitive Rathke's pouch (Figure 10-29). Experimental evidence from a number of species indicates that in the early embryo the cells in Rathke's pouch originate in the anterior ridge of the neural plate.

The infundibular process is intimately related to the hypothalamus (see Figure 1-14), and certain hypothalamic neurosecretory neurons send their processes into the infundibular process, which ultimately becomes the **neural lobe of the hypophysis.** Throughout development, the histological structure of the infundibulum retains a neural character.

As development proceeds, Rathke's pouch elongates toward the infundibulum (see Figure 10-29). While its blind end partially enfolds the infundibulum like a double-layered cup, the stalk of Rathke's pouch begins to regress. The outer wall of the cup thickens and assumes a glandular appearance in the course of its differentiation into the **pars distalis** (anterior lobe) of the hypophysis. The inner layer of the cup, which is closely adherent to the neural lobe, becomes the **pars intermedia.** It remains separated from the anterior lobe by a slit-like **residual lumen,** which represents all that remains of the original lumen of Rathke's pouch.

With the progression of pregnancy, the hypophysis undergoes a phase of cytodifferentiation. Late in the fetal period, specific cell types begin to produce small amounts of hormones. Molecular cascades underlying the differentiation of specific cell types in the pituitary are being discovered (Box 10-2).

Although Rathke's pouch normally begins to lose its connections to the stomodeal epithelium by the end of the second month, portions of the tissue may occasionally persist along the pathway of the elongating stalk. If the tissue is normal, it is called a **pharyngeal hypophysis.** Sometimes, however, the residual tissue becomes neoplastic and forms hormone-secreting tumors called **craniopharyngiomas.**

The **optic cups** are major outpocketings of the diencephalic wall during early embryogenesis. (They and the optic nerves [cranial nerve II] are discussed in Chapter 12.)

Telencephalon

Development of the **telencephalon** is dominated by the tremendous expansion of the bilateral **telencephalic vesicles,** which ultimately become the cerebral hemispheres (see Figure 10-23). The walls of the telencephalic vesicles

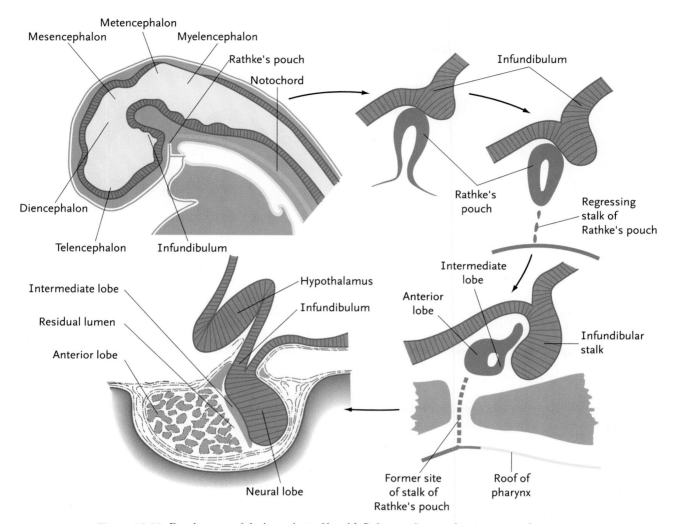

Figure 10-29 Development of the hypophysis. *Upper left,* Reference diagram showing a sagittal section through a **4-week-old** human embryo.

surround the expanded lateral ventricles, which are out-pocketings from the midline third ventricle located in the diencephalon (see Figure 10-35). Although the cerebral hemispheres first appear as lateral structures, the dynamics of their growth cause them to approach the midline over the roofs of the diencephalon and mesencephalon (Figure 10-30). The two cerebral hemispheres never actually meet in the dorsal midline because they are separated by a thin septum of connective tissue (part of the dura mater) known as the **falx cerebri.** Below this septum the two cerebral hemispheres are connected by the ependymal roof of the third ventricle.

Although the cerebral hemispheres expand greatly during the early months of pregnancy, their external surfaces remain smooth until the fourteenth week. With continued growth, the cerebral hemispheres undergo folding at several levels of organization. The most massive folding involves the large

---

BOX 10-2   Cytodifferentiation of Secretory Cells in the Adenohypophysis

Cytodifferentiation of four of the five major secretory cells in the adenohypophysis (thyrotrophs, gonadotrophs, lactotrophs, and somatotrophs) appears to depend on the expression of a Lim homeobox-containing gene (*Lhx3* in the mouse). Corticotrophs arise from a cell lineage that is independent of Lhx3. Lhx3 mutant mice do not form the anterior or intermediate lobes of the hypophysis. A transcriptional activator, **Pit-1,** a member of the POU homeodomain family, is expressed before the differentiation of any pituitary cell types, and it is required for the differentiation of cells of the somatotroph, lactotroph, and thyrotroph lineages. Further downstream, each cell type of the pituitary requires its own set of molecular activators so that it can differentiate.

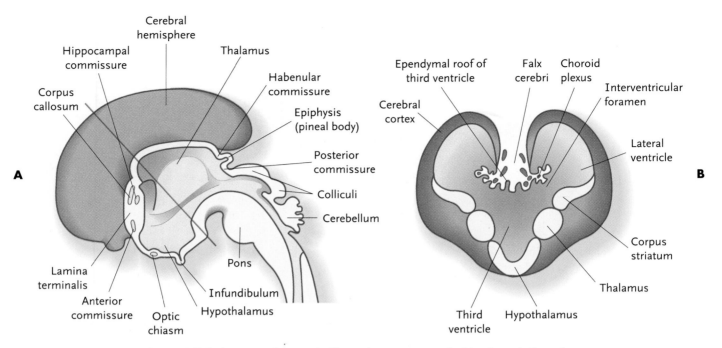

Figure 10-30 Early formation of the cerebral hemispheres in a **10-week-old** embryo. **A,** Sagittal section through the brain. **B,** Cross section through the level indicated by the red line in **A**. (Modified from Moore K, Persaud T: *The developing human,* ed 5, Philadelphia, 1993, WB Saunders.)

temporal lobes, which protrude laterally and rostrally from the caudal part of the cerebral hemispheres. From the fourth to the ninth month of pregnancy, the expanding temporal lobes and the frontal and parietal lobes completely cover areas of the cortex known as the **insula** (island) (Figure 10-31). While these major changes in organization are occurring, other precursors of major surface landmarks of the definitive cerebral cortex are being sculpted. Several major sulci and fissures begin to appear as early as the sixth month. By the eighth month the **sulci** (grooves) and **gyri** (convolutions) that characterize the mature brain take shape.

Internally, the base of each telencephalic vesicle thickens to form the comma-shaped **corpus striatum** (Figure 10-32). Located dorsal to the thalamus, the corpus striatum becomes more C-shaped as development progresses. With histodifferentiation of the cerebral cortex, many fiber tracts converge on the area of the corpus striatum, which becomes subdivided into two major nuclei: the **lentiform nucleus** and the **caudate nucleus.** These structures, which are components of the complex aggregation of nuclei known as the **basal ganglia,** are involved in the unconscious control of muscle tone and complex body movements.

Aside from the telencephalic vesicles, the other major component of the early telencephalon is the **lamina terminalis,** which forms its median rostral wall (Figures 10-33 and 10-35, *A*). Initially the two cerebral hemispheres develop separately, but toward the end of the first trimester of pregnancy, bundles of nerve fibers begin to cross from one cerebral hemisphere to the other. Many of these connections occur through the lamina terminalis.

The first set of connections to appear in the lamina terminalis becomes the **anterior commissure** (see Figure 10-23, *B*), which connects olfactory areas from the two sides of the brain. The second connection is the **hippocampal commissure (fornix).** The third commissure to take shape in the lamina terminalis is the corpus callosum, the most important connection between the right and left halves of the brain. It initially forms as a small bundle in the lamina terminalis but expands greatly to form a broad band connecting a large part of the base of the cerebral hemispheres (see Figure 10-33). Other commissures not related to the lamina terminalis are the **posterior** and **habenular commissures** (see Figure 10-30), which are located close to the base of the pineal gland, and the **optic chiasma,** the region in the diencephalon where parts of the optic nerve fibers cross to the other side of the brain.

Neuroanatomists subdivide the telencephalon into several functional components that are based on the phylogenetic development of this region. The oldest and most primitive component is called the **rhinencephalon** (also the **archicortex** and **paleocortex**). As the name implies, it is heavily involved in olfaction. The morphologically dominant cerebral hemispheres are called the **neocortex.** In early development, much of the telencephalon is occupied by rhinencephalic areas (Figure 10-34), but with the expansion of the cerebral hemispheres, the neocortex takes over as the component occupying most of the mass of the brain.

The **olfactory nerves** (cranial nerve I), arising from paired ectodermal placodes in the head, send fibers back into the **olfactory bulbs,** which are outgrowths from the rhinencephalon. A subpopulation of cells from the olfactory placode

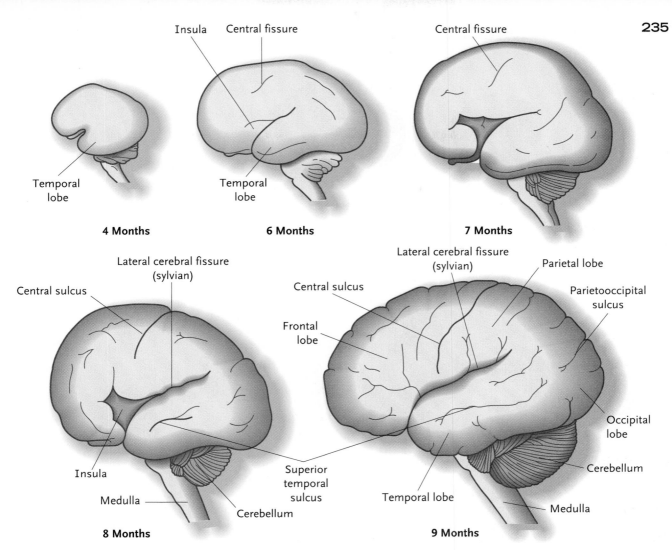

Figure 10-31 Lateral views of the developing brain.

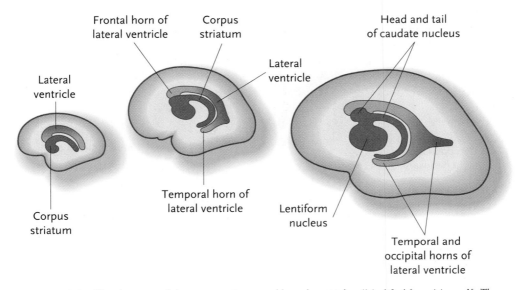

Figure 10-32 Development of the corpus striatum and lateral ventricles. (Modified from Moore K: *The developing human,* ed 4, Philadelphia, 1988, WB Saunders.)

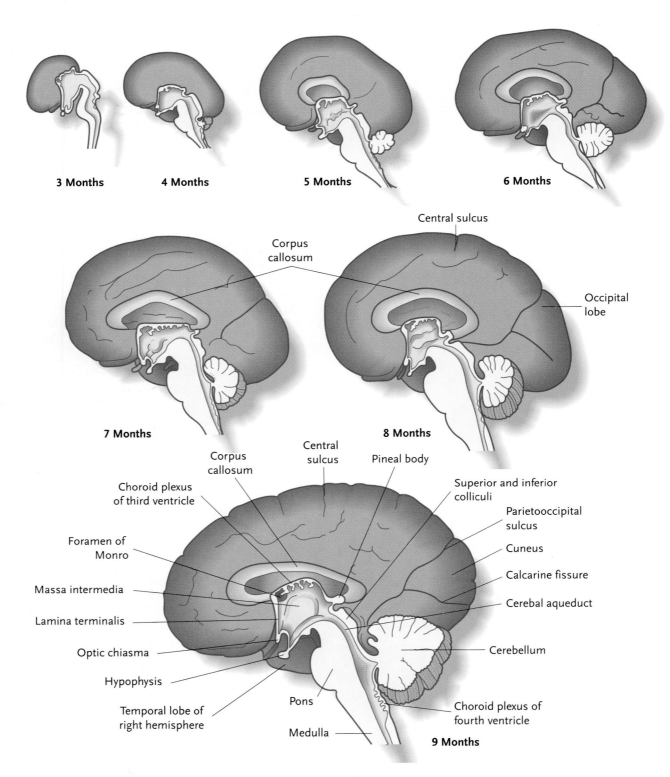

3 Months

4 Months

5 Months

6 Months

Central sulcus

Corpus callosum

Occipital lobe

7 Months

8 Months

Corpus callosum

Central sulcus

Pineal body

Superior and inferior colliculi

Choroid plexus of third ventricle

Parietooccipital sulcus

Foramen of Monro

Cuneus

Massa intermedia

Calcarine fissure

Lamina terminalis

Cerebal aqueduct

Optic chiasma

Cerebellum

Hypophysis

Temporal lobe of right hemisphere

Pons

Choroid plexus of fourth ventricle

Medulla

9 Months

Figure 10-33 Medial views of the developing brain.

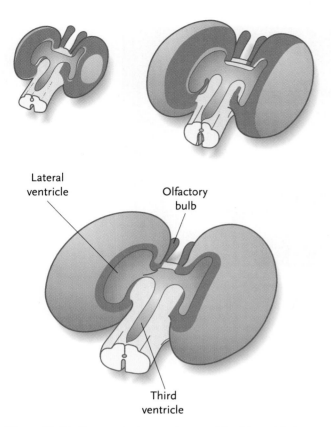

Lateral
ventricle

Olfactory
bulb

Third
ventricle

Figure 10-34 Decrease in the prominence of the rhinencephalic areas (*green*) of the brain as the cerebrum expands.

migrates along the olfactory nerve into the brain, ultimately settling in the hypothalamus, where these cells become the cells that secrete luteinizing hormone–releasing hormone.

VENTRICLES, MENINGES, AND CEREBROSPINAL FLUID FORMATION

The ventricular system of the brain represents an expansion of the central canal of the neural tube. As certain parts of the brain take shape, the central canal expands into well-defined **ventricles**, which are connected by thinner channels (Figure 10-35). The ventricles are lined by ependymal epithelium and filled with clear **cerebrospinal fluid**. Cerebrospinal fluid is formed in specialized areas called **choroid plexuses**, which are located in specific regions in the roof of the third, fourth, and lateral ventricles. Choroid plexuses are highly vascularized structures that project into the ventricles (see Figure 10-30, B) and secrete cerebrospinal fluid into the ventricular system.

Cerebrospinal fluid has a well-characterized circulatory path. As it forms, it flows from the lateral ventricles into the third and ultimately the fourth ventricle. Much of it then escapes through three small holes in the roof of the fourth ventricle and enters the **subarachnoid space** between two layers of meninges. A significant portion of the fluid leaves the skull and bathes the spinal cord as a protective layer.

If an imbalance exists between the production and resorption of cerebrospinal fluid or if its circulation is blocked, the fluid

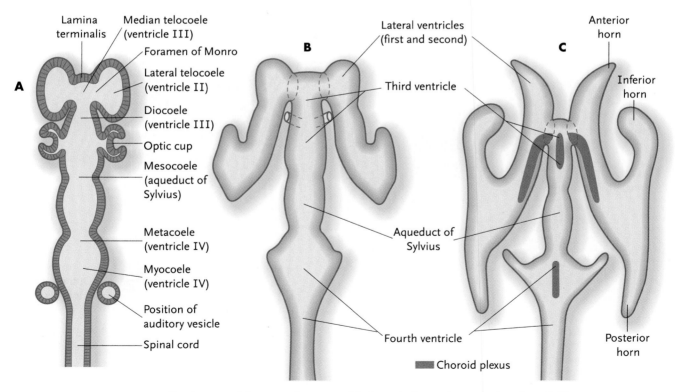

Figure 10-35 Development of the ventricular system of the brain. **A,** Section from an early embryo. **B,** Ventricular system during expansion of the cerebral hemispheres. **C,** Postnatal morphology of the ventricular system.

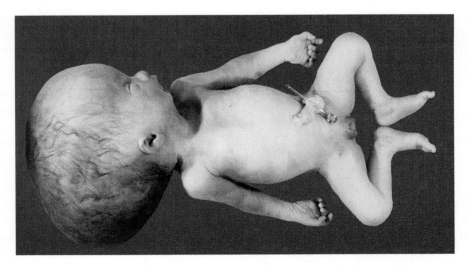

Figure 10-36 Fetus with pronounced hydrocephalus. (Courtesy M. Barr, Ann Arbor, Mich.)

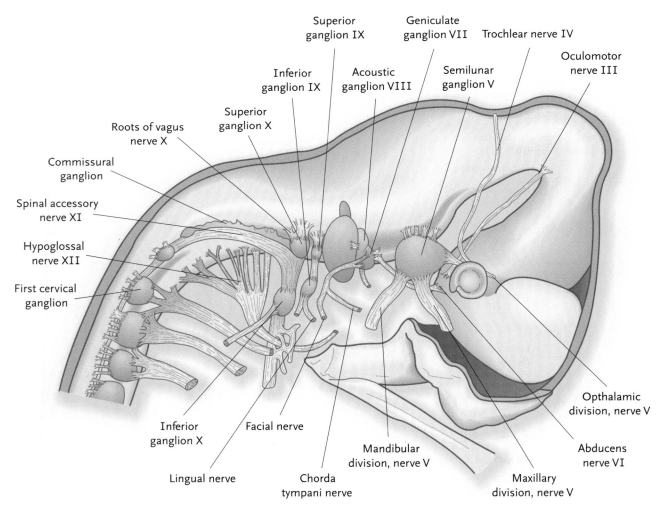

Figure 10-37 Reconstruction of the brain and cranial nerves of a 12-mm pig embryo.

may accumulate within the ventricular system of the brain and through increased mechanical pressure, result in a massive enlargement of the ventricular system. This in turn causes a thinning of the walls of the brain and a pronounced increase in the diameter of the skull, a condition known as **hydrocephalus** (Figure 10-36). The blockage of fluid can result from a congenital **stenosis** (narrowing) of the narrow parts of the ventricular system, or it can be the result of certain fetal viral infections.

A specific malformation leading to hydrocephalus is the **Arnold-Chiari malformation,** in which a tonguelike overgrowth of the cerebellum herniates into the foramen magnum, thereby mechanically preventing the escape of cerebrospinal fluid from the skull. This condition is often associated with some form of closure defect of the spinal cord or vertebral column (see Figure 12-40). At one time the Arnold-Chiari malformation was considered to result from traction of the spinal cord pulling the brain down into the foramen magnum, but a more contemporary hypothesis is that the reduced volume of a smaller-than-normal posterior fossa causes a caudal displacement of the hindbrain.

In the early fetal period, two layers of mesenchyme appear around the brain and spinal cord. The thick outer layer, which is of mesodermal origin, forms the tough **dura mater** as well as the membrane bones of the calvarium. A thin inner layer of neural crest origin later subdivides into a thin **pia mater,** which is closely apposed to the neural tissue, and a middle **arachnoid layer.** Spaces that form within the pia-arachnoid layer fill with cerebrospinal fluid.

CRANIAL NERVES

Although based on the same fundamental plan as the spinal nerves, the cranial nerves (Figure 10-37) have lost their regular segmental arrangement and have become highly specialized (Table 10-2). One of the major differences is the tendency of many cranial nerves to be either sensory (dorsal root based) or motor (ventral root based) rather than mixed, as is the case with the spinal nerves.

The cranial nerves can be subdivided into several categories on the basis of their function and embryological origin. Cranial nerves I and II (olfactory and optic) are often regarded as extensions of brain tracts rather than true nerves. Cranial nerves III, IV, VI, and XII are pure motor nerves that appear to have evolved from primitive ventral roots. Nerves V, VII, IX, and X are mixed nerves with both motor and sensory components, and each nerve supplies derivatives of a different pharyngeal arch (Table 10-2 and Figures 10-38 and 13-21).

The sensory components of the nerves supplying the pharyngeal arches (V, VII, IX, and X) and the auditory nerve (VIII) have a multiple origin from both the neural crest and the ectodermal placodes, which are located along the developing brain (see Figure 5-14). These nerves have complex, often multiple sensory ganglia. Neurons in some parts of the ganglia are of neural crest origin, and those of other parts or ganglia arise from placodal ectoderm. (Ectodermal placodes are discussed on p. 87.)

Text continued on p. 245

TABLE 10-2 Cranial Nerves

Cranial nerve	Associated component of central nervous system	Functional components	Distribution
Olfactory (I)	Telencephalon	Special sensory (olfaction)	Olfactory area of nose
Optic (II)	Diencephalon	Special sensory (vision)	Retina of eye
Oculomotor (III)	Mesencephalon	Motor, autonomic (minor)	Intraocular and four extraocular muscles
Trochlear (IV)	Mesencephalon	Motor	Superior oblique muscle of eye
Trigeminal (V)	Metencephalon	Sensory, motor (some)	Derivatives of branchial arch I
Abducens (VI)	Metencephalon	Motor	Lateral rectus muscle of eye
Facial (VII)	Metencephalon/myelencephalon junction	Motor Sensory (some) Autonomic (minor)	Derivatives of branchial arch II
Auditory (VIII)	Metencephalon/myelencephalon junction	Special sensory (hearing, balance)	Inner ear
Glossopharyngeal (IX)	Myelencephalon	Sensory, motor (some)	Derivatives of pharyngeal arch III
Vagus (X)	Myelencephalon	Sensory, motor, autonomic (major)	Derivatives of pharyngeal arch IV
Accessory (XI)	Myelencephalon Spinal cord	Motor Autonomic (minor)	Gut, heart, visceral organs Some neck muscles
Hypoglossal (XII)	Myelencephalon	Motor	Tongue muscles

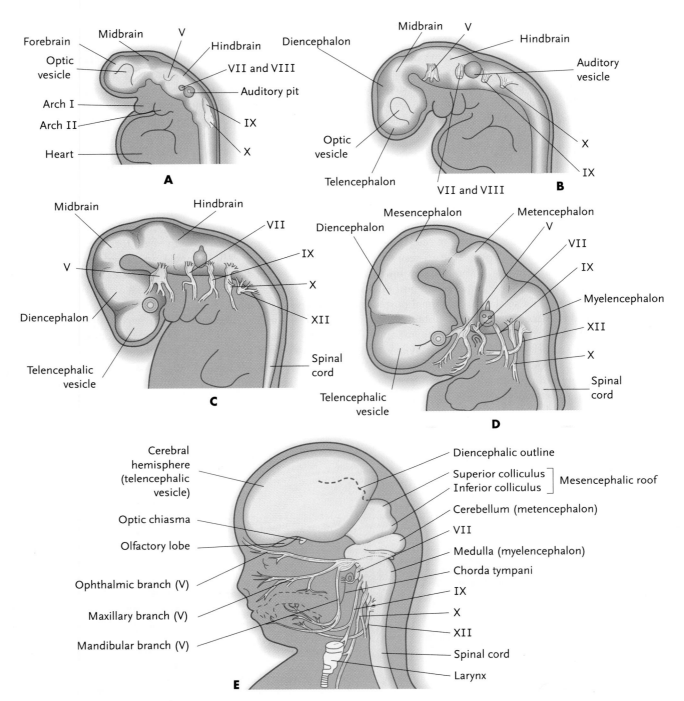

Figure 10-38 Development of the cranial nerves in human embryos. A, At 3½ weeks. B, At 4 weeks. C, At 5½ weeks. D, At 7 weeks. E, At 11 weeks.

CLINICAL CORRELATION 10-1
Congenital Malformations of the Nervous System

In an organ system as prominent and complex as the nervous system, it is not surprising that the brain and spinal cord are subject to a wide variety of congenital malformations. These range from severe structural anomalies resulting from incomplete closure of the neural tube to functional deficits caused by unknown factors acting late in pregnancy.

DEFECTS IN CLOSURE OF THE NEURAL TUBE
Failure of the neural tube to close occurs most commonly in the anterior and posterior neuropore, but failure to close in other locations is also possible. In this condition the spinal cord or brain in the affected area is splayed open, with the wall of the central canal or ventricular system constituting the outer surface. A number of the closure defects can be diagnosed by the detection of elevated levels of α-**fetoprotein** in the amniotic fluid or by ultrasound scanning. A closure defect of the spinal cord is called **rachischisis**, and a closure defect of the brain is called **cranioschisis.** A patient with cranioschisis dies. Rachischisis (Figures 10-39 and 10-40, A) is associated with

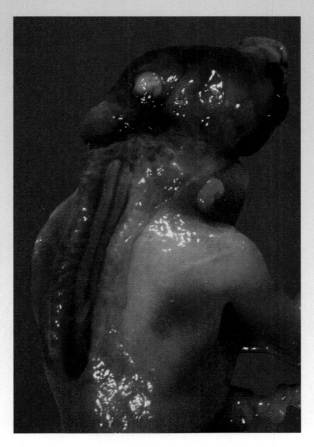

Figure 10-39 Fetus with a severe case of rachischisis. The brain is not covered by cranial bones, and the light-colored spinal cord is totally exposed. (Courtesy M. Barr, Ann Arbor, Mich.)

Continued

a wide variety of severe problems, including chronic infection, motor and sensory deficits, and disturbances in bladder function. These defects commonly accompany anencephaly (see Fig. 7-4), in which there is a massive deficiency of cranial structures.

OTHER CLOSURE DEFECTS

A defect in the formation of the bony covering overlying either the spinal cord or brain can result in a graded series of structural anomalies. In the spinal cord the simplest defect is called **spina bifida occulta** (Figure 10-40, *B*). The spinal cord and meninges re-

main in place, but the bony covering (neural arch) of one or more vertebrae is incomplete. Sometimes the defect goes unnoticed for many years. The neural arches are induced by the roof plate of the neural tube, with the mediation of Msx-2. Thus spina bifida occulta probably results from a local defect in induction. The site of the defect in the neural arches is often marked by a tuft of hair. This localized hair formation may result from exposure of the developing skin to other inductive influences from the neural tube or its coverings. Normally the neural arches act as a barrier to such influences.

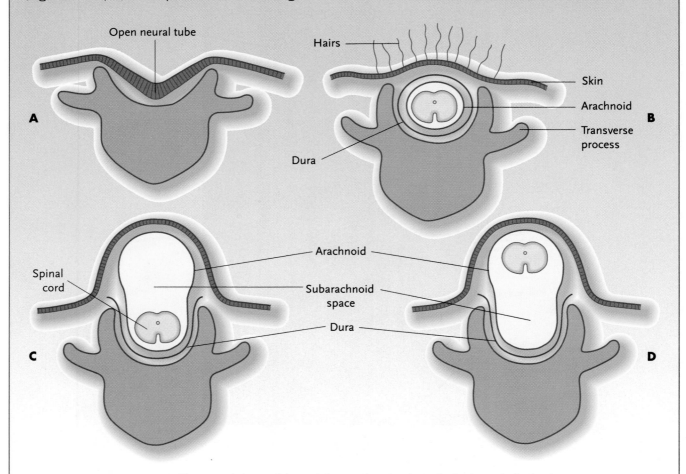

Figure 10-40 Varieties of closure defects of the spinal cord and vertebral column. **A,** Rachischisis. **B,** Spina bifida occulta, with hair growth over the defect. **C,** Meningocele. **D,** Myelomeningocele.

CLINICAL CORRELATION 10-1
Congenital Malformations of the Nervous System—cont'd

The next most severe category of defect is a **meningocele,** in which the dura mater may be missing in the area of the defect and the arachnoid layer bulges prominently beneath the skin (Figure 10-40, *C*). The spinal cord, however, remains in place, and neurological symptoms are often minor. The most severe condition is a **myelomeningocele,** in which the spinal cord bulges or is entirely displaced into the protruding subarachnoid space (Figures 10-40, *D,* and 10-41). Because of problems associated with displaced spinal roots, neurological problems are commonly associated with this condition.

A similar spectrum of anomalies is associated with cranial defects (Figures 10-42 and 10-43). A **meningocele** is typically associated with a small defect in the skull, whereas brain tissue alone **(meningoencephalocele)** or brain tissue containing part of the ventricular system **(meningohydroencephalocoele)** may protrude through a larger opening in the skull. Depending on the nature of the protruding tissue, these malformations may be associated with neurological deficits. The mechanical circumstances may also lead to secondary hydrocephalus in some cases.

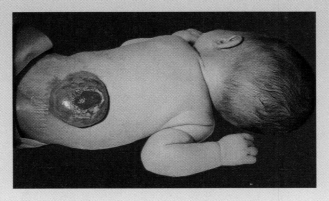

Figure 10-41 Infant with a myelomeningocele and secondary hydrocephalus. (Courtesy M. Barr, Ann Arbor, Mich.)

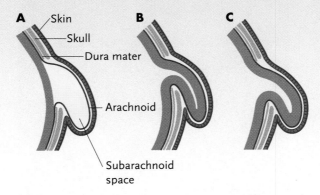

Figure 10-42 Herniations in the cranial region. **A,** Meningocele. **B,** Meningoencephalocele. **C,** Meningohydroencephalocele.

CLINICAL CORRELATION 10-1
Congenital Malformations of the Nervous System—cont'd

Microcephaly is a relatively uncommon condition characterized by the underdevelopment of both the brain and the cranium (see Figure 8-9). Although it can result from premature closure of the cranial sutures, in most cases, its etiology is uncertain.

Many of the functional defects of the nervous system are poorly characterized, and their etiology is not understood. Studies on mice with genetically based defects of movement or behavior caused by abnormalities of cell migration or histogenesis in certain regions of the brain suggest the probability of a parallel spectrum of human defects. A good example is **lissencephaly,** a condition characterized by a smooth brain surface instead of the gyri and sulci that characterize the normal brain. Underlying this gross defect is abnormal layering of cortical neurons in a manner reminiscent of the pathology seen in reeler mice (see p. 225). **Mental retardation** is common and can be attributed to many causes, both genetic and environmental. The timing of the insult to the brain may be late in the fetal period.

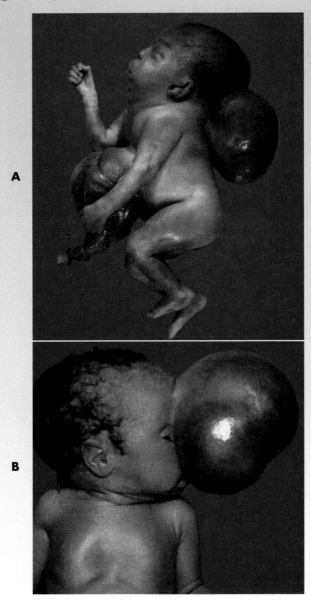

Figure 10-43 Fetuses with an occipital meningocele (**A**) and a frontal encephalocele (**B**). (Courtesy M. Barr, Ann Arbor, Mich.)

DEVELOPMENT OF NEURAL FUNCTION

During the first 5 weeks of embryonic development, there is no gross behavioral evidence of neural function. Primitive reflex activity can first be elicited at the sixth week, when touching the perioral skin with a fine bristle is followed by contralateral flexion of the neck. Over the next 6 to 8 weeks, the region of skin sensitive to tactile stimulation spreads from the face to the palms of the hands and the upper chest; by 12 weeks, the entire surface of the body except for the back and top of the head is sensitive. As these sensitive areas expand, the nature of the reflexes elicited matures from generalized movements to specific responses of more localized body parts. There is a general craniocaudal sequence of appearance of reflex movements.

Starting at the end of the fourth month the fetus begins a pattern of periods of activity followed by times of inactivity. Many women first become aware of fetal movements at this time. Between the fourth and fifth months, the fetus becomes capable of gripping firmly onto a glass rod. Although weak protorespiratory movements are possible, they cannot be sustained. The sucking reflex appears during the sixth month. Striking changes in the brain wave patterns take place at about 28 weeks, which is also a time when some prematurely born infants can sustain breathing and survive in an incubator.

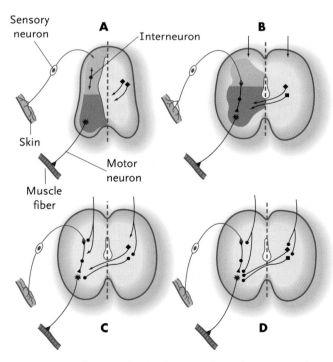

Figure 10-44 Stages in the development of neural circuitry. **A,** Presynaptic stage. **B,** Closure of the primary reflex circuit. **C,** Connections with longitudinal and lateral inputs. **D,** Completion of circuits and myelination. (Based on Bodian D. In Quartan GC, Melnechuk T, Adelman G, eds: *The neurosciences: second study program,* New York, 1970, Rockefeller University Press, pp 129-140.

Much of the behavioral development of fetuses after the sixth month has been revealed by observation of the behavior of prematurely born infants. Behavioral changes during the last trimester are more subtle and often reflect not only the establishment and completion of neural circuits but also their structural and functional maturation.

The development of functional circuitry can be illustrated by the spinal cord. Several stages of structural and functional maturation can be identified (Figure 10-44). The first is a pre-reflex stage, which is characterized by the initial differentiation (including axonal and dendritic growth) of the neurons according to a well-defined sequence, starting with motor and followed by sensory and finally including the interneurons that connect the two (see Figures 10-13 and 10-44, *A*). The second stage consists of closure of the primary circuit, which allows the expression of local segmental reflexes. While the local circuit is being set up, other axons are growing down descending tracts in the spinal cord or are crossing from the other side of the cord. When these axons make contact with the components of the simple reflex that was established in the second stage, the anatomical basis for intersegmental and cross-cord reflexes is set up. Later in the fetal period, these more complex circuits are completed, and the tracts are myelinated by oligodendrocytes.

The functional maturation of individual tracts, as indicated by their myelination, takes place over a broad time span and is not completed until early adulthood. Particularly in early postnatal life, the maturation of functional tracts in the nervous system can be followed by clinical neurological examination.

Myelination begins in the peripheral nervous system, with motor roots becoming myelinated before sensory roots (which occurs in the second through fifth months). Myelination begins in the spinal cord at about 11 weeks and proceeds according to a craniocaudal gradient. During the third trimester, myelination begins to occur in the brain, but there, in contrast to the peripheral nervous system, myelination is first seen in sensory tracts (e.g., in the visual system). Myelination in complex association pathways in the cerebral cortex occurs after birth. In the **corticospinal tracts,** the main direct connection between the cerebral cortex and the motor nerves emanating from the spinal cord, myelination extends caudally only to the level of the medulla by 40 weeks. Myelination continues after birth, and its course can be appreciated by the increasing mobility of infants during their first year of life.

CLINICAL VIGNETTE

An infant is born with rachischisis of the lower spine. During succeeding weeks, his head also begins to increase in size. Radiological imaging reveals that the infant's ventricular system is greatly dilated and the walls of the brain itself are thinned.

Assuming that the infant lives, what are some of the clinical problems that he faces in later life?

SUMMARY

- While the neural tube is closing, its open ends are the cranial and caudal neuropores. The newly formed brain consists of three parts: the prosencephalon, the mesencephalon, and the rhombencephalon. The prosencephalon later subdivides into the telencephalon and the diencephalon, and the rhombencephalon forms the metencephalon and myelencephalon.

- Within the neural tube, neuroepithelial cells undergo active mitotic proliferation. Their daughter cells form neuronal or glial progenitor cells. Among the glial cells, radial glial cells act as guide wires for the migration of neurons from their sites of origin to definite layers in the brain. Microglial cells arise from mesoderm.

- The neural tube divides into ventricular, intermediate, and marginal zones. Neuroblasts in the intermediate zone (future gray matter) send out processes that collect principally in the marginal zone (future white matter). The neural tube is also divided into a dorsal alar plate and a ventral basal plate. The basal plate represents the motor component of the spinal cord, and the alar plate is largely sensory.

- Through an induction by the notochord, mediated by sonic hedgehog, a floor plate develops in the neural tube. Further influences of sonic hedgehog, produced by both the notochord and floor plate, results in the induction of motoneurons in the basal plate.

- Much of the early brain is a highly segmented structure. This is reflected structurally in the rhombomeres and molecularly in the patterns of expression of homeobox-containing genes. Neurons and their processes developing within the rhombomeres follow specific rules of behavior with respect to rhombomere boundaries. Nerve processes growing from the spinal cord react to external cues provided by the environment of the somites. Neurons and neural crest cells can readily penetrate the anterior but not the posterior mesoderm of the somite.

- The midbrain and metencephalic structures are specified by a signaling center at the midbrain/hindbrain border. FGF-8 is one of the major signaling molecules.

- A peripheral nerve forms by the outgrowth of motor axons from the ventral horn of the spinal cord. The outgrowing axons are capped by a growth cone. This growing tip continually samples its immediate environment for cues that guide the amount and direction of axonal growth. The motor component of a peripheral nerve is joined by the sensory part, which is based on neural crest–derived cell bodies in dorsal root ganglia along the spinal cord. Axons and dendrites from the sensory cell bodies penetrate the spinal cord and also grow peripherally with the motor axons. Connections between the nerve and end organs are often mediated through trophic factors. Neurons that do not establish connections with peripheral end organs often die.

- The autonomic nervous system consists of two components: the sympathetic and parasympathetic nervous systems. Both components contain preganglionic neurons, which arise from the central nervous system, and postganglionic components, which are of neural crest origin. Typically, sympathetic neurons are adrenergic and parasympathetic neurons are cholinergic. However, the normal choice of transmitter can be overridden by environmental factors so that a sympathetic neuron, for example, can secrete acetylcholine.

- The spinal cord functions as a pathway for organized tracts of nerve processes as well as an integration center for local reflexes. During the fetal period, growth in the length of the spinal cord lags behind that of the vertebral column, pulling the nerve roots and leaving the end of the spinal cord as a cauda equina.

- Within the brain, the myelencephalon retains an organizational similarity to the spinal cord with respect to the tracts passing through, but centers that control respiration and heart rate also form at the site. The metencephalon contains two parts: the pons (which functions principally as a conduit) and the cerebellum (which integrates and coordinates many motor movements and sensory reflexes). In the cerebellum the gray matter forms on the outside. The ventral part of the mesencephalon is the region through which the major tracts of nerve processes that connect centers in the cerebral cortex with specific sites in the spinal cord pass. The dorsal part of the mesencephalon develops the superior and inferior colliculi, which are involved with the integration of visual and auditory signals, respectively.

- Both the diencephalon and the telencephalon represent modified alar plate regions. Many important nuclei and integrating centers develop in the diencephalon, among them the thalamus, hypothalamus, neural hypophysis, and pineal body. The eyes also arise as outgrowths from the diencephalon. In humans, the telencephalon ultimately overgrows other parts of the brain. Like the cerebellum, it is organized with the gray matter in layers outside the white matter. Neuroblasts migrate through the white matter to these layers by using radial glial cells as their guides.

- Within the central nervous system, the central canal expands to form a series of four ventricles in the brain. Specialized vascular plexuses form cerebrospinal fluid, which circulates throughout the central nervous system. Around the brain and spinal cord, two layers of mesenchyme form the meninges.

- The cranial nerves are organized on the same fundamental plan as the spinal nerves, but they have lost their regular segmental pattern and have become highly specialized. Some are purely motor, others are purely sensory, and still others are mixed.

- Many congenital malformations of the nervous system are based on incomplete closure of the neural tube or associated skeletal structures. In the spinal cord the spectrum of defects ranges from a widely open neural tube (rachischisis) to relatively minor defects in the neural arch over the cord (spina bifida occulta). A similar spectrum of defects is seen in the brain.

- Neural function appears in concert with the structural maturation of various components of the nervous system. The first reflex activity is seen in the sixth week. During successive weeks, the reflex movements become more complex, and spontaneous movements appear. Final functional maturation coincides with myelination of the tracts and is not completed until many years after birth.

REVIEW QUESTIONS

1. What molecule produced by the notochord is instrumental in inducing the floor plate of the neural tube?
   - A. Hoxa-5
   - B. Retinoic acid
   - C. Pax-3
   - D. Msx-1
   - E. Sonic hedgehog
2. The cell bodies of the motor neurons of a spinal nerve arise from the:
   - A. Basal plate
   - B. Marginal zone
   - C. Floor plate
   - D. Roof plate
   - E. Alar plate

3. A young patient with a tuft of hair over the lumbar region of the vertebral column undergoes surgery for a congenital anomaly in that region. During surgery, it was found that the dura and arachnoid layers over the spinal cord were complete but that the neural arches of several vertebrae were missing. What condition did the infant have?
    A. Meningocoele
    B. Meningomyelocoele
    C. Encephalocoele
    D. Spina bifida occulta
    E. Rachischisis
4. Growth cones adhere strongly to a substrate containing:
    A. Acetylcholine
    B. Laminin
    C. Epinephrine
    D. Norepinephrine
    E. Sonic hedgehog
5. Complete failure of the neural tube to close in the region of the spinal cord is:
    A. Spina bifida occulta
    B. Meningocele
    C. Cranioschisis
    D. Rachischisis
    E. Myelomeningocele
6. Rhombomeres are segmental divisions of the:
    A. Forebrain
    B. Midbrain
    C. Hindbrain
    D. Spinal cord
    E. None of the above
7. Pregnant women typically first become aware of fetal movements during what month of pregnancy?
    A. Second
    B. Third
    C. Fourth
    D. Sixth
    E. Eighth
8. Rathke's pouch arises from the:
    A. Diencephalon
    B. Stomodeal ectoderm
    C. Mesencephalon
    D. Pharyngeal endoderm
    E. Infundibulum
9. In the early days after birth, an infant does not pass fecal material and develops abdominal swelling. An anal opening is present. What is the probable condition?
10. What is the likely appearance of the spinal cord and brachial nerves in an infant who was born with the congenital absence of one arm (amelia)?

REFERENCES

Bally-Cuif L, Wassef M: Determination events in the nervous system of the vertebrate embryo, *Curr Opin Genet Dev* 5:450-458, 1995.
Black IB: Stages of neurotransmitter development of autonomic neurons, *Science* 215:1198-1204, 1982.
Bodian D: A model of synaptic and behavioral ontogeny. In Quartan GC, Melnechuk T, Adelman G, eds: *The neurosciences: second study program*, New York, 1970, Rockefeller University, pp 129-140.
Breedlove SM: Sexual dimorphism in the vertebrate central nervous system, *J Neurosci* 12:4133-4142, 1992.
Brown MC, Hopkins WG, Keynes RJ: *Essentials of neural development*, Cambridge, England, 1991, Cambridge University Press.
Bunge R, Johnson M, Ross CD: Nature and nurture in development of the autonomic neuron, *Science* 199:1409-1416, 1978.
Cameron RS, Rakić P: Glial cell lineage in the cerebral cortex: a review and synthesis, *Glia* 4:124-137, 1991.
Colello RJ, Pott U: Signals that initiate myelination in the developing mammalian nervous system, *Mol Neurobiol* 15:83-100, 1997.
Copp AJ and others: The embryonic development of mammalian neural tube defects, *Prog Neurobiol* 33:363-401, 1990.
Crossley PH, Martinez S, Martin GR: Midbrain development induced by FGF8 in the chick embryo, *Nature* 380:66-68, 1996.
Deutsch U, Gruss P: Murine paired domain proteins as regulatory factors of embryonic development, *Semin Dev Biol* 2:413-424, 1991.
Dubois PM, El Amraoui A: Embryology of the pituitary gland, *Trends Endocrinol Metab* 6:1-7, 1995.
Echelard Y and others: Sonic hedgehog, a member of a family of putative signaling molecules, is implicated in the regulation of CNS polarity, *Cell* 75:1417-1430, 1993.
Erickson J and others: Sonic hedgehog induces the differentiation of ventral forebrain neurons: a common signal for ventral patterning within the neural tube, *Cell* 81:747-756, 1995.
Ferrer I and others: Cell death and removal in the cerebral cortex during development, *Prog Neurobiol* 39:1-43, 1992.
Gassmann M, Lemke G: Neuregulins and neuregulin receptors in neural development, *Curr Biol* 7:87-92, 1997.
Gershon M: Genes and lineages in the formation of the enteric nervous system, *Curr Opin Neurobiol* 7:101-109, 1997.
Hajihosseini M, Tham TN, Dubois-Dalcq M: Origin of oligodendrocytes within the human spinal cord, *J Neurosci* 16:7981-7994, 1996.
Hooker D: *The prenatal origin of behavior*, Lawrence, Kan, 1952, University of Kansas Press.
Joyner AL: Engrailed, Wnt and Pax genes regulate midbrain-hindbrain development, *Trends Genet* 12:15-20, 1996.
Kageyama R, Nakanishi S: Helix-loop-helix factors in growth and differentiation of the vertebrate nervous system, *Curr Opin Genet Dev* 7:659-665, 1997.
Keynes R, Cook GMW: Axon guidance molecules, *Cell* 83:161-169, 1995.
Keynes RJ and others: Spinal nerve segmentation in higher vertebrates: axon guidance by repulsion and attraction, *Semin Neurosci* 8:339-345, 1996.
Landmesser LT, ed: *The assembly of the nervous system*, New York, 1989, Liss.
Landmesser LT: Growth cone guidance in the avian limb: a search for cellular and molecular mechanisms. In Letourneau PC, Kater SB, Macagno ER, eds: *The nerve growth cone*, New York, 1992, Raven, pp 373-385.
Le Douarin NM, Catala M, Batini C: Embryonic neural chimeras in the study of vertebrate brain and head development, *Int Rev Cytol* 175:241-309, 1997.
Lumsden A, Graham A: A forward role for hedgehog, *Curr Biol* 5:1347-1350, 1995.
Lumsden A, Keynes R: Segmental patterns of neuronal development in the chick hindbrain, *Nature* 337:424-428, 1989.
Lumsden A, Krumlauf R: Patterning the vertebrate neuraxis, *Science* 274:1109-1115, 1996.
Millet S and others: The caudal limit of OTX2 gene expression as a marker of the midbrain/hindbrain boundary: a study using in situ hybridization and chick/quail homotopic grafts, *Development* 122:3785-3797, 1996.
Moore K: *The developing human*, ed 4, Philadelphia, 1988, WB Saunders.
Müller F, O'Rahilly RO: The timing and sequence of appearance of neuromeres and their derivatives in staged human embryos, *Acta Anat* 158:83-99, 1997.
Norman MG: Malformations of the brain, *J Neuropath Exp Neurol* 55:133-143, 1996.
Oppenheim RW: Cell death during development of the nervous system, *Annu Rev Neurosci* 14:453-501, 1991.
O'Rahilly R, Gardner E: The timing and sequence of events in the development of the human nervous system during the embryonic period proper, *Z Anat Entwickl-Gesch* 134:1-12, 1974.

Orentas DM, Miller RH: The origin of spinal cord oligodendrocytes is dependent on local influences from the notochord, *Dev Biol* 177:43-54, 1996.

Parks JS, Adess ME, Brown MR: Genes regulating hypothalamic and pituitary development, *Acta Paediatr Suppl* 423:28-32, 1997.

Purves D, Lichtman JW: *Principles of neural development*, Sunderland, Mass, 1985, Sinauer Associates.

Rakić P: Radial versus tangential migration of neuronal clones in the developing cerebral cortex, *Proc Natl Acad Sci USA* 92:11323-11327, 1995.

Rakić P: Specification of cerebral cortical areas, *Science* 241:170-176, 1988.

Rao MS, Landis SC, Patterson PH: The cholinergic neuronal differentiation factor from heart cell conditioned medium is different from the cholinergic factors in sciatic nerve and spinal cord, *Dev Biol* 139:65-74, 1990.

Redies C: Cadherin expression in the developing vertebrate CNS: from neuromeres to brain nuclei and neural circuits, *Exp Cell Res* 220:243-256, 1995.

Robinson SR, Smotherman WP: Fundamental motor patterns of the mammalian fetus, *J Neurobiol* 23:1574-1600, 1992.

Rothman TP and others: The effect of back-transplants of the embryonic gut wall on growth of the neural tube, *Dev Biol* 124:331-346, 1987.

Rubenstein JLR and others: The embryonic vertebrate forebrain: the prosomeric model, *Science* 266:578-580, 1994.

Sadler T: *Langman's medical embryology*, ed 6, 1990, Williams & Wilkins.

Seitanidou T and others: Krox-20 is a key regulator of rhombomere-specific gene expression in the developing hindbrain, *Mech Dev* 65:31-42, 1997.

Serafini T and others: Netrin-1 is required for commissural axon guidance in the developing nervous system, *Cell* 87:1001-1014, 1996.

Sheng HZ and others: Multistep control of pituitary organogenesis, *Science* 278:1809-1812, 1997.

Sheng HZ and others: Specification of pituitary cell lineages by the LIM homeobox gene *Lhx3*, *Science* 272:1004-1007, 1996.

Shimamura K, Rubenstein JLR: Inductive interactions direct early regionalization of the mouse forebrain, *Development* 124:2709-2718, 1997.

Smith J: Ontogeny of the autonomic nervous system. In Gootman PM, ed: *Developmental neurobiology of the autonomic nervous system*, Clifton, NJ, 1986, Humana, pp 1-28.

Tanabe Y, Jessell TM: Diversity and pattern in the developing spinal cord, *Science* 274:1115-1123, 1996.

Tarozzo G, Peretto P, Fasolo A: Cell migration from the olfactory placode and the ontogeny of the neuroendocrine compartments, *Zool Sci* 12:367-383, 1995.

Tessier-Lavigne M, Goodman CS: The molecular biology of axon guidance, *Science* 274:1123-1133, 1996.

Theil T and others: Segmental expression of the EpphA4 (Sek-1) receptor tyrosine kinase in the hindbrain is under direct transcriptional control of Krox-20, *Development* 125:443-452, 1998.

Tosney KW: Cells and cell-interactions that guide motor axons in the developing chick embryo, *Bioessays* 13:17-23, 1991.

Vettivel S: Vertebral level of the termination of the spinal cord in human fetuses, *J Anat* 179:149-161, 1991.

Zorick TS, Lemke G: Schwann cell differentiation, *Curr Opin Cell Biol* 8:870-876, 1996.

11

NEURAL CREST

Although its existence has been recognized for over a century, not until adequate methods of marking neural crest cells became available—first with isotopic labels and subsequently with stable biological markers, monoclonal antibodies, intracellular dyes, and genetic markers—did the neural crest become one of the most widely studied components of the vertebrate embryo. The majority of studies on the neural crest have been conducted on the avian embryo because of its accessibility and the availability of specific markers. Research conducted on mammalian embryos suggests that except for relatively minor structural details, information learned from birds can be directly applied to mammalian embryos. Congenital malformations of the neural crest are presented in Clinical Correlation 11-1 located at the end of this chapter.

ORIGINS OF THE NEURAL CREST

The neural crest originates from cells located along the lateral margins of the neural plate. Neural crest cells are specified as the result of an inductive action by the nonneural ectoderm (possibly mediated by bone morphogenetic protein-4 [BMP-4] and BMP-7) on the lateral cells of the neural plate. The induced neural crest cells express **slug**, a transcription factor of the zinc finger family, which characterizes cells that break away from an embryonic epithelial layer and subsequently migrate as mesenchymal cells.*

Neural crest cells break from the neural plate or neural tube by changing their shape and properties from those of typical neuroepithelial cells to those of mesenchymal cells. In the head region, incipient neural crest cells send out processes that penetrate the basal lamina underlying the neuroepithelium well before neural tube closure (Figure 11-1). After the basal lamina is further degraded, the neural crest cells, which by this time have assumed a mesenchymal morphology, pass

*Slug is also expressed during gastrulation by cells of the epiblast after they have entered the walls of the primitive streak and are about to leave as mesenchymal cells of the mesodermal germ layer.

through the remnants of the basal lamina and embark on a remarkable series of migrations.

Another significant change accompanying the epithelial-to-mesenchymal transformation of the neural crest cells is a loss of cell-to-cell adhesiveness. This is accompanied by the loss of cell adhesion molecules (CAMs) characteristic of the neural tube (e.g., N-CAM and N-cadherin) on the neural crest cells during their migratory phase. After neural crest cells have completed their migrations and differentiated into certain structures (such as spinal ganglia), CAMs are often reexpressed.

In the trunk, neural crest cells do not leave the neuroepithelium until after the neural tube has formed. They do not, however, have to contend with penetrating a basal lamina because the dorsal part of the neural tube does not form a basal lamina until after migration of the crest cells.

MIGRATIONS OF THE NEURAL CREST

After leaving the neuroepithelium, the neural crest cells first encounter a relatively cell-free environment rich in extracellular matrix molecules (Figure 11-2). In this environment, they undergo extensive migrations along several well-defined pathways. These migrations are determined by both intrinsic properties of the neural crest cells and features of the external environment encountered by the migrating cells.

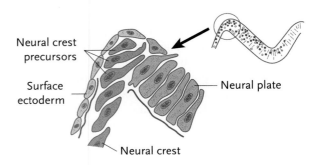

Figure 11-1 Early migration of neural crest cells from the lateral margin of the neural plate.

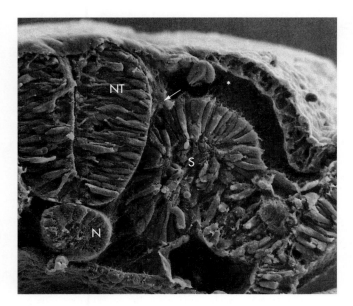

Figure 11-2 Scanning electron micrograph of a chick embryo, showing the early migration of neural crest cells *(arrow)* out of the neural tube *(NT)*. The subectodermal pathway of neural crest migration (*) is relatively cell free but contains a fine mesh of extracellular matrix molecules. *N*, Notochord; *S*, somite. (Courtesy K. Tosney, Ann Arbor, Mich.)

Because of the lack of suitable markers, the pathways of migration of neural crest cells in mammals have still not been completely mapped. However, data suggest that the pathways are similar to those in the chick. The availability of stable cellular and monoclonal antibody markers has made chimeric chick/quail embryos the object of intense investigation regarding the migrations and differentiation of neural crest cells.

Only generalizations can be made about the specific controls underlying the migrations of neural crest cells. Permissive factors are substrates containing fibronectin, laminin, and type IV collagen (Figure 11-3). Attachment to and migration over these substrate molecules is mediated by the family of attachment proteins called **integrins**. Organized basal laminae (e.g., those of the surface ectoderm and ventral neural tube) act as barriers that guide migrating crest cells along their surfaces. Other extracellular matrix molecules, notably **chondroitin sulfate–rich proteoglycans**, are not good substrates for migrating crest cells. Few neural crest cells are seen in areas that contain high concentrations of chondroitin sulfate (e.g., the sclerotome of the somites). The distribution of migrating neural crest cells in the somites illustrates this principle well. Neural crest cells enter only the anterior parts of the somites, where many of them settle to form the sensory ganglia. They do not penetrate the posterior regions of the somites, which have elevated concentrations of chondroitin sulfate. Neural crest cells in the trunk and the head follow different pathways of migration.

DIFFERENTIATION OF NEURAL CREST CELLS

Neural crest cells ultimately differentiate into an astonishing array of adult structures (Table 11-1). What controls their differentiation is one of the principal questions of neural crest biology. Two different hypotheses have been proposed. According to one, all neural crest cells are equal in developmental potential, and their ultimate differentiation is entirely determined by the environment through which they migrate and into which they finally settle. The other suggests that premigratory crest cells are already programmed for different developmental fates and that certain stem cells are favored while others are inhibited from further development during migration. Recent research indicates that the real answer can be found somewhere between these two positions.

Increasing evidence shows a correlation between the time of migration of neural crest cells from the neural tube and their developmental potential. For example, the cells that first begin to migrate have the potential to differentiate into many different types of cells. Crest cells that begin to migrate later are capable of forming only derivatives characteristic of more dorsal locations (e.g., spinal ganglia) but not sympathetic neurons or adrenal medullary cells. Those that leave the neural tube last are restricted to the dorsalmost pathway of migration and can form only pigment cells.

Several experiments have shown that the fates of neural crest cells are not irreversibly fixed along a single pathway. One type of experiment involves the transplantation of neural crest cells from one part of the body to another. For example, many neural crest cells from the trunk differentiate into sympathetic neurons that produce **norepinephrine** as the transmitter. In the cranial region, however, neural crest cells give rise to parasympathetic neurons, which produce **acetylcholine**. If thoracic neural crest cells are transplanted into the head, some cells differentiate into cholinergic parasympathetic neurons instead of the adrenergic sympathetic neurons normally produced. Conversely, cranial neural crest cells grafted into the thoracic region respond to their new environment by forming adrenergic sympathetic neurons. A more striking example is the conversion of cells of the periocular neural crest mesenchyme, which in birds would normally form cartilage, into neurons if they are associated with embryonic hindgut tissue in vitro. Many of the regional influences on the differentiation of local populations of neural crest cells are now recognized to be interactions between the migrating neural crest cells and specific tissues that they encounter during migration. Some examples of tissue interactions that promote the differentiation of specific neural crest derivatives are given in Table 11-2.

The plasticity of differentiation of neural crest cells can be demonstrated by cloning single neural crest cells in culture. In the same medium and under apparently the same environmental conditions, the progeny of the single cloned cells fre-

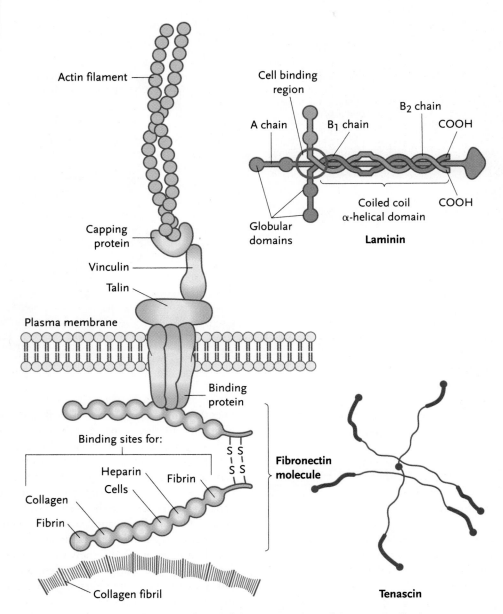

Figure 11-3 Structure of some of the common extracellular matrix molecules.

TABLE 11-1 Major Derivatives of the Neural Crest

	Trunk crest	Cranial crest
Nervous system		
Sensory nervous system	Spinal ganglia	Ganglia of trigeminal nerve (V), facial nerve (VII), glossopharyngeal nerve (superior ganglion) (IX), vagus nerve (jugular ganglion) (X)
Autonomic nervous system	Sympathetic chain ganglia, collateral ganglia: celiac and mesenteric	Parasympathetic ganglia: ciliary, ethmoidal, sphenopalatine, submandibular, visceral
	Parasympathetic ganglia: pelvic plexus, visceral	Satellite cells of sensory ganglia, Schwann cells of peripheral nerves, leptomeninges of prosencephalon and part of mesencephalon
	Satellite cells of sensory ganglia, Schwann cells of peripheral nerves, enteric glial cells	
Pigment cells	Melanocytes	Melanocytes
Endocrine and paraendocrine cells	Adrenal medulla, neurosecretory cells of heart and lungs	Carotid body (type I cells), parafollicular cells (thyroid)
Mesectodermal cells		
Skeleton	None	Cranial vault (squamosal and part of frontal), nasal and orbital, otic capsule (part), palate and maxillary, sphenoid (small contribution), trabeculae (part), visceral cartilages, external ear cartilage (part)
Connective tissue	None	Dermis and fat of skin; cornea of eye (fibroblasts of stroma and corneal endothelium); dental papilla (odontoblasts); connective tissue stroma of glands: thyroid, parathyroid, thymus, salivary, lacrimal; outflow tract (truncoconal region) of heart; cardiac semilunar valves; walls of aorta and aortic arch–derived arteries
Muscle	None	Ciliary muscles, dermal smooth muscles, vascular smooth muscle, minor skeletal muscle elements (?)

TABLE 11-2 Environmental Factors Promoting Differentiation of Neural Crest Cells

Neural crest derivative	Interacting structure
Bones of cranial vault	Brain
Bones of base of skull	Notochord, brain
Pharyngeal arch cartilages	Pharyngeal endoderm
Meckel's cartilage	Cranial ectoderm
Maxillary bone	Maxillary ectoderm
Mandible	Mandibular ectoderm
Palate	Palatal ectoderm
Otic capsule	Otic vesicle
Dentine of teeth	Oral ectoderm
Glandular stroma: thyroid, parathyroid, thymus, salivary	Local epithelium
Adrenal medullary chromaffin cells	Glucocorticoids secreted by adrenal cortex
Enteric neurons	Gut wall
Sympathetic neurons	Spinal cord, notochord, somites
Sensory neurons	Peripheral target tissue
Pigment cells	Extracellular matrix along pathway of migration

quently differentiate into neuronal and nonneuronal (e.g., pigment cell) phenotypes. Similarly, if individual neural crest cells are injected in vivo with a dye, over 50% of the injected cells give rise to progeny with two to four different phenotypes containing the dye. By exposing cloned neural crest precursor cells to specific environmental conditions in vitro, one can begin to understand the mechanisms that determine phenotype in vivo. For example, in one experiment, rat neural crest cells grown under standard in vitro conditions differentiated into neurons, but if they were exposed to **glial growth factor**, they differentiated into Schwann cells because the glial growth factor suppressed their tendency to differentiate into neurons. Similarly, the growth factors BMP-2 and BMP-4 cause cultured neural crest cells to differentiate into autonomic neurons, whereas exposure of these cells to transforming growth factor-β causes them to differentiate into smooth muscle.

Not all types of transformations among possible neural crest derivatives can occur. For example, crest cells from the trunk transplanted into the head cannot form cartilage or skeletal elements, although this is normal for cells of the cranial neural crest. Most experiments suggest that early neural crest cells segregate into intermediate lineages that preserve

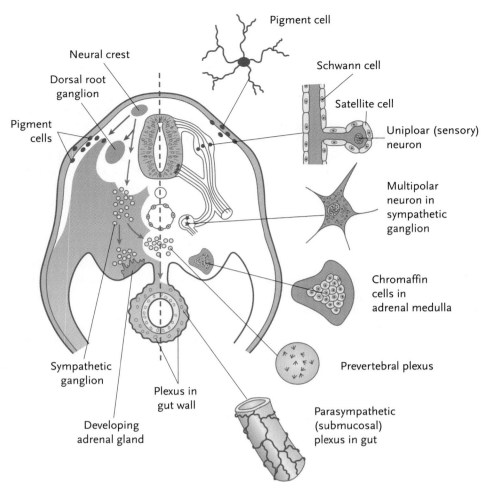

Figure 11-4 Major neural crest migratory pathways and derivatives in the trunk. *Left*, Pathways in the early embryo. The dorsolateral pathway is indicated by the green arrow; the ventral (sympathoadrenal) pathway is indicated by the red arrow; and the ventrolateral pathways is indicated by the purple arrow. *Right*, Derivatives of the trunk neural crest.

the option of differentiating into several but not all types of individual phenotypes. In the chick embryo, some neural crest cells are antigenically different from others even before they have left the neural tube.

A number of neural crest cells are bipotential, depending on signals from their local environment for cues to their final differentiation. One subline called the **sympathoadrenal lineage** forms adrenal medullary cells if exposed to adrenal glucocorticoid hormones. In contrast, if they are exposed first to **fibroblast growth factor (FGF)** and then to **nerve growth factor,** the same cells become sympathetic neurons. Similarly, cultured heart cells secrete a protein that converts postmitotic sympathetic neurons from an adrenergic (norepinephrine transmitter) phenotype to a cholinergic (acetylcholine-secreting) phenotype (see Figure 10-20). During normal development, the sympathetic neurons that innervate sweat glands are catecholaminergic until their axons actually contact the sweat glands. At that point, they become cholinergic. With such a great variety of neural crest derivatives, other devel-

opmental switches of one functional cell type to another are likely to be discovered.

TRUNK NEURAL CREST

The neural crest of the trunk extends from the level of the sixth somite to the most caudal somites. Within much of the trunk, three main migratory pathways of neural crest cells can be seen in cross section (Figure 11-4). One is a dorsolateral pathway between the ectoderm and the somites. The cells that elect this pathway disperse beneath the ectoderm and ultimately enter the ectoderm as pigment cells (**melanocytes**).

The second pathway of migration is a ventral one, along which the neural crest cells initially move into the space between the somites and the neural tube. It continues just under the ventromedial surface of the somite until the cells reach the dorsal aorta. Cells that follow this branch belong to the **sympathoadrenal lineage.** These cells contribute to the for-

mation of the adrenal medulla and elements of the sympathetic nervous system.

A third ventrolateral pathway leads into the anterior halves of the somites. The cells that follow this route form the segmentally arranged sensory ganglia.

The sympathoadrenal lineage is derived from a committed sympathoadrenal progenitor cell that has already passed a number of restriction points so that it can no longer form sensory neurons, glia, or melanocytes. This progenitor cell gives rise to four types of cellular progeny: (1) adrenal chromaffin cells, (2) small intensely fluorescent cells found in the sympathetic ganglia, (3) adrenergic sympathetic neurons, and (4) a small population of cholinergic sympathetic neurons.

Somewhat farther down this cellular lineage is a bipotential progenitor cell that can give rise to either adrenal chromaffin cells or sympathetic neurons. The bipotential progenitor cell already possesses some neuronal traits, but final differentiation depends on the environment surrounding these cells. In the presence of FGF and nerve growth factor in early sympathetic ganglia, these precursors differentiate into definitive sympathetic neurons. On the other hand, precursor cells in the developing adrenal medulla encounter glucocorticoids secreted by adrenal cortical cells. Under this hormonal influence, they lose their neuronal properties and differentiate into chromaffin cells. This differentiative choice, however, is not absolutely fixed, since chromaffin cells can be stimulated after birth to **transdifferentiate** into neurons if they are exposed to nerve growth factor in vitro.

The entire length of the gut is populated by neural crest–derived parasympathetic neurons and associated cells, the enteric glia. These arise from neural crest cells in the cervical (vagal) and sacral levels and undertake extensive migrations along the developing gut. Within the gut the neural crest cells form the **enteric nervous system,** which in many respects acts like an independent component of the nervous system. The number of enteric neurons nearly matches the number of neurons in the spinal cord, and most of them are not directly connected to the brain or spinal cord. This independence explains how the bowel can maintain reflex activity in the absence of input from the central nervous system.

Considerable evidence now suggests that neural crest cells are not committed to form gut-associated nervous tissue before leaving the spinal cord. If vagal crest is replaced by the neural crest of the trunk, which normally does not give rise to gut-associated derivatives, the gut is colonized by the transplanted trunk-level neural crest cells. Evidence that the pathways of migration affect differentiation is seen in the neurotransmitters produced by these transplanted crest cells. Parasympathetic neurons differentiated from trunk cells produce serotonin but not catecholamines in the gut. If they had differentiated in their normal sites in the trunk, these neurons would have produced catecholamines and not serotonin.

Despite the strong influence of the environment of the gut on the differentiation of neural crest cells exposed to its in-

fluences, neural crest cells retain a surprising degree of developmental flexibility. If crest-derived cells already in the gut of avian embryos are retransplanted into the trunk region of younger embryos, they seem to lose the memory of their former association with the gut. They enter the pathways (e.g., adrenal or peripheral nerve) common to trunk crest cells (except that they cannot enter pigment cell pathways) and differentiate accordingly.

Most neural crest precursors of gut-associated parasympathetic neurons express the basic helix-loop-helix transcription factor, **Mash 1,** which is also expressed in the precursors of sympathetic but not sensory neurons. Expression of Mash 1 in these cells is stimulated by the growth factors BMP-2 and BMP-4, and Mash 1 appears to maintain the competence of the postmigratory cells in the gut to differentiate into neurons. Other environmental factors are required for complete commitment of these cells to form autonomic neurons. There is recent evidence for a second population of late-appearing neural crest precursors of enteric neurons that do not express Mash 1.

Compared with the cranial neural crest, the trunk neural crest has a relatively limited range of differentiation options. The derivatives of the trunk neural crest are summarized in Table 11-1.

CRANIAL NEURAL CREST

The cranial neural crest is a major component of the cephalic end of the embryo. Comparative anatomical and developmental research suggests that the cranial neural crest may represent the major morphological substrate for the evolution of the vertebrate head. Largely because of the availability of precise cellular marking methods, the understanding of the cranial neural crest has increased dramatically. The majority of studies on the cranial neural crest have been conducted on avian embryos. Research on mammalian embryos, however, suggests that the properties and role of the neural crest in mammalian cranial development are quite similar to those in birds.

In the mammalian head, neural crest cells leave the future brain well before closure of the neural folds (Figure 11-5). Although the pathways of migration of the cranial neural crest in mammals are not nearly as well delineated as in birds, there nevertheless appear to be distinct but somewhat overlapping migratory territories in the embryonic mammalian head (Figure 11-6). Because of the distribution of primary mesenchymal cells and extracellular matrix molecules in the mammalian head, the neural crest cells migrate in diffuse streams throughout the cranial mesenchyme to reach their final destinations.

There is remarkable specificity in the relationship among the origins of the neural crest in the hindbrain, its ultimate destination within the pharyngeal arches, and the expression of certain gene products (Figures 11-7 and 11-8). The

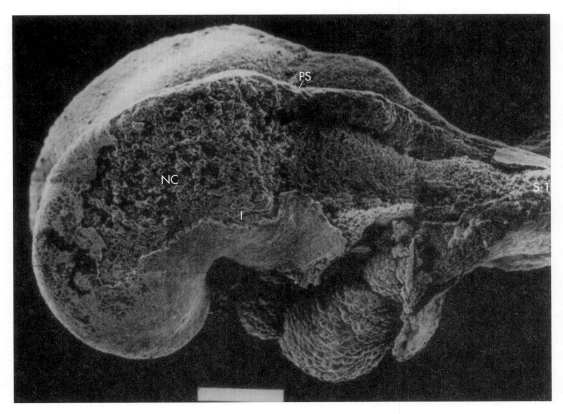

Figure 11-5 Neural crest migration in the head of a seven-somite rat embryo. In this scanning electron micrograph the ectoderm was removed from a large part of the side of the head, exposing migrating neural crest *(NC)* cells cranial (to the left) to the preotic sulcus *(PS)*. Many of the cells are migrating toward the first pharyngeal arch *(I)*. The area between the preotic sulcus and the first somite *(S-1)* is devoid of neural crest cells because in this region they have not begun to migrate from the closing neural folds. The white bar at the bottom represents 100 μm. (Based on Tan SS, Morriss-Kay G: *Cell Tissue Res* 204:403-416, 1985.)

neural crest associated with rhombomere 2 migrates into and forms the bulk of the first pharyngeal arch, that of rhombomere 4 into the second arch, and that of rhombomere 6 into the third arch. Neural crest cells do not appear to migrate directly lateral from rhombomeres 3 and 5. Some investigators feel that neural crest does not form in rhombomeres 3 and 5 or that neural crest cells do form but then undergo apoptosis. Intravital microscopic studies suggest that neural crest cells do form in these rhombomeres but that as they leave the rhombomeres, they turn sharply and join the migration pathways of the neural crest cells migrating from adjacent rhombomeres.

A close correlation exists between the pattern of migration of the rhombomeric neural crest cells and the expression of products of the *Hoxb* gene complex. *Hoxb-2*, *Hoxb-3*, and *Hoxb-4* products are expressed in a regular sequence in both the neural tube and the neural crest–derived mesenchyme of pharyngeal arches 2, 3, and 4. *Hoxb* is not expressed in rhombomere 2 or in the first pharyngeal arch mesenchyme. Only after the pharyngeal arches become populated with neural crest cells does the ectoderm overlying the arches express a similar pattern of *Hoxb* gene products (see Figure 11-8). These

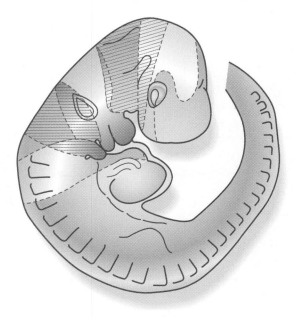

Figure 11-6 Major cranial neural crest migration routes in the mammal. (Based on Morriss-Kay G, Tuckett F: *J Craniofac Genet Dev Biol* 11:181-191, 1991.)

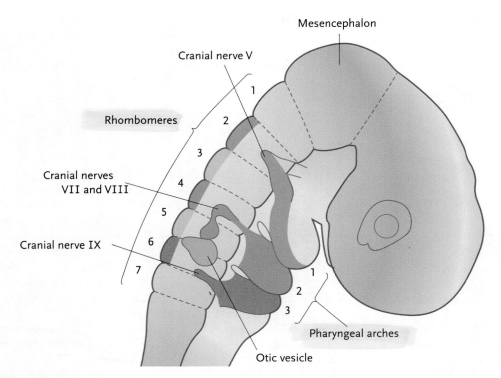

Figure 11-7 Migration paths of neural crest cells from rhombomeres 2, 4, and 6 into the first three pharyngeal arches.

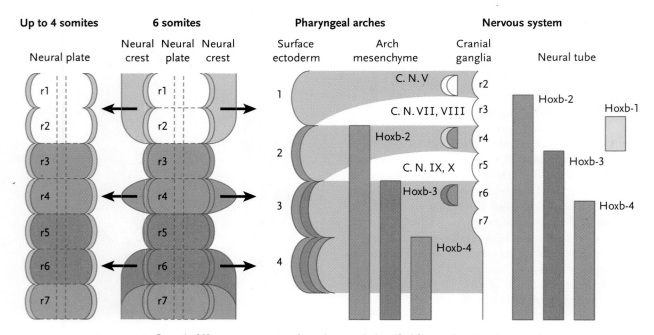

Figure 11-8 Spread of *Hox* gene expression from the neural plate (*far left*) into the migrating neural crest (*middle*) and into tissues of the pharyngeal arches (*right*). Arrows in the middle diagram indicate directions of neural crest migration. *C. N.*, Cranial nerve; *r*, rhombomere. (Modified from Hunt P and others: *Development* I[suppl]:187-196, 1991.)

Hoxb genes may play a role in positionally specifying the neural crest cells with which they are associated. Furthermore, interactions between the neural crest cells and the surface ectoderm of the pharyngeal arches may specify the ectoderm of the arches.

In the posterior part of the pharynx, a circumpharyngeal crest passes behind the sixth pharyngeal arch (Figure 11-9). Ventral to the pharynx it sweeps cranially, providing the pathway through which the hypoglossal nerve (XII) and its associated skeletal muscle precursor cells pass. The muscles innervated by the hypoglossal nerve and the hypopharyngeal muscles are the only somite-derived skeletal muscles whose connective tissue cells originate in the neural crest.

A major difference between cells of the cranial neural crest and those of the trunk is that the neural crest cells are patterned with level-specific instructions in the head, whereas those of the trunk do not appear to have imprinted level-specific instructions. Specifically, if neural crest cells that normally give rise to structures characteristic of pharyngeal arch 1 are transplanted to the level of pharyngeal arch 3, ectopic arch 1 structures (e.g., a supernumerary jaw) are formed at the level of arch 3. Similar level shifts of transplanted trunk neural crest do not result in the formation of abnormal structures.

In both avian and mammalian embryos an S-shaped **circumpharyngeal crest** migration pathway (see Figure 11-9) marks the rough boundary between cranial and trunk structures. In this region the dorsal somites (trunk) and ventral pharyngeal arches (cranial) overlap along the craniocaudal axis. The circumpharyngeal crest marks the pathway of migration of enteric crest cells toward the gut and cardiac neural crest cells into the cardiac outflow tract (see Figure 11-9). A disturbance in this area can result in cardiac septation defects (**aorticopulmonary septum**) as well as glandular and craniofacial malformations.

The **DiGeorge syndrome**, which is associated with a deletion on chromosome 22, is characterized by hypoplasia and reduced function of the thymus, thyroid, and parathyroid glands and cardiovascular defects, such as persistent truncus arteriosus and abnormalities of the aortic arches. Hoxa-3 mutant mice show a similar spectrum of pharyngeal defects. The common denominator for this constellation of pathology is a defect of the cranial neural crest supplying the third and fourth pharyngeal arches and cardiac outflow tract. Similar defects have been described in human embryos exposed to excessive amounts of retinoic acid early in embryogenesis.

Cranial neural crest cells differentiate into a wide variety of cell and tissue types (see Table 11-1), including connective tissue and skeletal tissues. These tissues constitute much of the soft and hard tissues of the face (Figure 11-10). (Specific details of morphogenesis of the head are presented in Chapter 13.)

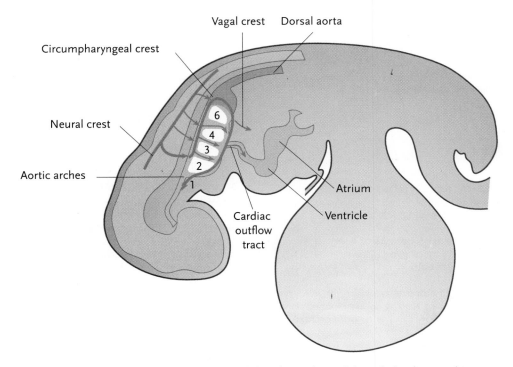

Figure 11-9 Migration of cranial neural crest cells (*green lines* and *arrows*) through the pharyngeal region and into the aortic arches and the outflow tract of the heart.

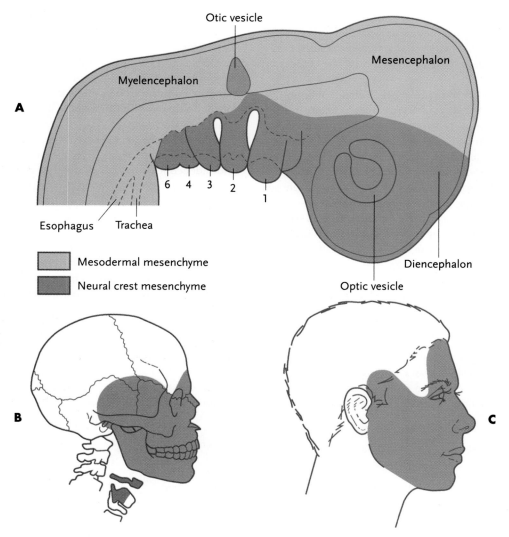

Figure 11-10 Neural crest distribution in the human face and neck. A, In the early embryo. B and C, In the adult skeleton and dermis.

BOX 11-1 Major Neurocristopathies

DEFECTS OF MIGRATION OR MORPHOGENESIS

Trunk Neural Crest
Hirschsprung's disease (aganglionic colon)

Cranial Neural Crest
Aorticopulmonary septation defects of heart
Anterior chamber defects of eye
Cleft lip, cleft palate, or both
Frontonasal dysplasia
DiGeorge syndrome (hypoparathyroidism, thyroid deficiency, thymic dysplasia leading to immunodeficiency, defects in cardiac outflow tract and aortic arches)
Certain dental anomalies

Trunk and Cranial Neural Crest
CHARGE association
Waardenburg's syndrome

TUMORS AND PROLIFERATION DEFECTS

Pheochromocytoma: tumor of chromaffin tissue of adrenal medulla
Neuroblastoma: tumor of adrenal medulla, autonomic ganglia, or both
Medullary carcinoma of thyroid: tumor of parafollicular (calcitonin-secreting) cells of thyroid
Carcinoid tumors—tumors of enterochromaffin cells of digestive tract
Neurofibromatosis (von Recklinghausen's disease): peripheral nerve tumors

GENETIC DEFECT INVOLVING NEURAL CREST CELLS

Albinism

CLINICAL CORRELATION 11-1
Neurocristopathies

Because of the complex developmental history of the neural crest, a variety of congenital malformations are associated with its defective development. These have commonly been subdivided into two main categories—defects of migration or morphogenesis and tumors of neural crest tissues (Box 11-1). Some of these defects involve only a single component of the neural crest; others affect multiple components and are recognized as syndromes.

Several syndromes or associations of defects are understandable only if the wide distribution of derivatives of the neural crest is recognized. For example, one association called **CHARGE** consists of *c*oloboma (see Chapter 12), *h*eart disease, *a*tresia of nasal choanae, *r*etardation of development, *g*enital hypoplasia in males, and anomalies of the *e*ar.

Types I and III of **Waardenburg's syndrome**, which is caused by Pax-3 mutations, involve various combinations of pigmentation defects (commonly a white stripe in the hair and other pigment anomalies in the skin), deafness, cleft palate, and **ocular hypertelorism** (increased space between the eyes). One variant (type I) of Waardenburg's syndrome is also characterized by hypoplasia of the limb muscles, which is not surprising considering the important association between Pax-3 and myogenic cells migrating into the limb buds from the somites. Pax-3 is similarly expressed in migrating cardiac neural crest cells, but is downregulated when the cells settle in the walls of the cardiac outflow tract or aortic arches. Cardiovascular defects in these areas are also seen in Pax-3 mutants.

Neurofibromatosis (von Recklinghausen's disease) is a common genetic disease manifested by multiple tumors of neural crest origin. Common features are **café au lait spots** (light brown pigmented lesions) on the skin, multiple (often hundreds) **neurofibromas** (peripheral nerve tumors), occasional gigantism of a limb or digit, and various other conditions. Neurofibromatosis occurs in approximately 1 of 3000 live births, and the gene is a very large one and subject to a high mutation rate.

Because of the massive contribution of the neural crest to the face and other parts of the head and neck, various malformations in the craniofacial region involve neural crest derivatives. A wide spectrum of facial abnormalities lumped together under the term **frontonasal dysplasia** (see Chapter 13) heavily involve neural crest–derived tissues.

CLINICAL VIGNETTE

A newborn is diagnosed as having an incomplete separation between the aorta and pulmonary artery (a mild form of persistent truncus arteriosus). Later, after corrective heart surgery, she has more colds and sore throats than her siblings. After testing, her physician tells the parents that there is evidence of immunodeficiency. The doctor also tells the parents that it would be a good idea to check her levels of parathyroid hormone.

What is the basis for this suggestion?

SUMMARY

- The neural crest arises from neuroepithelial cells along the lateral border of the neural plate. Having left the neural tube, neural crest cells migrate to peripheral locations throughout the body. Some substrates, such as those containing chondroitin sulfate molecules, are not favorable for neural crest cell migration.
- Neural crest cells differentiate into many types of adult cells, such as sensory and autonomic neurons, Schwann cells, pigment cells, and adrenal medullary cells. Cells from the cranial neural crest also differentiate into bone, cartilage, dentin, dermal fibroblasts, selected smooth muscle, the connective tissue stroma of pharyngeal glands, and several regions of the heart and great vessels.
- The control of differentiation of neural crest cells is diverse, with some cells being determined before they begin to migrate and others responding to environmental cues along their paths of migration. Trunk neural crest cells cannot differentiate into skeletal elements.
- Neural crest cells in the trunk follow three main paths of migration: (1) a dorsolateral pathway for pigment cells, (2) a ventral path for cells of the sympathoadrenal lineage, and (3) a ventrolateral pathway leading through the anterior halves of the somites for sensory ganglion–forming cells.
- Cells of the cranial neural crest form many tissues of the facial region. In the pharyngeal region the pathways of crest cell migration are closely correlated with regions of expression of products of the *Hoxb* gene complex. Cells of the cranial crest are patterned with level-specific instructions, whereas those of the trunk crest are not.
- Several genetic diseases and syndromes are associated with disturbances of the neural crest. Neurofibromatosis is often characterized by multiple tumors and pigment disturbances. Disturbances of the cardiac neural crest can result in septation defects in the heart and outflow tract.

REVIEW QUESTIONS

1. Which of these cell and tissue types arises from cranial but not trunk neural crest cells?
   A. Sensory ganglia
   B. Adrenal medulla
   C. Melanocytes
   D. Schwann cells
   E. None of the above

2. Which molecule is a poor substrate for migrating neural crest cells?
   A. Laminin
   B. Chondroitin sulfate
   C. Fibronectin
   D. Type IV collagen
   E. Hyaluronic acid

3. Neural crest cells arise from the:
   A. Somite
   B. Dorsal nonneural ectoderm
   C. Neural tube
   D. Splanchnic mesoderm
   E. Yolk sac endoderm

4. A 6-month-old infant exhibits multiple congenital defects, including a cleft palate, deafness, ocular hypertelorism, and a white forelock but otherwise dark hair on his head. The probable diagnosis is:
   A. CHARGE association
   B. von Recklinghausen's disease
   C. Hirschsprung's disease
   D. Waardenburg's syndrome
   E. None of the above

5. What molecule is involved in the migration of neural crest cells from the neural tube?
   A. Slug
   B. BMP-2
   C. Mash 1
   D. Norepinephrine
   E. Glial growth factor

6. Which is not a derivative of the neural crest?
   A. Sensory neurons
   B. Motor neurons
   C. Schwann cells
   D. Adrenal medulla
   E. Dental papilla

7. What maintains the competence of neural crest cells to differentiate into autonomic neurons?
   A. Sonic hedgehog
   B. Acetylcholine
   C. Mash 1
   D. Glial growth factor
   E. Transforming growth factor-β

8. If trunk neural crest cells are transplanted into the cranial region, they can form all of the following types of cells except:
   A. Pigment cells
   B. Schwann cells
   C. Sensory neurons
   D. Cartilage
   E. Autonomic neurons

9. How does the segmental distribution of the spinal ganglia occur?

10. What are three major differences between cranial and trunk neural crest?

REFERENCES

Anderson DJ: Cellular and molecular biology of neural crest lineage determination, *Trends Genet* 13:276-280, 1997.

Anderson DJ: Development and plasticity of a neural crest–derived neuroendocrine sublineage. In Landmesser LT, ed: *The assembly of the nervous system*, New York, 1989, Liss, pp 17-36.

Barald KF: Culture conditions affect the cholinergic development of an isolated subpopulation of chick mesencephalic neural crest cells, *Dev Biol* 135:349-366, 1989.

Birgbauer E and others: Rhombomeric origin and rostrocaudal reassortment of neural crest cells revealed by intravital microscopy, *Development* 121:935-945, 1995.

Bronner-Fraser M, Fraser SE: Cell lineage analysis of the avian neural crest, *Development* 2(suppl):17-22, 1991.

Conway SJ, Henderson DJ, Copp AJ: Pax3 is required for cardiac neural crest migration in the mouse: evidence from the splotch (Sp2H) mutant, *Development* 124:505-514, 1997.

Epstein JA: Pax3, neural crest and cardiovascular development, *Trends Cardiovasc Med* 6:255-261, 1996.

Erickson CA: Control of pathfinding by the avian trunk neural crest, *Development* 103(suppl):63-80, 1988.

Erickson CA: Morphogenesis of the neural crest. In Browder LW, ed: *Developmental biology*, vol 2, New York, 1986, Plenum, pp 481-543.

Erickson CA, Loring JF, Lester SM: Migratory pathways of HNK-1–immunoreactive neural crest cells in the rat embryo, *Dev Biol* 134:112-118, 1989.

Gershon MD: Genes and lineages in the formation of the enteric nervous system, *Curr Opin Neurobiol* 7:101-109, 1997.

Hall BK, Hörstadius S: *The neural crest*, London, 1988, Oxford University Press.

Hunt P, Wilkinson D, Krumlauf R: Patterning the vertebrate head: murine Hox 2 genes mark distinct subpopulations of premigratory and migratory cranial neural crest, *Development* 112:43-50, 1991.

Imai H and others: Contribution of early-emigrating midbrain crest cells to the dental mesenchyme of mandibular molar teeth in rat embryos, *Dev Biol* 176:151-165, 1996.

Johnston MC, Vig KWL, Ambrose LJH: Neurocristopathy as a unifying concept: clinical correlations. In Riccardi VM, Mulvihill JJ, eds: *Neurofibromatosis (von Recklinghausen disease)*, New York, 1981, Raven, pp 97-104.

Jones MC: The neurocristopathies: reinterpretation based upon the mechanism of abnormal morphogenesis, *Cleft Palate J* 27:136-140, 1990.

Kirby ML, Waldo KL: Neural crest and cardiovascular patterning, *Circ Res* 77:211-215, 1995.

Kuratani S: Spatial distribution of postotic crest cells defines the head/trunk interface of the vertebrate body: embryological interpretation of peripheral nerve morphology and evolution of the vertebrate head, *Anat Embryol* 195:1-13, 1997.

Kuratani SC, Kirby ML: Initial migration and distribution of the cardiac neural crest in the avian embryo: an introduction to the concept of the circumpharyngeal crest, *Am J Anat* 191:215-227, 1991.

Kuratani SC, Kirby ML: Migration and distribution of circumpharyngeal crest cells in the chick embryo, *Anat Rec* 234:263-280, 1992.

Lallier T, Bronner-Fraser M: The role of the extracellular matrix in neural crest migration, *Semin Dev Biol* 1:35-44, 1990.

Le Douarin N: *The neural crest*, Cambridge, England, 1982, Cambridge University Press.

Liem KF and others: Dorsal differentiation of neural plate cells induced by BMP-mediated signals from epidermal ectoderm, *Cell* 82:969-979, 1995.

Lumsden A: Multipotent cells in the avian neural crest, *Trends Neurosci* 12:81-83, 1989.

Lumsden A, Guthrie S: Alternating patterns of cell surface properties and neural crest cell migration during segmentation of the chick hindbrain, *Development* 2(suppl):9-15, 1991.

Manley NR, Capecci MR: The role of Hoxa-3 in mouse thymus and thyroid development, *Development* 121:1989-2003, 1995.

Morell R and others: Three mutations in the paired homeodomain of PAX3 that cause Waardenburg syndrome type 1, *Hum Hered* 47:38-41, 1997.

Morriss-Kay G, Tan S-S: Mapping cranial neural crest cell migration pathways in mammalian embryos, *Trends Genet* 3:257-261, 1987.

Morriss-Kay G, Tuckett F: Early events in mammalian craniofacial morphogenesis, *J Craniofac Genet Dev Biol* 11:181-191, 1991.

Newgreen DF, Erickson CA: The migration of neural crest cells, *Int Rev Cytol* 103:89-143, 1986.

Nieto MA and others: Control of cell behavior during vertebrate development by *Slug*, a zinc finger gene, *Science* 264:835-839, 1994.

Noden DM: Origins and patterning of craniofacial mesenchymal tissues, *J Craniofac Genet Dev Biol* 2(suppl):15-31, 1986.

Noden DM: The role of the neural crest in patterning of avian cranial skeletal, connective and muscle tissues, *Dev Biol* 96:144-165, 1983.

Oakley PA and others: Glycoconjugates mark a transient barrier to neural crest migration in the chicken embryo, *Development* 120:103-114, 1994.

Osumi-Yamashita N, Eto K: Mammalian cranial neural crest cells and facial development, *Dev Growth Differentiation* 32:454-459, 1990.

Patterson PH: Control of cell fate in a vertebrate neurogenic cell lineage, *Cell* 62:1035-1038, 1990.

Quevedo C, Holstein TJ: Molecular genetics and the ontogeny of pigment patterns in mammals, *Pigment Cell Res* 5:328-334, 1992.

Scammbler PJ: DiGeorge syndrome and related birth defects, *Semin Dev Biol* 5:303-310, 1994.

Sechrist J and others: Segmental migration of the hindbrain neural crest does not arise from its segmental generation, *Development* 118:691-703, 1993.

Selleck MAJ and others: Origins of neural crest diversity, *Dev Biol* 159:1-11, 1993.

Shah NM and others: Glial growth factor restricts mammalian neural crest stem cells to a glial fate, *Cell* 77:349-360, 1994.

Tan SS, Morriss-Kay G: The development and distribution of the cranial neural crest in the rat embryo, *Cell Tissue Res* 240:403-416, 1985.

Weston JA: Phenotypic diversification in neural crest–derived cells: the time and stability of commitment during early development, *Curr Topics Dev Biol* 20:195-210, 1986.

12

SENSE ORGANS

The sense organs arise in large measure from thickened placodes of cells in the ectodermal germ layer (see Figure 5-14). Forming largely in response to secondary inductions by the central nervous system, the ectodermal placodes can be subdivided into two groups. One group gives rise to a diverse array of sense organs such as the inner ear, the lens of the eye, and the olfactory sensory epithelium. The other group of placodes, which is closely associated with the pharyngeal arches, produces sensory neurons that combine with neural crest–derived neurons to form the sensory ganglia of many of the cranial nerves.

This chapter concentrates on the development of the eyes and ears, the most complex and important sense organs in humans. Discussion of the organs of smell and taste is deferred to Chapter 13, since their development is intimately associated with that of the face and pharynx. The sensory components of the cranial nerves are discussed in Chapter 10.

EYE

The eye is a very complex structure that originates from constituents derived from a number of sources, including the wall of the diencephalon, the overlying surface ectoderm, and migrating cranial neural crest mesenchyme. Two basic themes occur throughout ocular development. One is an ongoing series of inductive signals that result in the initial establishment of the major components of the eye. The other is the coordinated differentiation of many of these components.

For normal vision to occur, many complex structures within the eye must properly relate to neighboring structures. For example, the cornea and lens must both become transparent and properly aligned to provide an appropriate pathway for light to reach the retina. The retina in turn must be configured to both receive concrete visual images and transmit patterned visual signals to the proper parts of the brain through neural processes extending from the retina into the optic nerve.

Early Events in the Establishment of the Eye

The early eye fields are Pax-6–expressing areas on either side of the diencephalon. (See later section for further discussion of Pax-6 in the development of the eye.) An influence from the prechordal plate (probably sonic hedgehog) represses Pax-6 in the ventral midline and keeps the two optic fields separate. In the absence of the influence of the prechordal plate, forebrain tissue is deficient, the optic fields converge, and **cyclopia** results (see Figure 7-16).

Development of the eye is first evident at about 22 days' gestation, when the lateral walls of the diencephalon begin to bulge out as **optic grooves** (Figure 12-1). Within a few days the optic grooves enlarge to form **optic vesicles**, which terminate very close to the overlying surface ectoderm. Apposition of the outer wall of the optic vesicle to the surface ectoderm is essential for the transmission of an important inductive message that stimulates the surface ectodermal cells to thicken and begin forming the lens (Figure 12-2).

The interaction between the optic vesicle and overlying ectoderm was one of the first recognized inductive processes. It was initially characterized by deletion and transplantation experiments conducted on amphibian embryos. When the optic vesicles were removed early, the surface ectoderm differentiated into ordinary ectodermal cells instead of lens fibers. Conversely, when optic vesicles were combined with certain types of ectoderm other than eye, the ectoderm was stimulated to form lens fibers. Subsequent research on amphibian embryos has shown that a series of preparatory inductions from neural plate and underlying mesoderm condition the ectoderm for its final induction into lens by the optic vesicle. In mammals an important mechanism underlying the severe **microphthalmia** (tiny eyes) or **anophthalmia** (absence of eyes) seen in the *small eye* and *fidget* mutants is an interference in the apposition of optic vesicles and surface ectoderm, which interferes with lens induction.

The paired box gene, **Pax-6,** plays a prominent role throughout early eye development and at a number of later

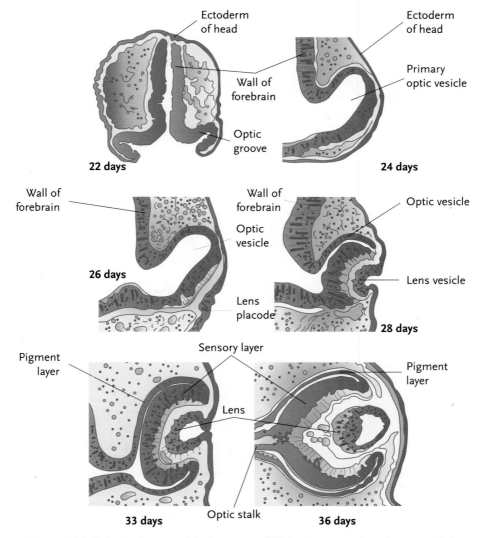

Figure 12-1 Early development of the human eye. (All drawings are made to the same scale.)

stages of development of the retina and lens. Pax-6 is initially expressed in both the lens and nasal placodes as well as much of the diencephalon. In *Drosophila*, Pax-6 has been called a *master gene* for eye development; that is, it can turn on the cascade of an estimated 2500 genes that guide development of the eye. The power of Pax-6 is shown by the formation of ectopic eyes on antennae and legs in *Drosophila* when the gene is improperly expressed. In the absence of Pax-6 expression (*eyeless* mutant), eyes do not form. In the *small eye* mutation, the mammalian equivalent of *eyeless*, the early optic vesicle forms, but, as previously noted, eye development does not progress because the surface ectoderm is unable to respond to the inductive signal emitted by the optic vesicle. The recent identification in humans of two genes (*Eya* [eyes absent] and *Six* [sine oculis]) that are activated by Pax-6 in *Drosophila* strongly suggests that despite major differences in the structure and development of the

vertebrate and insect eye, the basic genetic apparatus has been conserved throughout phylogeny. In mice, **Eya-1 and Eya-2** are expressed in the lens placodes and appear to be required for placodal induction and early differentiation, but in the absence of Pax-6 function, they are not expressed, and eye development fails to proceed.

As the process of lens induction occurs, the outer face of the optic vesicle begins to flatten and ultimately becomes concave. This results in the transformation of the optic vesicle to the **optic cup** (see Figure 12-1). Meanwhile, the induced lens ectoderm thickens and invaginates to form a **lens vesicle**, which detaches from the surface epithelium from which it originated (Figures 12-1 and 12-3). Then the lens vesicle takes over and becomes the primary agent of a new inductive reaction by acting on the overlying surface ectoderm and causing it to begin corneal development (see Figure 12-2).

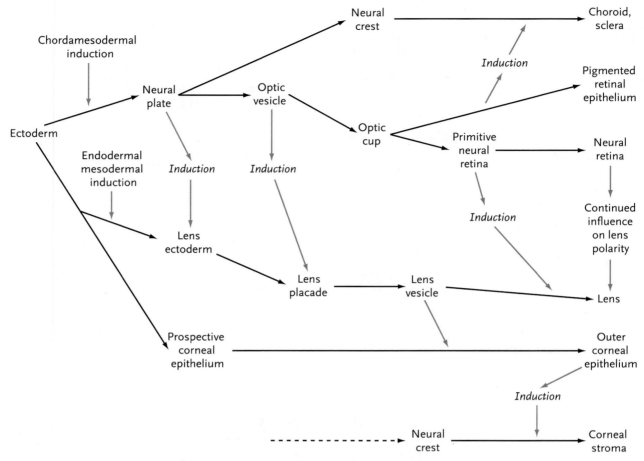

Figure 12-2 Flow chart of major inductive events and tissue transformations in eye development. Inductive events are indicated by colored arrows.

Formation of the optic cup is an asymmetrical process that occurs at the ventral margin of the optic vesicle rather than at its center. This results in the formation of a gap called the *choroid fissure,* which is continuous with a groove in the **optic stalk** (Figure 12-4). During much of early ocular development, the choroid fissure and optic groove form a channel through which the **hyaloid artery** passes into the posterior chamber of the eye. The optic stalk initially represents a narrow neck that connects the optic cup to the diencephalon, but as development progresses, it is invaded by neuronal processes emanating from the ganglion cells of the retina. After these processes have made their way to the appropriate regions of the brain, the optic stalk is properly known as the **optic nerve.** Later in development the choroid fissure closes, and no trace of it is seen in the normal iris. Nonclosure of the choroid fissure results in the anomaly of coloboma (see p. 276). Another paired box gene, **Pax-2,** is expressed in nonneuronal cells of the optic stalk and the early optic nerve while it is being invaded by retinal axons. The Pax-2–expressing cells provide guidance cues to outgrowing retinal

axons that pass through the optic nerve and optic chiasm and enter the contralateral optic tract. Coloboma and visual disturbances are frequently seen in individuals carrying mutant *Pax-2* genes. In *Pax-2* mutant mice, retinal axons do not cross the midline through the optic chiasm, but rather remain in the ipsilateral optic tract.

Formation of the Lens

From the earliest stages, formation of the lens depends on genetic instructions provided by Pax-6. The surface ectoderm of the head requires the action of Pax-6 for the induction of the lens placode, although this is by no means the only gene involved. The influence of Pax-6 continues until late in lens development, when it controls the activity of the genes for the lens crystallin proteins.

When it is breaking off from the surface ectoderm, the lens vesicle is roughly spherical and has a large central cavity (see Figure 12-1). At the end of the sixth week the cells at the inner pole of the lens vesicle begin to elongate in an early step to-

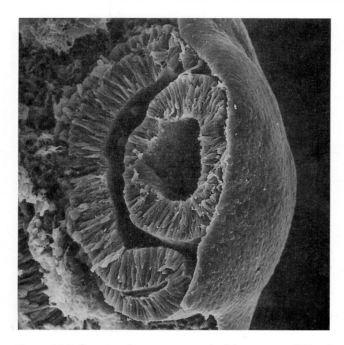

Figure 12-3 Scanning electron micrograph of the optic cup (*left*) and lens vesicle (*center*) in the chick embryo. (Courtesy K. Tosney, Ann Arbor, Mich.)

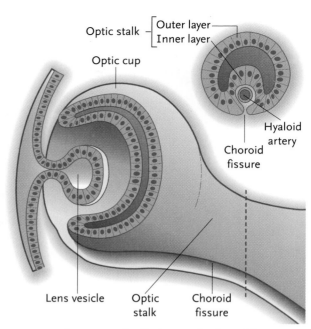

Figure 12-4 Optic cup and stalk showing the choroid fissure containing the hyaloid artery. The cross section (*top*) is taken from the level of the dashed line.

ward their transformation into the long, transparent cells called **lens fibers** (Figure 12-5).

Differentiation of the lens is a very precise and well-orchestrated process involving several levels of organization. At the cellular level, relatively nonspecialized lens epithelial cells undergo a profound transformation into transparent, elongated cells that contain large quantities of specialized **crystallin proteins.** At the tissue level the entire lens is responsive to signals from the retina and other structures of the eye so that its shape and overall organization are best adapted for the transmission of undistorted light rays from the corneal entrance to the light-receiving cells of the retina.

At the cellular level, cytodifferentiation of the lens consists of the transformation of mitotically active lens epithelial cells into elongated postmitotic lens fiber cells. Up to 90% of the soluble protein in these postmitotic cells consists of crystallin proteins. The mammalian lens contains three major crystallin proteins: α, β, and γ.

The formation of crystallin-containing lens fibers begins with the elongation of epithelial cells from the inner pole of the lens vesicle (see Figure 12-1). These cells make up the fibers of the **lens nucleus** (Figure 12-6). The remainder of the lens fibers arise from the transformation of the cuboidal cells of the anterior lens epithelium. During embryonic life, mitotic activity is spread throughout the outer lens epithelial cells. Around the time of birth, mitotic activity ceases in the central region of this epithelium, leaving a germinative ring of mitotically active cells around the cen-

tral region. Daughter cells from the germinative region move into the equatorial region of cellular elongation, where they cease to divide and take on the cytological characteristics of ribonucleic acid–producing (RNA-producing) cells and begin to form crystallin messenger RNAs. These cells soon elongate tremendously, fill up with crystallins, and transform into secondary lens fibers that form concentric layers around the primary fibers of the lens nucleus. The midline region where secondary lens fibers from opposite points on the equator join is recognized as the anterior and posterior **lens suture** (see Figure 12-5, *D*). With this arrangement, the lens fibers toward the periphery are successively younger. As long as the lens grows, new secondary fibers move in from the equator onto the outer cortex of the lens.

The crystallin proteins show a very characteristic pattern and sequence of appearance, with the α-crystallins appearing first in the morphologically undifferentiated epithelial cells. Synthesis of β-crystallins is seen when the lens fibers begin to elongate, whereas the expression of γ-crystallins is restricted to terminally differentiated lens fiber cells. Each of the crystallin protein families contains several members. They show different patterns of activation (some members of a family being coordinately activated) and different patterns of accumulation. There are often pronounced interspecies differences in patterns of crystallin expression. These presumably facilitate the optical clearing of the lens to allow the efficient transmission of light, but many details remain to be elucidated.

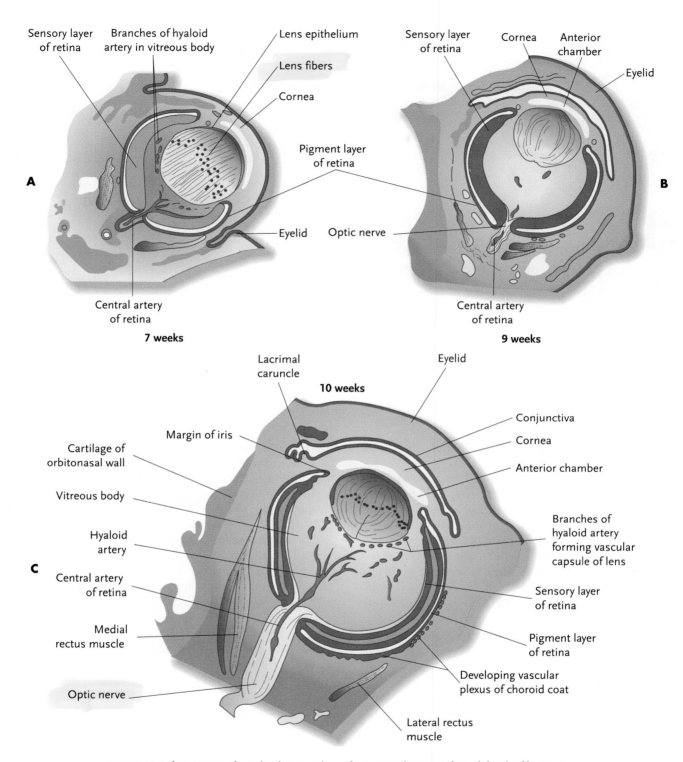

Figure 12-5 Later stages of eye development drawn from coronal sections through heads of human embryos. **A,** At **7 weeks. B,** At **9 weeks. C,** At **10 weeks.** (Modified from Carlson B: *Patten's foundations of embryology*, ed 6, New York, 1996, McGraw-Hill.)

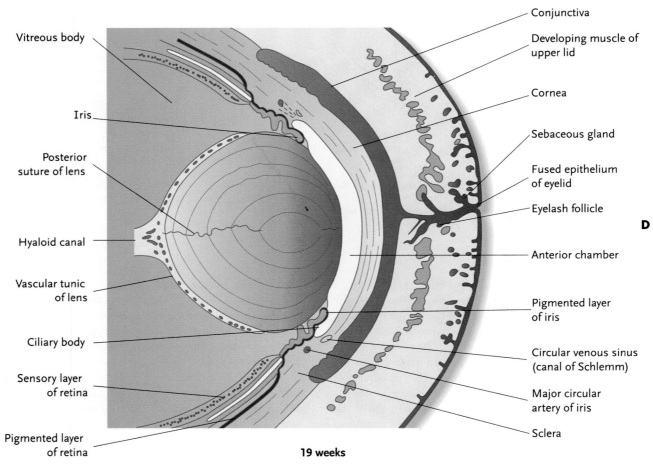

19 weeks

Figure 12-5—cont'd D, At 19 weeks. (Modified from Carlson B: *Patten's foundations of embryology*, ed 6, New York, 1996, McGraw-Hill.)

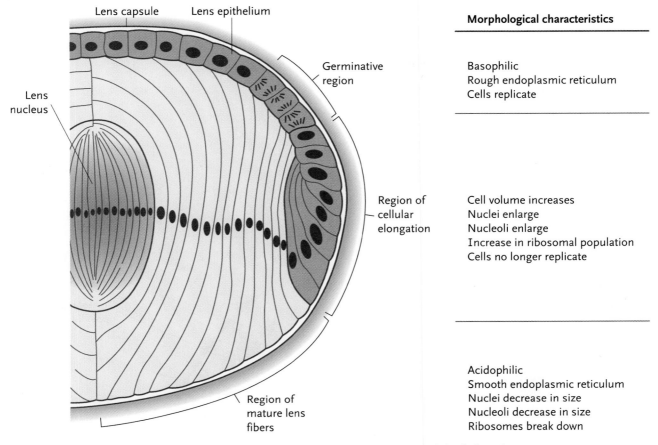

Figure 12-6 Organization of the vertebrate lens. As the lens grows, epithelial cells from the germinative region stop dividing, elongate, and differentiate into lens fiber cells that produce lens crystallin proteins. (After Papaconstantinou J: *Science* 156:338-346, 1967.)

Throughout much of its life the lens is under the influence of the retina. After induction of the lens, secretions of the retina, of which **fibroblast growth factor (FGF)** is a major component, accumulate in the vitreous humor behind the lens and stimulate the formation of lens fibers. A striking example of the continued influence of the retina on lens morphology is seen after a developing lens is rotated so that its outer pole faces the retina. Very rapidly and presumably under the influence of retinal secretions, the low epithelial cells of the former outer pole begin to elongate and form an additional set of lens fibers (Figure 12-7). A new lens epithelium forms on the corneal side of the rotated lens. Such structural adaptations are striking evidence of a mechanism that ensures correct alignment between the lens and the rest of the visual system throughout development.

Formation of the Cornea

Formation of the cornea is the result of the last of the series of major inductive events in eye formation (see Figure 12-2),

with the lens vesicle acting on the overlying surface ectoderm. This induction results in the transformation of a typical surface ectoderm, consisting of a basal layer of cuboidal cells and a superficial periderm, to a transparent, multilayered structure with a complex extracellular matrix and cellular contributions from several sources.

The inductive influence of the lens stimulates a change in the basal ectodermal cells. They increase in height, largely as a result of the elaboration of secretory organelles (e.g., Golgi apparatus) on the basal ends of the cells. As these changes are completed, the cells begin to secrete epithelially derived collagen types I, II, and IX to form the **primary stroma** of the cornea (Figure 12-8).

Using the primary stroma as a basis for migration, neural crest cells around the lip of the optic cup migrate centrally between the primary stroma and the lens capsule. Although mesenchymal in morphology during their migration, these cells become transformed into a cuboidal epithelium called the **corneal endothelium** once their migration is completed. At this point the early cornea consists of (1) an outer

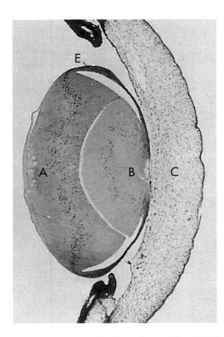

Figure 12-7 Section through the lens of an 11-day-old chick embryo. At 5 days the lens was surgically reversed so that the anterior epithelial cells (*E*) faced the vitreous body and retina. The formerly low epithelial cells elongated to form new lens fibers (*A*). Because of the reversal of the polarity of the equatorial zone of the lens, new epithelial cells were added over the original mass of lens fibers (*B*) onto the corneal face of the reversed lens. *C*, Cornea. (From DeHaan RL, Ursprung H, eds: *Organogenesis*, New York, 1965, Holt, Rinehart, Winston.)

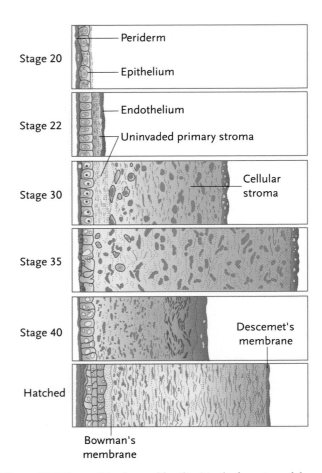

Figure 12-8 Stages (Hamburger-Hamilton) in the formation of the cornea in the chick embryo. (Based on studies by Hay ED, Revel JP: *Monogr Devel Biol* 1:1-144, 1969.)

epithelium, (2) a still acellular primary stroma, and (3) an inner endothelium.

After the corneal endothelium has formed a continuous layer, its cells synthesize large amounts of **hyaluronic acid** and secrete it into the primary stroma. Because of its pronounced water-binding capacities, hyaluronic acid causes the primary stroma to swell greatly. This provides a proper substrate for the second wave of cellular migration into the developing cornea (Figure 12-9). These cells, also of neural crest origin, are fibroblastic in nature. They migrate and proliferate in the hyaluronate-rich spaces between layers of collagen in the primary corneal stroma. The migratory phase of cellular seeding of the primary corneal stroma ceases when these cells begin to produce large amounts of **hyaluronidase,** which breaks down much of the hyaluronic acid in the primary stroma. In other parts of the embryo (e.g., limb bud), there is also a close correlation between high amounts of hyaluronic acid and cellular migration and a cessation of migration with its removal. With the removal of hyaluronic acid, the cornea decreases in thickness. Once the migratory fibroblasts have settled, the primary corneal stroma is considered to have been transformed into the **secondary stroma.**

The fibroblasts of the secondary stroma contribute to its organization by secreting coarse collagen fibers to the stromal matrix. Nevertheless, prominent layers of acellular matrix continue to be secreted by both epithelial and endothelial cells of the cornea. These secretions provide the remaining layers that constitute the mature cornea. Listed from outside in, they are (1) the outer epithelium, (2) **Bowman's membrane,** (3) the secondary stroma, (4) **Descemet's membrane,** and (5) the corneal endothelium (see Figure 12-8).

The final developmental changes in the cornea involve the formation of a transparent pathway free from optical distortion, through which light can enter the eye. A major change is a great increase in transparency, from about 40% to 100% transmission of light. This is accomplished by removing much of the water from the secondary stroma. The initial removal of water occurs with the degradation of much of the water-binding hyaluronic acid. The second phase of dehydration is mediated by **thyroxine,** which is secreted into the blood by the maturing thyroid gland. Thyroxine acts on the corneal endothelium by causing it to pump sodium from the secondary stroma into the anterior

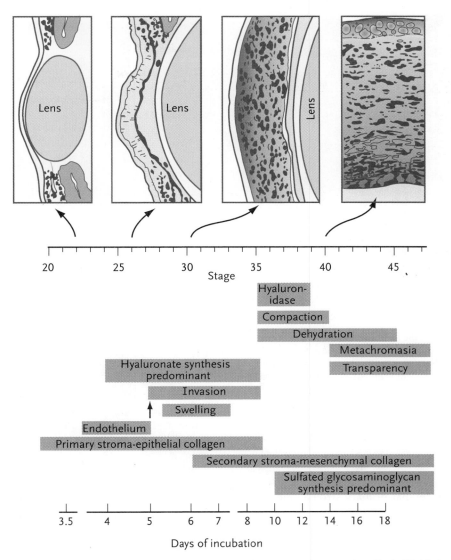

Figure 12-9 Major events in corneal morphogenesis in the chick embryo. (Based on Toole BP, Trelstad RL: *Dev Biol* 26:28-35, 1971; and on studies by Hay ED, Revel JP: *Monogr Devel Biol* 1:1-144, 1969.)

chamber of the eye. Water molecules follow the sodium ions, thus effectively completing the dehydration of the corneal stroma. The role of the thyroid gland in this process was demonstrated in two ways. When relatively mature thyroid glands were transplanted onto the extraembryonic membranes of young chick embryos, allowing thyroid hormone to gain access to the embryonic circulation via the blood vessels supplying the membrane (**chorioallantoic membrane**), premature dehydration of the cornea took place. Conversely, the application of thyroid inhibitors retarded the clearing of the cornea.

The other late event in the cornea is a pronounced change in its radius of curvature in relation to that of the eyeball as a whole. This morphogenetic change, which involves a number

of mechanical events, including intraocular fluid pressure, allows the cornea to work with the lens in bringing light rays into focus on the retina. If irregularities develop in the curvature of the cornea during its final morphogenesis, the individual develops **astigmatism**, which causes distortions in the visual image.

Retina and Other Derivatives of the Optic Cup

While the lens and cornea are taking shape, profound changes are also occurring in the optic cup (see Figure 12-1). The inner layer of the optic cup thickens, and the epithelial cells begin a long process of differentiation into neu-

rons and light receptor cells of the **neural retina**. The outer layer of the optic cup remains relatively thin and ultimately becomes transformed into the **pigment layer of the retina** (see Figure 12-5). At the same time, the outer lips of the optic cup undergo a quite different transformation into the iris and ciliary body, which are involved in controlling the amount of light that enters the eye and the curvature of the lens, respectively.

The neural retina is a multilayered structure; its embryonic development can be appreciated only after its adult organization is understood (Figure 12-10). When seen in cross section under a microscope, the neural retina consists of alternating light- and dense-staining strips that correspond to layers rich in nuclei or cell processes, respectively. The direct sensory pathway in the neural retina is a chain of three neurons that traverse the thickness of the retina. The first element of the chain is the light receptor cell, either a **rod** or a **cone**. A light ray that enters the eye passes through the entire thickness of the neural retina until it impinges on the outer segment of a rod or cone cell (photoreceptor) in the extreme outer layer of the retina. The nucleus of the stimulated rod and cone cell is located in the **outer nuclear layer**. The photoreceptor cell sends a process toward the **outer plexiform layer**, where it synapses with a process from a bipolar cell located in the **inner nuclear layer**. The other process from the bipolar neuron leads into the **internal plexiform layer** and synapses with the third neuron in the chain, the **ganglion cell**. The bodies of the ganglion cells, which are located in the **ganglion cell layer**, send out long processes that course through the innermost **nerve fiber layer** toward their exit site from the eye, the optic nerve, through which they reach the brain.

If all light signals were processed only through the simple three-link series of neurons in the retina, visual acuity would be much less than it actually is. Many levels of integration have occurred by the time a visual pattern is stored in the visual cortex of the brain. The first is in the neural retina. At synaptic sites in both the inner and outer plexiform layers of the retina, other cells such as **horizontal** and **amacrine cells** (see Figure 12-10) are involved in the horizontal redistribution of the simple visual signal. This facilitates the integration of components of a visual pattern. Another prominent cell type in the retina is the **Müller glial cell**, which sends processes to almost all layers of the retina and appears to play a role similar to that of astrocytes in the central nervous system.

Neural retina

From the original columnar epithelium of the inner sensory layer of the optic cup (see Figure 12-5), the primordium of the neural retina takes on the form of a mitotically active, thickened pseudostratified columnar epithelium organized in a manner similar to that of the early neural tube. During the

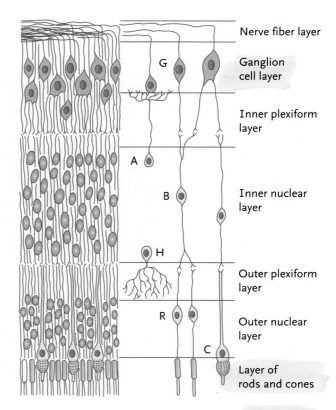

Figure 12-10 Tissue and cellular organization of the neural retina of a human fetus. *A*, Amacrine cell; *B*, bipolar cell; *C*, cone; *G*, ganglion cell; *H*, horizontal cell; *R*, rod.

early stages of development of the retina, its polarity becomes fixed according to the same axial sequence as that seen in the limbs (see Chapter 9). The nasotemporal (anteroposterior) axis is fixed first; this is followed by fixation of the dorsoventral axis. Finally, radial polarity is established.

As the number of cells in the early retina increases, the differentiation of cell types begins. There are two major gradients of differentiation in the retina. The first proceeds roughly linearly from the inner to the outer layers of the retina. The second moves horizontally from the center toward the periphery of the retina.

Differentiation in the first gradient begins with the appearance of ganglion cells and the early definition of the ganglion layer (Figure 12-11). As the ganglion cells differentiate, the surrounding cells are prevented from premature differentiation by the activity of the **Notch** gene. A major function of Notch is to maintain populations of cells in the nondifferentiated state until the appropriate local cues for their further differentiation appear. With the later differentiation of the horizontal and amacrine cells, the inner and outer nuclear layers take shape. As the cells within the nuclear layers send out processes, the inner and outer plexiform layers become better defined. The bipolar neurons and

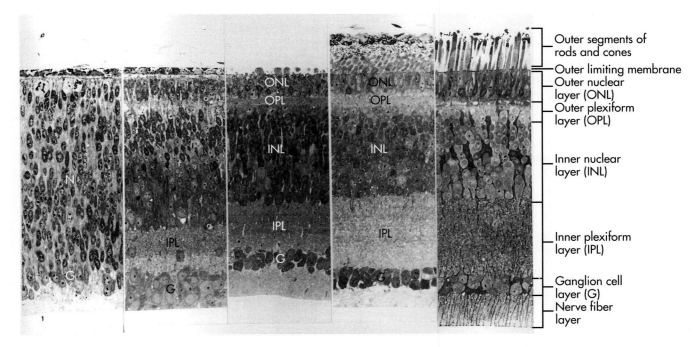

Figure 12-11 Progressive development of retinal layers in the chick embryo. At the far left, the ganglion cell layer begins to take shape from the broad neuroblast layer *(N)*. With time, further layers take shape until all layers of the retina are represented *(far right)*. (From Sheffield J, Fischman D: *Zeitschr f Zellforsch* 194:405-418, 1970.)

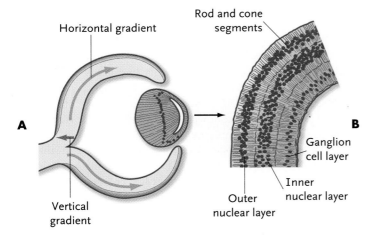

Figure 12-12 A, Horizontal and vertical gradients in the differentiation of layers of the neural retina. **B,** Segment of the embryonic neural retina showing the major cellular layers.

the rod and cone cells differentiate last, thus completing the first gradient.

The horizontal gradient of differentiation of the neural retina is based on the outward spread of the first vertical gradient from the center to the periphery of the retina (Figure 12-12). The retina cannot grow from within. Thus during the phase of growth in the human eye (or throughout life in the case of continuously growing animals such as fish),

developmentally immature retinal precursor cells along the edge of the retina undergo mitosis as an ever-expanding concentric ring on the periphery of the retina. Just inside the ring of mitosis, cellular differentiation takes place in a manner corresponding roughly to that of the vertical gradient.

Cell lineage experiments involving the use of retroviral or other tracers (such as horseradish peroxidase) introduced into neuronal precursors in the early retina have revealed two significant cellular features of retinal differentiation. First, progeny of a single labeled cell are distributed in a remarkably straight radial pattern following the vertical axis of retinal differentiation. There seems to be little lateral mixing among columns of retinal cells (Figure 12-13). The second cellular feature of retinal differentiation is that a single labeled precursor cell can give rise to more than one type of differentiated retinal cell.

A later stage in retinal differentiation is the growth of axons from the ganglion cells along the innermost layer of the retina toward the optic stalk. Once the axons reach the optic stalk, they grow into it, following cues provided by Pax-2–expressing cells, and make their way toward the visual centers of the brain. During this axonal ingrowth, the axons use various local and positional cues to make very precise connections with the brain. Much of the basic research on the development of retinal connections with the brain has been conducted on fish and amphibian embryos. In general, the lessons learned on these forms are applicable to development of the human visual system.

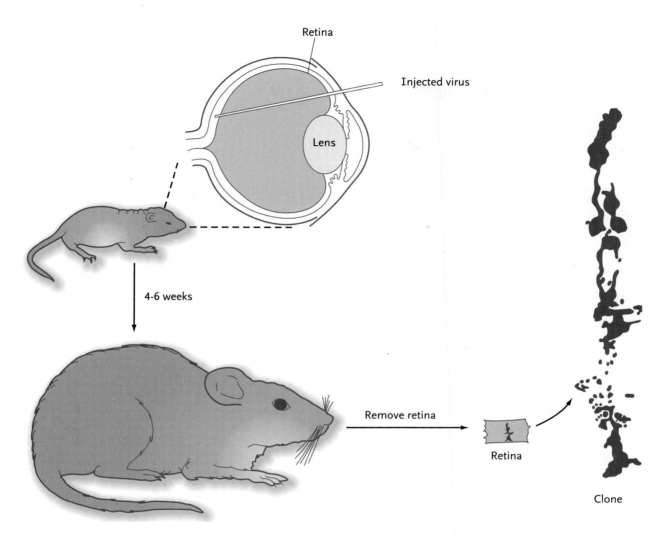

Figure 12-13 Experiment illustrating the origins and lineages of retinal cells in the rat. *Top,* Injection of a retroviral vector that includes the gene for β-galactosidase into the space between the neural and pigmented retinal layers. About 4 to 6 weeks later, the retinas were removed, fixed, and histochemically reacted for β-galactosidase activity. The drawing at the right illustrates a vertical clone of cells derived from a virally infected precursor cell. Several cell types (rods, a bipolar cell, and a Müller glial cell) constituted this clone. (Modified from Turner DL, Cepko CL: *Nature* 328:131-136, 1987.)

Iris and ciliary body

At the lip of the optic cup where the developing neural and pigment retinas meet, differentiation of the **iris** and **ciliary body** occurs. Rather than being sensory in function, these structures are involved in modulating the amount and character of light that ultimately impinges on the retina. The iris partially encircles the outer part of the lens, and through contraction or relaxation, it controls the amount of light passing through the lens. The iris contains an inner unpigmented epithelial layer and an outer pigmented layer, which are continuous with the neural and pigmented layers of the retina, respectively (Figure 12-14). The **stroma of the iris,** which is superficial to the outer pigmented layer of the iris, is of neural crest origin and secondarily migrates into the iris. Within the stroma of the iris lie the primordia of the **sphincter pupillae** and **dilator pupillae** muscles. These muscles are unusual because they are of neurectodermal origin; they seem to arise from the anterior epithelial layer of the iris.

Between the iris and neural retina lies the ciliary body, a muscle-containing structure that is connected to the lens by radial sets of fibers called the **suspensory ligament of the lens.** By contractions of the ciliary musculature acting through the suspensory ligament, the ciliary body modulates the shape of the lens in focusing light rays on the retina. Normal development of the ciliary body depends on an appropriate amount of intraocular fluid pressure. If some of the fluid of the developing eye is shunted off, a defective ciliary body results.

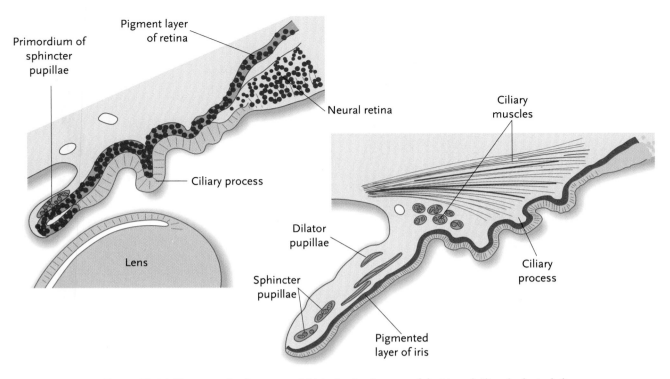

Figure 12-14 Two stages (earlier stage at left) in the development of the iris and ciliary body, including the sphincter and dilator pupillae muscles.

Eye color results from levels and distribution of pigmentation in the iris. The bluish color of the iris in most newborns is caused by the intrinsic pigmentation of the outer pigmented layer of the iris. Pigment cells also appear in the iridial stroma in front of the pigmented epithelium. The greater the density of pigment cells in this area, the browner the eye color. Definitive pigmentation of the eye gradually develops over the first 6 to 10 months of postnatal life.

Vitreous Body and Hyaloid Artery System

During early development of the retina, a loose mesenchyme invades the cavity of the optic cup and forms a loose fibrillar mesh along with a gelatinous substance that fills the space between the neural retina and lens. This material is called the **vitreous body.**

During much of embryonic development the vitreous body is supplied by the hyaloid artery and its branches (Figure 12-15). The hyaloid artery enters the eyeball through the choroid fissure of the optic stalk (see Figure 12-4), passes through the retina and vitreous body, and terminates in branches to the posterior wall of the lens. As development progresses, the portions of the hyaloid artery (as well as its branches supplying the lens) in the vitreous body regress through apoptosis of their endothelial cells, leaving a **hyaloid**

canal. The more proximal part of the hyaloid arterial system persists as the **central artery of the retina** and its branches.

Choroid Coat and Sclera

Outside the optic cup lies a layer of mesenchymal cells, largely of neural crest origin. Reacting to an inductive influence from the pigmented epithelium of the retina, these cells differentiate into structures that provide vascular and mechanical support for the eye. The innermost cells of this layer differentiate into a highly vascular tunic called the **choroid coat** (see Figure 12-5, C) and the outermost cells form a white, densely collagenous covering known as the **sclera.** The opaque sclera, which serves as a tough outer coating of the eye, is continuous with the cornea. The extraocular muscles, which provide gross movements to the eyeball, attach to the sclera.

Eyelids and Lacrimal Glands

The eyelids first become apparent during the seventh week as folds of skin that grow over the cornea (Figures 12-5 and 12-16, A). Once their formation has commenced, the eyelids rapidly grow over the eye until they meet and fuse with one another by the end of the ninth week (Figure 12-16, B). The

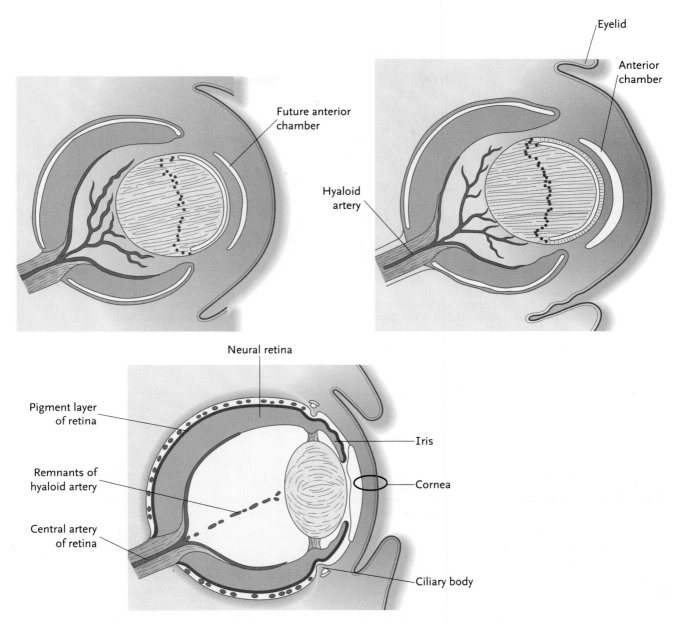

Figure 12-15 Stages in development and regression of the hyaloid artery in the embryonic eye.

temporary fusion involves only the epithelial layers of the eyelids, resulting in a persisting epithelial lamina between them. Before the eyelids reopen, eyelashes and the small glands that lie along the margins of the lids begin to differentiate from the common epithelial lamina. Although signs of loosening of the epithelial union of the lids can be seen in the sixth month, reopening of the eyelids normally does not occur until well into the seventh month of pregnancy.

The space between the front of the eyeball and the eyelids is known as the **conjunctival sac.** Multiple epithelial buds grow from the lateral surface ectoderm at about the time when the eyelids fuse. These buds differentiate into the lacrimal glands, which produce a watery secretion that bathes the outer surface of the cornea when mature. This secretion ultimately passes into the nasal chamber by way of the **nasolacrimal duct** (see Chapter 13). The lacrimal glands are not fully mature at birth, and newborns typically do not produce tears when crying. The glands begin to function in lacrimation at about 6 weeks.

Despite the many types of malformations of the eye and visual system, the incidence of most individual types of defects is uncommon. Examples of a few of the many ocular malformations are given in Clinical Correlation 12-1.

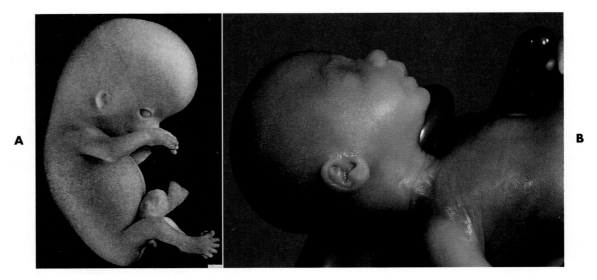

Figure 12-16 A, Head of a human embryo approximately **47 days old.** Upper and lower eyelids have begun to form. The external ear is still low set and incompletely formed. **B,** A **5½-month-old** (200 crown-rump length) human embryo. The upper and lower eyelids are fused and the external ear is better formed. Note the receding chin. (**A** From Streeter G: *Carnegie contributions to embryology*, No. 230, 165-196, 1951; **B** EH 1196 from the Pattern Embryological Collection at the University of Michigan, courtesy A. Burdi, Ann Arbor, Mich.)

CLINICAL CORRELATION 12-1
Congenital Malformations of the Eye

ANOPHTHALMOS AND MICROPHTHALMOS
Anophthalmos, the absence of an eye, is very rare and can normally be attributed to lack of formation of the optic vesicle. Since this structure acts as the inductive trigger for much of subsequent eye development, many local inductive interactions involved in the formation of eye structures fail to occur. **Microphthalmos,** which can range from an eyeball that is slightly smaller than normal to one that is almost vestigial, can be associated with genetic defects (e.g., aniridia) or various other causes, including intrauterine infections (Figure 12-17, *A*).

COLOBOMA OF THE IRIS
Nonclosure of the choroid fissure of the iris during the sixth or seventh week results in its persistence as a defect called **coloboma iridis** (Figure 12-17, *B*). The location of colobomas of the iris (typically at the 5 o'clock position in the right eye and the 7 o'clock position in the left) marks the position of the embryonic choroid fissure.

CONGENITAL CATARACT
Cataract is a condition characterized by opacity of the lens of the eye. Not so much a structural malformation as a dysplasia, congenital cataracts first came into prominence as one of the triad of defects resulting from exposure of the embryo to the rubella virus.

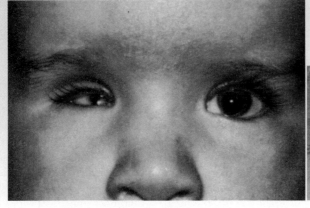

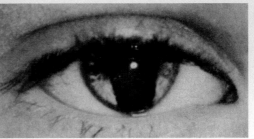

Figure 12-17 A, Microphthalmos of the right eye. **B,** Congenital coloboma of the iris. The fissure is in the region of closure of the choroid fissure. (**A** from Smith B: *Ophthalmic plastic and reconstructive surgery*, vol 2, St Louis, 1987, Mosby. **B** from Newell F: *Ophthalmology: principles and concepts*, St Louis, 1986, Mosby.)

EAR

The ear is a complex structure consisting of three major subdivisions: the external, middle, and internal ear. The **external ear** consists of the **pinna** (auricle), the **external auditory meatus** (external ear canal), and the outer layers of the **tympanic membrane** (eardrum) and functions principally as a sound-collecting apparatus. The middle ear acts as a transmitting device. This function is served by the chain of three middle ear ossicles, which connect the inner side of the tympanic membrane to the oval window of the inner ear. Other components of the middle ear are the middle ear cavity (**tympanic cavity**), the **auditory tube** (eustachian tube), the middle ear musculature, and the inner layer of the tympanic membrane. The inner ear contains the primary sensory apparatus, which is involved with both hearing and balance. These functions are served by the **cochlea** and **vestibular apparatus,** respectively.

From an embryological standpoint the ear has a dual origin. The inner ear arises from a thickened ectodermal placode at the level of the rhombencephalon. The structures of the middle and external ear are derivatives of the first and second pharyngeal arches and the intervening first pharyngeal cleft and pharyngeal pouch.

Development of the Inner Ear

Development of the ear begins with preliminary inductions of the surface ectoderm, first by the notochord (chordameso-derm) and then by the paraxial mesoderm (Figure 12-18). These inductions prepare the ectoderm for a third induction, in which the rhombencephalon induces the adjacent surface ectoderm to thicken and form the **otic placode** (Figure 12-19). Late in the fourth week, possibly under the influence of **FGF-3** secreted by the adjacent rhombencephalon, the otic placode invaginates and then separates from the surface ectoderm to form the **otic vesicle,** or **otocyst.** Even at the earliest stages of development of the otocyst, the localized expression of certain molecules presages the formation of specific morphological derivatives of the otocyst.

The otic vesicle soon begins to elongate, forming a dorsal vestibular region and a ventral cochlear region (Figure 12-20, A). The paired box gene, *Pax-2*, is heavily involved in early development of the otic vesicle. In the absence of Pax-2 function, neither the cochlea nor the spiral ganglion form. Quite early, the **endolymphatic duct** arises as a short, fingerlike projection from the dorsomedial surface of the otocyst (Figure 12-20, B). FGF-3, secreted by rhombomeres 5 and 6, appears to be necessary for normal development of the endolymphatic duct. At about 5 weeks, the appearance of two ridges in the vestibular portion of the otocyst foreshadows the formation of two of the **semicircular ducts** (Figure 12-20, C). As the ridges expand laterally, an area of programmed cell death inside the ridge converts the flangelike structures to canals by setting up a zone of resorption (Figure 12-20, C). The epithelial precursors of the semicircular canals express the homeobox-containing

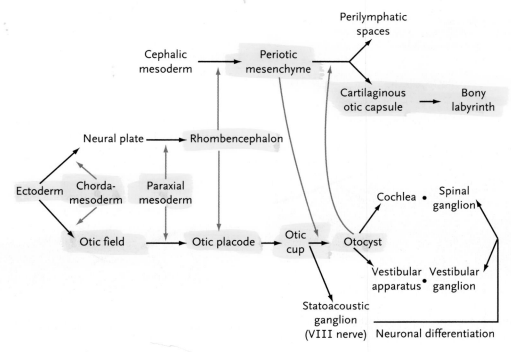

Figure 12-18 Flow chart of major inductive events and tissue transformations in the developing ear. Colored arrows refer to inductive events. (Based on McPhee JR, van de Water TR. In Jahn AF, Santos-Sacchi J, eds: *Physiology of the ear*, New York, 1988, Raven, pp 221-242.)

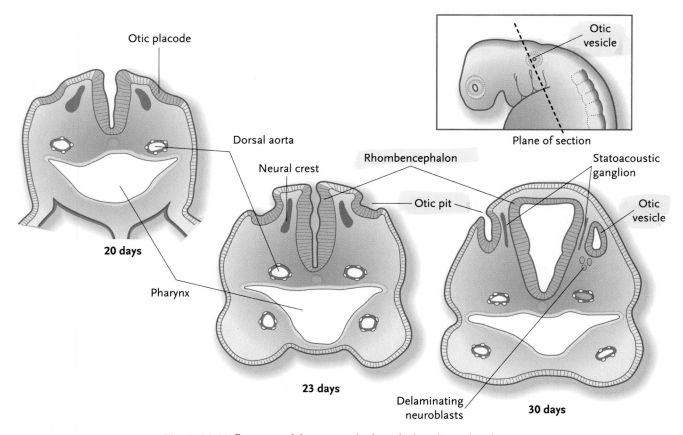

Figure 12-19 Formation of the otic vesicles from thickened otic placodes.

transcription factor genes **Nkx5-1 and Nkx5-2.** If these genes are inactivated in mice, semicircular canals fail to form. Thus the development of the two main parts of the inner ear is under separate genetic control: Pax-2 for the auditory portion (cochlea) and Nkx5 for the vestibular portion (semicircular canals). The cochlear part of the otocyst begins to elongate in a spiral, having attained one complete revolution at 8 weeks and two revolutions by 10 weeks (Figure 12-20, *C* through *F*). The last half turn of the cochlear spiral (a total of 2½ turns) is not completed until 25 weeks.

The inner ear (membranous labyrinth) is encased in a capsule of skeletal tissue that begins as a condensation of mesodermal mesenchyme around the developing otocyst at 6 weeks' gestation. The process of encasement of the otocyst begins with an induction of the surrounding mesenchyme by the epithelium of the otocyst (see Figure 12-18). This induction stimulates the mesenchymal cells, mainly of mesodermal origin, to form a cartilaginous matrix (starting at about 8 weeks). The capsular cartilage then serves as a template for the later formation of the true bony labyrinth. The conversion from the cartilaginous to the bony labyrinth occurs between 16 and 23 weeks' gestation.

The sensory neurons that make up the eighth cranial nerve (specifically the **statoacoustic ganglion**) arise from cells that

migrate out from a portion of the medial wall of the otocyst (see Figure 12-19). The cochlear part (**spiral ganglion**) of the eighth nerve fans out in close association with the sensory cells (collectively known as the **organ of Corti**) that develop within the cochlea. Neural crest cells invade the developing statoacoustic ganglion and ultimately form the satellite and supporting cells within it. The sensory cells of the organ of Corti are also derived from the epithelium of the otocyst. They undergo a very complex pattern of differentiation (Figure 12-21). The generation of sensory neuroblast precursors in the inner ear appears to use the **Notch pathway** to control the proportion of epithelial cells that differentiate into neuroblasts in a manner similar to that described for the differentiation of ganglion cells in the early retina (see p. 271). As in other sensory systems, highly regulated developmental controls ensure precise matching between sensory cells designed to receive sound waves at different frequencies or gravitational information and the neurons that transmit the signals to the brain.

Development of the Middle Ear

Formation of the middle ear is intimately associated with developmental changes in the first and second pharyngeal arches (see Chapter 13). Both the **middle ear cavity** and the

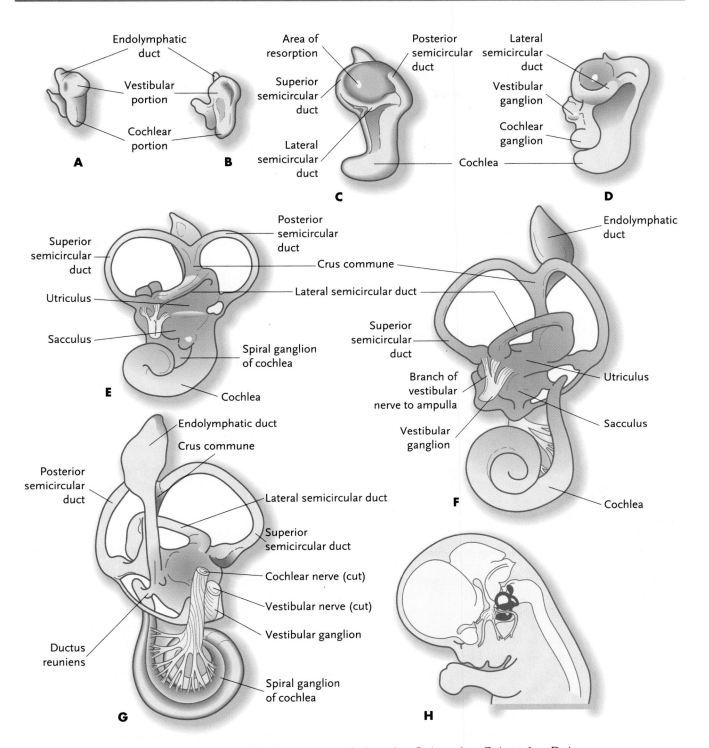

Figure 12-20 Development of the human inner ear. **A**, At **28 days**. **B**, At **33 days**. **C**, At **38 days**. **D**, At **41 days**. **E**, At **50 days**. **F**, At **56 days**, lateral view. **G**, At **56 days**, medial view. **H**, Central reference drawing at **56 days**. (From Carlson B: *Patten's foundations of embryology*, ed 6, New York, 1996, McGraw-Hill.)

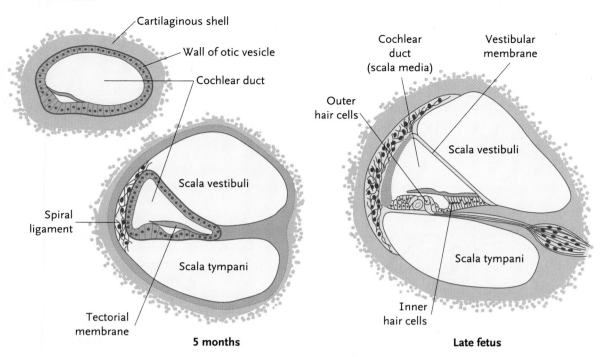

Figure 12-21 Cross sections through the developing organ of Corti.

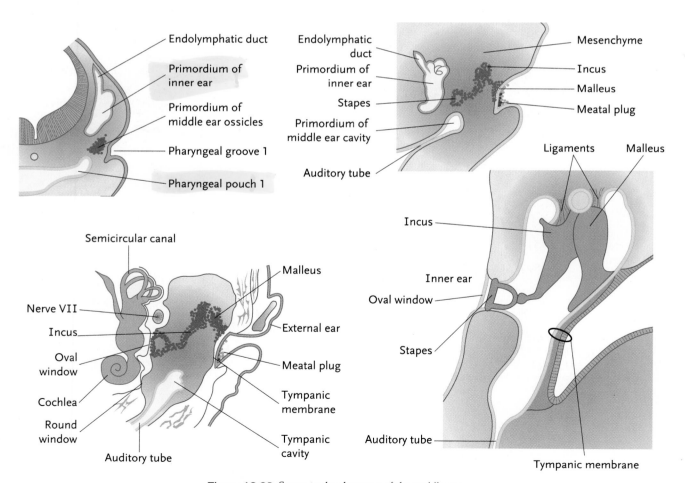

Figure 12-22 Stages in development of the middle ear.

auditory tube arise from an expansion of the first pharyngeal pouch called the **tubotympanic sulcus** (Figure 12-22). Such an origin ensures that the entire middle ear cavity and auditory tube are lined with an endodermally derived epithelium.

By the end of the second month of pregnancy, the blind end of the tubotympanic sulcus (pharyngeal pouch 1) approaches the innermost portion of the first pharyngeal cleft. Nonetheless, these two structures are still separated by a mass of mesenchyme. Later the endodermal epithelium of the tubotympanic sulcus becomes more closely apposed to the ectoderm lining the first pharyngeal cleft, but they are always separated by a thin layer of mesoderm. This complex, containing tissue from all three germ layers, becomes the **tympanic membrane** (eardrum). During fetal life, a ring-shaped bone, called the **tympanic ring,** supports the tympanic membrane. Experiments have shown that the tympanic ring is actively involved in morphogenesis of the tympanic membrane.

Just dorsal to the end of the tubotympanic sulcus, a conspicuous condensation of mesenchyme of neural crest origin appears at 6 weeks and gradually takes on the form of the middle

ear ossicles. These ossicles, which lie in a bed of very loose embryonic connective tissue, extend from the inner layer of the tympanic membrane to the oval window of the inner ear. Although the middle ear cavity is surrounded by the developing temporal bone, the future middle ear cavity remains filled with loose mesenchyme until late in pregnancy. During the eighth and ninth month, programmed cell death and other resorptive processes gradually clear the middle ear cavity, leaving the auditory ossicles suspended within it. Even at the time of birth, remains of the middle ear connective tissue may dampen the free movement of the auditory ossicles. Free movement of the auditory ossicles is acquired within 2 months after birth. Coincident with the removal of the connective tissue of the middle ear cavity is the expansion of the endodermal epithelium of the tubotympanic sulcus, which ultimately lines the entire middle ear cavity.

The middle ear ossicles themselves have a dual origin. According to comparative anatomical evidence, the **malleus** and **incus** arise from mesoderm of the first pharyngeal arch, whereas the **stapes** originates from second arch mesoderm (Figure 12-23). However, on the basis of

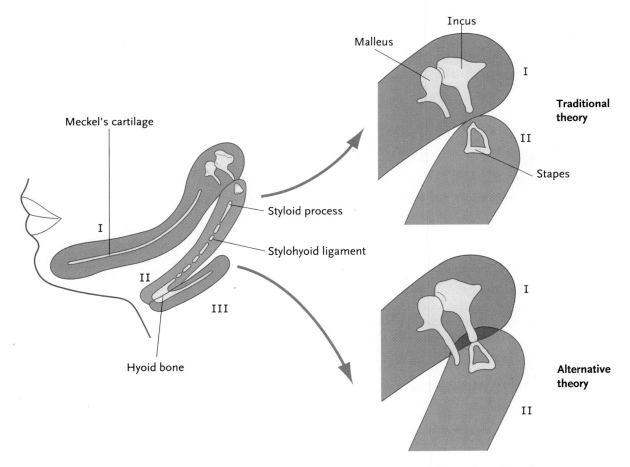

Figure 12-23 Two theories of the formation of the middle ear ossicles. According to the traditional theory, the malleus and incus are derived from arch I and the stapes from arch II. According to an alternative theory based on pathological data, parts of the malleus and incus may also arise from arch II. (After McPhee JR, van de Water TR. In Jahn AF, Santos-Sacchi J, eds: *Physiology of the ear,* New York, 1988, Raven, pp 221-242.)

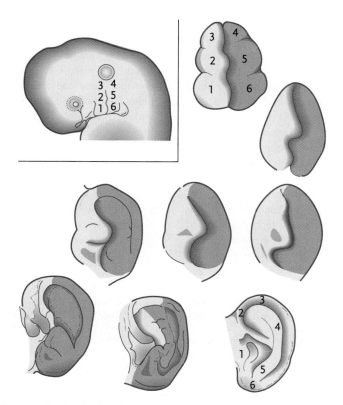

Figure 12-24 Stages in development of the external ear. Components derived from the mandibular arch (I) are unshaded; those derived from the hyoid arch (II) are shaded.

studies of certain human genetic disorders, a second hypothesis has been proposed. According to this, only the head of the malleus and the body of the incus arise from first arch mesoderm, and the remainder of these bones, plus the stapes, are of second arch origin.

Two middle ear muscles help modulate the transmission of auditory stimuli through the middle ear. The **tensor tympani muscle,** which is attached to the malleus, is derived from first arch mesoderm and is correspondingly innervated by the trigeminal nerve (V). The **stapedius muscle** is associated with the stapes, is of second arch origin, and is innervated by the facial nerve (VII), which supplies derivatives of that arch.

Development of the External Ear

The external ear (pinna) is derived from mesenchymal tissue of the first and second pharyngeal arches that flank the first (hyomandibular) pharyngeal cleft. During the second month, three nodular masses of mesenchyme (**auricular hillocks**) take shape along each side of the first pharyngeal cleft (Figure 12-24). The auricular hillocks enlarge asymmetrically and ultimately coalesce to form a recog-

nizable external ear. During its formation, the pinna shifts from the base of the neck to its normal adult location on the side of the head. Because of its intimate association with the pharyngeal arches and its complex origin, the external ear is a sensitive indicator of abnormal development in the pharyngeal region. Other anomalies of the first and second arches are often attended by misshapen or abnormally located external ears.

The external auditory meatus takes shape during the end of the second month by an inward expansion of the first pharyngeal cleft. Early in the third month the ectodermal epithelium of the forming meatus proliferates, forming a solid mass of epithelial cells called the **meatal plug** (see Figure 12-22). Late during the fetal period (at 28 weeks), a channel within the meatal plug extends the existing external auditory meatus to the level of the tympanic membrane.

The external ear and external auditory meatus are very sensitive to drugs. Exposure to agents such as streptomycin, thalidomide, and salicylates during the first trimester can cause agenesis or atresia of both of these structures. Congenital malformations of the ear are discussed in Clinical Correlation 12-2.

CLINICAL CORRELATION 12-2
Congenital Malformations of the Ear

The ear is subject to a wide variety of genetically based defects, ranging from those that affect the function of specific hair cells in the inner ear to those that produce gross malformations of the middle and external ear. Defects of the middle and external ear are often associated with genetic conditions that affect broader areas of cranial tissues or regions. Therefore many malformations involving the first or second pharyngeal arches are also accompanied by malformations of the ear and reduced acuity of hearing.

CONGENITAL DEAFNESS

Many disturbances of development of the ear can lead to hearing impairments, which affect one in every 1000 newborns. Conditions such as **rubella** can lead to maldevelopment of the organ of Corti, causing inner ear deafness. Abnormalities of the middle ear ossicles or ligaments, which can be associated with anomalies of the first and second arches, can interfere with transmission, resulting in middle ear deafness. Agenesis or major atresias of the external

ear can cause deafness by interfering with the primary collection of sound waves.

The very recent surge of molecular studies on the development of the inner ear has identified in both mice and humans a variety of mutants of the inner ear that could lead to deficits in hearing, equilibrium, or both. Such mutants, such as mutations of Pax-3 causing variants of the Waardenburg's syndrome (see p. 259), can affect development at levels from gross morphogenesis to specific cellular defects in the cochleosaccular complex.

AURICULAR ANOMALIES

Because of the multiple origins of its components, there is great variety in the normal form of the pinna. Variations include obvious malformations such as **auricular appendages**, or **sinuses** (Figure 12-25). Many malformations of the external ears are not functionally important but are associated with other developmental anomalies such as malformations of the kidneys and pharyngeal arches.

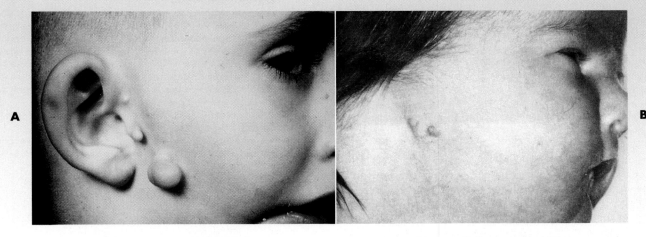

Figure 12-25 A, Auricular anomalies and tags associated with the mandibular arch (I) component of the external ear. **B**, Anotia. The external ear is represented only by a couple of small tags. (Courtesy M. Barr, Ann Arbor, Mich.)

SUMMARY

- The eye begins as an outpocketing (optic groove) of the lateral wall of the diencephalon. The optic grooves enlarge to form the optic vesicles, which induce the overlying ectoderm to form the lens primordium. The optic stalk, which connects the optic cup to the diencephalon, forms a groove containing the hyaloid artery, which supplies the developing eye. The paired box gene *Pax-6* acts as a master control gene for eye development.

- Under the influence of Pax-6, the lens forms from an ectodermal thickening that invaginates to form a lens vesicle. The cells of the inner wall of the lens vesicle elongate and synthesize lens-specific crystallin proteins. In the growing lens the inner epithelium forms a spherical mass of banana-shaped lens fibers (epithelial cells). The anterior lens epithelium consists of cuboidal

CLINICAL VIGNETTE

A pediatrician is asked to examine a young boy who has arrived from a country with poor access to medical care. The boy has low-set, misshapen ears, an underslung lower jaw, and a severe hearing deficit. The boy's teeth are also poorly aligned.

What is the common denominator for this set of conditions?

The doctor also orders an imaging study of the boy's kidneys and urinary tract. Why did she do that?

epithelial cells. The overall polarity of the lens is under the influence of the retina.

- The cornea is formed through induction of the surface ectoderm by the lens. After induction, the basal ectodermal cells secrete an extracellular matrix that serves as a substrate for the migration of neural crest cells forming the corneal endothelial layer. The corneal endothelial cells secrete large amounts of hyaluronic acid into the early cornea. This permits the migration of a second wave of neural crest cells into the cornea. These fibroblast-like cells secrete collagen fibers into the coarse corneal stroma matrix. Under the influence of thyroxine, water is removed from the corneal matrix, and it becomes transparent.

- The neural retina differentiates from the inner layer of the optic cup. The outer layer forms the pigment layer of the retina. The neural retina is a complex multilayered structure with three layers of neurons connected by cellular processes. Cellular differentiation in the neural retina follows both vertical and horizontal gradients. Cell processes grow from retinal neurons through the optic stalk to make connections with optic centers within the brain.

- The iris and ciliary body form from the outer edge of the optic cup. Sphincter and dilator pupillae muscles form within the iris. Eye color is related to the levels and distribution of pigmentation within the iris. Outside the optic cup, mesenchyme differentiates into a vascular choroid coat and a tough collagenous sclera. Eyelids begin as folds of skin that grow over the cornea and then fuse, closing off the eyes. The eyelids reopen late in the seventh month.

- The developing eyes are sensitive to a number of teratogens and intrauterine infections. Exposure to these can cause microphthalmia or congenital cataracts. Nonclosure of the choroid fissure results in coloboma.

- The inner ear arises by an induction of the surface ectoderm by the developing hindbrain. Steps in its formation include ectodermal thickening (placode), invagination to form an otic vesicle, and later, growth and morphogenesis into auditory (cochlea) and vestibular (semicircular canals) portions. Normal development of the cochlea depends on the proper expression of Pax-2, whereas Nkx5 is required for the formation of the semicircular canals.

- Development of the middle ear is associated with the first pharyngeal cleft and the arches on either side. Middle ear ossicles and associated muscles take shape within the middle ear cavity.

- The external ear arises from six modular masses of mesenchyme that take shape in the pharyngeal arch tissue surrounding the first pharyngeal cleft.

- Congenital deafness can occur after a number of intrauterine disturbances such as a rubella infection. Structural anomalies of the external ear are common.

REVIEW QUESTIONS

1. Neural crest–derived cells constitute a significant component of which tissue of the eye?
   - A. Neural retina
   - B. Lens
   - C. Optic nerve
   - D. Cornea
   - E. None of the above

2. The otic placode arises through an inductive message given off by the:
   - A. Telencephalon
   - B. Rhombencephalon
   - C. Infundibulum
   - D. Diencephalon
   - E. Mesencephalon

3. What molecule plays a role in guidance of advancing retinal axons through the optic nerve?
   - A. Pax-2
   - B. FGF-3
   - C. Bone morphogenetic protein-4
   - D. Pax-6
   - E. Bone morphogenetic protein-7

4. Surface ectoderm is induced to become corneal epithelium by an inductive event originating in the:
   - A. Optic cup
   - B. Chordamesoderm
   - C. Optic vesicle
   - D. Lens vesicle
   - E. Neural retina

5. The second pharyngeal arch contributes to the:
   - A. Cochlea, ear lobe
   - B. Auditory tube, incus
   - C. Stapes, ear lobe
   - D. Auditory tube, stapes
   - E. Otic vesicle, stapes

6. During a routine physical examination, an infant was found to have a small segment missing from the lower part of one iris. What is the diagnosis, what is the basis for the condition, and why might the infant be sensitive to bright light?

7. Why does a person sometimes get a runny nose while crying?

8. What extracellular matrix molecule is often associated with migrations of mesenchymal cells, and where does such an event occur in the developing eye?

9. Why is the hearing of a newborn often not as acute as it is a few months later?

10. Why are malformations or hypoplasia of the lower jaw commonly associated with abnormalities in the shape or position of the ears?

REFERENCES

Ahmad I, Zagouras P, Artavanis-Tsakonas S: Involvement of Notch-1 in mammalian retinal neurogenesis: association of Notch-1 activity with both immature and terminally differentiated cells, *Mech Dev* 53:73-85, 1995.

Alvarez G, Schwarz M, Gruss P: Pax-2 in the chiasm, *Cell Tissue Res* 290:197-200, 1997.

Anniko M: Embryonic development of vestibular sense organs and their innervation. In Romand R, ed: *Development of auditory and vestibular systems*, New York, 1983, Academic, pp 375-423.

Anson BJ, Hanson JS, Richany SF: Early embryology of auditory ossicles and associated structures in relation to certain anomalies observed clinically, *Ann Otol Rhinol Laryngol* 69:427-447, 1960.

Barishak YR: *Embryology of the eye and its adnexae*, Basel, Switzerland, 1992, Karger.

Carlson B: *Patten's foundations of embryology*, ed 6, New York, 1996, McGraw-Hill.

Corwin J, ed: Developmental biology of the ear, *Semin Cell Dev Biol* 8:215-284, 1997.

Coulombre AJ, Coulombre JL: The role of intraocular pressure in the development of the chick eye. III. Ciliary body, *Am J Ophthalmol* 44:85-92, 1957.

Coulombre JL, Coulombre AJ: Lens development: fiber elongation and lens orientation, *Science* 142:1489-1490, 1963.

Cvekl A, Piatigorsky J: Lens development and crystallin gene expression: many roles for Pax-6, *BioEssays* 18:621-630, 1996.

DeHaan RL, Ursprung H, eds: *Organogenesis*, New York, 1965, Holt, Rinehart, Winston.

England M: *Life before birth*, ed 2, St Louis, 1996, Mosby-Wolfe.

Fekete DM: Cell fate specification in the inner ear, *Curr Opin Neurobiol* 6:533-541, 1996.

Fekete DM and others: Involvement of programmed cell death in morphogenesis of the vertebrate inner ear, *Development* 124:2451-2461, 1997.

Fini ME, Strissel KJ, West-Mays JA: Perspectives on eye development, *Dev Genet* 20:175-185, 1997.

Fritsch B, Barald KF, Lomax MI: Early embryology of the vertebrate ear. In Rubel EW, Popper AN, Fay RR, eds: *Development of the auditory system*, New York, 1997, Springer, pp 80-145.

Graw J: Genetic aspects of embryonic eye development in vertebrates, *Dev Genet* 18:181-197, 1996.

Hadrys T and others: Nkx5-1 controls semicircular canal formation in the mouse inner ear, *Development* 125:33-39, 1998.

Hanson JR, Anson BJ, Strickland EM: Branchial sources of auditory ossicles in man, *Arch Otolaryngol* 76:200-215, 1962.

Harris WA, Holt CE: Early events in the embryogenesis of the vertebrate visual system: cellular determination and pathfinding, *Annu Rev Neurosci* 13:155-169, 1990.

Hay ED: Development of the vertebrate cornea, *Int Rev Cytol* 63:263-322, 1980.

Hyatt GA, Dowling JE: Retinoic acid: a key molecule for eye and photoreceptor development, *Invest Ophthalmol Vis Sci* 38:1471-1475, 1997.

Jakobiec FA, ed: *Ocular anatomy, embryology and teratology*, Philadelphia, 1982, Harper & Row.

Lang RA: Apoptosis in mammalian eye development: lens morphogenesis, vascular regression and immune privilege, *Cell Death Differen* 4:12-20, 1997.

Lewis WH: Experimental studies on the development of the eye in amphibia. I. On the origin of the lens, *Am J Anat* 3:505-536, 1904.

MacDonald R, Wilson SW: Pax proteins and eye development, *Curr Opin Neurobiol* 6:49-56, 1996.

Mallo M: Embryological and genetic aspects of middle ear development, *Int J Dev Biol* 42:11-22, 1998.

Mann I: *The development of the human eye*, ed 3, New York, 1964, Grune & Stratton.

McKay IJ, Lewis J, Lumsden A: The role of FGF-3 in early inner ear development: an analysis in normal and kreisler mutant mice, *Dev Biol* 174:370-378, 1996.

McPhee JR, van de Water TR: Structural and functional development of the ear. In Jahn AF, Santos-Sacchi J, eds: *Physiology of the ear*, New York, 1988, Raven, pp 221-242.

Newell F: *Ophthalmology: principles and concepts*, St Louis, 1986, Mosby.

Nishimura Y, Kumoi T: The embryologic development of the human external auditory meatus, *Acta Otolaryngol* 112:496-503, 1992.

Noden DM, van de Water TR: The developing ear: tissue origins and interactions. In Ruben RW and others, eds: *The biology of change in otolaryngology*, Amsterdam, 1986, Elsevier Science, pp 15-46.

Noden DM, van de Water TR: Genetic analysis of mammalian ear development, *Trends Neurosci* 15:235-237, 1992.

O'Rahilly R: The timing and sequence of events in the development of the human eye and ear during the embryonic period proper, *Anat Embryol* 168:87-99, 1983.

Otteson DC and others: Pax2 expression and retinal morphogenesis in the normal and Krd mouse, *Dev Biol* 193:209-224, 1998.

Piatigorsky J: Lens differentiation in vertebrates, *Differentiation* 19:134-153, 1981.

Quinn JC, West JD, Kaufman MH: Genetic background effects on dental and other craniofacial abnormalities in homozygous small eye (Pax6Sey/Pax6Sey) mice, *Anat Embryol* 196:311-321, 1997.

Rubel EW: Ontogeny of auditory system function, *Annu Rev Physiol* 46:213-229, 1984.

Smith B: *Ophthalmic plastic and reconstructive surgery*, vol 2, St Louis, 1987, Mosby.

Spemann H: *Embryonic development and induction*, New Haven, Conn, 1938, Yale University.

Stark MR and others: Neural tube–ectoderm interactions are required for trigeminal placode formation, *Development* 124:4287-4295, 1997.

Steel KP, Brown SDM: Genes and deafness, *Trends Genet* 10:428-435, 1994.

Streeter GC: Development of the auricle in the human embryo, *Contr Embryol Carnegie Inst* 14:111-138, 1922.

Toole BP, Trelstad RL: Hyaluronate production and removal during corneal development in the chick, *Dev Biol* 26:28-35, 1971.

Torres M, Gomez-Pardo E, Gruss P: Pax2 contributes to inner ear patterning and optic nerve trajectory, *Development* 122:3381-3391, 1996.

Traboulsi EI: Developmental genes and ocular malformation syndromes, *Am J Ophthalmol* 115:105-107, 1993.

van de Water TR: Determinants of neuron-sensory receptor cell interaction during development of the inner ear, *Hear Res* 22:265-277, 1986.

Wride MA: Cellular and molecular features of lens differentiation: a review of recent advances, *Differentiation* 61:77-93, 1996.

Xu P-X and others: Mouse Eya homologues of the *Drosophila* eyes absent gene require Pax6 for expression in lens and nasal placode, *Development* 124:219-231, 1997.

13

HEAD AND NECK

Among the earliest vertebrates the cranial region consisted of two principal components: (1) a **chondrocranium** associated with the brain and the major sense organs (nose, eye, ear) and (2) a **viscerocranium**, a series of branchial (pharyngeal) arches associated with the oral region and the pharynx (Figure 13-1, *A*). As vertebrates became more complex, the contributions of the neural crest to the head became much more prominent, and the face and many dermal (intramembranously formed) bones of the skull (**dermocranium**) were added. With the early evolution of the face, the most anterior of the branchial arches underwent a transformation to form the upper and lower jaws as well as two of the middle ear bones, the malleus and the incus. Along with an increase in complexity of the face (Figure 13-1, *B*) came a corresponding increase in complexity of the forebrain (the telencephalon and diencephalon). From both structural and molecular aspects, the rostral part of the head shows distinctly different characteristics from the pharyngeal region, as follows:

1. The pharyngeal region and hindbrain are highly segmented (see Figure 13-3), whereas segmentation is much less evident in the forebrain and rostral part of the head.
2. Structural segmentation in the pharyngeal region is associated with complex segmental patterns of gene expression (see Figure 10-10).
3. Formation of the forebrain and associated structures of the rostral part of the head depends on the actions of specific genes (e.g., *Lim-1* [see Figure 4-11], *Emx-1*, *Emx-2*, *Otx-1*, and *Otx-2*) and inductive signaling by the prechordal mesoderm.
4. Much of the connective tissue and skeleton of the rostral (phylogenetically newer) part of the head is derived from the neural crest. Neural crest cells are also prominent contributors to the ventral part of the pharyngeal region.

In previous chapters the development of certain components of the head (e.g., the nervous system, neural crest, bones of the skull) has been detailed. The first part of this chapter provides an integrated view of early craniofacial development to show how the major components are interrelated. The remainder of the chapter concentrates on the development of the face, pharynx, and pharyngeal arch system. Clinical Correlations 13-1 and 13-2 present malformations associated with the head and neck. These are located later in the chapter.

EARLY DEVELOPMENT OF THE HEAD AND NECK

Development of the head and neck begins early in embryonic life and continues until the cessation of postnatal growth in the late teens. Cephalization begins with the rapid expansion of the rostral end of the neural plate. Very early the future brain is the dominant component of the craniofacial region. Beneath the brain, the face, which does not take shape until later in embryogenesis, is represented by the **stomodeum** (Figure 13-2). In the early embryo the stomodeum is sealed off from the primitive gut by the **oropharyngeal membrane,** which breaks down by the end of the first embryonic month (see Figure 5-28). Surrounding the stomodeum are several tissue prominences that constitute the building blocks of the face (see Figure 13-5). In the rostral midline is the frontonasal prominence, which is populated by mesenchymal cells derived from forebrain and some midbrain neural crest. On either side of the frontonasal prominence, ectodermal nasal placodes develop into horseshoe-shaped structures, each consisting of a nasomedial process, also derived from forebrain neural crest, and a nasolateral process, derived from midbrain neural crest. Further caudally, the stomodeum is bounded by maxillary and mandibular processes, which are filled with neural crest–derived mesenchyme originating from the first two rhombomeres.

The future cervical region is dominated by the pharyngeal apparatus, consisting of a series of pharyngeal pouches, arches, and clefts. Many components of the face, ears, and

286

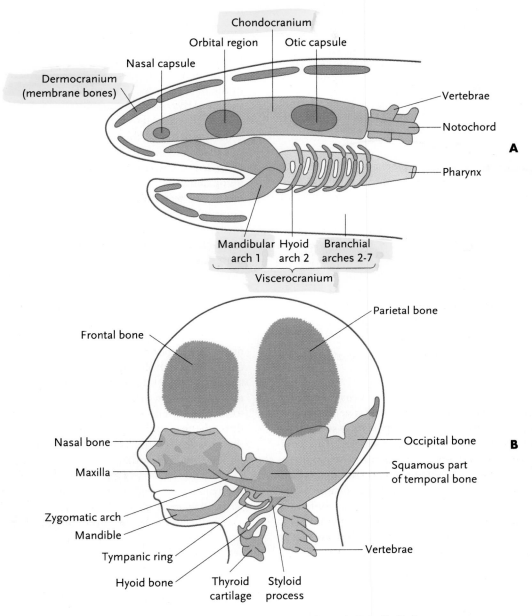

Figure 13-1 Organization of the major components of the vertebrate skull. **A,** Skull of a primitive aquatic vertebrate, showing the chondrocranium (*green*), the viscerocranium (*orange*), and the dermocranium (*brown*). **B,** Human fetal head, showing the distribution of the same components of the cranial skeleton.

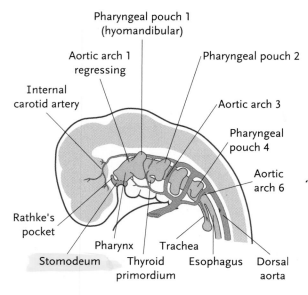

Figure 13-2 Basic organization of the pharyngeal region of the human embryo at the end of the **first month**.

glands of the head and neck arise from the pharyngeal region. Also prominent are the paired ectodermal placodes (see Figure 5-14), which form much of the sensory tissue of the cranial region.

Tissue Components and Segmentation of the Early Craniofacial Region

The early craniofacial region consists of a massive neural tube beneath which lie the notochord and a ventrally situated pharynx (see Figure 13-2). The pharynx is surrounded by a series of pharyngeal arches. Many of the tissue components of the head and neck are organized segmentally. Figure 13-3 illustrates the segmentation of the tissue components of the head. As discussed in earlier chapters, distinct patterns of expression of certain homeobox-containing genes are associated with morphological segmentation in some cranial tissues, particularly the central nervous system (see Figure 10-10). The chain of events between segmental patterns of gene expression and the appearance of morphological segmentation in parts of the cranial region remains incompletely understood.

Early Cellular Migrations and Tissue Displacements in the Craniofacial Region

Early craniofacial development is characterized by a number of massive migrations and displacements of cells and tissues. The neural crest is the first tissue to exhibit massive migratory behavior, with cells migrating from the nervous system even before closure of the cranial neural tube (see Chapter 11). Ini-

tially, segmental groups of neural crest cells are segregated, especially in the pharyngeal region (see Figure 13-3). However, these populations of cells become confluent during their migrations through the pharyngeal arches. Experiments suggest that the neural crest cells have received some morphogenetic instructions before they commence their migrations. For example, when the presumptive neural crest cells of the second and third pharyngeal arches of avian embryos were replaced with first arch neural crest cells, a duplicate set of first arch structures (essentially the entire lower jaw apparatus) was formed at a level caudal to that of the normal lower jaw of the host embryo.

The early cranial mesoderm consists mainly of the **paraxial** and **prechordal mesoderm** (see Figure 13-3). Mesenchymal cells originating in the paraxial mesoderm form the connective tissue and skeletal elements of the caudal part of the cranium and the dorsal part of the neck. Somitomere-derived myogenic cells from paraxial mesoderm undergo extensive migrations to form the bulk of the muscles of the cranial region. Like their counterparts in the trunk and limbs, these myogenic cells integrate with local connective tissue to form muscles. Another similarity with the trunk musculature is that morphogenetic control appears to reside within the connective tissue elements of the muscles rather than in the myogenic cells themselves. In the face and ventral pharynx, this connective tissue is of neural crest origin.

The prechordal mesoderm, which emits important forebrain inductive signals in the early embryo, is a transient mass of cells located in the midline, rostral to the tip of the notochord. Although the fate of these cells is controversial, some investigators feel that the myoblasts contributing to the extraocular muscles take origin from these cells. On their way to the eye, cells of the prechordal mesoderm may pass through the rostralmost somites. Other investigators feel that the extraocular muscles have a purely somitomeric origin.

The **lateral mesoderm** is not well defined in the cranial region. Transplantation experiments have shown that it gives rise to endothelial and smooth muscle cells and at least in birds, to some portions of the laryngeal cartilages.

Another set of tissue displacements of importance in the cranial region is the joining of cells derived from the ectodermal placodes with those of the neural crest to form parts of sense organs and ganglia of certain cranial nerves (see Figure 5-14).

FUNDAMENTAL ORGANIZATION OF THE PHARYNGEAL REGION

Because many components of the face are derived from the pharyngeal region, an understanding of the basic organization of this region is important. In the 1-month-old embryo the pharyngeal part of the foregut contains four lateral pairs of endodermally lined outpocketings called **pharyngeal**

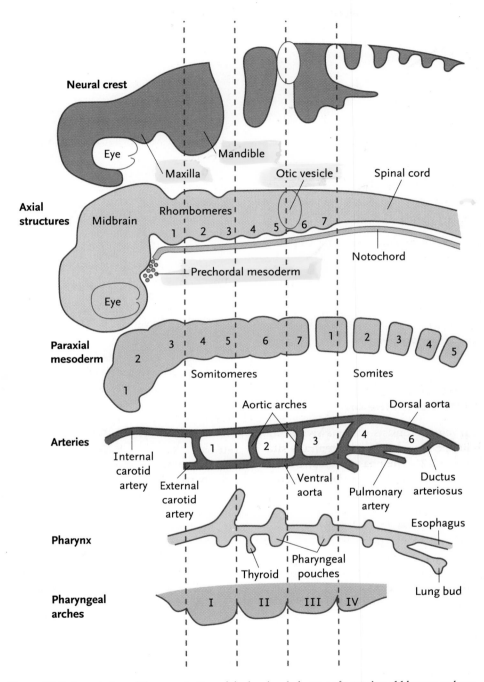

Figure 13-3 Lateral view of the organization of the head and pharynx of a **30-day-old** human embryo, with individual tissue components separated but in register through the dashed lines. (Based on Noden DM: *Brain Behav Evol* 38:190-225, 1991.)

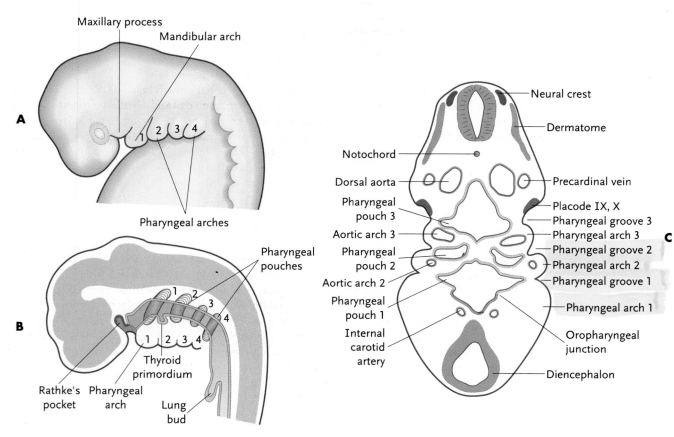

Figure 13-4 A and B, Superficial and sagittal views of the head and pharynx of a human embryo during the **fifth week**. C, Cross section through the pharyngeal region of a human embryo of the same age. Because of the strong C curvature of the head and neck of the embryo, a single section passes through the levels of both the forebrain (*bottom*) and hindbrain (*top*).

pouches and an unpaired ventral midline diverticulum, the **thyroid primordium** (Figure 13-4). If the contours of the ectodermal covering over the pharyngeal region are followed, bilateral pairs of inpocketings called **pharyngeal grooves** that almost make contact with the lateralmost extent of the pharyngeal pouches are seen (Figure 13-4, C).

Alternating with the pharyngeal grooves and pouches are paired masses of mesenchyme called **pharyngeal (branchial) arches.** Central to each pharyngeal arch is a prominent artery called an **aortic arch,** which extends from the ventral to the dorsal aorta (see Chapter 16 and Figure 13-2). The mesenchyme of the pharyngeal arches is of dual origin. The mesenchyme of the incipient musculature originates from mesoderm, specifically the somitomeres. Much of the remaining pharyngeal arch mesenchyme, especially that of the ventral part, is derived from the neural crest, whereas mesoderm makes varying contributions to the dorsal pharyngeal arch mesenchyme. The early formation of the pharyngeal arches is closely associated with the spread of expression of products of the **Hoxb** gene family from the rhombomeres of the neural tube to the pharyngeal arch mesenchyme and ultimately the overlying ectoderm (see Figure 11-8).

DEVELOPMENT OF THE FACIAL REGION

Formation of the Face and Jaws

Structures of the face and jaws originate from several primordia that surround the stomodeal depression of the 4- to 5-week-old human embryo (Figure 13-5). These primordia consist of an unpaired **frontonasal prominence;** paired **nasomedial processes,** which are components of the horseshoe-shaped olfactory (nasal) primordia; and paired **maxillary processes** and **mandibular prominences,** both components of the first pharyngeal arches. The primordia that form the face are now recognized to have distinctly different developmental properties. According to present understanding, the neural crest cells, which constitute the bulk of the mesenchyme of these primordia, become endowed with specific morphogenetic information before they migrate into the facial primordia. The nature of this information and the way it is used remain poorly understood. The upper jaw contains neural crest cells derived from the forebrain and midbrain, whereas the lower jaw contains mesenchymal cells derived from midbrain and hindbrain (rhombomeres 1 and 2) neural crest.

As in the limb buds, outgrowth of the facial primordia depends on mesenchymal-ectodermal interactions, although the site of the interaction is not marked by an apical ectodermal thickening as it is in the limb bud. Recombination experiments in birds have shown that the mesenchyme from all three facial primordia (frontonasal mass, maxillary, and mandibular primordia) can maintain the thickened apical ectodermal ridge of the limb bud. **Sonic hedgehog** and **fibroblast growth factor (FGF),** which have recently been iden-

tified in the ectoderm at the tips of the frontonasal and maxillary processes, may act, respectively, as morphogenetic organizer and stimulus for mesenchymal outgrowth in the facial primordia. The homeobox-containing gene **Msx-1** is expressed in the rapidly proliferating mesenchyme at the tips of the facial primordia. The parallel with expression of Msx-1 in the progress zone of the limb suggests that similar mechanisms act in both outgrowing limb and facial primordia. **Retinoic acid** is also heavily involved in the early development of the face. Both the deficiency and the excess of retinoic acid cause striking facial anomalies, with an excess of retinoic acid inhibiting outgrowth of the frontonasal and nasomedial processes. Retinoic acid is known to influence the expression of 3–paralogues of the *Hox* genes, but its exact position in the sequences of gene expression involved in the control of facial development remains poorly understood.

Through differential growth between 4 and 8 weeks (see Figure 13-5), the nasomedial and maxillary processes become relatively more prominent and ultimately fuse to form the upper lip and jaw (Figure 13-6). As this is occurring, the frontonasal prominence, which was a prominent tissue bordering the stomodeal area in the 4- and 5-week-old embryo, is displaced without contributing significantly to the upper jaw as the two nasomedial processes merge. The merged nasomedial processes form the **intermaxillary segment,** which is a precursor for (1) the **philtrum** of the lip, (2) the **premaxillary component** of the upper jaw, and (3) the **primary palate.**

Between the maxillary process and the nasal primordium (nasolateral process) is a **nasolacrimal groove** (nasooptic furrow) that extends to the developing eye (see Figure 13-5). The ectoderm of the floor of the nasolacrimal groove thickens to form a solid epithelial cord, which detaches from the groove. The epithelial cord then undergoes canalization and forms the **nasolacrimal duct** and near the eye, the **lacrimal sac.** The nasolacrimal duct extends from the medial corner of the eye to the nasal cavity (inferior meatus) and in postnatal life acts as a drain for lacrimal fluid. This connection explains why people can get a runny nose when crying. Meanwhile, the expanding nasomedial process fuses with the maxillary process, and over the region of the nasolacrimal groove, the nasolateral process merges with the superficial region of the maxillary process. The region of fusion of the nasomedial and maxillary processes is marked by an epithelial seam, called the **nasal fin.** Mesenchyme soon penetrates the nasal fin, resulting in a continuous union between the nasomedial and maxillary processes.

The lower jaw is formed in a simpler manner. The bilateral mandibular prominences enlarge, and their medial components merge in the midline, forming the point of the lower jaw. The midline dimple that is seen in the lower jaw of some individuals is a reflection of variation in the degree of merging of the mandibular prominences. A prominent cartilaginous rod called **Meckel's cartilage** differentiates within the lower jaw (see Figure 13-22, *D*). Derived from neural

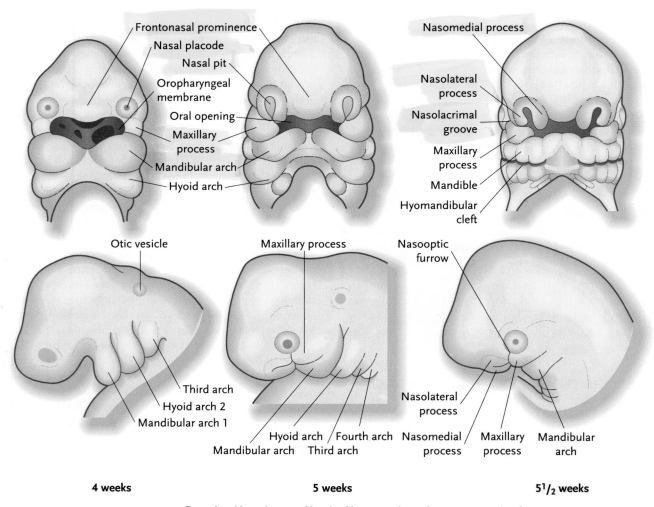

Figure 13-5 Frontal and lateral views of heads of human embryos from **4** to **8 weeks** of age.

crest cells of the first pharyngeal arch, Meckel's cartilage forms the basis around which the membrane bones (which form the definitive skeleton of the lower jaw) are laid down. Experimental evidence indicates that the rodlike shape of Meckel's cartilage is related to the inhibition of further chondrogenesis by the surrounding ectoderm. If the ectoderm is removed around Meckel's cartilage, large masses of cartilage form instead of a rod. These properties are similar to the inhibitory interactions between ectoderm and chondrogenesis in the limb bud.

Shortly after the basic facial structures take shape, they are invaded by mesodermal cells associated with the first and second pharyngeal arches. These cells form the muscles of mastication (first arch derivatives, which are innervated by cranial nerve V) and the muscles of facial expression (second arch derivatives, which are innervated by cranial nerve VII).

Although the basic structure of the face is established between the fourth and eighth weeks, changes in the propor-

tionality of the various regions continue until well after birth. In particular, the midface remains underdeveloped during embryogenesis and even early postnatal life.

Formation of the Palate

The early embryo possesses a common oronasal cavity, but in mammals the **palate** forms between the sixth and tenth weeks to separate the oral from the nasal cavity. The palate is derived from three primordia: an unpaired **median palatine process** and a pair of **lateral palatine processes** (Figure 13-7).

The median palatine process is an ingrowth from the newly merged nasomedial processes. As it grows, the median palatine process forms a triangular bony structure called the **primary palate**. In postnatal life the skeletal component of the primary palate is referred to as the **premaxillary component of the maxilla**. The four upper incisor teeth arise from this structure (Figure 13-8).

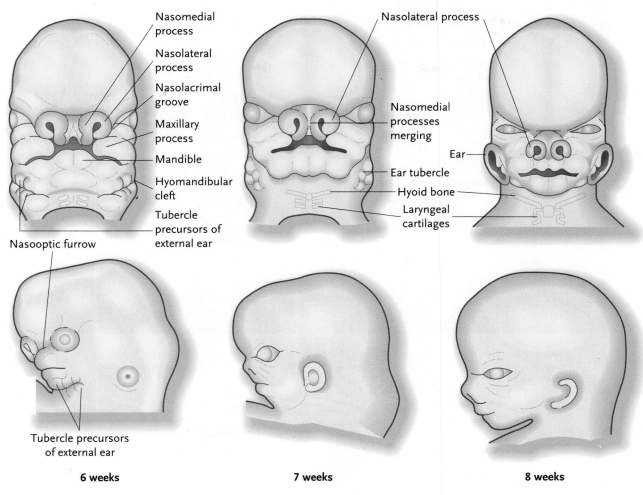

Figure 13-5—cont'd

The lateral palatine processes, which are the precursors of the **secondary palate**, first appear during the sixth week. At first they grow downward on either side of the tongue (Figure 13-9). At the apical border of the outgrowing palatal shelves, ectodermal thickenings reminiscent of the apical ectodermal ridge of the limb bud can sometimes be seen (Figure 13-10). Outgrowth of the palatal shelves appears to involve both ectodermal-mesenchymal interactions and the actions of specific growth factors, such as **epidermal growth factor** and **transforming growth factor-α** on the mesenchymal cells. During the seventh week, the lateral palatine processes (**palatal shelves**) dramatically dislodge from their positions alongside the tongue and become oriented perpendicularly to the maxillary processes. The apices of these processes meet in the midline and begin to fuse.

Despite many years of investigation, the mechanism underlying the elevation of the palatine shelves remains obscure. Swelling of the extracellular matrix of the palatal shelves appears to impart a resiliency that allows them to approximate one another within minutes or hours of their becoming dislodged from along the tongue. There is speculation that the dislodgment, which occurs during a period when the head is growing in height but not width, may be precipitated by hiccuping of the embryo. When elevation of the palatal shelves occurs, opening of the jaw, swallowing, and sucking have normally not yet occurred.

Another structure involved in formation of the palate is the **nasal septum** (see Figures 13-7 and 13-9). This midline structure, which is a downgrowth from the frontonasal prominence, reaches the level of the palatal shelves when the latter fuse to form the definitive secondary palate. Rostrally, the nasal septum is continuous with the primary palate.

At the gross level, the palatal shelves fuse in the midline, but rostrally they also join the primary palate. The midline point of the fusion of the primary palate with the two palatal shelves is marked by the **incisive foramen** (see Figure 13-8).

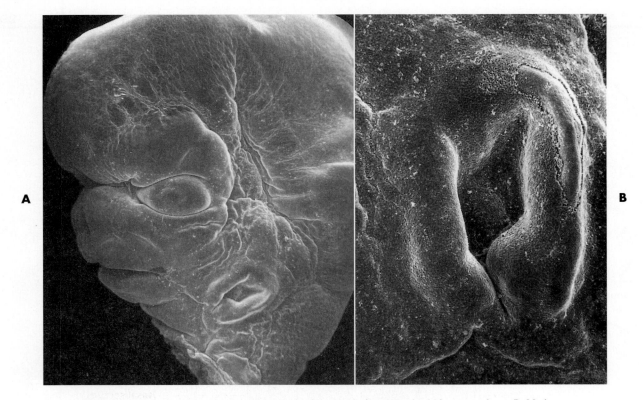

Figure 13-6 **A,** Scanning electron micrograph of the head of an **8-week-old** human embryo. **B,** Higher magnification of the ear, which is located in the neck in **A.** (From Jirásek JE: *Atlas of human prenatal morphogenesis,* Amsterdam, 1983, Martinus Nijhoff.)

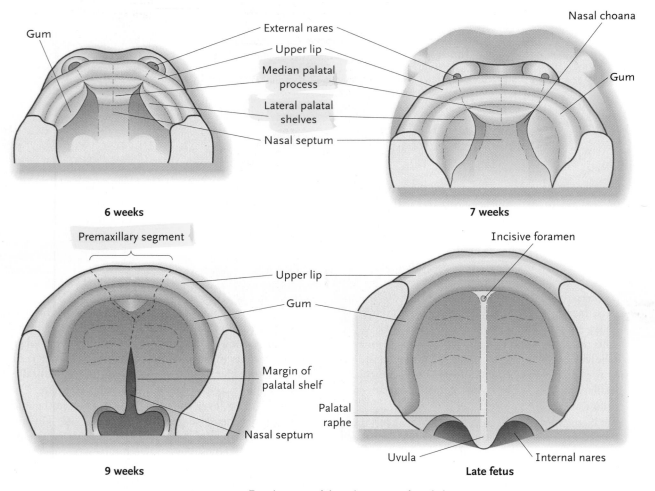

Figure 13-7 Development of the palate as seen from below.

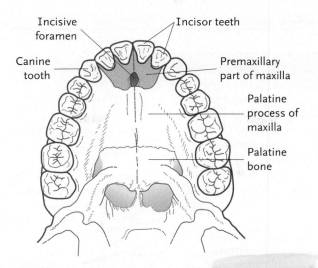

Figure 13-8 Postnatal bony palate, showing the premaxillary segment.

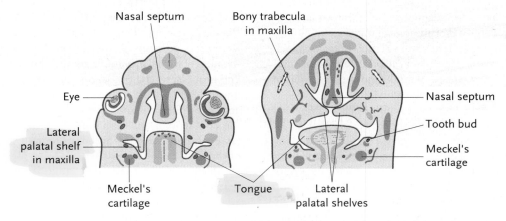

Figure 13-9 Frontal sections through the human head, showing fusion of the palatal shelves. (From Patten B: *Human embryology*, ed 3, New York, 1968, McGraw-Hill.)

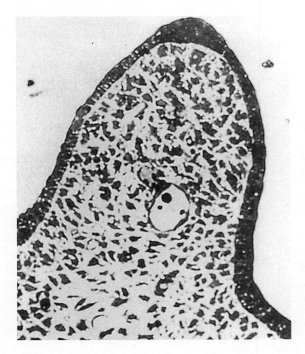

Figure 13-10 Histological section through a palatal shelf of a mouse embryo showing organization (including an apical ectodermal thickening) similar to that of a limb bud. (From Carlson B: *Patten's foundations of embryology*, ed 3, New York, 1974, McGraw-Hill.)

Because of its clinical importance, fusion of the palatal shelves has been investigated intensively. When the palatal shelves first make midline contact, each is covered throughout by a homogeneous epithelium. During the process of fusion, however, the midline epithelial seam disappears. The epithelium on the nasal surface of the palate differentiates into a ciliated columnar type, whereas the epithelium takes on a stratified squamous form on the oral surface of the palate. Significant developmental questions include the following:

1. What causes the disappearance of the midline epithelial seam?
2. What signals result in the diverse pathways of differentiation of the epithelium on either side of the palate?

The disappearance of the midline epithelial seam after the approximation of the palatal shelves involves several fundamental developmental processes (Figure 13-11). Some of the epithelial cells at the fusion seam undergo apoptosis and disappear. Others undergo a morphological transformation into mesenchymal cells through the action of growth factors, such as transforming growth factor-β. Still other epithelial cells may migrate out from the plane of fusion and become inserted into the epithelium lining the oral cavity.

Experiments involving the in vitro culture of a single palatal shelf of a number of species have shown clearly that all aspects of epithelial differentiation (cell death in the midline and different pathways of differentiation on the oral and nasal surfaces) can occur in the absence of contact with the opposite palatal shelf. These different pathways of differentiation are not intrinsic to the regional epithelia but are mediated by the underlying neural crest–derived mesenchyme. The mechanism underlying this regional specification of the epithelium remains little understood. According to one model, the underlying mesenchyme produces growth factors that influence the production and regional distribution of extracellular matrix molecules (e.g., type IX collagen). The way these events are received and interpreted by the epithelial cells is unknown.

Formation of the Nose and Olfactory Apparatus

The human olfactory apparatus first becomes visible at the end of the first month as a pair of thickened ectodermal **nasal placodes** located on the frontal aspect of the head (Figure 13-12, *A*). Like the formation of the lens placodes, the formation of the nasal placodes requires the expression of **Pax-6**. In the absence of Pax-6 expression, neither the nasal nor the lens placodes form. The nasal placodes originate from the anterolateral edge of the neural plate before its closure.

Soon after their formation, the nasal placodes form a surface depression (the **nasal pits**) surrounded by horseshoe-shaped elevations of mesenchymal tissue with the open ends facing the future mouth (see Figure 13-5). The two limbs of the mesenchymal elevations are the **nasomedial** and **nasolateral processes**. As the nasal primordia merge toward the midline during the sixth and seventh weeks, the nasomedial processes form the tip and crest of the nose along with part of the nasal septum, and the nasolateral processes form the wings (**alae**) of the nose. The frontonasal process contributes to part of the bridge of the nose.

Meanwhile, the nasal pits continue to deepen toward the oral cavity and form substantial cavities themselves (see Figure 13-12). By 6½ weeks only a thin **oronasal membrane** separates the oral from the nasal cavities. The oronasal membrane soon breaks down, making the nasal cavities continuous with the oral cavity through openings behind the primary palate called **nasal choanae**. With the fusion of the lateral palatal shelves, the nasal cavity is considerably lengthened and ultimately communicates with the upper pharynx.

During the third month, shelflike structures called **nasal conchae** form on the lateral wall of the nasal cavity. These structures increase the surface area available for conditioning the air within the nasal cavity. Late in fetal life and for several years after birth the paranasal sinuses form as outgrowths from the walls of the nasal cavities. The size and shape of these structures have a significant impact on the form of the face during its postnatal growth period.

Around midpregnancy, a pair of epithelial invaginations into each side of the nasal septum near the palate can be seen. These diverticula, known as **vomeronasal organs**, reach a maximum size of about 6 to 8 mm at around the sixth fetal month and then begin to regress completely or leave small cystic structures. In most mammals and many other vertebrates the vomeronasal organs, which are lined with a modified olfactory epithelium, remain prominent and appear to be involved in the olfaction of food in the mouth or sexual olfactory stimuli (e.g., pheromones).

The dorsalmost epithelium of the nasal pits undergoes differentiation as a highly specialized olfactory epithelium (see Figure 13-12). Beginning in the embryonic period and throughout life, the olfactory epithelium is able to form prim-

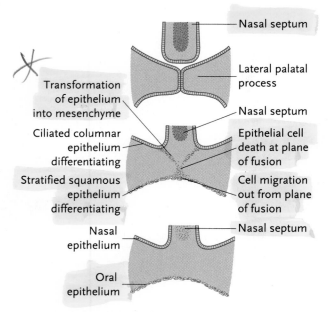

Figure 13-11 Developmental processes associated with fusion of the palatal shelves and the nasal septum.

itive sensory bipolar neurons, which send axonal projections toward the olfactory bulb of the brain. Preceding axonal ingrowth, some cells break free from this epithelium and migrate toward the brain. Some of these cells may synthesize a substrate for the ingrowth of the olfactory axons. Other cells migrating from the olfactory placode synthesize luteinizing hormone–releasing hormone and become translocated to the hypothalamus. Cells of the olfactory placode also form supporting (sustentacular) cells and glandular cells in the olfactory region of the nose. Physiological evidence demonstrates that the olfactory epithelium is capable of some function in late fetal life but that full olfactory function is not attained until after birth.

Formation of the Salivary Glands

Starting in the sixth week the **salivary glands** originate as solid, ridgelike thickenings of the oral epithelium (Figure 13-13). Extensive epithelial shifts in the oral cavity make it difficult to determine the germ layer origins of the salivary gland epithelium. The parotid glands are probably derived from ectoderm, whereas the submandibular and sublingual glands are thought to be derived from endoderm.

As with other glandular structures associated with the digestive tract, the development of salivary glands depends on a continuing series of epitheliomesenchymal interactions. The basal lamina that surrounds the early epithelial lobular ingrowths differs in composition depending on the growth potential of the region. Around the stalk and in clefts, the basal lamina contains types I and IV collagen and a basement membrane-1 (BM-1) proteoglycan. These components are not found in the regions of the lobules that undergo further growth. Under the influence of the surrounding mesenchyme, the basal lamina in growing regions loses the collagens and proteoglycans that are associated with stable structures (e.g., stalks, clefts). In addition to alterations in the basal lamina,

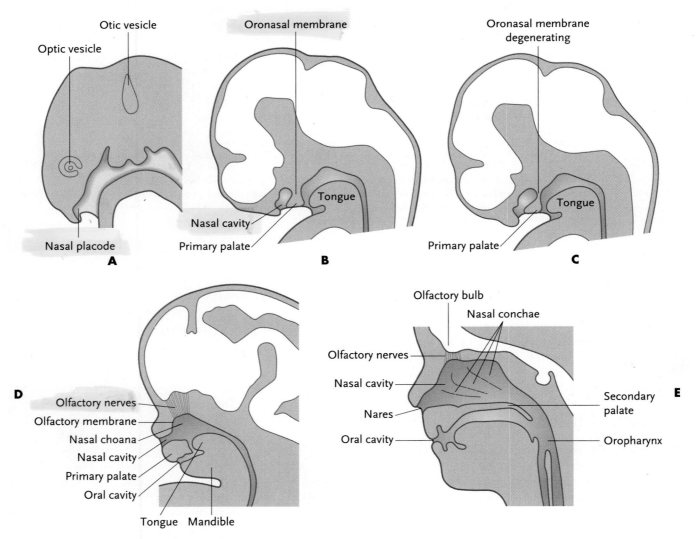

Figure 13-12 Sagittal sections through embryonic heads with special emphasis on development of the nasal chambers. A, At **5 weeks.** B, At **6 weeks.** C, At **6½ weeks.** D, At **7 weeks.** E, At **12 weeks.**

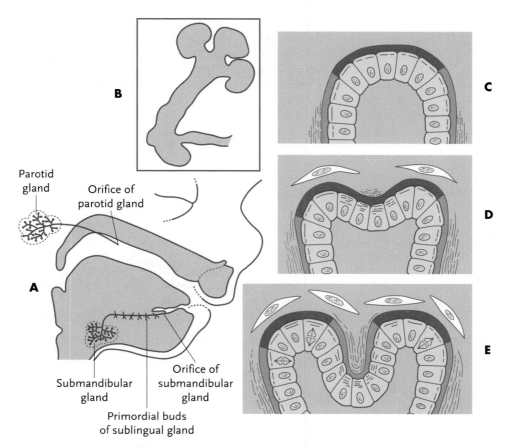

Figure 13-13 Development of the salivary glands. **A,** Salivary gland development in an **11-week-old** human embryo. **B,** Development of salivary gland epithelium in vitro. **C,** Accumulation of newly synthesized glycosaminoglycans (*dark green*) in the basal lamina at the end of a primary lobule. **D,** Early cleft formation is associated with the contraction of bundles of microfilaments in the apices of the epithelial cells lining the cleft. Collagen fibers (*wavy lines*) are lined up lateral to the lobule and in the newly forming cleft. **E,** As the cleft deepens, glycosaminoglycan synthesis is reduced in the cleft, and collagen deposition continues. (**C** through **E** show the relationship between disposition of the extracellular matrix and lobulaton of the glandular primordium.)

branching is associated with the local contraction of ordered microfilaments within the apices of epithelial cells at the branch points. Continued growth at the tips of lobules of the glands is supported by high levels of mitotic activity of the epithelium and the deposition of newly synthesized glycosaminoglycans in the area. The structural and functional differentiation of the epithelium of the salivary gland continues throughout fetal life.

Formation of the Teeth

A tooth is a highly specialized extracellular matrix consisting of two principal components—enamel and dentin—each secreted by a different embryonic epithelium. Tooth development is a highly orchestrated process involving intimate interactions between the epithelia that produce the dentin and enamel. Extending a common theme of development into the macroscopic dimension, teeth undergo an **isoform transition,**

with the postnatal replacement of the deciduous teeth by their permanent adult counterparts.

Stages of tooth development

Tooth development begins with the migration of neural crest cells into the regions of the upper and lower jaws. Some of these neural crest–derived mesenchymal cells are specified for tooth formation. They act on the overlying oral ectoderm, which thickens into C-shaped bands (**dental laminae**) in the upper and lower jaws. The appearance of the dental laminae during the sixth week is the first manifestation of a series of ectodermal-mesenchymal interactions that continues until tooth formation is virtually completed.

Although each tooth has a specific time sequence and morphology of development, certain general developmental stages are common to all teeth (Figure 13-14). As the dental lamina grows into the neural crest mesenchyme, epithelial

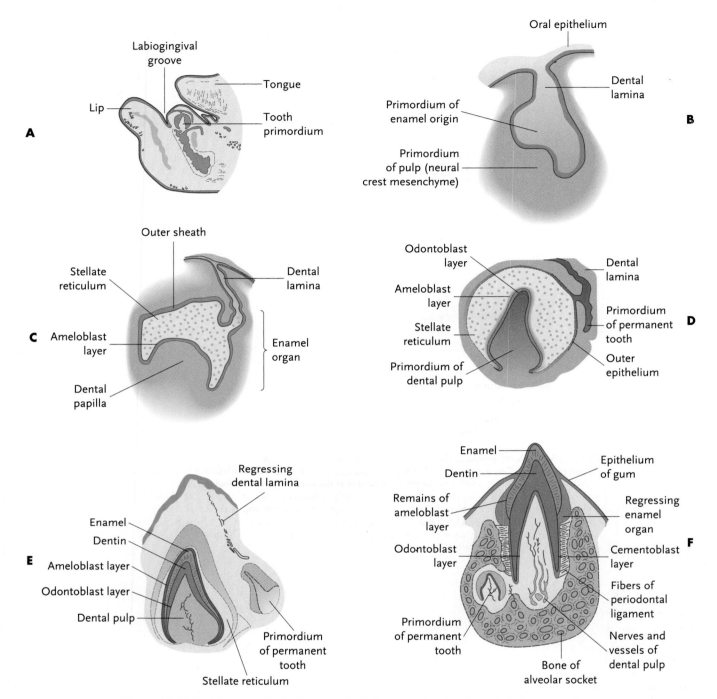

Figure 13-14 Development of a deciduous tooth. **A,** Parasagittal section through the lower jaw of a **14-week-old** human embryo showing the relative location of the tooth primordium. **B,** Tooth primordium in the bud stage in a **9-week-old** embryo. **C,** Tooth primordium at the cap stage in an **11-week-old** embryo, showing the enamel organ. **D,** Central incisor primordium at the bell stage in a **14-week-old** embryo before deposition of enamel or dentin. **E,** Unerupted incisor tooth in a term fetus. **F,** Partially erupted incisor tooth showing the primordium of a permanent tooth near one of its roots. (After Patten B: *Human embryology,* ed 3, New York, 1968, McGraw-Hill.)

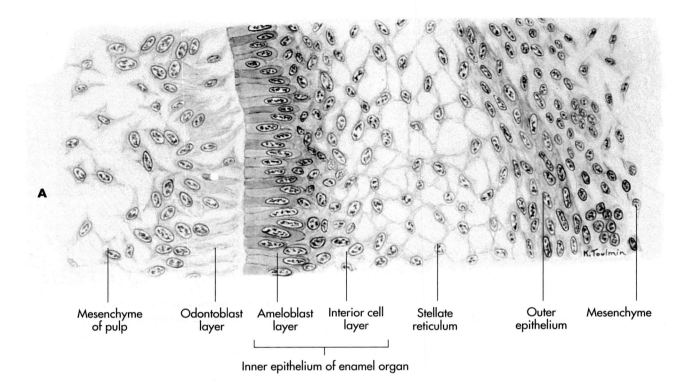

A

Mesenchyme of pulp   Odontoblast layer   Ameloblast layer   Interior cell layer   Stellate reticulum   Outer epithelium   Mesenchyme

Inner epithelium of enamel organ

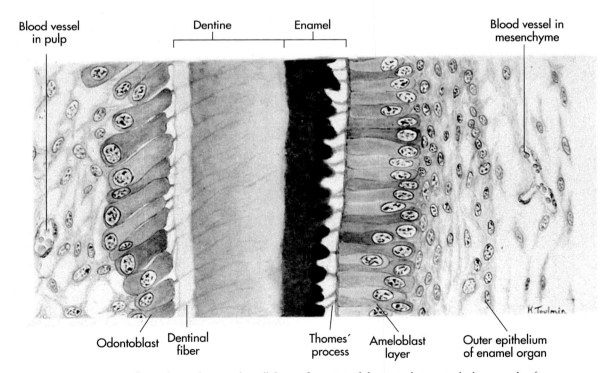

B

Blood vessel in pulp   Dentine   Enamel   Blood vessel in mesenchyme

Odontoblast   Dentinal fiber   Thomes' process   Ameloblast layer   Outer epithelium of enamel organ

Figure 13-15 Pig embryos showing the cellular configuration of the enamel organ and adjacent pulp of forming teeth before and after the beginning of deposition of enamel and dentin. **A,** Stage equivalent to a **4-month-old** human embryo. **B,** Stage equivalent to a **5-month-old** human embryo. (After Patten B: *Human embryology,* ed 3, New York, 1968, McGraw-Hill.)

primordia of the individual teeth begin to take shape as **tooth buds.** In keeping with their interactive mode of development, the tooth buds are associated with condensations of mesenchymal cells. The tooth bud soon expands, passing through a mushroom-shaped **cap stage** before entering the **bell stage.**

By the bell stage the tooth primordium already has a complex structure, even though it has not formed any components of the definitive tooth. The epithelial component, called the **enamel organ,** is still connected to the oral epithelium by an irregular stalk of dental lamina, which soon begins to degenerate. The enamel organ consists of an **outer sheath** of epithelium, a mesenchymelike **stellate reticulum,** and an inner epithelial **ameloblast layer.** Ameloblasts are the cells that begin to secrete the enamel of the tooth. Within the concave surface of the enamel organ is a condensation of neural crest mesenchyme called the **dental papilla.** Cells of the dental papilla opposite the ameloblast layer become transformed into columnar epithelial cells called **odontoblasts** (Figure 13-15). These cells secrete the dentin of the tooth. Attached to the dental lamina close to the enamel organ is a small bud of the permanent tooth (see Figure 13-14, *E* and *F*). Although delayed, it goes through the same developmental stages as the deciduous tooth.

Late in the bell stage the odontoblasts and ameloblasts begin to secrete precursors of dentin and enamel, beginning first at the future apex of the tooth. Over several months the definitive form of the tooth takes shape (see Figure 13-14). Meanwhile, a condensation of mesenchymal cells forms around the developing tooth. Cells of this structure, called the **dental sac,** produce specialized extracellular matrix components (**cementum** and the **periodontal ligament**) that provide the tooth a firm attachment to the jaw. While these events are occurring, the tooth elongates and begins to erupt through the gums (**gingiva**).

Tissue interactions in tooth development

Tissue recombination experiments have shown that the thickened ectoderm of the dental lamina initiates tooth development. The ectodermal cells express the transcription factor **Lef-1** (lymphoid enhancer factor-1), which in a still unknown manner drives the ectodermal cells to produce the signaling molecules **bone morphogenetic protein (BMP-4), FGF-8,** and **sonic hedgehog** (Figure 13-16). These ectodermal signals act on the underlying neural crest–derived mesenchyme, causing it to take part in tooth formation. Determination of the dental mesenchyme is reflected in the expression of a number of characteristic molecules, including the transcription factors **Msx-1, Msx-2,** and **Egr-1** (early growth response-1), the extracellular matrix molecules **tenascin** and **syndecan,** which promote cohesion of the mesenchymal cells; and **BMP-4.**

If the overlying ectoderm is separated from the neural crest mesenchyme, the mesenchyme does not become determined to form a tooth. The role of BMP-4 in the initial induction of the dental mesenchyme was demonstrated by adding a small bead soaked in BMP-4 to a small mass of cultured neural crest mesenchyme (Figure 13-16, *B*). Under the influence of the BMP-4 released from the bead, the mesenchyme began to express Msx-1, Msx-2, Egr-1, and BMP-4. The mesenchyme did not, however, produce tenascin or syndecan, showing that other signals in addition to BMP-4 are required to achieve the full inductive response.

With the initial induction of the dental mesenchyme, that tissue itself becomes the next prime mover in tooth development. Inductive signals emanating from the dental mesenchyme next act on the ectoderm of the dental ledge, now in the late bud to early cap stage. Recombination experiments have shown that the dental mesenchyme determines the specific form of the tooth. When molar mesenchyme is combined in vitro with incisor epithelium, a molar tooth takes shape, whereas combining incisor mesenchyme with molar epithelium results in the formation of an incisor.

Under the inductive influence of the dental mesenchyme, now called the *dental papilla,* a new signaling center, called the **enamel knot,** forms in the overlying ectoderm (see Figure 13-16). Cells of the enamel knot produce several signaling molecules, including **sonic hedgehog, FGF-4, BMP-2, BMP-4,** and **BMP-7.** These signals are transmitted laterally through the epithelium of the dental cap and also back to the mesenchyme of the dental papilla, and they appear to stimulate the proliferation and differentiation of the ameloblastic and odontoblastic epithelia. Ultimately the cells of the enamel knot undergo apoptosis, which has been postulated to be the mechanism that terminates the inductive signaling from this structure.

Formation of dentin and enamel

Late in their differentiation, odontoblasts withdraw from the cell cycle, elongate, and start secreting **predentin** from their apical surfaces, which face the enamel organ. The production of predentin signals a shift in the patterns of synthesis from type III collagen and fibronectin to type I collagen and other molecules (e.g., **dentin phosphoprotein, dentin osteocalcin**) that characterize the dentin matrix. The first dentin is laid against the inner surface of the enamel organ at the apex of the tooth (see Figure 13-15, *B*). With the secretion of additional dentin, the accumulated material pushes the odontoblastic epithelium from the odontoblast-ameloblast interface.

Terminal differentiation of the ameloblasts occurs after the odontoblasts begin to secrete predentin. In response to inductive signals from the odontoblasts, the ameloblasts withdraw from the cell cycle and begin a new pattern of synthesis, producing two classes of proteins: **amelogenins** and **enamelins.** About 5% of enamel consists of organic matrix, and amelogenins account for about 90% of this, with enamelins constituting most of the remainder. Enamelins are secreted before the amelogenins, and they may serve as nuclei for the formation of crystals of **hydroxyapatite,** the dominant inorganic component of enamel.

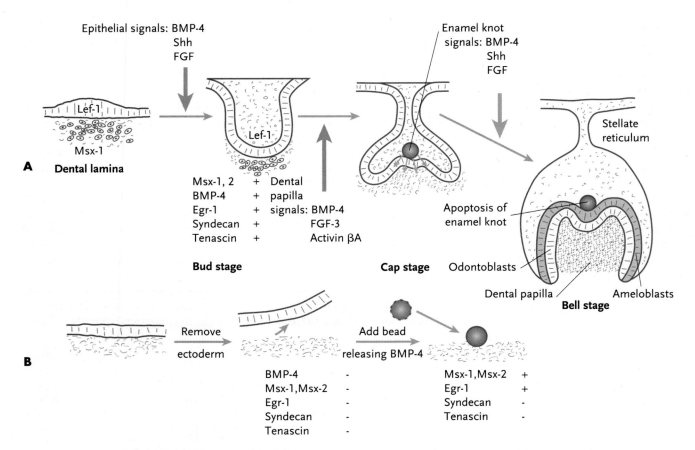

Figure 13-16 A, Inductive interactions during tooth development. Molecules associated with the green arrow represent components of the signal from dental lamina ectoderm to underlying neural crest mesenchyme; molecules associated with the violet arrow are signals from the dental papilla to the overlying ectoderm; molecules associated with the pink arrow are signals from the enamel knot to dental papilla. **B,** In vitro experiment showing that a bead releasing BMP-4 can induce dental mesenchyme to express specific markers (Msx-1, Msx-2, and Egr-1).

TABLE 13-1   Usual Times of Eruption and Shedding of Deciduous and Permanent Teeth

Teeth	Eruption	Shedding
DECIDUOUS		
Central incisors	6-8 mo	6-7 yr
Lateral incisors	7-10 mo	7-8 yr
Canines	14-18 mo	10-12 yr
First molars	12-16 mo	9-11 yr
Second molars	20-24 mo	10-12 yr
PERMANENT		
Central incisors	7-8 yr	
Lateral incisors	8-9 yr	
Canines	12-13 yr	
First premolars	10-11 yr	
Second premolars	11-12 yr	
First molars	6-7 yr	
Second molars	12-13 yr	
Third molars	15-25 yr	

The amelogenin genes are located on the X and Y chromosomes in humans. Enamel genes have been highly conserved during vertebrate phylogeny. It has been suggested that in early vertebrates, enamel once served as part of an electroreceptor apparatus.

Tooth eruption and replacement

Each tooth has a specific time of eruption and replacement (Table 13-1). With the growth of the root, the enamel-covered crown pushes through the oral epithelium. The sequence of eruption begins with the central incisor teeth, usually a few months after birth, and continues generally stepwise until the last of the deciduous molars forms at the end of the second year. A total of 20 deciduous teeth are formed.

Meanwhile, the primordium of the permanent tooth is embedded in a cavity extending into the bone on the lingual side of the alveolar socket in which the tooth is embedded (see Figure 13-14, F). As the permanent tooth develops, its increasing size causes resorption of the root of the deciduous tooth. When a sufficient amount of the root is destroyed, the deciduous tooth falls out, leaving room for the permanent tooth to take its place. The sequence of eruption of the permanent teeth is the same as that of the deciduous teeth, but an additional 12 permanent teeth (for a total of 32) are formed without deciduous counterparts.

The formation and eruption of teeth are important factors in midfacial growth, much of which occurs after birth. Tooth development and the corresponding growth of the jaw to accommodate the teeth, along with the development of the paranasal sinuses, account for much of the tissue mass of the midface.

CLINICAL CORRELATION 13-1
Malformations of the Face and Oral Region

CLEFT LIP AND PALATE

Cleft lip and cleft palate are relatively common malformations, with an incidence of approximately 1 in 1000 and 1 in 2500 births, respectively. Numerous combinations and degrees of severity exist, ranging from a unilateral cleft lip to a bilateral cleft lip associated with a fully cleft palate.

Structurally, **cleft lip** results from the lack of fusion of the maxillary and nasomedial processes. In the most complete form of the defect, the entire premaxillary segment is separated from both max-

illae, resulting in bilateral clefts that run through the lip and the upper jaw between the lateral incisors and the canine teeth (Figure 13-17). The point of convergence of the two clefts is the incisive foramen (see Figure 13-8). The premaxillary segment commonly protrudes past the normal facial contours when viewed from the side. The mechanism frequently underlying cleft lip is hypoplasia of the maxillary process, preventing contact between the maxillary and nasomedial processes from being established.

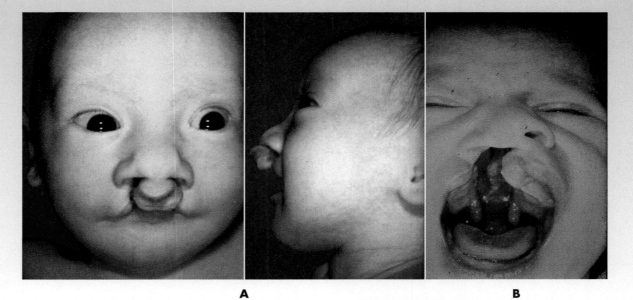

A   **B**

Figure 13-17 **A**, Front and lateral views of an infant with bilateral cleft lip and palate. On the lateral view, note how the premaxillary segment is tipped outward. **B**, Unilateral cleft lip and complete cleft palate. Note the duplicated uvula at the back of the oral cavity. (Courtesy A. Burdi, Ann Arbor, Mich.)

Continued

CLINICAL CORRELATION 13-1
Malformations of the Face and Oral Region—cont'd

Cleft palate results from incomplete or absent fusion of the palatal shelves (Figures 13-17, *B*, and 13-18). The extent of palatal clefting ranges from involvement of the entire length of the palate to something as minor as a bifid uvula. As with cleft lip, cleft palate is usually multifactorial. Some chromosomal syndromes (such as trisomy 13) are characterized by a high incidence of clefts. In other cases, cleft lip and palate can be linked to the ac-

tion of a chemical teratogen (e.g., anticonvulsant medications). Experiments on mice have shown that the incidence of cleft palate after exposure to a dose of cortisone is strongly related to the genetic background of the mouse. The higher incidence of cleft palate in females may be related to the palatal shelves in females fusing about a week later than they do in males, thus prolonging the susceptible period.

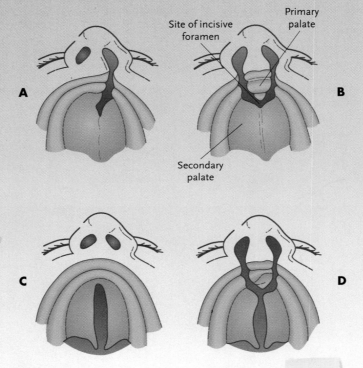

Figure 13-18 Common varieties of cleft lip and palate. **A,** Unilateral cleft passing through the lip and between the premaxilla (primary palate) and secondary palate. **B,** Bilateral cleft lip and palate similar to that seen in the patient in Figure 13-17, *A.* **C,** Midline palatal cleft. **D,** Bilateral cleft lip and palate continuous with a midline cleft of the secondary palate.

CLINICAL CORRELATION 13-1
Malformations of the Face and Oral Region—cont'd

OBLIQUE FACIAL CLEFT

This rare defect results when the nasolateral process fails to fuse with the maxillary process, usually resulting from hypoplasia of one of the tissue masses (Figure 13-19, A). It frequently manifests as an epithelially lined fissure running from the upper lip to the medial corner of the eye.

MACROSTOMIA (LATERAL FACIAL CLEFT)

An even rarer condition called **macrostomia** (Figure 13-19, B) results from hypoplasia or poor merging of the maxillary and mandibular processes. As the name implies, this condition manifests as a very large mouth on one or both sides. In severe cases the cleft can reach almost to the ears.

MEDIAN CLEFT LIP

Another rare anomaly, **median cleft lip**, results from incomplete merging of the two nasomedial processes (Figure 13-19, C).

HOLOPROSENCEPHALY

Holoprosencephaly includes a broad spectrum of defects, all based on defective formation of the forebrain (prosencephalon) and structures whose normal formation depends on influences from the forebrain. The defect arises in early pregnancy when the forebrain is taking shape, and the brain defects usually involve archencephalic structures (e.g., the olfactory system). Because of the influence of the brain on surrounding structures, primary defects of the forebrain often manifest externally as facial malformations, typically a reduction in tissue of the frontonasal process.

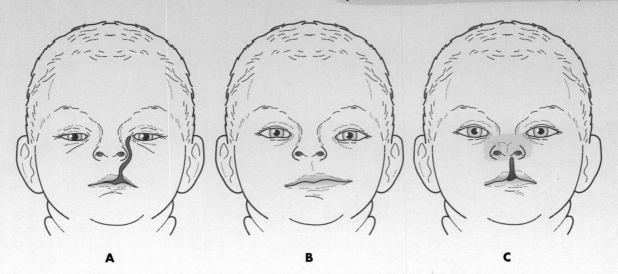

A   **B**   **C**

Figure 13-19 Varieties of facial clefts. **A,** Oblique facial cleft combined with a cleft lip. **B,** Macrostomia. **C,** Medial cleft lip with a partial nasal cleft.

Continued

CLINICAL CORRELATION 13-1
Malformations of the Face and Oral Region—cont'd

In extreme cases, holoprosencephaly can take the form of cyclopia (see Figure 7-16), in which the near absence of upper and midfacial tissue results in a convergence and fusion of the optic primordia. Reduction defects of the nose can also be components of this condition. The nose can be either absent or represented by a tubular **proboscis** (or two such structures), sometimes even located above the eye. Midline defects of the upper lip can also be attributed to holoprosencephaly (see Figure 13-19, *C*).

Some cases of holoprosencephaly (e.g., **Meckel's syndrome,** which includes midline cleft lip, olfactory bulb absence or hypoplasia, and nasal abnormalities) can be attributed to genetic causes. Meckel's syndrome is an autosomal recessive condition. Recent research has shown that several types of hereditary holoprosencephaly result from mutations of the **sonic hedgehog** gene, which normally induces the formation of a number of midline structures in the forebrain. In their absence, normally bilateral primordia, such as the optic fields, fuse, resulting in varying degrees of cyclopia. Exposure to an excess of retinoic acid, which causes misregulation of genes in the sonic hedgehog pathway, also causes holoprosencephaly in laboratory animals and possibly in humans as well. Most cases of holoprosencephaly appear to be multifactorial, although maternal consumption of alcohol during the first month of pregnancy is suspected to be a leading cause of this condition. Trisomies of chromosomes 13 and 18 are commonly associated with holoprosencephaly.

FRONTONASAL DYSPLASIA
Frontonasal dysplasia encompasses various nasal malformations that result from an excess of tissue in the frontonasal process. The spectrum of anomalies usually includes a broad nasal bridge and **hypertelorism** (an excessive distance between the eyes). In very severe cases the two external nares are separated, often by several centimeters, and a median cleft lip can also occur (Figure 13-20).

ABNORMALITIES OF THE TEETH
A wide variety of conditions affect the teeth. Some are abnormalities of pattern, which could be a reflection of abnormal morphogenetic instructions of the early neural crest or secondary to growth defects of the jaw. Abnormal morphogenesis of individual teeth is common, with frequent variations including extra or distorted roots, enamel "pearls" (small masses of enamel) along the tooth, and abnormally shaped crowns. At a different level are **amelogenesis imperfecta** and **dentinogenesis imperfecta.** These rare genetic conditions are characterized by a defect in expression of one or more matrix proteins of the enamel or dentin. Progress is being made in identifying the specific genes that are defective in these conditions. For example, a single point mutation in Msx-1 has been found in members of a family who lacked all permanent second premolars and third molars. Knockouts of many of the genes that are important in early tooth development result in deficient or absent tooth formation.

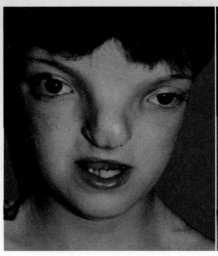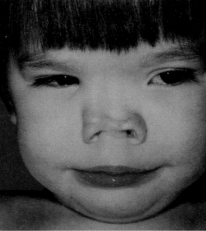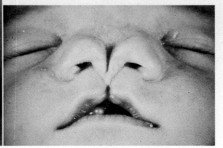

Figure 13-20 Varying degrees of frontonasal dysplasia. (Courtesy A. Burdi, Ann Arbor, Mich.)

DEVELOPMENT OF THE PHARYNX AND ITS DERIVATIVES

Considering the complexity of the structural arrangements of the embryonic pharynx, it is not surprising that a wide variety of structures originate in the pharyngeal region. This provides many opportunities for abnormal development, discussed in Clinical Correlation 13-2 at the end of this section. This section details aspects of later development that lead to the formation of specific structures. Adult derivatives of the regions of the pharynx and pharyngeal arches are summarized in Figure 13-21.

External Development of the Pharyngeal Region

Externally, the pharyngeal (branchial) region is characterized by four pharyngeal arches and grooves interposed between the arches (see Figure 13-4). These structures give rise to a diverse array of derivatives.

Pharyngeal arches

In addition to being packed with mesenchyme (mainly of neural crest origin except for the premuscle mesoderm, which migrates from the somitomeres), each pharyngeal arch is associated with a major artery (aortic arch) and a cranial nerve (see Figure 13-21). Each also contains a central rod of precartilaginous mesenchyme, which is transformed into characteristic adult skeletal derivatives. Understanding the relationship between the pharyngeal arches and their innervation and vascular supply is very important, since tissues often maintain their relationship with their original nerve as they migrate out or become displaced from their site of origin in the pharyngeal arch system.

The **first pharyngeal arch** (mandibular) contributes mainly to structures of the face (both mandibular and maxillary portions) and ear (see Figure 13-21). Its central cartilaginous rod, Meckel's cartilage, is a prominent component of the embryonic lower jaw until it is surrounded by locally formed intramembranous bone, which forms the definitive jaw. During

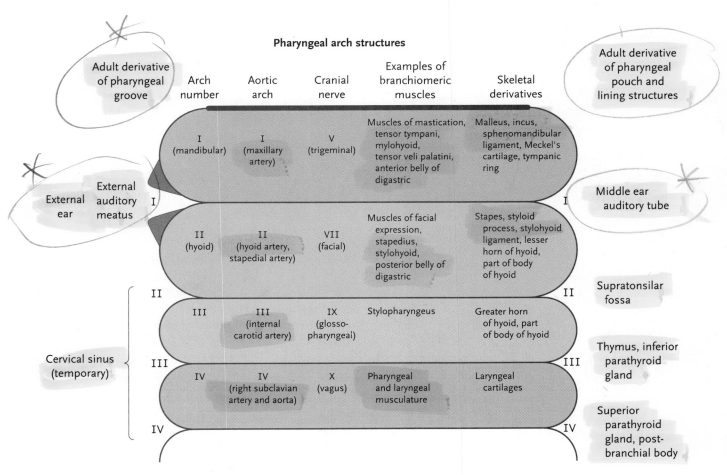

Figure 13-21 Pharyngeal derivatives.

later development the distal part of Meckel's cartilage undergoes resorption because of extensive apoptosis of the chondrocytes. More dorsally, Meckel's cartilage forms the **sphenomandibular ligament**, the **anterior ligament of the malleus**, and the **malleus** (Figure 13-22). In addition, the **incus** arises from a primordium of the **quadrate cartilage**. The first arch musculature is associated with the masticatory apparatus,

the pharynx, and the middle ear. A common feature of these muscles is their innervation by the trigeminal nerve (V).

A signaling molecule, **endothelin-1** (ET-1), plays a prominent role in the development of the first pharyngeal arch. ET-1 is expressed principally in the epithelium covering the arch, and in its absence, most structures derived from this arch fail to form properly. ET-1 may play a role in the ep-

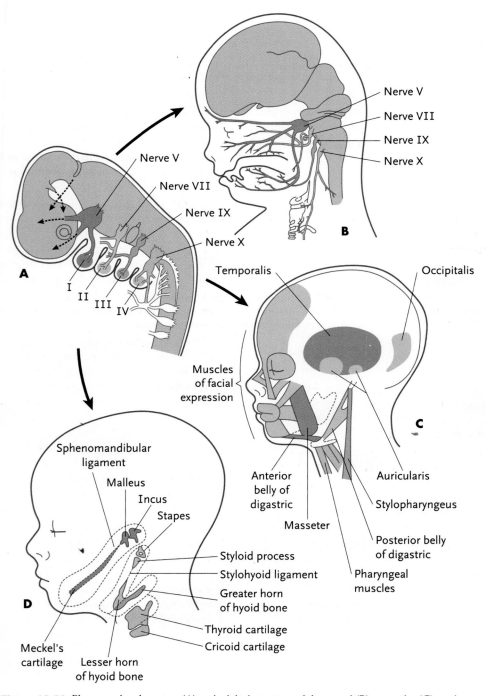

Figure 13-22 Pharyngeal arch system (**A**) and adult derivatives of the neural (**B**), muscular (**C**), and skeletal (**D**) components of the arches.

ithelial–neural crest signaling that is important in the elaboration of first arch derivatives.

The **second pharyngeal arch** (hyoid) also forms a string of skeletal structures from the body of the hyoid bone to the **stapes** of the middle ear. Although much of the second arch mesoderm migrates to the face to form the **muscles of facial expression,** additional muscles become associated with other second arch skeletal derivatives, a good example being the **stapedius muscle,** which is associated with the stapes bone. These second arch muscles are innervated by the facial nerve (VII).

Patterning of the second pharyngeal arch is strongly influenced by the homeobox gene *Hoxa-2.* When this gene is knocked out in mice, skeletal derivatives of the second arch fail to form. Interestingly, the second arch in such mutant animals contains mirror image duplicates of many of the bones of the first arch skeleton. One possible explanation for this phenomenon is that the formation of first arch structures is a default condition for the second arch, but that this is overridden by the influence of Hoxa-2.

The **third** and **fourth pharyngeal arches** are otherwise unnamed. The third arch gives rise to structures related to the hyoid bone and upper pharynx. The third arch skeleton becomes the greater horn of the hyoid bone. The one muscular derivative (stylopharyngeus) of the third arch is innervated by the glossopharyngeal nerve (IX). The fourth arch gives rise to certain muscles and cartilages of the larynx and lower pharynx. The muscles are innervated by the vagus nerve (X), which also grows into the thoracic and abdominal cavities.

Pharyngeal grooves

The first pharyngeal groove is the only one that persists as a recognizable adult structure: the **external auditory meatus.** Grooves II and III become covered by the enlarged external portion of the second arch (a phylogenetic homologue of the operculum [gill cover] of fish). The enlargement of the second arch is caused by the presence of a signaling center in the ectoderm at its tip; such a signaling center is not present in arches 3 or 4. As in the facial primordia, this signaling center produces sonic hedgehog, FGF-8, and BMP-7, which stimulate growth of the underlying mesenchyme. During the period of their overshadowing by the hyoid (second) arch, grooves II and III are collectively known as the **cervical sinus** (Figure 13-23). As development progresses, the posterior ectoderm of the second arch fuses with ectoderm of a swelling (cardiac swelling) just posterior to the fourth arch, causing the cervical sinus to disappear and the external contours of the neck become smooth.

Pharynx and pharyngeal pouches

The embryonic pharynx is directly converted to the smooth-walled pharynx of the adult. Of greater developmental interest is the fate of the pharyngeal pouches and their lining epithelium.

As with their corresponding first pharyngeal clefts, the **first pharyngeal pouches** become intimately involved in the formation of the ear. The end of each pouch expands to become the **tympanic cavity** of the middle ear, and the remainder becomes the **auditory (eustachian) tube,** which connects the middle ear with the pharynx (see Figure 12-22).

The **second pharyngeal pouches** become shallower and less conspicuous as development progresses. Late in the fetal period, patches of lymphoid tissue form aggregations in the walls to create the **palatine (faucial) tonsils.** The pouches themselves are represented only as the **supratonsillar fossae.**

The **third pharyngeal pouch** is a more complex structure, consisting of a solid, dorsal epithelial mass and a hollow, elongated ventral portion (see Figure 13-23). By the fifth week of gestation, cells identifiable as **parathyroid** tissue can be recognized in the endoderm of the solid dorsal mass. The ventral elongation of the third pouch differentiates into the epithelial portion of the **thymus gland.** The primordia of both the thymus and the parathyroid glands lose their connection with the third pharyngeal pouch and migrate caudally from their site of origin. Although the parathyroid III primordia initially comigrate with the thymic primordia, they ultimately continue to migrate toward the midline. There they join with the thyroid gland, passing the parathyroid primordia of the fourth pouch to form the **inferior parathyroid glands.** The third pharyngeal pouch disappears.

The **fourth pharyngeal pouch** is organized somewhat like the third, with a solid, bulbous, dorsal parathyroid IV primordium. It also contains a small ventral epithelial outpocketing, which contributes a minor component to the thymus in some species. In humans the thymic component of the fourth pouch is vestigial. At the ventralmost part of each fourth pouch is another structure called the **postbranchial (ultimobranchial) body** (see Figure 13-23).

Uncertainty surrounds the cellular origins and composition of the postbranchial bodies. Although according to one view the postbranchial bodies arise purely from pharyngeal endoderm, recent data suggest that neural crest cells migrate into the postbranchial bodies and ultimately become the secretory component of these structures.

As with their counterparts from the third pouch, the parathyroid IV primordia lose their connection with the fourth pouch and migrate toward the thyroid gland as the **superior parathyroid glands.** The postbranchial bodies also migrate toward the thyroid, where they become incorporated as **parafollicular** or **C cells.** The parafollicular cells, which are of neural crest origin, produce the polypeptide hormone **calcitonin,** which acts to reduce the concentration of calcium in the blood. The parathyroid glands produce **parathyroid hormone,** which causes an increase in blood calcium levels.

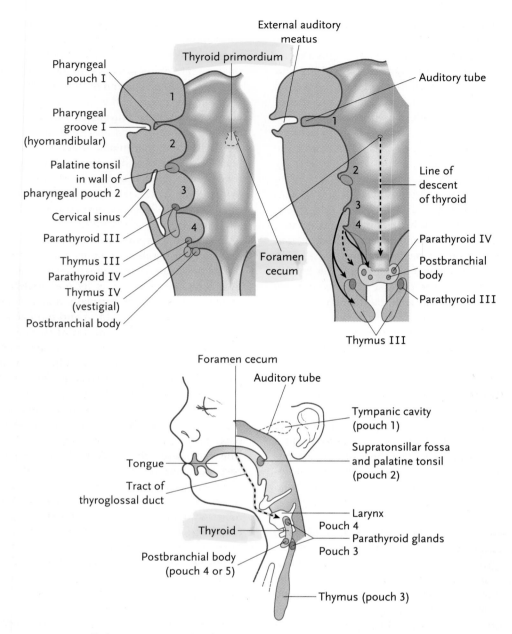

Figure 13-23 Embryonic origins and pathways of primordia of glands derived from the pharyngeal pouches and the floor of the pharynx.

Midline structures arising from the pharynx

An unpaired primordium of the **thyroid gland** appears in the ventral midline of the pharynx between the first and second pouches (see Figure 13-23). Starting during the fourth week as an endodermal thickening just caudal to the median tongue bud (tuberculum impar), the thyroid primordium soon elongates to form a prominent downgrowth called the **thyroid diverticulum.** Caudal extension of the thyroid diverticulum continues during pharyngeal development. During its caudal migration, the tip of the thyroid diverticulum expands and bifurcates to form the thyroid gland itself, which consists of two main lobes connected by an isthmus. For some time the gland remains connected to its original site of origin by a narrow **thyroglossal duct.** By about the seventh week, when the thyroid has reached its final location at the level of the second and third tracheal cartilages, the thyroglossal duct has largely regressed. Nevertheless, in almost half the population the distal portion of the thyroglossal duct persists as the **pyramidal lobe of the thyroid.** The original site of the thyroid primordium persists as the **foramen cecum,** a small blind pit at the base of the tongue.

The thyroid gland undergoes histodifferentiation and begins functioning relatively early in embryonic development. By the tenth week of gestation, follicles containing some colloid material are evident, and a few weeks thereafter the gland begins to synthesize noniodinated **thyroglobulin.** Secretion of **triiodothyronine,** one of the forms of thyroid hormone, is detectable by late in the fourth month.

Thymus and lymphoid organs

The paired endodermal thymic primordia begin to migrate from their pharyngeal pouch origins during the sixth week. Their path of migration takes them through a substrate of mesenchymal cells until they reach the area of the future mediastinum behind the sternum. By the end of their migration, the two closely apposed thymic lobes are still epithelial structures. Soon, however, they become invested with a capsule of neural crest–derived connective tissue, which also forms septa among the endodermal epithelial cords. In the absence of neural crest the thymus fails to develop. Thus an interaction between the neural crest and endodermal components of the thymic primordia conditions the latter for subsequent differentiation of thymic structure and function.

At about 9 to 10 weeks' gestation, blood-borne thymocyte precursors (**prothymocytes**), which originate in the hematopoietic tissue, begin to invade the epithelial thymus, presumably in response to the secretion of peptides by the thymus. Within the thymus the prothymocytes force apart the epithelial cells, causing them to form a spongy **epithelial reticulum.** Under the influence of the thymic epithelium the prothymocytes proliferate and redistribute, forming the cortical and medullary regions of the thymus. By 14 to 15 weeks, blood vessels grow into the thymus, and a week later, some epithelial cells aggregate into small, spherical **Hassal's corpuscles.** At this point the overall organization of the thymus is the same as that of adults. Functionally, the action of various **thymic hormones** causes the thymus to condition or instruct the prothymocytes migrating into it to become competent members of the **T lymphocyte** family. The T lymphocytes leave the thymus and populate other lymphoid organs (e.g., lymph nodes, spleen) as fully functional immune cells.

The T lymphocytes are principally involved in **cellular immune responses.** Another population of lymphocytes that also originates in the bone marrow is instructed to become **B lymphocytes,** which are the mediators of **humoral immune responses.** B lymphocyte precursors (**pro B cells**) must also undergo conditioning to become fully functional, but their conditioning does not occur in the thymus. In birds, the pro B cells pass through a cloacal lymphoid organ known as the **bursa of Fabricius,** where conditioning occurs. Humans do not possess a bursa, but its functional equivalent, although still not defined, is assumed to exist. B lymphocyte conditioning is thought to occur in the bone marrow; in early embryos, conditioning possibly occurs in the liver.

The thymus and the bursa or mammalian equivalent are commonly referred to as **central lymphoid organs.** The lymphoid structures that are seeded by B and T lymphocytes are called **peripheral lymphoid organs.** (Figure 13-24 shows the development and function of the lymphoid system.)

Formation of the tongue

The tongue begins to take shape from a series of ventral swellings in the floor of the pharynx about the same time as the palate forms in the mouth. Major shifts in the positions of tissues of the tongue occur, making the characteristics of the adult form difficult to comprehend without knowledge of the basic elements of its embryonic development.

In 5-week-old embryos the tongue is represented by a pair of **lateral lingual swellings** in the ventral regions of the first pharyngeal arches and two median unpaired swellings. The **tuberculum impar** is located between the first and second arches, and the **copula** (yoke) unites the second and third arches (Figure 13-25, *A* and *B*). The foramen cecum, which marks the original location of the thyroid primordium, serves as a convenient landmark delineating the border between the original tuberculum impar and the copula. Caudal to the copula is another swelling that represents the **epiglottis.**

Growth of the body of the tongue is accomplished by a great expansion of the lateral lingual swellings, with a minor contribution by the tuberculum impar (Figure 13-25, *C* and *D*). The root of the tongue is derived from the copula along with additional ventromedial tissue between the third and fourth pharyngeal arches.

Because of its innervation by the hypoglossal nerve (XII), the musculature of the tongue is assumed to arise from the **occipital (postotic) myotomes** and to have migrated a considerable distance into the lingual swellings, retaining its original nerve supply. The general sensory innervation of the tongue accurately reflects the pharyngeal arch origins of the epithelium. Thus the lingual epithelium over the body of the tongue is innervated by the trigeminal nerve (V) in keeping with the first arch origins of the lateral lingual swellings. Correspondingly, the root of the tongue is innervated by the glossopharyngeal nerve (IX—third arch) and vagus nerve (X—fourth arch). The epithelium of the second arch is overgrown by that of the third arch; therefore there is no general sensory innervation of the tongue by the seventh nerve.

The seventh (facial) and ninth nerves innervate the taste buds. The contribution of the seventh nerve is facilitated by its chorda tympani branch, which joins with the lingual branch of the trigeminal nerve and thus has access to the body of the tongue. Taste buds, which appear during the seventh week of gestation, result from an interaction between the lingual epithelium and special visceral afferent fibers of nerves VII and IX. Considerable evidence indicates that the fetus is able to taste, and it has been postulated that the fetus uses the taste function to monitor its intraamniotic environment.

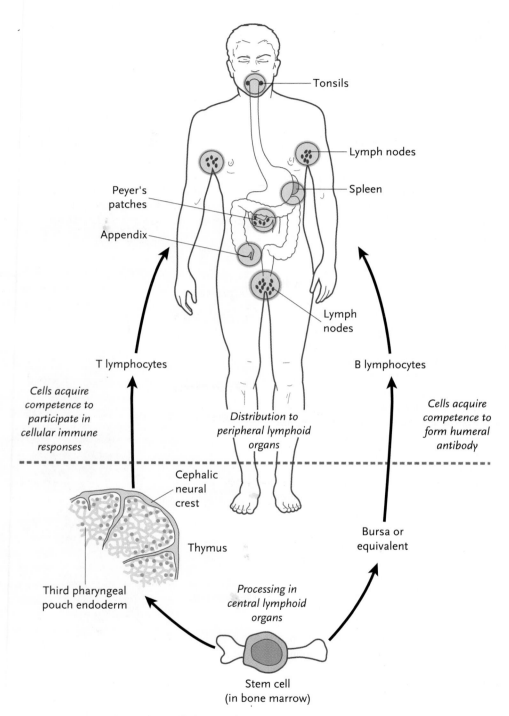

Figure 13-24 Embryonic development of the lymphoid system.

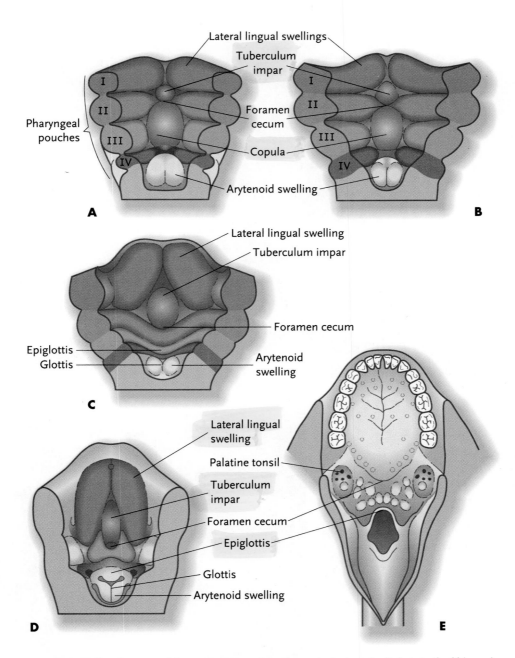

Figure 13-25 Development of the tongue as seen from above. **A,** At **4 weeks. B,** Late in the **fifth week. C,** Early in the **sixth week. D,** Middle of the **seventh week. E,** Adult.

SYNDROMES INVOLVING THE FIRST PHARYNGEAL ARCH

Several syndromes involve hypoplasia of the mandible and other structures arising from the first pharyngeal arch. However, the mechanisms underlying the hypoplasia are not clear. Certainly, a number of syndromes have a genetic basis. Whether hypoplasia of first arch–derived structures in humans is related to deficiencies of endothelin-1 function (see p. 308) remains to be determined. Hypoplasia of the lower face has also been associated with the ingestion of isotretinoin (a vitamin A derivative used for the treatment of acne) during early pregnancy.

The **Pierre Robin syndrome** involves extreme **micrognathia** (small mandible), cleft palate, and associated defects of the ear. An imbalance often exists between the size of the tongue and the very hypoplastic jaw, which can lead to respiratory distress caused by mechanical interference of the pharyngeal airway by the relatively large tongue. Although many cases of Pierre Robin syndrome are sporadic, others appear to have a genetic basis.

Treacher Collins syndrome (mandibulofacial dysostosis) is typically inherited as an autosomal dominant condition. It includes a wide variety of anomalies, not all of which are found in the same patient. Common components of the syndrome include hypoplasia of the mandible and facial bones, malformations of the external and middle ears, high or cleft palate, faulty dentition, and coloboma-type defects of the lower eyelid (Figure 13-26).

The most extreme form of first arch hypoplasia is **agnathia,** in which the lower jaw basically fails to form (Figure 13-27). In severe agnathia the external ears remain in the ventral cervical region and may even join in the ventral midline.

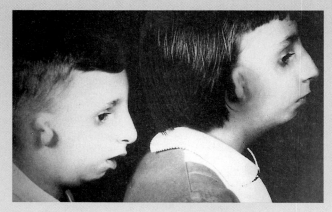

Figure 13-26 Siblings with Treacher Collins syndrome. (Courtesy A. Burdi, Ann Arbor, Mich.)

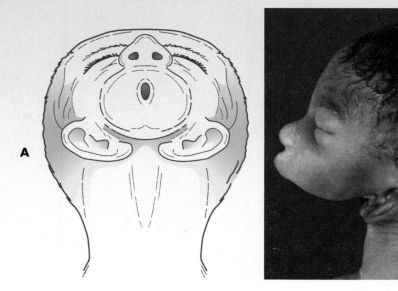

A   **B**

Figure 13-27 Agnathia. **A,** Ventral view of the upturned face of an infant. **B,** Lateral view of the face of a fetus with agnathia. Note the cervical location of the external ears. (Courtesy M. Barr, Ann Arbor, Mich.)

CLINICAL CORRELATION 13-2
Anomalies and Syndromes Involving the Pharynx and Pharyngeal Arches—cont'd

LATERAL CYSTS, SINUSES, AND FISTULAS

Structural malformations such as lateral cysts, sinuses, and fistulas can be related directly to the abnormal persistence of pharyngeal grooves, pharyngeal pouches, or both. A **cyst** is a completely enclosed, epithelially lined cavity that may be derived from the persistence of part of a pharyngeal pouch, a pharyngeal groove, or a cervical sinus. A **sinus** is closed on one end and open to the outside or to the pharynx. A **fistula** (Latin for "pipe") is an epithelially lined tube that is open at both ends—in this case to the outside and to the pharynx.

The postnatal location of these structures accurately marks the location of their embryonic precursors. External openings of fistulas are typically found anterior to the sternocleidomastoid muscle in the neck (Figure 13-28). Fistulas from remnants of pharyngeal grooves II or III may result from incomplete closure of the cervical sinus by tissue of the hyoid arch. Although present from birth, cervical cysts are often not manifested until after puberty. At that time they expand because of increased amounts of secretions by the epithelium that lines the inner surface of the cyst, corresponding to maturational changes in the normal epidermis.

Preauricular sinuses or **fistulas,** which are found in a triangular region in front of the ear, are also common. These structures are assumed to represent persistent clefts between preauricular hillocks on the first and second arches. True fistulas **(cervicoaural fistulas)** represent persisting ventral portions of the first pharyngeal groove. These extend from a pharyngeal opening to somewhere along the auditory tube or even the external auditory meatus.

THYROGLOSSAL DUCT REMNANTS

Various abnormal structures can persist along the pathway of the thyroglossal duct. **Ectopic thyroid tissue** can be found anywhere along the pathway of migration of the thyroid primordium from the foramen cecum in the tongue to the isthmus of the normal thyroid gland (Figure 13-29). This fact must be considered in the clinical diagnosis or surgical treatment of carcinomas and other conditions affecting thyroid tissue. Less common are midline cysts or sinuses involving the former thyroglossal duct (Figure 13-30). Because of their location, they can usually be easily distinguished from their lateral cervical counterparts.

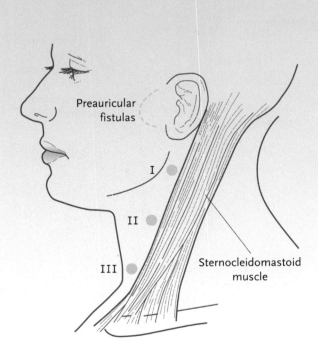

Figure 13-28 Common locations of lateral cervical (branchial) cysts and sinuses (*red circles*) and preauricular fistulas. The roman numerals refer to the cervical cleft origin of the cysts.

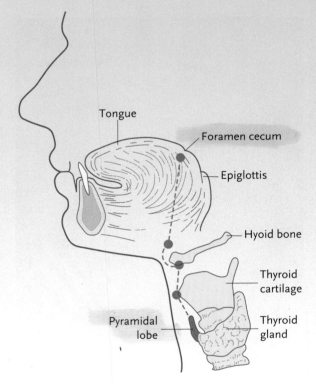

Figure 13-29 Common locations (*red circles*) of thyroglossal duct remnants.

Continued

CLINICAL CORRELATION 13-2
Anomalies and Syndromes Involving the Pharynx and Pharyngeal Arches—cont'd

MALFORMATIONS OF THE TONGUE

The most common malformation of the tongue is **ankyloglossia** (tongue-tie). This condition is caused by less-than-normal regression of the **frenulum,** the thin midline tissue that connects the ventral surface of the tongue to the floor of the mouth. Less common malformations of the tongue are **macroglossia** and **microglossia,** which are characterized by hyperplasia and hypoplasia of lingual tissue, respectively.

ECTOPIC PARATHYROID OR THYMIC TISSUE

Because of their extensive migrations during early embryogenesis, parathyroid glands and components of the thymus gland are often found in abnormal sites (Figure 13-31). Typically, this displacement is not ac-

companied by functional abnormalities, but awareness of the possibility of ectopic tissue or even supernumerary parathyroid glands is important for the surgeon.

DIGEORGE SYNDROME

DiGeorge syndrome is a cranial neural crest deficiency and is manifest by immunological defects and hypoparathyroidism (see Box 11-1). The underlying pathological condition is failure of differentiation of the thymus and parathyroid glands. Associated anomalies are malformations of first arch structures and defects of the outflow tract of the heart, which contains an important cranial neural crest contribution as well. Hoxa-3 mutant mice exhibit many of the characteristics of the human DiGeorge syndrome.

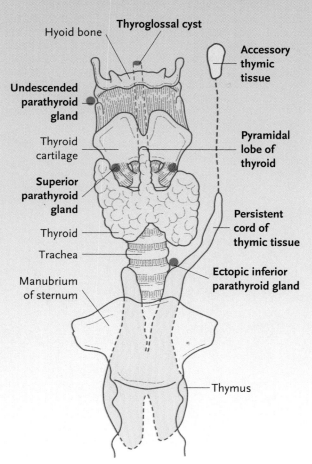

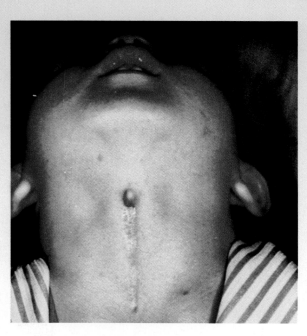

Figure 13-30 Individual with a thyroglossal duct sinus in the ventral midline of the neck. (Courtesy A. Burdi, Ann Arbor, Mich.)

Figure 13-31 Locations where abnormally positioned pharyngeal glands or portions of glands can be found.

CLINICAL VIGNETTE

A nervous-looking 23-year-old woman came to her physician complaining of feeling too hot, losing too much weight, and sweating more than she had previously. On physical examination, her skin was warm and fine in texture, she had a fine tremor of her fingers, and her eyes bulged slightly. As part of the diagnostic follow-up, she was given a dose of radioactive iodine; then scanning was performed to localize the iodine. The scans showed that most of the radioactive iodine was localized to a small mass of tissue at the base of the tongue. A neoplastic growth in the tissue mass was diagnosed, but the location of the mass was attributed to a congenital malformation.

Explain the embryological basis for the location of the neoplastic growth.

SUMMARY

- The early craniofacial region arises from the rostral portions of the neural tube, the notochord, and the pharynx, which is surrounded by a series of paired aortic arches. Between the aortic arches and the overlying ectoderm are large masses of neural crest and mesodermally derived mesenchyme. A number of these components show evidence of anatomical segmentation or segmental patterns of gene expression.

- Massive migrations of segmental groups of neural crest cells provide the mesenchyme for much of the facial region. The musculature of the craniofacial region is derived from somitomeric mesoderm or the occipital somites. The connective tissue component of the facial musculature is of neural crest origin.

- The pharyngeal (branchial) region is organized around paired mesenchymal pharyngeal arches, which alternate with endodermally lined pharyngeal pouches and ectodermally lined pharyngeal grooves.

- The face and lower jaw arise from an unpaired frontonasal prominence and paired nasomedial, maxillary, and mandibular processes. Through differential growth and fusion, the nasomedial processes form the upper jaw and lip, and the frontonasal prominence forms the upper part of the face. The expanding mandibular processes merge to form the lower jaw and lip. A nasolacrimal groove between the nasolateral and maxillary processes ultimately becomes canalized to form the nasolacrimal duct, which connects the orbit to the nasal cavity.

- The palate arises from the fusion of an unpaired median palatine process and paired lateral palatine processes. The former forms the primary palate, and the latter forms the secondary palate.

- The olfactory apparatus begins as a pair of thickened ectodermal nasal placodes. As these sink to form nasal pits, they are surrounded by horseshoe-shaped nasomedial and nasolateral processes. The former form the bridge and septum of the nose, and the nasolateral processes form the alae of the nose. The deepening nasal pits break into the oral cavity, and only later are the nasal cavities separated from the oral cavity by the palate.

- The salivary glands arise as epithelial outgrowths of the oral epithelium. Through a series of continuing interactions with the surrounding mesenchyme, the expanding glandular epithelium branches and differentiates.

- Teeth form from interactions between oral ectoderm (dental lamina) and neural crest mesenchyme. A developing tooth is first a tooth bud, which then passes through a cap and bell stage. Late in the bell stage, ectodermal cells (ameloblasts) of the epithelial enamel organ begin to form enamel, and the neural crest–derived epithelium (odontoblasts) begins to secrete dentin. Precursors of the permanent teeth form dental primordia along the more advanced primary teeth.

- Malformations of the face are relatively common. Many, such as cleft lip and cleft palate, represent the persistence of the structural arrangements that are normal for earlier embryonic stages. Others, such as holoprosencephaly and hypertelorism, result from growth disturbances in the frontonasal process. Most facial malformations appear to be multifactorial in origin, involving both genetic susceptibility and environmental causes.

- Components of the pharynx (pharyngeal grooves, pharyngeal arches, and pharyngeal pouches) give rise to a wide variety of structures. The first arch gives rise to the upper and lower jaws and associated structures. The first groove and pouch, along with associated mesenchyme from the first and second arches, form the many structures of the external and middle ear. The second, third, and fourth pharyngeal grooves become obliterated and form the outer surface of the neck, and the components of the second through fourth arches form the pharyngeal skeleton and much of the musculature and connective tissue of the pharyngeal part of the neck. The endoderm of the third and fourth pouches forms the thymus and parathyroid glands. The thyroid gland arises from an unpaired ventral endodermal outgrowth of the upper pharynx.

- The tongue originates from multiple ventral swellings in the floor of the pharynx. The bulk of the tongue comes from the paired lateral lingual swellings in the region of the first pharyngeal arches. The unpaired tuberculum impar and copula also contribute to the formation of the tongue. The tongue musculature, along with the hypoglossal nerve (cranial nerve XII), which supplies the muscles, arises from the occipital somites. General sensory innervation of the tongue (from cranial nerves V, IX, and X) corresponds with the embryological origin of the innervated part of the tongue. Cranial nerves VII and IX innervate the taste buds on the tongue.

- Many malformations of the lower face and jaw are related to hypoplasia of the first pharyngeal arches. Cysts, sinuses, and fistulas of the neck are commonly caused by abnormal persistence of pharyngeal grooves or pouches. Ectopic glandular tissue (thyroid, thymus, or parathyroid) is explained by the persistence of tissue rests along the pathway of migration of the glands. Certain syndromes (e.g., DiGeorge syndrome), which seemingly affect disparate organs, can be attributed to neural crest defects.

REVIEW QUESTIONS

1. The facial (VII) nerve supplies muscles derived from which pharyngeal arch?
    A. First
    B. Second
    C. Third
    D. Fourth
    E. Sixth

2. Cleft lip results from lack of fusion of the:
   A. Nasomedial and nasolateral processes
   B. Nasomedial and maxillary processes
   C. Nasolateral and maxillary processes
   D. Nasolateral and mandibular processes
   E. Nasomedial and mandibular processes

3. In cases of holoprosencephaly, defects of facial structures are typically secondary to defects of the:
   A. Pharynx
   B. Oral cavity
   C. Forebrain
   D. Eyes
   E. Hindbrain

4. Meckel's cartilage is a prominent structure in the early formation of the:
   A. Upper jaw
   B. Hard palate
   C. Nasal septum
   D. Soft palate
   E. Lower jaw

5. An early induction in tooth development consists of the ectoderm of the dental epithelium acting on the underlying neural crest mesenchyme. Which of the following molecules is an important mediator of the inductive stimulus?
   A. BMP-4
   B. Tenascin
   C. Hoxb-13
   D. Msx-1
   E. Syndecan

6. A 15-year-old boy with mild acne developed a tender boil along the anterior border of the sternocleidomastoid muscle. What embryological condition would be included in a differential diagnosis?

7. The physician of the 15-year-old boy determined that the boy had a congenital cyst that needed to be removed surgically. What should the surgeon consider during removal of the cyst?

8. Why does a person sometimes get a runny nose when crying?

9. A woman who took an anticonvulsant drug during the tenth week of pregnancy gave birth to an infant with bilateral cleft lip and cleft palate. She sued the physician, blaming the facial malformations on the drug, and you are called in as an expert witness for the defense. What would be the basis for your case?

10. A woman who averaged three mixed drinks a day during pregnancy gave birth to an infant who was mildly retarded and who had a small notch in an upturned upper lip and a reduced olfactory sensitivity. What is the basis for this constellation of defects?

REFERENCES

Balling R and others: Craniofacial abnormalities induced by ectopic expression of the homeobox gene *Hox-1.1* in transgenic mice, *Cell* 58:337-347, 1989.

Belloni E and others: Identification of sonic hedgehog as a candidate gene responsible for holoprosencephaly, *Nature Genet* 14:353-356, 1996.

Bockman DE, Kirby ML: Dependence of thymus development on derivatives of the neural crest, *Science* 223:498-500, 1984.

Bradley RB, Mistretta CM: Fetal sensory receptors, *Physiol Rev* 55:352-382, 1975.

Brickell P, Thorogood P: Retinoic acid and retinoic acid receptors in craniofacial development, *Semin Cell Dev Biol* 8:437-443, 1997.

Burdi AR: Sexual differences in closure of the human palatal shelves, *Cleft Palate J* 6:1-7, 1969.

Diewert VM, Wang K-Y: Recent advances in primary palate and midface morphogenesis research, *Crit Rev Oral Biol Med* 4:111-130, 1992.

Dixon MJ: Treacher Collins syndrome: an example of a craniofacial development defect, *Semin Dev Biol* 5:283-291, 1994.

Farbman AI: Developmental neurobiology of the olfactory system. In Ferguson MJ, Honig LS: Epithelial-mesenchymal interactions during vertebrate palatogenesis, *Curr Top Dev Biol* 19:137-163, 1984.

Gans C, Northcutt RG: Neural crest and the origin of vertebrates: a new head, *Science* 220:268-274, 1983.

Gendron-Maguire M and others: Hoxa-2 mutant mice exhibit homeotic transformation of skeletal elements derived from cranial neural crest, *Cell* 75:1317-1331, 1993.

Getchell TV and others, eds: *Smell and taste in health and disease*, New York, 1991, Raven, pp 19-33.

Grindley JC, Davidson DR, Hill RE: The role of Pax-6 in eye and nasal development, *Development* 121:1433-1442, 1995.

Grobstein C: Epithelio-mesenchymal specificity in the morphogenesis of mouse submandibular rudiments in vitro, *J Exp Zool* 124:383-413, 1953.

Hanken J, Hall BK, eds: *The skull*, vol 1, *Development*, Chicago, 1993, University of Chicago Press.

Helms JA and others: Sonic hedgehog participates in craniofacial morphogenesis and is down-regulated by teratogenic doses of retinoic acid, *Dev Biol* 187:25-35, 1997.

Hieda Y, Nakanishi Y: Epithelial morphogenesis in mouse embryonic submandibular gland: its relationship to the tissue organization of epithelium and mesenchyme, *Dev Growth Differentiation* 39:1-8, 1997.

Hunt P and others: Homeobox genes and models for patterning the hindbrain and branchial arches, *Development* 1(suppl):187-196, 1991.

Jirásek JE: *Atlas of human prenatal morphogenesis*, Amsterdam, 1983, Martinus Nijhoff.

Kollar EJ: Tooth development and dental patterning. In Connelly T, Brinkley L, Carlson B, eds: *Morphogenesis and pattern formation*, New York, 1981, Raven, pp 87-102.

Kumoi T, Nishimura Y, Shiota K: The embryonic development of the human anterior nasal aperture, *Acta Otolaryngol* 113:93-97, 1993.

Kuratani S, Matsuo I, Aizawa S: Developmental patterning and evolution of the mammalian viscerocranium: genetic insights into comparative morphology, *Dev Dynam* 209:139-155, 1997.

Kurihara Y and others: Elevated blood pressure and craniofacial abnormalities in mice deficient in endothelin-1, *Nature* 368:703-710, 1994.

Maas R, Bei M: The genetic control of early tooth development, *Crit Rev Oral Biol Med* 8:4-39, 1997.

Manley NR, Capecchi MR: The role of Hoxa-3 in mouse thymus and thyroid development, *Development* 121:1989-2003, 1995.

Matsuo I and others: Mouse Otx2 functions in the formation and patterning of rostral head, *Genes Dev* 9:2646-2658, 1995.

Mazzola RF: Congenital malformations in the frontonasal area: their pathogenesis and classification, *Clin Plast Surg* 3:573-609, 1976.

Mina M and others: Experimental analysis of *Msx-1* and *Msx-2* gene expression during chick mandibular morphogenesis, *Dev Dynam* 202:195-214, 1995.

Mombaerts P, ed: Development of the olfactory system, *Semin Cell Dev Biol* 8:151-213, 1997.

Muenke M: Holoprosencephaly as a genetic model for normal craniofacial development, *Semin Dev Biol* 5:293-301, 1994.

Noden DM: Cell movements and control of patterned tissue assembly during craniofacial development, *J Craniofac Genet Dev Biol* 11:192-213, 1991.

Noden DM: Vertebrate craniofacial development: the relation between ontogenetic process and morphological outcome, *Brain Behav Evol* 38:190-225, 1991.

Osumi-Yamashita N: Retinoic acid and mammalian craniofacial morphogenesis, *J Biosci* 21:313-327, 1996.

Patten B: *Human embryology*, ed 3, New York, 1968, McGraw-Hill.

Richman JM, Tickle C: Epithelial-mesenchymal interactions in the outgrowth of limb buds and facial primordia in chick embryos, *Dev Biol* 154:299-308, 1992.

Richman JM and others: Effect of fibroblast growth factors on outgrowth of facial mesenchyme, *Development* 189:135-147, 1997.

Rijli FM and others: A homeotic transformation is generated in the rostral branchial region of the head by disruption of *Hoxa-2*, which acts as a selector gene, *Cell* 75:1333-1349, 1993.

Ruch JV, Lesot H, Begue-Kirn C: Odontoblast differentiation, *Int J Dev Biol* 39:51-68, 1995.

Salzer GM, Zenker W: Das juxtaorale Organ, *Bibl Anat* 3:1-113, 1962.

Sperber GH: *Craniofacial embryology*, ed 4, London, 1989, Butterworth.

Stock DW, Weiss KM, Zhao Z: Patterning of the mammalian dentition in development and evolution, *BioEssays* 19:481-490, 1997.

Stricker M and others, eds: *Craniofacial malformations*, Edinburgh, 1990, Churchill Livingstone.

Tan SS, Morriss-Kay G: The development and distribution of the cranial neural crest in the rat embryo, *Cell Tissue Res* 240:403-416, 1985.

Thesleff I, Nieminen P: Tooth morphogenesis and cell differentiation, *Curr Opin Cell Biol* 8:844-850, 1996.

Thesleff I and others: Molecular mechanisms of cell and tissue interactions during early tooth development, *Anat Rec* 245:151-161, 1996.

Thorogood P, Tickle C, eds: Craniofacial development, *Development* 103(suppl):1-257, 1988.

Wall NA, Hogan BLM: Expression of bone morphogenetic protein-4 (BMP-4), bone morphogenetic protein-7 (BMP-7), fibroblast growth factor-8 (FGF-8) and sonic hedgehog (SHH) during branchial arch development in the chick, *Mech Dev* 53:383-392, 1995.

Whiting J: Craniofacial abnormalities induced by the ectopic expression of homeobox genes, *Mutation Res* 396:97-112, 1997.

Zeichner-David M and others: Control of ameloblast differentiation, *Int J Dev Biol* 39:69-92, 1995.

Zimmerman EF, ed: Palate development: normal and abnormal, cellular and molecular aspects, *Curr Top Dev Biol* 19:1-243, 1984.

14

DIGESTIVE AND RESPIRATORY SYSTEMS AND BODY CAVITIES

The initial formation of the digestive system by the lateral folding of the endodermal germ layer into a tube is described in Chapter 5. From the simple tubular gut, development of the digestive system can be viewed at several levels, ranging from the elongation and gross twistings and foldings of the digestive tube itself, to the series of inductions and tissue interactions that provide the basis for development of the digestive glands, to the biochemical maturation of the secretory and absorptive epithelia associated with the digestive tract. Clinical Correlations 14-1 to 14-3 discuss malformations associated with the digestive system.

Formation of the respiratory system begins with a very unimposing ventral outpocketing of the foregut. Soon, however, this outpocketing embarks on a unique course of development while still following some of the basic patterns of epithelial-mesenchymal interactions characteristic of other gut-associated glands. Initially, both the digestive and respiratory systems form in a common body cavity, but functional considerations later necessitate the division of this primitive body cavity. Clinical Correlation 14-4 presents malformations associated with the respiratory system. Clinical Correlation 14-5 discusses malformations related to other body cavities.

DIGESTIVE SYSTEM

Chapter 5 describes the formation of the primitive endodermal digestive tube, which is bounded at its cephalic end by the **oropharyngeal membrane** and at its caudal end by the **cloacal plate** (see Figure 5-25). Because of its intimate relationship with the yolk sac through the **yolk stalk,** the gut can be divided into a **foregut,** an open-bottomed **midgut,** and a **hindgut.** As early as the end of the first month, small endodermal diverticula, which represent primordia of the major digestive glands, can be identified (Figure 14-1). (Development of the pharynx and its glandular derivatives is discussed in Chapter 13.)

Formation of the gut tube proper involves continuous elongation, herniation past the body wall, rotation and folding for efficient packing into the body cavity, and histogenesis and functional maturation. While these processes are occurring, the primordial digestive glands and respiratory structures are growing in complex branching patterns as a result of continuous epithelial-mesenchymal interactions. These interactions also occur in the developing digestive tube itself, with specific regional mesenchymal influences determining the character of the epithelium lining that part of the digestive tract.

Formation of the Esophagus

Just caudal to the most posterior pharyngeal pouches of the 4-week-old embryo the pharynx becomes abruptly narrowed, and a small ventral outgrowth (lung bud) appears (see Figure 5-25). The region of foregut just caudal to the lung bud is the **esophagus.** This segment is initially very short, with the stomach seeming to reach almost to the pharynx. In the second month of development, during which the gut elongates considerably, the esophagus assumes nearly postnatal proportions in relation to the location of the stomach.

Although the esophagus grossly resembles a simple tube, it undergoes a series of striking differentiative changes at the tissue level. In its earliest stages the endodermal lining epithelium of the esophagus is stratified columnar. By the eighth week the epithelium has partially occluded the lumen of the esophagus, and large vacuoles appear (Figure 14-2). In succeeding weeks the vacuoles coalesce, and the esophageal lumen recanalizes but with a multilayered ciliated epithelium. During the fourth month, this epithelium finally becomes replaced with the stratified squamous epithelium that characterizes the mature esophagus.

Deeper in the esophageal wall, layers of muscle also differentiate in response to inductive signals from the gut endoderm. Very early (5 weeks' gestation) the primordium of

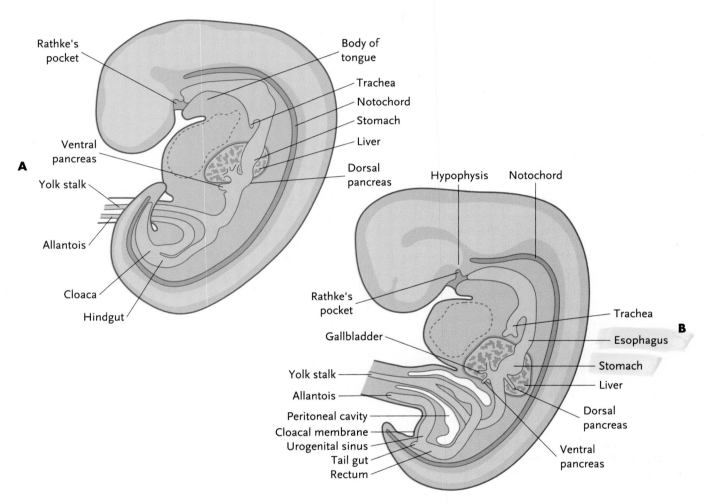

Figure 14-1 Early stages in the formation of the digestive tract as seen in sagittal section. **A,** Early in the **fifth week. B,** Early in the **sixth week.**

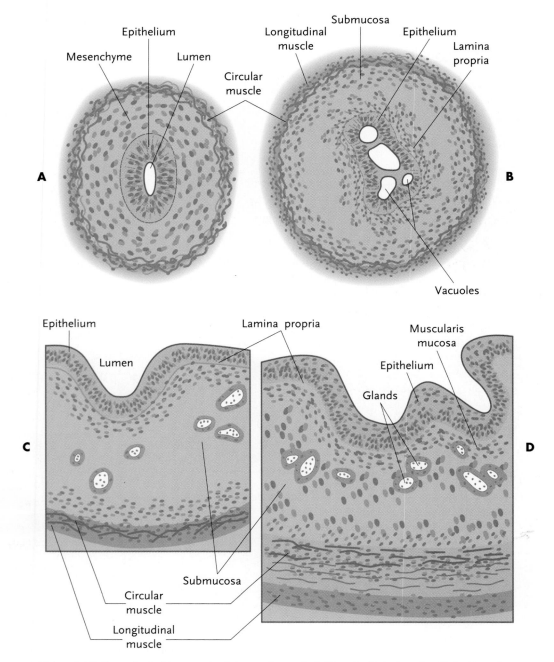

Figure 14-2 Stages in the histogenesis of the esophagus. A, At 7 weeks. B, At 8 weeks. C, At 12 weeks. D, At 34 weeks.

the inner circular muscular layer of esophagus is recognizable, and by 8 weeks the outer longitudinal layer of muscle begins to take shape. The esophageal wall contains both smooth and skeletal muscle. The smooth muscle cells differentiate from the local splanchnic mesoderm associated with the gut. Experiments on mouse embryos suggest that the skeletal muscle cells in the esophageal wall arise by the di-

rect transformation of existing smooth muscle cells into skeletal muscle.* All esophageal musculature is innervated by the vagus nerve (X).

*The direct transformation of one differentiated cell type to another is called **transdifferentiation**. Transdifferentiation is rare in vertebrates, occurring in processes such as regeneration of the lens from the dorsal iris or neural retina from pigmented retina in amphibians.

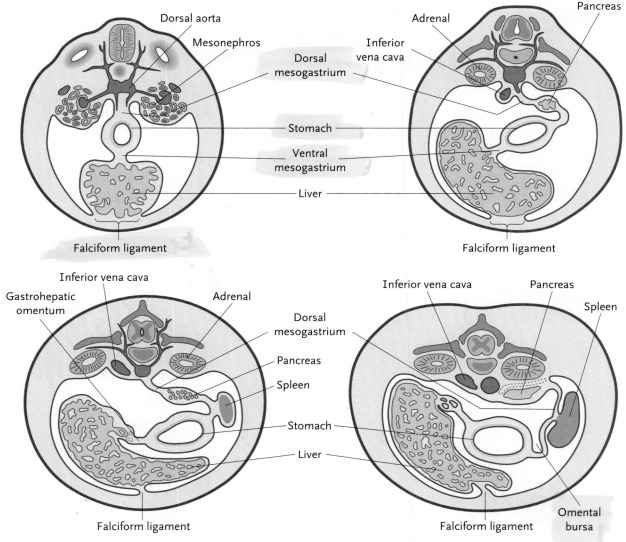

Figure 14-3 Cross sections through the level of the developing stomach, showing changes in the relationships of the mesenteries as the stomach rotates.

Formation of the Stomach

Very early in the formation of the digestive tract the **stomach** is recognizable as a dilated region with a shape remarkably similar to that of the adult stomach (see Figure 14-1). The early stomach is suspended from the dorsal body wall by a portion of the dorsal mesentery called the **dorsal mesogastrium.** It is connected to the ventral body wall by a ventral mesentery that also encloses the developing liver (Figure 14-3).

When the stomach first appears, its concave border faces ventrally, and its convex border faces dorsally. Two concomitant positional shifts bring the stomach to its adult configuration. The first is an approximately 90-degree rotation about its craniocaudal axis so that its originally dorsal convex border faces left and its ventral concave border faces right. The other positional shift consists of a minor tipping of the caudal (pyloric) end of the stomach in a cranial direction so that the long axis of the stomach is positioned somewhat diagonally across the body (Figure 14-4).

During rotation of the stomach, the dorsal mesogastrium is carried with it, leading to the formation of a pouchlike structure called the **omental bursa** (*bursa* comes from a Latin word meaning "sac" or "pouch"). Both the spleen and the tail of the pancreas are embedded in the dorsal mesogastrium (see Figure 14-3). As the stomach rotates, the dorsal mesogastrium and the omental bursa that it encloses enlarge dramatically. Soon, part of the dorsal mesogastrium, which becomes the **greater**

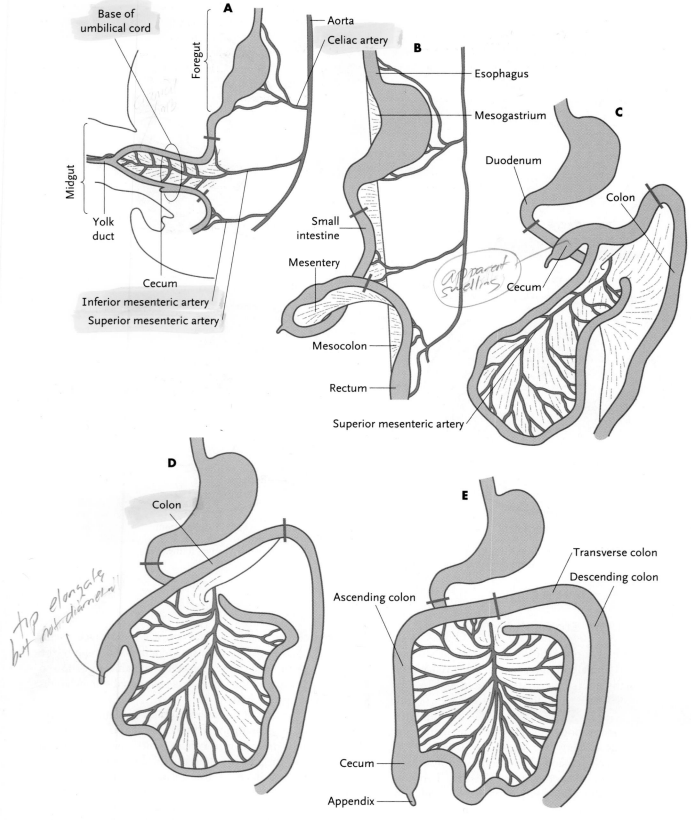

Figure 14-4 Stages in the development and rotation of the gut. **A,** At **5 weeks. B,** At **6 weeks. C,** At **11 weeks. D,** At **12 weeks. E,** Fetal period. Areas between the green lines represent the midgut, which is supplied by the superior mesenteric artery.

omentum, overhangs the transverse colon and portions of the small intestines as a large, double flap of fatty tissue (Figure 14-5). The two sides of the greater omentum ultimately fuse, obliterating the omental bursa within the greater omentum. The rapidly enlarging liver occupies an increasingly large portion of the ventral mesentery.

At the histological level the **gastric mucosa** begins to take shape late in the second month with the appearance of folds (**rugae**) and the first **gastric pits.** During the early fetal period, the individual cell types that characterize the gastric mucosa begin to differentiate. Biochemical and cytochemical studies have shown the gradual functional differentiation of specific cell types during the late fetal period. In most mammals, including humans, cells of the gastric mucosa begin to secrete hydrochloric acid shortly before birth.

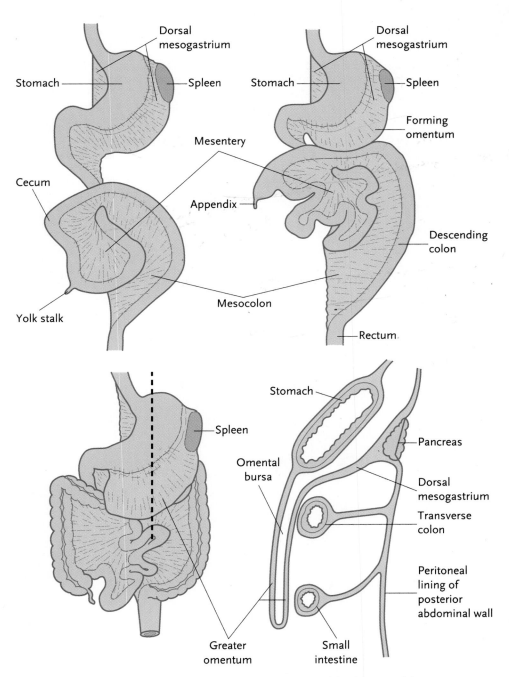

Figure 14-5 Stages in the rotation of the stomach and intestines and development of the greater omentum. A section through the level of the dashed line (*lower left*) is shown (*lower right*).

CLINICAL CORRELATION 14-1
Malformations of the Esophagus and Stomach

ESOPHAGUS

The most common anomalies of the esophagus are associated with abnormalities of the developing respiratory tract (see p. 347). Other rather rare anomalies are **stenosis** and **atresia** of the esophagus. Stenosis is usually attributed to abnormal recanalization of the esophagus after epithelial occlusion of its lumen. Atresia of the esophagus is most commonly associated with abnormal development of the respiratory tract. In both of these conditions, impaired swallowing by the fetus can lead to an excessive accumulation of amniotic fluid (**polyhydramnios**). Just after birth a newborn with these anomalies commonly has difficulty swallowing milk, and regurgitation and choking while drinking are indications for examination of the patency of the esophagus.

STOMACH
Pyloric Stenosis

Pyloric stenosis, which appears to be more physiological than anatomical, consists of hypertrophy of the circular layer of smooth muscle that surrounds the pyloric (outlet) end of the stomach. The hyper-

trophy causes a narrowing (stenosis) of the pyloric opening and impedes the passage of food. Several hours after a meal the infant violently vomits (**projectile vomiting**) the contents of that meal. The enlarged pyloric end of the stomach can often be palpated on physical examination. Although pyloric stenosis is commonly treated by a simple surgical incision through the layer of circular smooth muscle of the pylorus, the hypertrophy sometimes diminishes untreated by several weeks after birth. The pathogenesis of this defect remains unknown, but it seems to have a genetic basis. Pyloric stenosis is more common in males than in females, and the incidence has been reported as from 1 in 200 to 1 in 1000 infants.

Heterotopic Gastric Mucosa

Heterotopic gastric mucosa has been found in a variety of otherwise normal organs (Figure 14-6). This condition is often of clinical significance because if the heterotopic mucosa secretes hydrochloric acid, ulcers can form in unexpected locations.

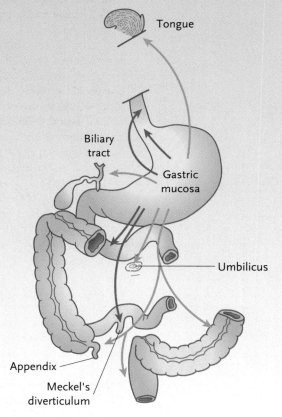

Tongue

Biliary tract

Gastric mucosa

Umbilicus

Appendix

Meckel's diverticulum

Figure 14-6 Locations of heterotopic gastric tissue. The red arrows point to the most frequently occurring sites. The pink arrows indicate less common sites of occurrence. (Based on Gray SW, Skandalakis JE: *Embryology for surgeons*, Philadelphia, 1972, WB Saunders.)

Formation of the Intestines

The intestines are formed from the posterior part of the foregut, the midgut, and the hindgut (Table 14-1). Two points of reference are useful in understanding the gross transformation of the primitive gut tube from a relatively straight cylinder to the complex folded arrangement characteristic of the adult intestinal tract. The first is the yolk stalk, which extends from the floor of the midgut to the yolk sac. In the adult the site of attachment of the yolk stalk is on the small intestine about 2 feet cranial to the junction between small and large intestine (**ileocecal junction**). On the dorsal side of the primitive gut an unpaired ventral branch of the aorta, the **superior mesenteric artery,** and its branches feed the midgut (see Figure 14-4). The superior mesenteric artery itself serves as a pivot point about which later rotation of the gut occurs.

As early as the fifth week, rapid growth of the gut tube causes it to buckle out in a hairpinlike loop. The major change that causes the intestines to assume their adult positions is a counterclockwise rotation of the caudal limb of the intestinal loop (with the yolk stalk attachment and superior mesenteric artery as reference points) around the

cephalic limb from its ventral aspect. The main consequence of this rotation is to bring the future colon across the small intestine so that it can readily assume its C-shaped position along the ventral abdominal wall (see Figure 14-4). Behind the colon the small intestine undergoes a great elongation and becomes packed in its characteristic position in the abdominal cavity.

The rotation and other positional changes of the gut occur partly because the length of the gut increases more than the length of the embryo. From almost the first stages the volume of the expanded gut tract is greater than the body cavity can accommodate. Consequently, the developing intestines herniate into the body stalk (the umbilical cord after further development) (Figure 14-7). Intestinal herniation begins as early as the sixth or seventh week of embryogenesis. By the tenth week the abdominal cavity has enlarged sufficiently to accommodate the intestinal tract, and the herniated intestinal loops begin to move through the intestinal ring back into the abdominal cavity. Coils of small intestine return first. As they do, they force the distal part of the colon, which was never herniated, to the left side of the peritoneal cavity, thus establishing the definitive position of the descending colon. After the small intestine has taken its intraabdominal position, the herniated proximal part of the colon also returns, with its cecal end swinging to the right and downward (see Figure 14-4).

During these coilings, herniations, and return movements, the intestines are suspended from the dorsal body wall by a mesentery (Figure 14-8). As the intestines assume their definitive positions within the body cavity, their mesenteries follow. Parts of the mesentery associated with the duodenum and colon (**mesoduodenum** and **mesocolon**) fuse with the peritoneal lining of the dorsal body wall.

Starting in the sixth week the primordium of the **cecum** becomes apparent as a swelling in the caudal limb of the midgut (see Figure 14-4). In succeeding weeks the cecal enlargement becomes so prominent that the distal small intestine enters the colon at a right angle.

The tip of the cecum elongates, but its diameter does not increase in proportion to the rest of the cecum. This wormlike appendage is aptly called the **vermiform appendix.**

Partitioning of the cloaca

In the early embryo the caudal end of the hindgut terminates in the endodermally lined **cloaca,** which in lower vertebrates serves as a common termination for the digestive and urogenital systems. The cloaca also includes the base of the allantois, which later expands as a common **urogenital sinus** (see Chapter 15). A **cloacal (proctodeal) membrane** consisting of apposed layers of ectoderm and endoderm acts as a barrier between the cloaca and an ectodermal depression known as the **proctodeum** (Figure 14-9). A shelf of mesodermal tissue called the **urorectal septum** is situated between the hindgut and the base of the allantois. During the sixth and seventh weeks, the

TABLE 14-1 Derivatives of Regions of the Primitive Gut

Blood supply	Adult derivatives
FOREGUT	
Celiac artery (lower esophagus to duodenum)	Pharynx
	Esophagus
	Stomach
	Upper duodenum
	Glands of pharyngeal pouches, respiratory tract, liver and gallbladder, pancreas
MIDGUT	
Superior mesenteric artery	Lower duodenum
	Jejunum and ileum
	Cecum and vermiform appendix
	Ascending colon
	Cranial half of transverse colon
HINDGUT	
Inferior mesenteric artery	Caudal half of transverse colon
	Descending colon
	Rectum
	Superior part of anal canal

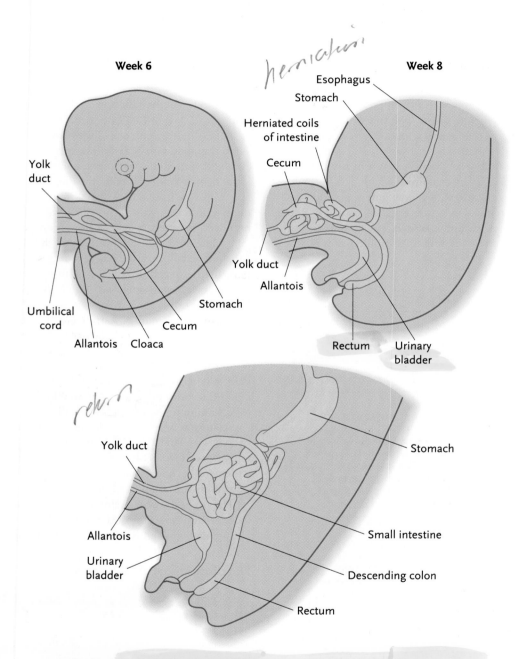

Week 6

herniation

Week 8

Esophagus

Stomach

Herniated coils
of intestine

Cecum

Yolk
duct

Yolk duct

Allantois

Umbilical
cord

Allantois   Cloaca

Stomach

Cecum

Rectum   Urinary
bladder

return

Yolk duct

Stomach

Allantois

Small intestine

Urinary
bladder

Descending colon

Rectum

Figure 14-7   Stages of herniation of the intestines into the body stalk and their return.

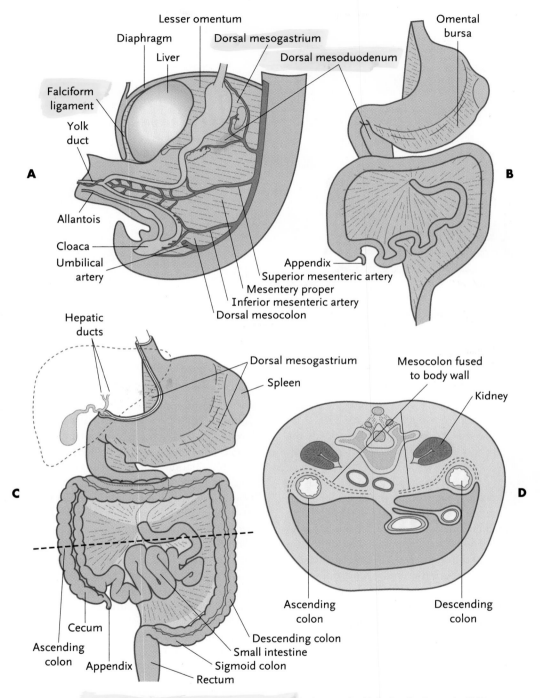

Figure 14-8 Stages in the development of the mesenteries. **A**, At **5 weeks**. **B**, In the **third month**. **C**, During the late fetal period. **D**, Cross section through the dashed line in **C**. In **C**, the shaded areas represent regions where the mesentery is fused to the dorsal body wall.

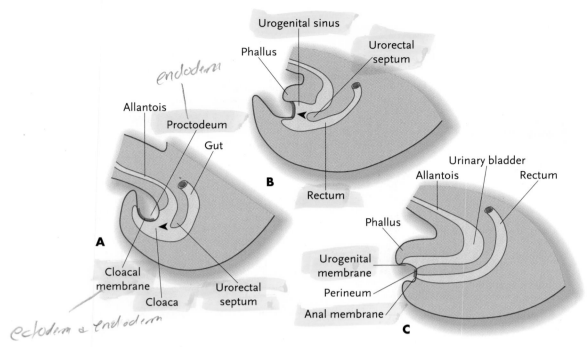

endoderm

ectoderm & endoderm

Figure 14-9 Stages in the subdivision of the common cloaca by the urorectal septum. A, In the **fifth week**. B, In the **sixth week**. C, In the **eighth week**.

urorectal septum grows toward the cloacal membrane. At the same time, lateral mesodermal ridges extend into the cloaca. The combined ingrowth of the lateral ridges and growth of the urorectal septum toward the cloacal membrane divide the cloaca into the **rectum** and **urogenital sinus** (Figure 14-9, *B*). Double mutants of *Hoxa-13* and *Hoxd-13* result in the absence of cloacal partitioning along with hypodevelopment of the phallus (genital tubercle). Once the cloaca becomes partitioned, the cloacal membrane also becomes subdivided into an **anal membrane**, which blocks the end of the hindgut, and a **urogenital membrane**, which seals the urogenital sinus from the exterior. By the end of the eighth week the anal membrane ruptures and affords free access between the hindgut and the exterior of the body. The area where the urorectal septum and lateral mesodermal folds fuse with the cloacal membrane becomes the **perineal body**, which represents the partition between the digestive and urogenital systems.

Histogenesis of the intestinal tract

Shortly after its initial formation the intestinal tract consists of a simple layer of columnar endodermal epithelium surrounded by a layer of splanchnopleural mesoderm. Three major phases are involved in the histogenesis of the intestinal epithelium: (1) an early phase of epithelial proliferation and morphogenesis, (2) an intermediate period of cellular differentiation in which the distinctive cell types characteristic of

the intestinal epithelium appear, and (3) a final phase of biochemical and functional maturation of the different types of epithelial cells. The mesenchymal wall of the intestine also differentiates into several layers of highly innervated smooth muscle and connective tissue. An overall craniocaudal gradient of differentiation is present within the developing intestine.

Early in the second month the epithelium of the small intestine begins a phase of rapid proliferation that results in the epithelium temporarily occluding the lumen by 6 to 7 weeks' gestation. Within a couple of weeks, recanalization of the intestinal lumen has occurred. At about this time, small, cracklike secondary lumina appear beneath the surface of the multilayered epithelium, and aggregates of mesoderm push into the epithelium. A combination of coalescence of the secondary lumina with continued mesenchymal upgrowth beneath the epithelium results in the formation of numerous fingerlike **intestinal villi**, which greatly increase the absorptive surface of the intestinal surface. By this time the epithelium has transformed from a stratified into a simple columnar type.

With the formation of villi, pitlike **intestinal crypts** also form at the base of the villi. The crypts contain **epithelial stem cells**, which have a high rate of mitosis and serve as the source of epithelial cells for the entire intestinal surface (Figure 14-10). Experimental evidence suggests that all of the epithelial cells in a single crypt have a monoclonal origin (e.g., all are derived from a single precursor cell in the embryo). Autoradiographic studies on postnatal individuals have shown that over 3 to 4 days, ep-

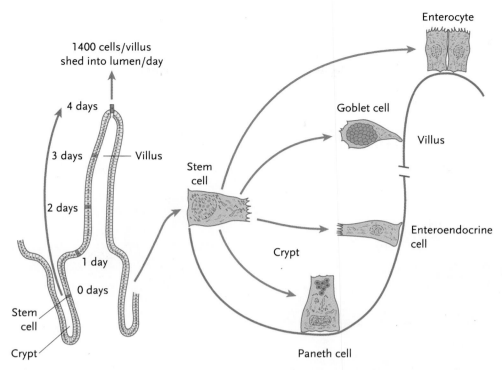

Figure 14-10 Differentiation of intestinal epithelial cells from stem cells located in the crypts. The time scale shows the typical course of migration of daughter cells starting with their generation from the stem cell population to their being shed from the villus into the intestinal lumen.

ithelial cells originating in the crypts migrate up the villus and are ultimately shed from the tips of the villi. The intestinal epithelium is continuously renewed by this mechanism.

Shortly after the formation of the crypts, individual epithelial stem cells within them begin to form each of the four types of mature epithelial cells found in the intestinal epithelial lining.* By the end of the second trimester of pregnancy, all cell types found in the adult intestinal lining have differentiated, but many of these cells do not possess adult functional patterns. A number of specific biochemical patterns of differentiation are present as early as 12 weeks' gestation and mature during the fetal period. For example, **lactase,** an enzyme that breaks down the disaccharide **lactose** (milk sugar), is one of the digestive enzymes synthesized in the fetal period in anticipation of the early postnatal period during which the newborn subsists principally on the mother's milk. Further biochemical differentiation of the intestine occurs after birth, often in response to specific dietary patterns.

Histodifferentiation of the intestinal tract is not an isolated property of the individual tissue components of the intestinal wall. During the early embryonic period and sometimes into postnatal life the epithelial and mesodermal components of the intestinal wall communicate by inductive interactions. In-

terspecies recombination experiments show that the gut mesoderm exerts a regional influence on intestinal epithelial differentiation (e.g., whether the epithelium differentiates into a duodenal or colonic phenotype). Once regional determination is set, however, the controls for biochemical differentiation of the epithelium are inherent. This pattern of inductive influence and the epithelial reaction are very similar to those outlined earlier for dermal-epidermal interactions in the developing skin (see Chapter 8).

Final enzymatic differentiation of intestinal absorptive cells is strongly influenced by glucocorticoids, and the underlying mesoderm appears to mediate this hormonal effect. In a converse inductive influence the intestinal endoderm induces the differentiation of smooth muscle from mesenchymal cells in the wall of the intestine. The mechanism of the interactions between mesenchyme and endoderm are not completely understood. In some cases the mesoderm may exert its effects directly on the endoderm, whereas in other cases extracellular matrix molecules secreted by the mesodermal cells may mediate the inductive interactions.

Although the intestine develops many functional capabilities during the fetal period, no major digestive function occurs until feeding begins after birth. The intestines of the fetus contain a greenish material called **meconium** (see Figure 17-9), which is a mixture of lanugo hairs and vernix caseosa sloughed from the skin, desquamated cells from the gut, bile secretion, and other materials swallowed with the amniotic fluid.

*For a number of years, it was thought that the peptide hormone-secreting cells in the intestinal tract were derived from neural crest. This assertion has not been supported by transplantation and marking experiments.

Text continued on p. 337

CLINICAL CORRELATION 14-2
Malformations of the Intestinal Tract

DUODENAL STENOSIS AND ATRESIA

Duodenal stenosis and atresia typically result from absent or incomplete recanalization of the duodenal lumen after it is plugged by endothelium. These malformations are rare.

VITELLINE DUCT REMNANTS

The most common family of anomalies of the intestinal tract is some form of persistence of the **vitelline (yolk) duct.** The most common member of this family is **Meckel's diverticulum,** which is present in 2% to 4% of the population. A typical Meckel's diverticulum is a blind pouch a few centimeters long located on the antimesenteric border of the ileum about 50 cm cranial from the ileocecal junction (Figure 14-11, A and E). This structure represents the persistent proximal portion of the yolk stalk. Simple Meckel's diverticula are often asymptomatic, but they occasionally become inflamed or contain ectopic tissue (e.g., gastric, pancreatic, or even endometrial tissue), which can cause ulceration.

In some cases a ligament connects a Meckel's diverticulum to the umbilicus (Figure 14-11, B), or a simple vitelline ligament that may have an associated persisting **vitelline artery** can connect the intestine to the umbilicus. Occasionally the intestine rotates about such a ligament, causing a condition known as **volvulus** (Figure 14-11, D). This can lead to strangulation of the bowel.

A persistent vitelline duct can take the form of a **vitelline fistula** (Figure 14-11, C), which constitutes a direct connection between the intestinal lumen and the outside of the body via the umbilicus. Rarely, a **vitelline duct cyst** is present along the length of a vitelline ligament.

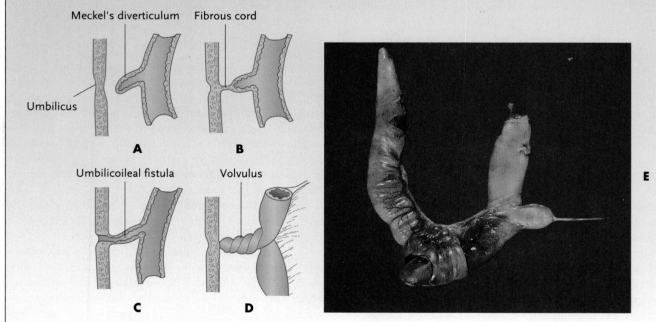

Figure 14-11 Varieties of vitelline duct remnants. A, Meckel's diverticulum. B, Fibrous cord connecting a Meckel's diverticulum to the umbilicus. C, Umbilicoileal (vitelline) fistula. D, Volvulus caused by rotation of the intestine around a vitelline duct remnant. E, Meckel's diverticulum protruding at the left from a segment of ileum. The bowel above the diverticulum is reddish because of an associated intussusception just above the Meckel's diverticulum (Photo 2681 from the Arey-DaPeña Pediatric Pathology Photographic Collection, Human Development Anatomy Center, National Museum of Health and Medicine, Armed Forces Institute of Pathology, Washington, DC.)

CLINICAL CORRELATION 14-2
Malformations of the Intestinal Tract—cont'd

OMPHALOCELE

Omphalocele represents the failure of return of the intestinal loops into the body cavity during the tenth week. After birth, the intestinal loops can be easily seen within an almost transparent sac consisting of amnion on the outside and peritoneal membrane on the inside (Figure 14-12). The incidence of omphalocele is approximately 1 in 3500 births, but half of the infants with this condition are stillborn.

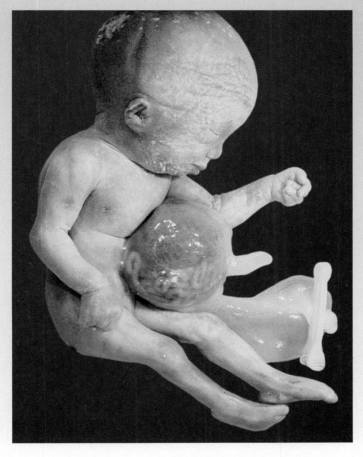

Figure 14-12 Omphalocele in a stillborn. Loops of small intestine can be clearly seen through the nearly transparent amniotic membrane that covers the omphalocele. (Courtesy M. Barr, Ann Arbor, Mich.)

Continued

CLINICAL CORRELATION 14-2
Malformations of the Intestinal Tract—cont'd

CONGENITAL UMBILICAL HERNIA

In congenital umbilical hernia, which is especially common in premature infants, the intestines return normally into the body cavity, but the musculature (rectus abdominis) of the ventral abdominal wall fails to close the umbilical ring, allowing a varying amount of omentum or bowel to protrude through the umbilicus. In contrast to omphalocele, the protruding tissue in an umbilical hernia is covered by skin rather than amniotic membrane.

Both omphalocele and congenital umbilical hernia are associated with closure defects in the ventral abdominal wall. If these defects are large, they may be accompanied by massive protrusion of abdominal contents or with other closure defects such as exstrophy of the bladder (see Chapter 15).

ABNORMAL ROTATION OF THE GUT

Sometimes the intestines undergo no or abnormal rotation as they return to the abdominal cavity. This can result in a wide spectrum of anatomical anomalies (Figure 14-13). In most cases these are asymptomatic, but occasionally, they can lead to volvulus or another form of strangulation of the gut.

INTESTINAL DUPLICATIONS, DIVERTICULA, AND ATRESIA

As with the esophagus and duodenum, the remainder of the intestinal tract is susceptible to various anomalies that seem to be based on incomplete recanalization of the lumen after the stage of temporary blocking of the lumen by epithelium during the first trimester. Some of the variants of these conditions are shown in Figure 14-14.

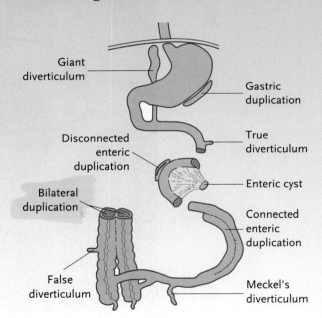

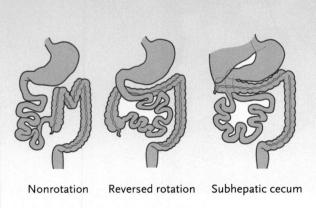

Nonrotation   Reversed rotation   Subhepatic cecum

Figure 14-13 Types of abnormal rotations of the gut.

Figure 14-14 Types of diverticula and duplications that can occur in the digestive tract. (Based on Gray SW, Skandalakis JE: *Embryology for surgeons*, Philadelphia, 1972, WB Saunders.)

CLINICAL CORRELATION 14-2
Malformations of the Intestinal Tract—cont'd

AGANGLIONIC MEGACOLON (HIRSCHSPRUNG'S DISEASE)

The basis of aganglionic megacolon, which is manifested by great dilatation of certain segments of the colon, is the absence of parasympathetic ganglia in the affected walls of the colon. This has been attributed to the defective migration of neural crest cells into that portion of the hindgut early in the second month of pregnancy. Evidence from mutant mice developing aganglionic segments of the bowel strongly suggests that the environment of the gut wall inhibits the migration of neural crest cells into the affected segment of gut. This was shown by experiments in which crest cells from mutant mice were capable of colonizing normal gut, but normal crest cells could not migrate into gut segments of mutant mice. The accumulation of laminin in the gut wall as the result of overproduction of **endothelin-3** serves as a stop signal for neural crest migration. The distal colon is the most affected region for aganglionosis, but in a small

number of cases, aganglionic segments extend as far cranially as the ascending colon. Estimates of the frequency of megacolon vary widely—from 1 in 1000 to 1 in 30,000 births.

IMPERFORATE ANUS

Imperforate anus includes a spectrum of anal defects that can range from a simple membrane covering the anal opening (persistence of the anal membrane) to atresia of varying lengths of the anal canal, rectum, or both structures. Grossly, all are characterized by the absence of an anal opening (Figure 14-15). Any examination of a newborn must include a determination of the presence of an anal opening. Of considerable importance when considering the surgical treatment of imperforate anus is the extent of the atretic segment. Treatment of a persistent anal membrane can be trivial, whereas more extensive defects, especially those involving the anal musculature, constitute very challenging surgical problems.

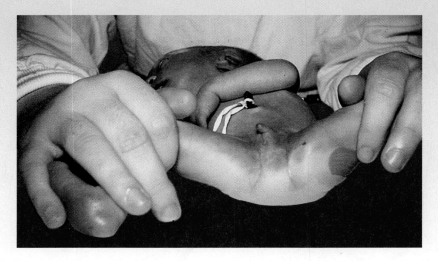

Figure 14-15 Anal atresia in a newborn. No trace of an anal opening is seen. (Courtesy M. Barr, Ann Arbor, Mich.)

Continued

CLINICAL CORRELATION 14-2
Malformations of the Intestinal Tract—cont'd

HINGUT FISTULAS

In many cases, anal atresia is accompanied by a fistula linking the patent portion of the hindgut to another structure in the region of the original urogenital sinus region. Common types of fistulas connect the hindgut with the vagina, the urethra, or the bladder, and others may lead to the surface in the perineal area (Figure 14-16).

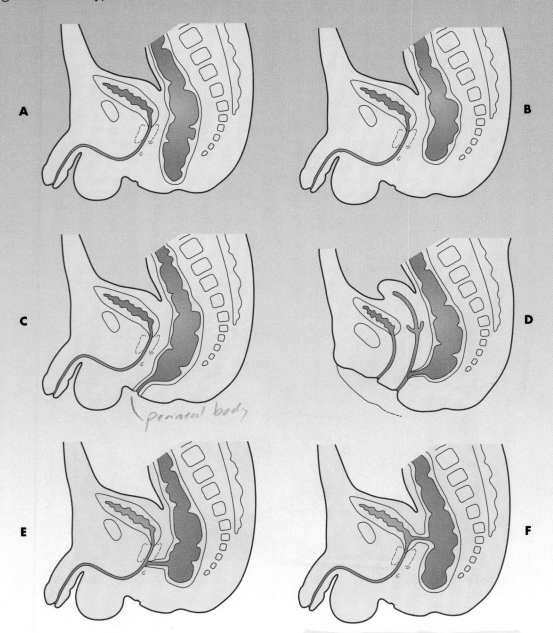

Figure 14-16 Varieties of hindgut fistulas and atresias. **A,** Persistent anal membrane. **B,** Anal atresia. **C,** Anoperineal fistula. **D,** Rectovaginal fistula. **E,** Rectourethral fistula. **F,** Rectovesical fistula.

Glands of the Digestive System

The glands of the digestive system arise through inductive processes between the early epithelial outgrowths and the surrounding mesenchyme. The various glandular epithelia have considerably different requirements in the types of mesenchyme that can support their development. For example, in tissue recombination experiments, pancreatic epithelium undergoes typical development when juxtaposed with mesenchyme from almost any source. The development of salivary gland epithelium, on the other hand, is supported by mesenchyme from lung or accessory sexual glands but not by many other types of mesenchyme. Inductive support of hepatic (liver) epithelium follows a distinctive pattern. Normal epithelial development is supported by mesenchyme derived from lateral plate or intermediate mesoderm, but axial mesenchyme (either somitic or neural crest) fails to support hepatic differentiation. The inductive properties of certain glandular mesenchymes may be correlated with different modes of vascularization of these mesenchymes (see p. 403).

Formation of the liver

Early in the third week an endodermal hepatic diverticulum arises from the floor of the foregut and grows into the mesenchyme of the **septum transversum** (see Figure 5-25). The hepatic diverticulum is the manifestation of a series of inductive processes that have already begun to take place (Figure 14-17). The original hepatic diverticulum branches into many hepatic cords, which are closely associated with splanchnic mesoderm of the septum transversum. The mesoderm supports continued growth and proliferation of the hepatic endoderm. This occurs in part through the actions of **hepatic growth factor**, which is bound by the receptor molecule, c-**met**, located on the surface of the endodermal hepatocytes. A number of experimental studies have shown that mesoderm from either the splanchnopleural or somatopleural components of the lateral plate mesoderm can support further hepatic growth and differentiation, whereas paraxial mesoderm has only a limited capacity to support hepatic development.

In addition to cords of hepatic endoderm, a system of bile drainage ducts forms in the developing liver. Near the area where the hepatic ducts become confluent, a dilatation foreshadows the further development of the **gallbladder** (Figure 14-18). The hepatic cords form a series of loosely packed and highly irregular sheets that alternate with mesodermally lined **sinusoids**, through which blood percolates and exchanges nutrients with the **hepatocytes**. The developing liver is richly vascularized, with many major vessels passing through it in the embryonic period (see Figure 16-11).

The entire liver soon becomes too large to be contained in the septum transversum, and it protrudes into the ventral mesentery within the abdominal cavity. As it continues to expand, the rapidly growing liver remains covered by a glistening, translucent layer of mesenteric tissue that now serves as the connective tissue capsule of the liver. Between the liver and the ventral body wall is a thin, sickle-shaped piece of ventral mesentery: the **falciform ligament**. The ventral mesentery between the liver and the stomach is the **lesser omentum** (see Figure 14-3).

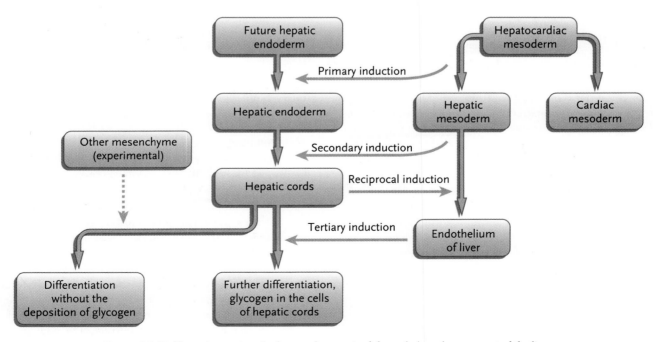

Figure 14-17 Tissue interactions in the morphogenesis of the endodermal component of the liver.

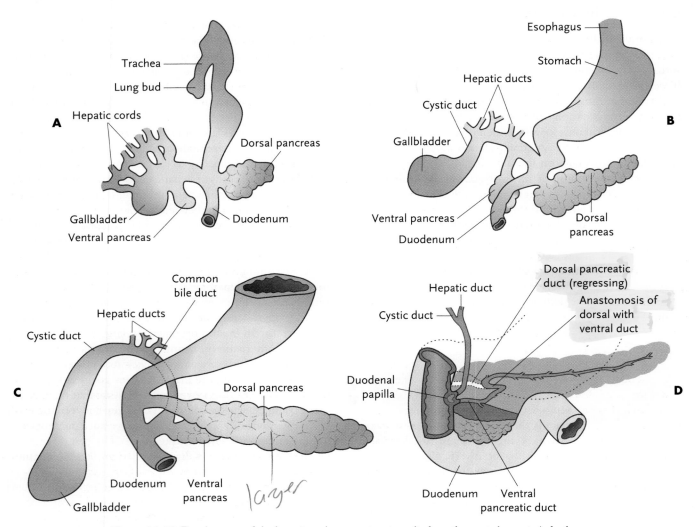

Figure 14-18 Development of the hepatic and pancreatic primordia from the ventral aspect. **A,** In the **fifth week. B,** In the **sixth week. C,** In the **seventh week. D,** In the late fetus, showing fusion of the dorsal and ventral pancreatic ducts and regression of the distal portion of the dorsal duct.

Development of hepatic function. Development of the liver is not only a matter of increasing its mass and structural complexity. As the liver develops, its cells gradually acquire the capacity to perform the many biochemical functions characterizing the mature, functioning liver. One characteristic major function of the liver is to produce the plasma protein **serum albumin.** The messenger ribonucleic acid (mRNA) for albumin has been detected in mammalian hepatocytes during the earliest stages of their ingrowth into the hepatic mesoderm, and it appears to depend on the earlier expression of the transcription factor, **hepatic nuclear factor-3.**

A major function of the adult liver is the synthesis and storage of **glycogen,** which serves as a carbohydrate reserve. As the fetal period progresses, the liver actively stores glycogen. This function is strongly stimulated by adrenocortical hormones and is indirectly stimulated by the anterior pi-

tuitary. Similarly, the fetal period includes the functional development of the system of enzymes involved in the synthesis of urea from nitrogenous metabolites. By birth, these have attained full functional capacity.

A major function of the embryonic liver is the production of blood cells. After yolk sac hematopoiesis, the liver is one of the chief sites of intraembryonic blood formation. Hematopoietic cells, seeding the liver from origins in other sites, appear in small clusters among the hepatic parenchymal cells.

At approximately 12 weeks' gestation the hepatocytes begin to produce **bile** largely through the breakdown of hemoglobin. The bile drains down the newly formed bile duct system and is stored in the gallbladder. As bile is released into the intestines, it stains the other intestinal contents a dark green, which is one of the characteristics of meconium.

Formation of the pancreas

Shortly after the hepatic primordium first appears, two pancreatic buds begin to grow out of the dorsal and ventral walls of the foregut (see Figure 5-25). The dorsal bud is a direct outgrowth from the duodenal endoderm; the ventral bud arises from the endoderm of the hepatic diverticulum (see Figure 14-18). The dorsal pancreatic bud is induced from the dorsal gut endoderm by the notochord, which early in development is directly opposed to the endoderm (see Figure 4-7, C). The ventral pancreatic bud appears to be induced by the hepatic mesoderm. During the earliest stages of pancreatic bud formation, the homeodomain-containing transcription factor **Pdx-1** is expressed. When this gene is eliminated by targeted mutagenesis, development of the pancreatic buds ceases. Another early expressed LIM-homeodomain gene, **Islet-1**, is required for the formation of dorsal pancreatic mesoderm and the formation of islets. Expression of both of these genes (as well as *Pax-6*) in the dorsal pancreatic bud is eliminated in the absence of a notochordal influence, but interestingly, their expression in the ventral pancreatic bud is unaffected by removal of the notochord.

During the phase of early growth, the dorsal pancreas becomes considerably larger than the ventral pancreas. At about the same time the duodenum rotates to the right and forms a C-shaped loop, carrying the ventral pancreas and common bile duct behind it and into the dorsal mesentery. The ventral pancreas soon makes contact and fuses with the dorsal pancreas.

Both the dorsal and the ventral pancreas possess a large duct. After fusion of the two pancreatic primordia, the main duct of the ventral pancreas makes an anastomotic connection with the duct of the dorsal pancreas. The portion of the dorsal pancreatic duct between the anastomotic connection and the duodenum normally regresses, leaving the main duct of the ventral pancreas (**duct of Wirsung**) the definitive outlet from the pancreas into the duodenum (see Figure 14-18).

The pancreas is a dual organ with both endocrine and exocrine functions. The exocrine portion consists of large numbers of **acini**, which are connected to a secretory duct system. The endocrine component consists of roughly a million richly vascularized **islets of Langerhans**, which are scattered among the acini.

Once established, the pancreatic primordia grow through several epithelial-mesenchymal interactions of the type typically seen in the development of glands associated with the gut. During the phase of outgrowth, the glandular epithelium of the pancreas takes shape by the sequential budding of cords of cells derived from the population of pancreatic founder cells (Figure 14-19). From the cellular cords, both the acini and their ducts differentiate. Tissue recombination experiments, conducted both in vitro and in vivo, have shown that the presence of mesenchyme is necessary for the formation

of acini but that ducts can form in the absence of mesenchyme if the endodermal precursor cells are exposed to a gel rich in basement membrane material. Although the presence of mesenchyme is required for the differentiation of acini, the mesenchyme need not be of pancreatic origin. In vitro, pancreatic endoderm combined with salivary gland mesoderm differentiates even better than that exposed to pancreatic mesenchyme. This shows that in the case of the pancreas the inductive influence of the mesenchyme is permissive, rather than instructive.

Differentiation of the acini is divided into three phases (see Figure 14-19). The first, called the **predifferentiated state**, occurs while the pancreatic primordia are first taking shape. A population of pancreatic founder cells that exhibits virtually undetectable levels of digestive enzyme activity is established. As the pancreatic buds begin to grow outward, the epithelium undergoes a transition into a second, **protodifferentiated state**. During this phase, the exocrine cells synthesize low levels of many hydrolytic enzymes that they will ultimately produce. After the main period of outgrowth, the pancreatic acinar cells pass through another transition before attaining a third, **differentiated state**. By this time, they have acquired an elaborate protein-synthesizing apparatus, and the inactive forms of the polypeptide digestive enzymes are stored in the cytoplasm as **zymogen granules**. Glucocorticoid hormones from the fetal adrenal cortex stimulate increased production of a number of digestive enzymes.

Development of the islets of Langerhans follows a somewhat different course from that of the acini. They are formed from groups of epithelial cells that break away from the acinar epithelial cells during the second (protodifferentiated) phase of acinar cell development. The sequence of appearance of the various types of islet cells is well defined. The first to differentiate (at 8 to 9 weeks) are the α-cells, which secrete **glucagon**. This is followed by the appearance of β-cells, which secrete **insulin**. During the second phase of pancreatic differentiation (protodifferentiated state) the levels of glucagon synthesis considerably exceed those of insulin. Even later, a third population of islet cells (δ-cells) begins to secrete **somatostatin** and a fourth population (**PP-cells**) secretes **pancreatic polypeptide**. By the third phase of pancreatic development, secretory granules are evident in the cytoplasm of most islet cells. Insulin and glucagon are present in the fetal circulation by the end of the fifth month of gestation. Although for many years it was thought that pancreatic islets were derived, at least in part, from the ductal system, recent research has shown that islets can form in the absence of both ducts and pancreatic mesenchyme. This suggests that the formation of islets may actually be a default mechanism for pancreatic endoderm that has not been exposed to mesoderm. The expression of glucagon and insulin in very early pancreatic bud endoderm supports such a concept.

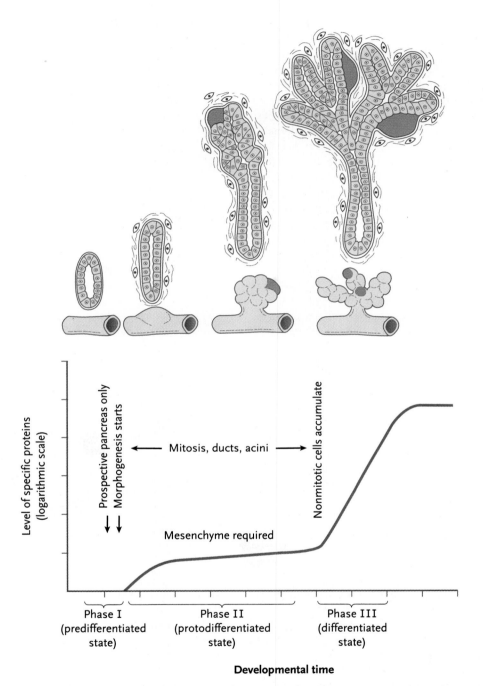

Figure 14-19 Stages of structural and functional differentiation of the pancreas. The green areas represent primitive islets. (Modified from Pictet R, Rutter W: *Handbook of physiology*, section 7: *Endocrinology*, vol 1, Washington, DC, 1972, American Physiological Society, pp 25-66.)

CLINICAL CORRELATION 14-3
Anomalies of the Liver and Pancreas

Many minor variations in the shape of the liver or bile ducts occur, but these normally have no functional significance. One of the most serious malformations involving the liver is **biliary atresia**. This can involve any level from the tiny bile canaliculi to the major bile-carrying ducts. Newborns with this condition typically develop severe **jaundice** shortly after birth. Some cases can be treated surgically; for others, a liver transplant is necessary.

On rare occasions a ring of pancreatic tissue completely encircles the duodenum, forming an **annular pancreas** (Figure 14-20). This can sometimes cause obstruction of the duodenum after birth. The cause of annular pancreas is not established, but the most commonly accepted explanation is that outgrowths from a bifid ventral pancreas may encircle the duodenum from both sides.

Heterotopic pancreatic tissue can occasionally be found along the digestive tract, and it occurs most frequently in the duodenum or mucosa of the stomach (Figure 14-21). About 6% of Meckel's diverticula contain heterotopic pancreatic tissue.

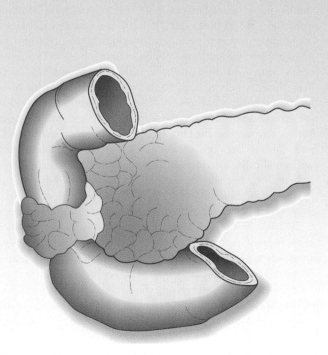

Figure 14-20 Annular pancreas encircling the duodenum.

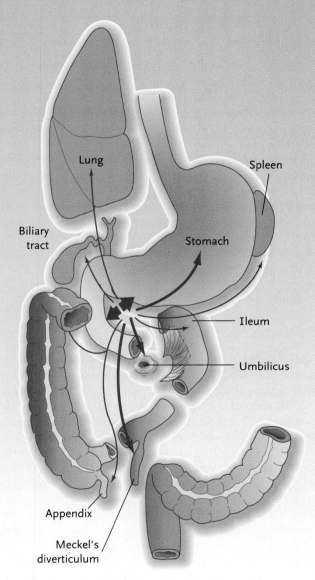

Figure 14-21 Most common locations in which heterotopic pancreatic tissue can be found. The thickness of the arrows corresponds to the frequency of heterotopic tissue in that location. (Based on Gray SW, Skandalakis JE: *Embryology for surgeons*, Philadelphia, 1972, WB Saunders.)

RESPIRATORY SYSTEM

The respiratory system is first seen during the fourth week as an inconspicuous midline **laryngotracheal groove** in the ventral midline at the posterior limit of the pharyngeal region. By the fifth week of gestation, further outgrowth has transformed the laryngotracheal groove into a well-defined **respiratory diverticulum** (see Figure 5-25) that grows into the splanchnic mesoderm almost parallel to the esophagus. Through a series of interactions with the surrounding mesoderm, the respiratory diverticulum elongates into a tracheal portion and begins to form the first of 23 sets of bifurcations (**lung buds**) that continue into postnatal life.

Formation of the Larynx

During the fourth and fifth weeks of gestation, a rapid proliferation of the fourth and sixth pharyngeal arch mesenchyme around the site of origin of the respiratory bud converts the opening slit from the esophagus into a T-shaped **glottis** bounded by two lateral **arytenoid swellings** and a cranial **epiglottis**. The mesenchyme surrounding the laryngeal orifice ultimately differentiates into the **thyroid, cricoid**, and **arytenoid cartilages**, which form the skeletal supports of the **larynx**. Like the esophagus, the lumen of the larynx undergoes a temporary epithelial occlusion. In the process of recanalization during the ninth and tenth weeks, a pair of lateral folds and recesses forms the structural basis for the **vocal cords** and adjacent **laryngeal ventricles**. The somitomere-derived musculature of the larynx is innervated by branches of the vagus nerve (X), that associated with the fourth arch is innervated by the **superior laryngeal nerve**, and that of the sixth arch is innervated by the **recurrent laryngeal nerve**.

Formation of the Trachea and Bronchial Tree

After its initial appearance, the respiratory diverticulum undergoes considerable elongation before a pair of bronchial buds appears at the end. The straight portion of the respiratory diverticulum is the primordium of the trachea. The bronchial buds, which ultimately become the primary bronchi, give rise to additional buds—three on the right and two on the left. These buds become the **secondary**, or **stem, bronchi**, and their numbers presage the formation of the three lobes of the right lung and the two lobes of the left (Figure 14-22). From this point, each secondary bronchial bud undergoes a long series of branchings until a maximum 23 successive orders of branching have occurred. Morphogenesis of the lung continues after birth, and stabilization of the morphological pattern of the lungs does not occur until about 8 years of age. An array of *Hox* genes (*Hoxa-3* to *Hoxa-5* and *Hoxb-3* to *Hoxb-6*) is expressed early in the developing respiratory tract. Combinatorial patterns of expression of *Hox* genes may be involved in regional specification of the respiratory tract.

The mesoderm surrounding the endoderm controls the extent of branching within the respiratory tract. Numerous tissue recombination experiments have shown that the mesoderm surrounding the trachea inhibits branching, whereas that surrounding the bronchial buds promotes branching. If tracheal endoderm is combined with bronchial mesoderm, abnormal budding is induced. Conversely, tracheal mesoderm placed around bronchial endoderm inhibits bronchial budding. Mesoderm of certain other organs such as salivary glands can promote budding of the bronchial endoderm, but a pattern of branching characteristic of the mesoderm is induced. A mesoderm capable of promoting or sustaining budding must maintain a high rate of proliferation of the epithelial cells. Generally, the pattern of the epithelial organ is largely determined by the mesoderm. Structural and functional differentiation of the epithelium is a specific property of the epithelial cells, but the epithelial phenotype corresponds to the region dictated by the mesoderm.

The basic principles underlying pulmonary branching are similar to those operating in the development of the salivary glands and pancreas. At points of branching, epithelial cell proliferation is reduced, and the deposition of types I and III collagen, fibronectin, and proteoglycans stabilizes the morphology of the branching point and more proximal ductal regions. On the other hand, heightened epithelial cell proliferation characterizes the rapidly expanding portions of the epithelial buds (Figure 14-23).

The activities of many molecules contribute to lung morphogenesis, but a truly coherent hierarchy of molecular control has not yet been laid out. Several growth factors, including **fibroblast growth factor-10 (FGF-10)** produced by local mesenchyme (splanchnic mesoderm), seem to be involved in stimulating the initial outgrowth of endodermal buds in the developing lung. The tips of the epithelial buds produce **sonic hedgehog**, which appears to induce the expression of **bone morphogenetic protein-4 (BMP-4)** and to repress FGF-10 in the surrounding mesenchyme. In this most distal area, the basal lamina surrounding the lung epithelium is porous, allowing direct contact between processes of the epithelial and mesenchymal cells. The protooncogene, **N-myc**, is also involved in branching because if its expression is inhibited, branching fails to occur. N-myc activity is inhibited by high concentrations of transforming growth factor-β1, and the presence of high concentrations of this factor along the walls of established bronchi may explain, in part, the lack of branching in these areas. The concurrent presence of the epithelial cell–associated proteoglycan, **syndecan**, is important for maintaining the stability of epithelial sheets along the ducts. Interacting with the extracellular matrix protein, **tenascin**, it is found along already formed ducts but not in areas where branching is occurring in terminal saccular regions of the developing airway.

As with branching morphogenesis, the formation and maintenance of epithelially lined ducts involve a special set of molecular components. Hoxb-5 is expressed during the early development of smaller bronchioles (e.g., terminal bronchioles) but not in the components of the lung that will be involved in actual respiratory exchange (i.e., respiratory bron-

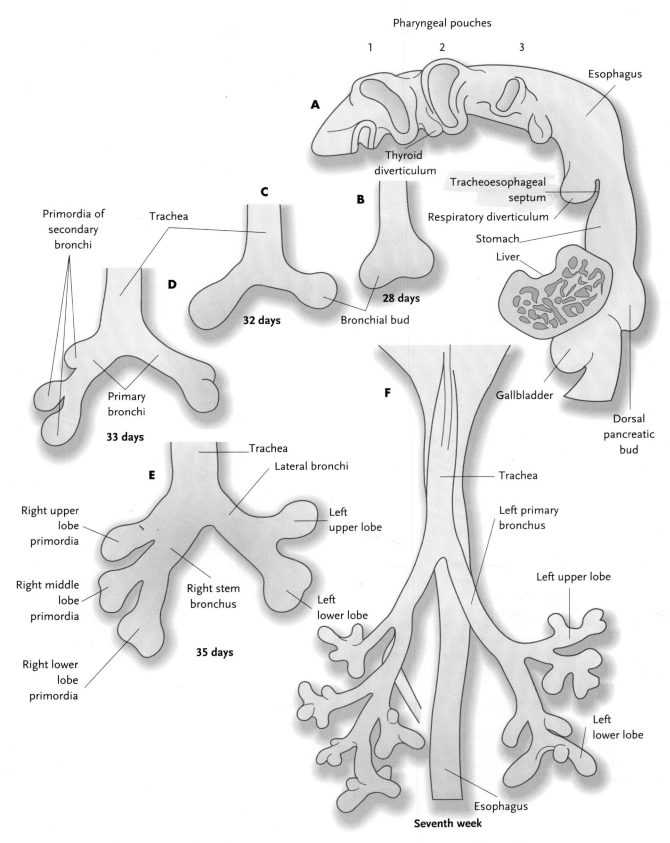

Figure 14-22 Development of the major branching patterns of the lungs. **A,** Lateral view of the pharynx, showing the respiratory diverticulum in a **4-week-old** embryo. **B,** At **4 weeks. C,** At **32 days. D,** At **33 days. E,** At the end of the **fifth week. F,** Early in the **seventh week.**

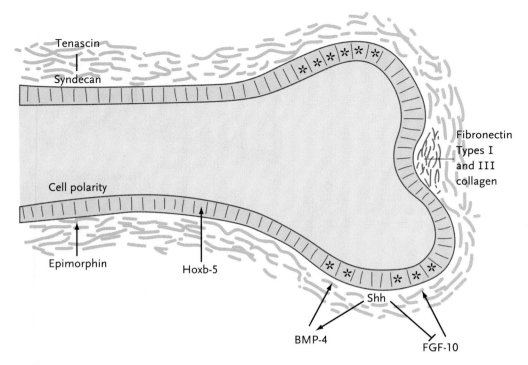

Figure 14-23 Molecular aspects of branching and duct formation in the developing lung. Asterisks indicate mitotic epithelial cells. *BMP,* Bone morphogenetic protein; *FGF,* fibroblast growth factor.

chioles, alveolar ducts, alveoli). The protein **epimorphin** is important in the later formation of epithelial tubes. Epimorphin is located in the mesenchyme and appears to provide a signal that allows overlying epithelial cells to establish proper polarity or cell arrangements. In the embryonic lung the developing epithelial ducts become disorganized and do not form lumens if epimorphin is blocked by specific antibodies.

Stages in Lung Development

Embryonic stage (weeks 4 to 7)

The embryonic stage includes the initial formation of the respiratory diverticulum up to the formation of all major bronchopulmonary segments. During this period, the developing lungs grow into and begin to fill the bilateral **pleural cavities.** These represent the major components of the thoracic body cavity above the pericardium (Figure 14-24).

Pseudoglandular stage (weeks 8 to 16)

The pseudoglandular stage is the period of major formation and growth of the duct systems within the bronchopulmonary segments before their terminal portions form respiratory components. The histological structure of the lung resembles that of a gland (Figure 14-25), thus providing the basis for the designation of this stage. During this period, the pulmonary arterial system begins to form. The elongating vessels parallel the major developing ducts.

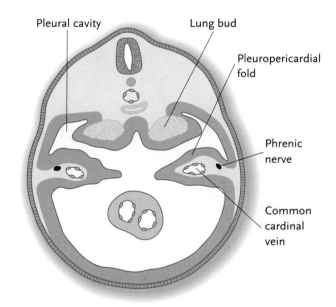

Figure 14-24 Cross section through the thorax showing the lung buds growing into the pleural cavities. The pleuropericardial folds separate the future pleural from the pericardial cavities.

Canalicular stage (weeks 17 to 26)

The canalicular stage is characterized by the formation of **respiratory bronchioles** as the result of budding of the terminal components of the system of bronchioles that formed during the pseudoglandular stage. The other major

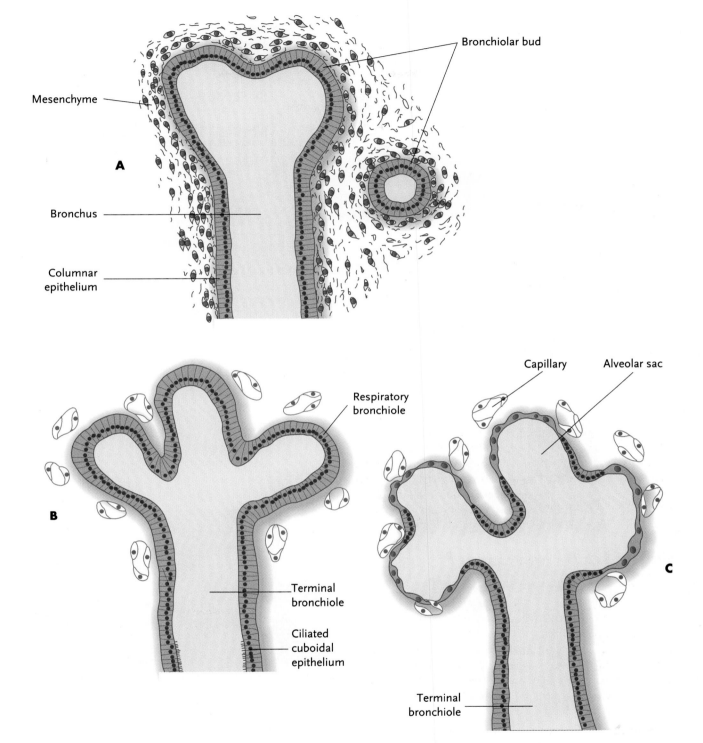

Mesenchyme

Bronchiolar bud

Bronchus

Columnar epithelium

A

Respiratory bronchiole

Terminal bronchiole

Ciliated cuboidal epithelium

B

Capillary

Alveolar sac

Terminal bronchiole

C

Figure 14-25 Stages in histogenesis of the lungs. **A,** Pseudoglandular phase (up to **17 weeks**). **B,** Canalicular phase (**17** to **26 weeks**). **C,** Terminal sac phase (**26 weeks** to birth).

CLINICAL CORRELATION 14-4
Malformations of the Respiratory System

TRACHEOESOPHAGEAL FISTULAS
The most common family of malformations of the respiratory tract is related to abnormal separation of the tracheal bud from the esophagus during early development of the respiratory system. Many common anatomical varieties of tracheoesophageal fistulas exist (Figure 14-26), but virtually all involve the stenosis or atresia of a segment of trachea or esophagus and an abnormal connection between them. These are manifested early after birth by the newborn's choking or regurgitation of milk when feeding.

TRACHEAL OR PULMONARY ATRESIA
These rare malformations are incompatible with life. They are probably caused by fundamental defects in the epithelial-mesenchymal interactions on which formation of the respiratory system depends.

GROSS MALFORMATIONS OF THE LUNGS
Because of their structural complexity, the lungs are subject to several structural variations or malformations (e.g., abnormal lobation). These are usually asymptomatic but can be foci of chronic respiratory

infection. Recognition of the possibility of these variations from normal is important for the pulmonary surgeon.

RESPIRATORY DISTRESS SYNDROME (HYALINE MEMBRANE DISEASE)
Respiratory distress syndrome is often manifested in infants born prematurely and is characterized by labored breathing. In infants who die of this condition, the lungs are underinflated, and the alveoli are partially filled with a proteinaceous fluid that forms a membrane over the respiratory surfaces (Figure 14-27). This is related to insufficiencies in the formation of surfactant by the type II alveolar cells.

CONGENITAL CYSTS IN THE LUNG
Abnormal cystic structures can form in the lung or other parts of the respiratory tract. These can range from large single cysts to numerous small cysts located throughout the parenchyma of the lung. They may be associated with polycystic kidneys. If the cysts are numerous, they can cause respiratory distress.

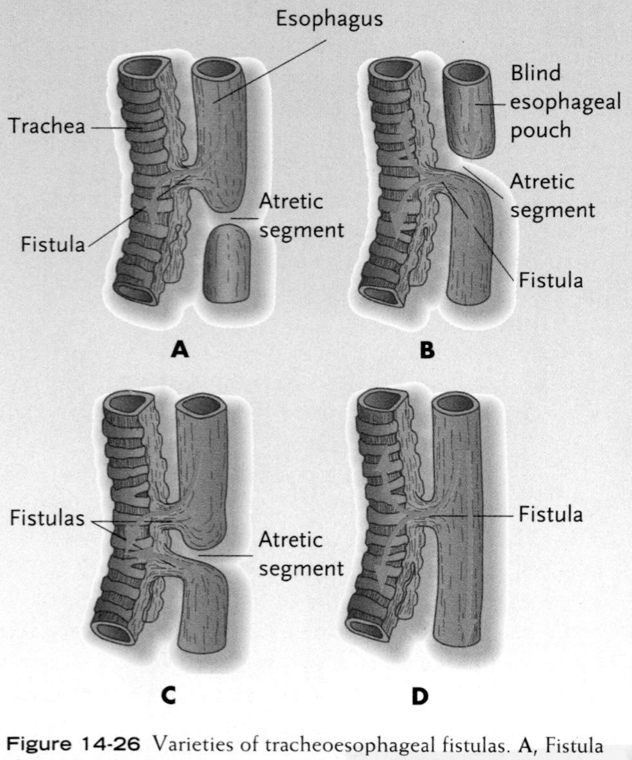

Figure 14-26 Varieties of tracheoesophageal fistulas. A, Fistula above the atretic esophageal segment. B, Fistula below the atretic esophageal segment. C, Fistulas above and below the atretic esophageal segment. D, Fistula between the patent esophagus and the trachea.

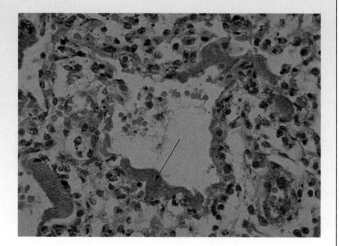
Figure 14-27 Photomicrograph from the lung of a newborn who died of hyaline membrane disease. The arrow points to the "membrane" that interferes with gas exchange. (Slide #427 from the Arey-DaPeña Pediatric Pathology Photographic Collection, Human Developmental Anatomy Center, National Museum of Health and Medicine, Armed Forces Institute of Pathology, Washington, DC.)

event during this stage is the intense ingrowth of blood vessels into the developing lungs and the close association of capillaries with the walls of the respiratory bronchioles (see Figure 14-25). Occasionally a fetus born toward the end of this period can survive with intensive care, but respiratory immaturity is the principal reason for poor viability.

Terminal sac stage (weeks 26 to birth)

During the terminal sac stage, the terminal air sacs (**alveoli**) bud off the respiratory bronchioles that largely formed during the canalicular stage. The epithelium lining the alveoli differentiates into two types of cells: **type I alveolar cells** (pneumocytes), across which gas exchange occurs after birth, and **type II secretory epithelial cells**. These latter cells form **pulmonary surfactant**, the material that spreads over the surface of the alveoli to reduce surface tension and facilitate expansion of the alveoli during breathing. Research involving specific markers of the epithelial cells has shown that the type II cells form first in the alveolar lining. After proliferation, some type II cells flatten, lose their characteristic secretory function, and undergo terminal differentiation into type I pneumocytes. Other type I cells may differentiate directly from a pool of epithelial precursor cells in the early alveolar lining. With increasing amounts of pulmonary surfactant being formed, the fetus has a correspondingly greater chance of survival if born prematurely. In the fetus the respiratory passageways in the lungs are filled with fluid (see Chapter 17). During the last 4 weeks of pregnancy, greatly increased formation of alveoli results in an exponential increase in the respiratory surface area of the lung. These weeks are sometimes referred to as the *alveolar period of lung development.*

Postnatal stage

At birth the mammalian lung is far from mature. An estimated 90% or more of the roughly 300 million alveoli found in the mature human lung are formed after birth. The major mechanism for this increase is the formation of secondary connective tissue septa that divide existing alveolar sacs. When they first appear, the secondary septa are relatively thick. In time, they transform into thinner mature septa capable of full respiratory exchange function.

BODY CAVITIES

Formation of the Common Coelom and Mesentery

As the lateral mesoderm of the early embryo splits and then folds laterally, the space between the somatic and splanchnic layers of mesoderm becomes the common **intraembryonic coelom** (Figure 14-28) (see Chapter 5). The same folding process that results in the completion of the ventral body

wall and the separation of the intraembryonic from the extraembryonic coelom also brings the two layers of splanchnic mesoderm around the newly formed gut as the **primary**, or **common, mesentery**. The primary mesentery suspends the gut from the dorsal body wall as the **dorsal mesentery** and attaches it to the ventral body wall as the **ventral mesentery**. This placement effectively divides the coelom into right and left components. Soon, however, most of the ventral mesentery breaks down and causes a confluence of the right and left halves of the coelom. In the region of the developing stomach and liver the ventral mesentery persists, forming the **ventral mesogastrium** and the falciform ligament of the liver (see Figure 14-3). Further cranially the tubular primordium of the heart is similarly supported by a **dorsal mesocardium** and briefly by a **ventral mesocardium**, which soon breaks down.

Formation of the Septum Transversum and Pleural Canals

A major factor in division of the common coelom into thoracic and abdominal components is the **septum transversum**. This septum grows from the ventral body wall as a semicircular shelf, separating the heart from the developing liver (Figure 14-29). During its early development, a major portion of the liver is embedded in the septum transversum. Ultimately, the septum transversum constitutes a significant component of the diaphragm (see p. 352).

The expanding septum transversum serves as a partial partition between the pericardial and peritoneal portions of the coelom. By the time the expanding edge of the septum transversum reaches the floor of the foregut, it has almost cut the common coelom into two parts. Two short channels located on either side of the foregut, however, connect the two major parts (Figure 14-30). Initially known as the **pleural (pericardioperitoneal) canals**, these channels represent the spaces into which the developing lungs grow. The pleural canals enlarge greatly as the lungs increase in size and ultimately form the **pleural cavities**.

The pleural canals are partially delimited by two paired folds of tissue: the pleuropericardial and pleuroperitoneal folds. The **pleuropericardial folds** (see Figure 14-24) are ridges of tissue associated with the common cardinal veins, which bulge into the dorsolateral wall of the coelom as they arch toward the midline of the thoracic portion of the coelom and enter the sinus venosus of the heart (Figure 14-31). Initially, the pleuropericardial folds are not large and cause only a narrowing at the junction of the pericardial cavity and pleural canals. However, as the lungs expand, the folds form prominent shelves that meet at the midline, forming the fibrous (parietal) layer of the pericardium.

Associated with the pleuropericardial folds are the paired **phrenic nerves**. These arise from joined branches of cervical roots 3, 4, and 5 and supply the muscle fibers of the diaphragm. With the shifts in positions of various components of the body

Text continued on p. 352

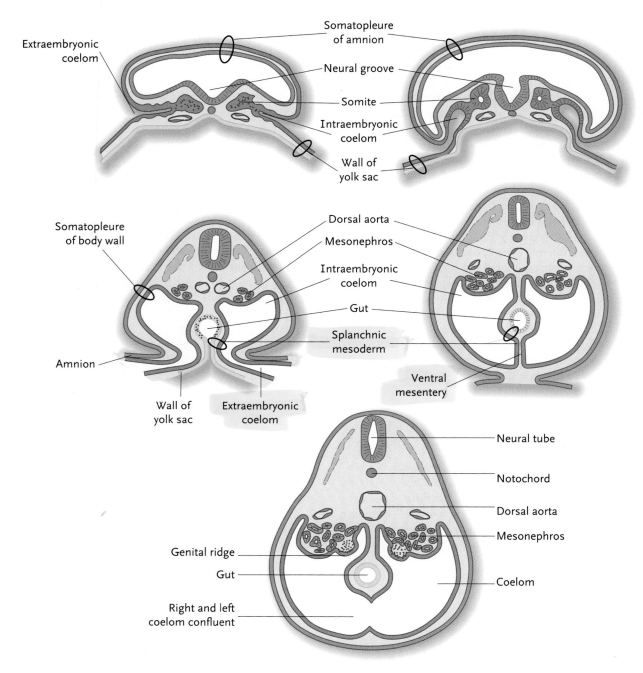

Figure 14-28 Early stages in the development of the coelom and mesenteries. (Modified from Carlson B: *Patten's foundations of embryology,* ed 6, New York, 1996, McGraw-Hill.)

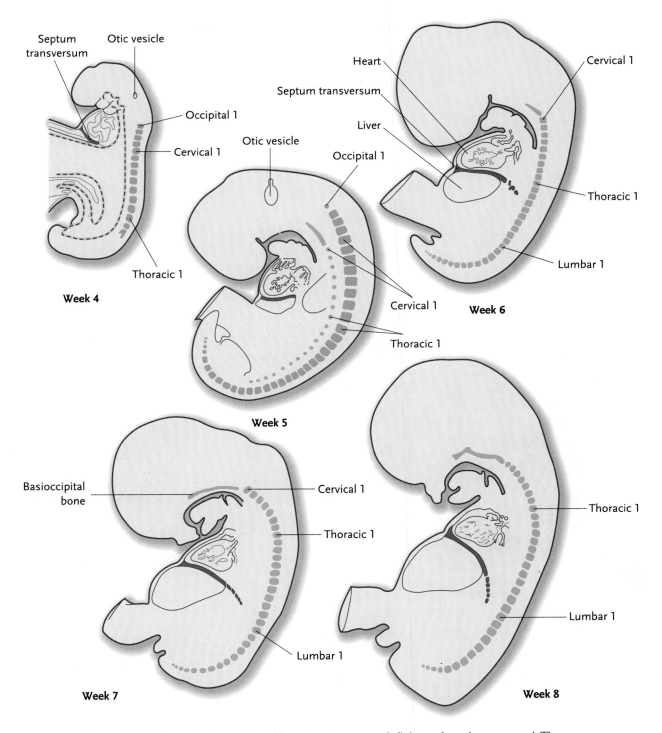

Figure 14-29 Changes in the position of the septum transversum (*red*) during the embryonic period. The gray repeating structures are somites. The orange repeating structures are elements of the axial skeleton.

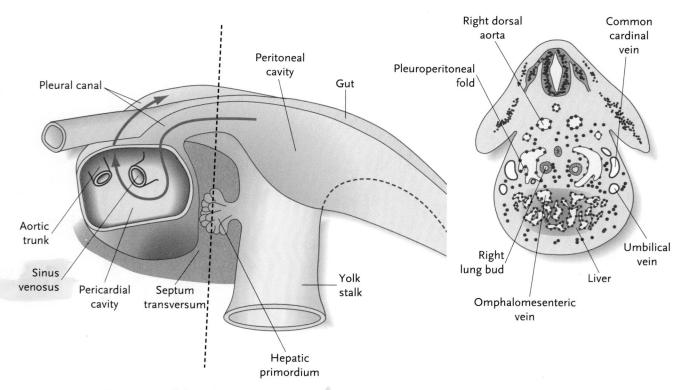

Figure 14-30 Relationships among the pericardial cavity, pleural canals, and peritoneal cavity. The red arrow passes from the left pleural cavity into the pericardial cavity and then into the right pleural canal. The dashed line on the left represents the level of the cross section on the right.

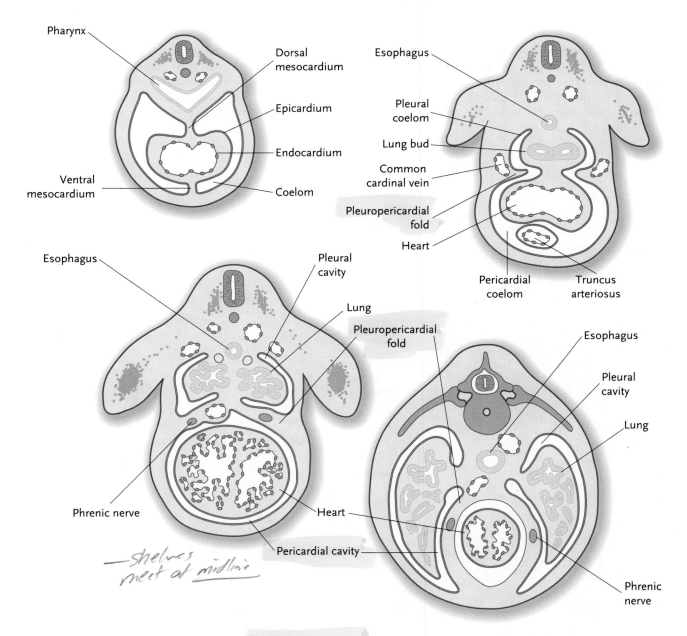

Figure 14-31 Development of the pleuropericardial folds. (Modified from Carlson B: *Patten's foundations of embryology,* ed 6, New York, 1996, McGraw-Hill.)

during growth, the diaphragm ultimately descends to the level of the lower thoracic vertebrae. As it does, it carries the phrenic nerves with it. Even in adults the pathway of the phrenic nerves through the fibrous pericardium is a reminder of their early association with the pleuropericardial folds.

At the caudal ends of the pleural canals, another pair of folds, the **pleuroperitoneal folds**, becomes prominent as the expanding lungs push into the mesoderm of the body wall. The pleuroperitoneal folds occupy successively greater portions of the pleural canal until they fuse with the septum transversum and the mesentery of the esophagus, effectively obliterating the pleural canal (Figure 14-32). All connections between the abdominal cavity and the thoracic cavity are thus eliminated.

Formation of the Diaphragm

The **diaphragm**, which separates the thoracic from the abdominal cavity in adults, is a composite structure derived from several embryonic components (see Figure 14-32). The large ventral component of the diaphragm arises from the septum transversum, which fuses with the ventral part of the esophageal mesentery. Converging on the esophageal mesentery from the dorsolateral sides are the pleuroperitoneal folds. These components form the bulk of the diaphragm. As the lungs continue to grow, their caudal tips excavate additional space in the body wall. The body wall mesenchyme separated from the body wall proper becomes a third component of the diaphragm by forming a thin rim of tissue along its dorsolateral borders.

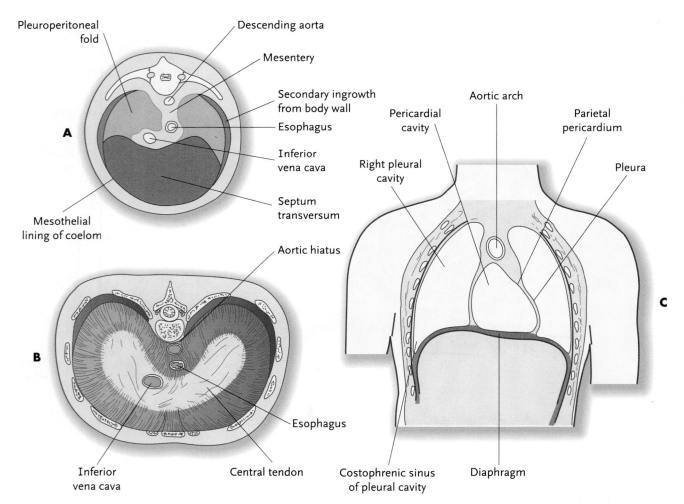

Figure 14-32 Stages in the formation of the diaphragm. **A,** Components making up the embryonic diaphragm. **B,** Adult diaphragm as seen from the thoracic side. **C,** Frontal section showing relations of the diaphragm to the pleural and pericardial cavities.

VENTRAL BODY WALL DEFECTS, ECTOPIA CORDIS, GASTROSCHISIS, AND OMPHALOCELE

The opposing sides of the body wall occasionally fail to fuse as the embryo assumes its cylindrical shape late in the first month. Several defective mechanisms such as hypoplasia of the tissues can account for these defects. A quantitatively minor defect in closure of the thoracic wall is manifested as **failure of sternal fusion** (Figure 14-33). If growth of the two sides of the thoracic wall is severely defective, the heart can form outside the thoracic cavity, resulting in **ectopia cordis** (Figure 14-34).

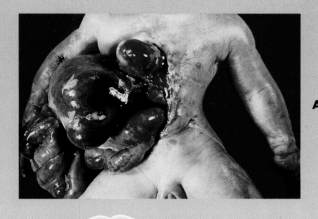

A

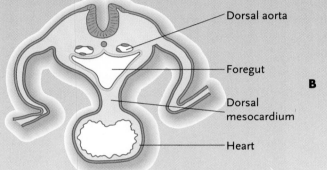

B

- Dorsal aorta
- Foregut
- Dorsal mesocardium
- Heart

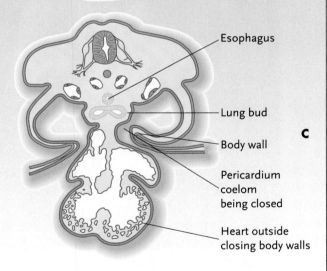

C

- Esophagus
- Lung bud
- Body wall
- Pericardium coelom being closed
- Heart outside closing body walls

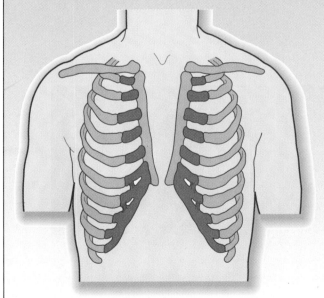

Figure 14-33 Failure of fusion of the paired components of the embryonic sternum.

Figure 14-34 Ectopia cordis. **A**, Fetus with a major ventral abdominal wall defect that combines gastroschisis and ectopia cordis. **B** and **C**, Cross sections illustrating the inability of the folding sides of the body wall to encompass the developing heart, resulting in ectopia cordis. (Courtesy M. Barr, Ann Arbor, Mich.)

Continued

CLINICAL CORRELATION 14-5
Malformations of the Body Cavities, Diaphragm, and Body Wall—cont'd

Closure defects of the ventral abdominal wall can lead to similar gross malformations. In many cases of omphalocele (see Figure 14-12), hypoplasia of the abdominal wall itself or deficiencies of abdominal musculature are evident. More serious cases involve evisceration of the abdominal contents through a fissure between the umbilicus and sternum **(gastroschisis)** (Figure 14-35). Caudal to the umbilicus, an associated closure defect of the urinary bladder (exstrophy of the bladder [see Figure 15-19]) is common.

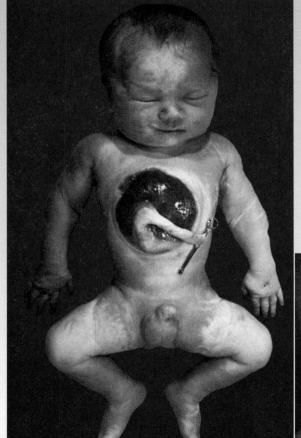

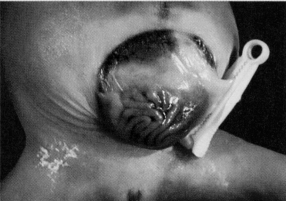

Figure 14-35 Defective closure of the ventral abdominal wall cranial (**A**) and caudal (**B**) to the umbilicus.(Courtesy M. Barr, Ann Arbor, Mich.)

CLINICAL CORRELATION 14-5
Malformations of the Body Cavities, Diaphragm, and Body Wall—cont'd

DIAPHRAGMATIC HERNIAS

Incomplete fusion or hypoplasia of one or more of the components of the diaphragm can lead to an open connection between the abdominal and thoracic cavities. If the defect is large enough, a variety of structures in the abdominal cavity (usually part of the stomach or intestines) can herniate into the thoracic cavity, or more rarely, thoracic structures can penetrate into the abdominal cavity. Minor cases of herniation can cause digestive symptoms. In the case of major defects, herniation of massive portions of the intestines can press against the heart or lungs and interfere with their function. Some common sites of defects in the diaphragm are shown in Figure 14-36.

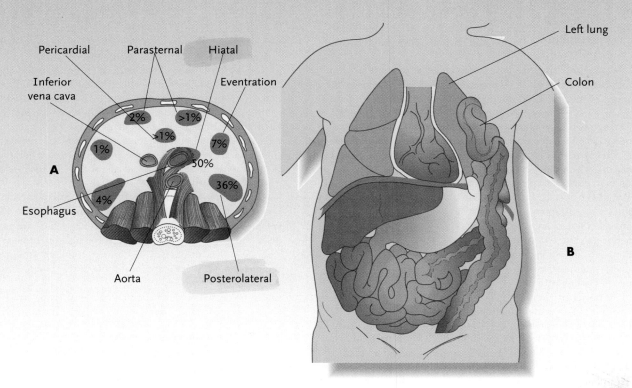

Figure 14-36 A, Common sites of diaphragmatic hernias. Percentages of occurrence are indicated. B, Diaphragmatic hernia with intestines entering the left pleural cavity and compressing the left lung.

CLINICAL VIGNETTE

A 14-year-old girl was troubled for several years with moderately severe upper abdominal pains that recurred on a fairly regular basis at roughly monthly intervals. After passing through several pediatric and medical clinics without obtaining relief, she was sent to a psychiatrist, who also could not resolve her symptoms. Finally, an astute physician suspected that her symptoms might be caused by a congenital anomaly. Further testing and ultimately surgery proved this suspicion to be correct.

What was the diagnosis?

SUMMARY

- The digestive system arises from the primitive endodermally lined gut tube, which is bounded cranially by the oropharyngeal membrane and caudally by the cloacal membrane. The gut is divided into foregut, midgut, and hindgut segments, with the midgut opening into the yolk sac. Development of virtually all parts of the gut depends on epithelial-mesenchymal interactions. Responding to such interactions, primordia of the respiratory system, the liver, the pancreas, and other digestive glands bud out from the original gut tube.

- The esophagus takes shape as a simple tubular structure between the pharynx and stomach. At one stage the epithelium occludes the lumen of the esophagus; the lumen later recanalizes. The developing stomach is suspended from a dorsal and ventral mesogastrium. Through two types of rotation, the stomach attains its adult position. Common malformations of the stomach are pyloric stenosis, which interferes with emptying of the stomach, and ectopic gastric mucosa, which can produce ulcers in unexpected locations.

- As they grow, the intestines form a hairpin loop that herniates into the body stalk. Further growth of the small intestine causes small intestinal loops to accumulate in the body stalk. While the intestines retract into the body cavity, they rotate around the superior mesenteric artery. This results in the characteristic positioning of the colon around the small intestine in the abdominal cavity. During these changes in position, parts of the dorsal mesentery fuse with the peritoneal lining of the dorsal body wall. In the posterior part of the gut the urorectal septum partitions the cloaca into the rectum and urogenital sinus.

- During its differentiation, the lining of the intestinal tract passes through phases of (1) epithelial proliferation, (2) cellular differentiation, and (3) biochemical and functional maturation. Like the esophagus, the small intestine goes through a period of occlusion of the lumen by the epithelium. At later stages, intestinal crypts located at the base of villi contain epithelial stem cells, which supply the entire intestinal epithelial surface with various epithelial cells.

- The intestinal tract is subject to a variety of malformations, including local stenosis, atresia, duplications, diverticula, and abnormal rotation. Incomplete resorption of the vitelline duct can give rise to Meckel's diverticulum, vitelline duct ligaments, cysts, or fistulas. Omphalocele is the failure of the intestines to return to the body cavity from the body stalk. Aganglionic megacolon is caused by the failure of parasympathetic neurons to populate the distal part of the colon. Failure of the anal membrane to break down

(imperforate anus) may be associated with fistulas connecting the digestive tract to various regions of the urogenital system.

- Digestive glands arise as epithelial diverticula from the gut. Their formation and further outgrowth are based on inductive interactions with the surrounding mesenchyme. The primordium of the liver arises in the septum transversum, but as it expands, it protrudes into the ventral mesentery. As it develops, the liver acquires the capacity to synthesize and secrete serum albumin and to store glycogen among other biochemical functions. The pancreas grows out as dorsal and ventral pancreatic buds that ultimately fuse to form a single pancreas. Within the pancreas the epithelium forms exocrine components, which secrete digestive enzymes, and endocrine components (islets of Langerhans), which secrete insulin and glucagon.

- The respiratory system arises as a ventral outgrowth from the gut just caudal to the pharynx. Through epithelial-mesenchymal interactions the tip of the respiratory diverticulum undergoes up to 23 sets of dichotomous branchings. Other interactions with the surrounding mesenchyme stabilize the tubular parts of the respiratory tract by inhibiting branching. Lung development goes through several stages: (1) the embryonic stage, (2) the pseudoglandular stage, (3) the canalicular stage, (4) the terminal sac stage, and (5) the postnatal stage.

- Important malformations of the respiratory tract include tracheoesophageal fistulas, which result in abnormal connections between the trachea and esophagus. Atresia of components of the respiratory system is rare, but anatomical variations in the morphology of the lungs are common. Respiratory distress syndrome, commonly seen in premature infants, is related to insufficiencies in the formation of pulmonary surfactant by type II alveolar cells.

- In its most basic condition the intraembryonic coelom is separated into right and left components by the dorsal and ventral mesenteries, which suspend the gut. Except for the region of the stomach and liver, the ventral mesentery disappears. In the region of the heart the dorsal mesocardium persists, and the ventral mesocardium disappears.

- The septum transversum divides the coelom into thoracic and abdominal regions, which are connected by pleural canals. The developing lungs grow into the pleural canals, which are partially delimited by paired pleuropericardial and pleuroperitoneal folds. The definitive diaphragm is formed from (1) the septum transversum, (2) pleuroperitoneal folds, and (3) ingrowths from body wall mesenchyme.

- Quantitative deficiencies in ventral body wall tissue can result in abnormalities ranging from failure of sternal fusion to ectopia cordis in the thorax and omphalocele to gastroschisis and/or exstrophy of the bladder in the abdomen. Defects in the diaphragm are diaphragmatic hernias and can result in the intestines herniating into the thoracic cavity.

REVIEW QUESTIONS

1. Which condition is most closely associated with a disturbance of neural crest?
    A. Anal atresia
    B. Meckel's diverticulum
    C. Omphalocoele
    D. Volvulus
    E. Aganglionic megacolon

2. Meckel's diverticulum is most commonly located in the:
   A. Ileum
   B. Ascending colon
   C. Jejunum
   D. Transverse colon
   E. Duodenum
3. The primordium of which structure is located in the septum transversum?
   A. Dorsal pancreas
   B. Lung
   C. Liver
   D. Thymus
   E. Spleen
4. The yolk stalk is most closely associated with which artery?
   A. Celiac
   B. Umbilical
   C. Superior mesenteric
   D. Aorta
   E. Inferior mesenteric
5. The dorsal pancreatic bud is initially induced from the gut endoderm by the:
   A. Liver
   B. Notochord
   C. Lung bud
   D. Yolk sac
   E. None of the above
6. Splanchnic mesoderm acts as an inducer of all of the following tissues or organs except:
   A. Teeth
   B. Trachea
   C. Liver
   D. Lungs
   E. Pancreas
7. During its first feeding, a newborn begins to choke. What congenital anomalies should be included in the differential diagnosis?
8. A newborn took its first feeding of milk without incident but an hour later was crying in pain and vomited the milk with considerable force. Examination of revealed a hard mass near the midline in the upper region of the abdomen. What was the diagnosis?
9. An infant was noted to extrude a small amount of mucus and fluid from the umbilicus when crying or straining. This should make the physician think of what congenital anomaly in the differential diagnosis?
10. A newborn was given a cursory physical examination and was taken home by the mother 1 day after delivery. Several days later the mother brought the child to the clinic. The newborn was in obvious severe discomfort with a swollen abdomen. Physical examination revealed that an important congenital anomaly had been overlooked at the original examination. What was that anomaly?

REFERENCES

Alescio T, Cassini A: Induction in vitro of tracheal buds by pulmonary mesenchyme grafted on tracheal epithelium, *J Exp Zool* 150:83-94, 1962.

Avery ME, Wang N-S, Taeusch HW: The lung of the newborn infant, *Sci Am* 228:74-85, 1973.

Bellusci S and others: Evidence from normal expression and targeted misexpression that bone morphogenetic protein-4 (Bmp-4) plays a role in mouse embryonic lung morphogenesis, *Development* 122:1693-1702, 1996.

Bellusci S and others: Fibroblast growth factor 10 (FGF10) and branching morphogenesis in the embryonic mouse lung, *Development* 124:4867-4878, 1997.

Boyden EA: Development of the human lung, *Pract Pediatr* 4:1-17, 1975.

Brauker JH, Trautman MS, Bernfield M: Syndecan, a cell surface proteoglycan, exhibits a molecular polymorphism during lung development, *Dev Biol* 111:213-220, 1991.

Burri PH: Fetal and postnatal development of the lung, *Ann Rev Physiol* 46:617-628, 1984.

Cardoso WV: Transcription factors and pattern formation in the developing lung, *Am J Physiol (Lung Cell Mol Physiol 13)* 269:L429-L442, 1995.

Carlson B: *Patten's foundations of embryology*, ed 6, New York, 1996, McGraw-Hill.

Chytil F: Retinoids in lung development, *FASEB J* 10:986-992, 1996.

Colony PC: Successive phases of human fetal development. In Kretchmer N, Minkowski A, eds: *Nutritional adaptation of the gastrointestinal tract of the newborn*, New York, 1983, Raven, pp 3-28.

Duluc I and others: Fetal endoderm primarily holds the temporal and positional information required for mammalian intestinal development, *J Cell Biol* 126:211-221, 1994.

Gittes GK and others: Lineage-specific morphogenesis in the developing pancreas: role of mesenchymal factors, *Development* 122:439-447, 1996.

Gordon JI, Hermiston ML: Differentiation and self-renewal in the mouse gastrointestinal epithelium, *Curr Opin Cell Biol* 6:795-803, 1994.

Gray SW, Skandalakis JE: *Embryology for surgeons*, Philadelphia, 1972, WB Saunders.

Hilfer SR: Morphogenesis of the lung: control of embryonic and fetal branching, *Annu Rev Physiol* 58:93-113, 1996.

Hirai Y and others: Epimorphin: a mesenchymal protein essential for epithelial morphogenesis, *Cell* 69:471-481, 1992.

Hollinshead WH: Embryology and anatomy of the anal canal and rectum, *Dis Colon Rectum* 5:18-22, 1962.

Hollinshead WH: Embryology and surgical anatomy of the colon, *Dis Colon Rectum* 5:23-27, 1962.

Jackson CM: On the developmental topography of the thoracic and abdominal viscera, *Anat Rec* 3:361-396, 1909.

Jacobs-Cohen RJ and others: Inability of neural crest cells to colonize the presumptive aganglionic bowel of ls/ls mutant mice: requirement for a permissive environment, *J Comp Neurol* 255:425-438, 1987.

Kappen C: *Hox* genes in the lung, *Am J Respir Cell Mol Biol* 15:156-162, 1996.

Kedinger M and others: Epithelial-mesenchymal interactions in intestinal epithelial differentiation, *Scand J Gastroenterol* 23(suppl 151):62-69, 1988.

Kim SK, Hebrok M, Melton DA: Notochord to endoderm signaling is required for pancreas development, *Development* 124:4243-4252, 1997.

Le Douarin NM: An experimental analysis of liver development, *Med Biol* 53:427-455, 1975.

Lewis FT: The form of the stomach in human embryos with notes upon the nomenclature of the stomach, *Am J Anat* 13:477-503, 1912.

Mall FP: Development of the human coelom, *J Morphol* 12:395-453, 1897.

McGowan SE: Extracellular matrix and the regulation of lung development and repair, *FASEB J* 6:2895-2904, 1992.

McHugh KM: Molecular analysis of gastrointestinal smooth muscle development, *J Pediatr Gastroenterol Nutr* 23:379-394, 1996.

Moens CB and others: A targeted mutation reveals a role for N-*myc* in branching morphogenesis in the embryonic mouse lung, *Genes Dev* 6:691-704, 1992.

Mueller TS and others: Expression of avian Pax1 and Pax9 is intrinsically regulated in the pharyngeal endoderm, but depends on environmental influences in the paraxial mesoderm, *Dev Biol* 178:403-417, 1996.

O'Rahilly R: The timing and sequence of events in the development of the human digestive system and associated structures during the embryonic period proper, *Anat Embryol* 153:123-136, 1978.

O'Rahilly R, Boyden EA: The timing and sequence of events in the development of the human respiratory system during the embryonic period proper, *Z Anat Entwickl-Gesch* 141:237-250, 1973.

O'Rahilly R, Tucker JA: The early development of the larynx in staged human embryos, *Ann Otolaryngol Rhinol Laryngol* 82(suppl 7):1-27, 1973.

Patapoutian A, Wold BJ, Wagner RA: Evidence for developmentally programmed transdifferentiation in mouse esophageal muscle, *Science* 270:1818-1821, 1995.

Pictet R, Rutter WJ: Development of the embryonic endocrine pancreas. In *Handbook of physiology*, section 7: *Endocrinology*, vol 1, Washington, DC, 1972, American Physiological Society, pp 25-66.

Ponder BAJ and others: Derivations of mouse intestinal crypts from single progenitor cells, *Nature* 313:689-691, 1985.

Potten CS, Loeffler M: Stem cells: attributes, cycles, spirals, pitfalls and uncertainties—lessons for and from the crypt, *Development* 110:1001-1020, 1990.

Roberts DJ and others: Sonic hedgehog is an endodermal signal inducing *Bmp-4* and *Hox* genes during induction and regionalization of the chick hindgut, *Development* 121:3163-3174, 1995.

Schuger L and others: Amphiregulin in lung branching morphogenesis: interaction with heparan sulfate proteoglycan modulates cell proliferation, *Development* 122:1759-1767, 1996.

Simon-Assman P and others: Extracellular matrix components in intestinal development, *Experientia* 51:883-900, 1995.

Skandalakis LJ and others: Surgical embryology and anatomy of the pancreas, *Surg Clin North Am* 73:661-697, 1993.

Slack JMW: Developmental biology of the pancreas, *Development* 121:1569-1580, 1995.

Stephens FD: Embryology of the cloaca and embryogenesis of anorectal malformations, *Birth Defects Orig Artic Ser* 24:177-209, 1988.

Teitleman G, Lee JK: Cell lineage analysis of pancreatic islet cell development: glucagon and insulin precursors arise from catecholaminergic precursors present in the pancreatic duct, *Dev Biol* 121:454-466, 1987.

Thompson ABR, Keelan M: The development of the small intestine, *Can J Physiol Pharmacol* 64:13-29, 1986.

Volpe MAV and others: Hoxb-5 expression in the developing mouse lung suggests a role in branching morphogenesis and epithelial cell fate, *Histochem Cell Biol* 108:495-504, 1997.

Warot X and others: Gene dosage-dependent effects of the Hoxa-13 and Hoxd-13 mutations on morphogenesis of the terminal parts of the digestive and urogenital tracts, *Development* 124:4781-4791, 1997.

Wells LJ: Development of the human diaphragm and pleural sacs, *Carnegie Contr Embryol* 35:107-134, 1954.

Wells LJ, Boyden EA: The development of the human bronchopulmonary segments in human embryos of horizons XVII to XIX, *Am J Anat* 95:163-201, 1954.

Wessels NK: *Tissue interactions and development*, Menlo Park, Calif, 1977, WA Benjamin.

Yasugi S, Mizuno T: Mesenchymal-epithelial interactions in the organogenesis of the digestive tract, *Zool Sci* 7:159-170, 1990.

Yokouchi Y, Sakiyama J-I, Kuroiwa A: Coordinated expression of Abd-B subfamily genes of the HoxA cluster in the developing digestive tract of chick embryo, *Dev Biol* 169:76-89, 1995.

Zaret KS: Molecular genetics of early liver development, *Annu Rev Physiol* 58:231-251, 1996.

15

UROGENITAL SYSTEM

The urogenital system arises from the intermediate mesoderm of the early embryo (see Figure 5-15). Several major themes underlie the development of urinary and genital structures from this common precursor. The first is the interconnectedness of urinary and genital development, in which early components of one system are taken over by another during its later development. A second is the recapitulation during human ontogeny of kidney types (the equivalent of organ isoforms) that are terminal forms of the kidney in lower vertebrates. A third theme is the dependence of differentiation and maintenance of many structures in the urogenital system on epithelial-mesenchymal interactions. Finally, the sexual differentiation of many structures passes from an indifferent stage, in which male and female differences are not readily apparent, to a male or female pathway depending on the presence of specific promoting or inhibiting factors acting on the structure. Although phenotypic sex is genetically determined, genetic sex can be overridden by environmental factors, leading to a discordance between the two. Clinical Correlations 15-1 and 15-2 discuss abnormalities of the urinary and genital systems, respectively. These are found at the end of each section.

URINARY SYSTEM

The urinary system begins to take shape before any gonadal development is evident. Embryogenesis of the kidney begins with the formation of an elongated pair of excretory organs similar in structure and function to the kidneys of lower vertebrates. These early forms of the kidney are later supplanted by the definitive metanephric kidneys, but as they regress, certain components are retained to be reused by other components of the urogenital system.

Early Forms of the Kidney

The common representation of mammalian kidney development includes three successive phases beginning with the appearance of the **pronephros**, the developmental homo-

logue of the type of kidney found in only the lowest vertebrates. In human embryos the first evidence of a urinary system consists of the appearance of a few segmentally arranged sets of epithelial cords that differentiate from the anterior intermediate mesoderm at about 22 days' gestation. These structures are more appropriately called **nephrotomes**. The nephrotomes connect laterally with a pair of **primary nephric (pronephric) ducts**, which grow toward the cloaca (Figure 15-1). The molecular basis for the initiation of kidney development remains poorly understood, but knockout experiments have suggested that the homeodomain genes, **Lim-1** and **Pax-2**, are important in the earliest stages of kidney development.

As the primary nephric ducts extend caudally, they stimulate the intermediate mesoderm to form additional segmental sets of tubules. These tubules are structurally equivalent to the **mesonephric tubules** of fishes and amphibians. A typical mesonephric unit consists of a vascular **glomerulus**, which is partially surrounded by an epithelial glomerular capsule. The glomerular capsule is continuous with a contorted mesonephric tubule, which is surrounded by a mesh of capillaries (see Figure 15-1, B). Each mesonephric tubule empties separately into the continuation of the primary nephric duct, which becomes known as the **mesonephric (wolffian) duct**.

The formation of pairs of mesonephric tubules occurs along a craniocaudal gradient. The first four to six pairs of mesonephric tubules (as well as the pronephric tubules) appear to arise as outgrowths from the primary nephric ducts. Farther caudally, mesonephric tubules take shape separately in the intermediate mesoderm slightly behind the caudal extension of the mesonephric ducts. By the end of the fourth week of gestation the mesonephric ducts attach to the cloaca, and a continuous lumen is present throughout each. There is a difference in the developmental controls between the most cranial four to six pairs of mesonephric ducts and the remaining caudal ones. Knockouts for the **WT-1** (Wilms' tumor suppressor) gene result in the absence of posterior mesonephric tubules, whereas the cranial ones that bud off the pronephric duct form normally. As is the case in the for-

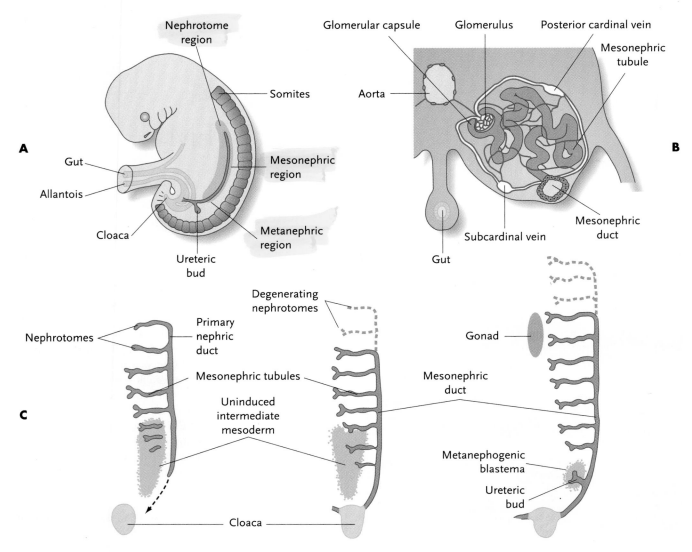

Figure 15-1 Early stages in the establishment of the urinary system. **A,** Subdivision of the intermediate mesoderm into areas that will form nephrotomes, mesonephros, and metanephros. **B,** Cross section through mesonephros showing a well-developed mesonephric tubule and its associated vasculature. **C,** Caudal progression of formation of the mesonephros and degeneration of the most cranial segments of the primitive kidney.

mation of the metanephros (see below), WT-1 appears to regulate the transformation from mesenchyme to epithelium during the early formation of renal (mesonephric) tubules. Very near its attachment site to the cloaca, the mesonephric duct develops an epithelial outgrowth called the **ureteric bud** (see Figure 15-1, *A*). Early in the fifth week the ureteric bud begins to grow into the most posterior region of the intermediate mesoderm. It then sets up a series of continuous inductive interactions leading to the formation of the definitive kidney, the **metanephros.**

Although there is evidence of urinary function in the mammalian mesonephric kidney, the physiology of the mesonephros has not been extensively .investigated. Urine formation in the mesonephros begins with a filtrate of blood

from the glomerulus into the glomerular capsule. This filtrate then flows into the tubular portion of the mesonephros, where the selective resorption of ions and other substances occurs. The return of resorbed materials to the blood is facilitated by the presence of a dense plexus of capillaries around the mesonephric tubules.

The structure of the human embryonic mesonephros is very similar to that of adult fishes and aquatic amphibians, and it functions principally to filter and remove body wastes. Because these species and the amniote embryo exist in an aquatic environment, there is little need to conserve water. Therefore the mesonephros does not develop a medullary region or an elaborate system for concentrating urine as the adult human kidney must.

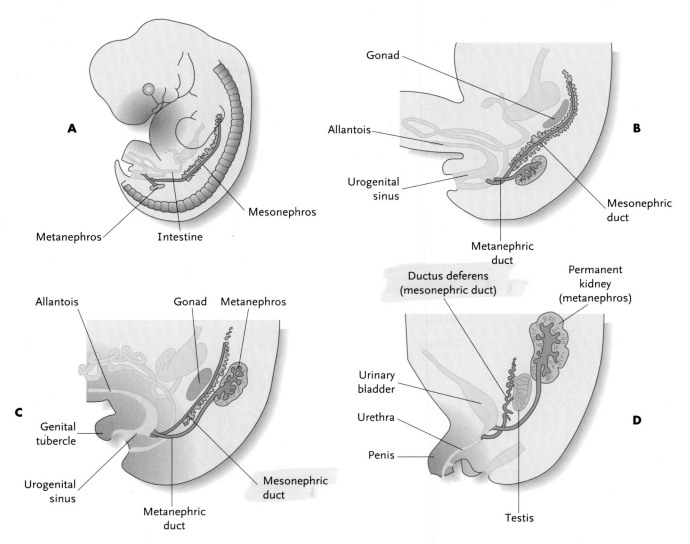

Figure 15-2 Stages in the formation of the metanephros. **A,** At **6 weeks. B,** At **7 weeks. C,** At **8 weeks. D,** At **3 months** (male).

The mesonephros is most prominent while the definitive metanephros is taking shape. Although it rapidly regresses as a urinary unit after the metanephric kidneys become functional, the mesonephric ducts and some of the mesonephric tubules persist in the male and become incorporated as integral components of the genital duct system (Figure 15-2)

Metanephros

Development of the metanephros begins early in the fifth week, when the ureteric bud (**metanephric diverticulum**) grows into the posterior portion of the intermediate mesoderm. Mesenchymal cells of the intermediate mesoderm condense around the metanephric diverticulum to form the **metanephrogenic blastema** (see Figure 15-1, C). Outgrowth of the ureteric bud from the mesonephric duct is a response to the secretion of **glial cell line–derived neurotrophic factor (GDNF)** by the undifferentiated mesenchyme of the metanephrogenic blastema (Figure 15-3). This inductive signal is bound by **c-Ret,** a member of the tyrosine kinase receptor superfamily, which is located in the plasma membranes of the epithelial cells of the early ureteric bud. The formation of GDNF in the metanephric mesenchyme is regulated by **WT-1.**

The morphological basis for the development of the metanephric kidney is the elongation and branching (up to 14 or 15 times) of the ureteric bud, which becomes the col-

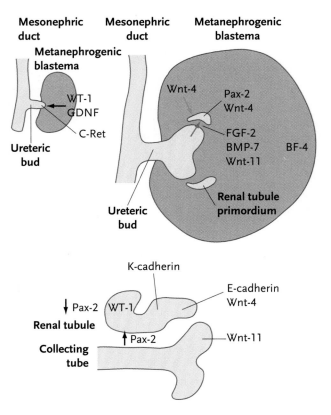

Figure 15-3 Molecular basis for the early formation of the metanephros and ureter. *BMP,* Bone morphogenetic protein; *FGF,* fibroblast growth factor; *GDNF,* glial cell line–derived neurotrophic factor.

lecting (**metanephric**) **duct** system of the metanephros, and the formation of renal tubules from mesenchymal condensations (metanephrogenic blastema) located around the tips of the branches. The mechanism underlying these events is a series of reciprocal inductive interactions between the tips of the branches of the metanephric ducts and the surrounding metanephrogenic blastemal cells. Without the metanephric duct system, tubules do not form; conversely, the metanephrogenic mesoderm acts on the metanephric duct system, inducing its characteristic branching. In response to the GDNF inductive signal by the metanephric mesenchyme, the epithelial cells of the ureteric bud produce **fibroblast growth factor (FGF-2), bone morphogenetic protein (BMP-7),** and **Wnt-11,** which induce the surrounding metanephric mesenchyme to begin to form the epithelial precursors of renal tubules. Tubule formation also requires a sequential inductive signal, **Wnt-4,** which is produced by the metanephric mesenchyme itself. This early induction patterns the metanephric mesenchyme into a tubular epithelial domain, in which the cells express Wnt-4 and Pax-2, and a stromal region, in which the mesenchymal cells express a winged helix transcription factor, **BF-2.**

The formation of individual functional tubules (**nephrons**) in the developing metanephros involves three mesodermal cell lineages: epithelial cells derived from the ureteric bud, mesenchymal cells of the metanephrogenic blastema, and ingrowing vascular endothelial cells. The earliest stage is the condensation of mesenchymal blastemal cells around the terminal bud of the ureteric bud (later to become the metanephric duct). The preinduced mesenchyme contains several interstitial proteins, such as types I and III collagen and fibronectin. As the mesenchymal cells condense after local induction by the branching tips of the ureteric bud, these proteins are lost and are replaced with epithelial-type proteins (type IV collagen, syndecan-1, laminin, and heparin sulfate proteoglycan), which are ultimately localized to the basement membranes (Figure 15-4).

As the terminal bud of the metanephric duct branches, the surrounding mesenchyme splits into two parts. A single condensation of mesenchymal cells goes through a defined series of stages to form a renal tubule. After a growth phase, mitotic activity within the rounded blastemal mesenchyme decreases, and the primordium of the tubule assumes a comma shape (Figure 15-5, *A*). Within the comma a group of cells farthest from the end of the metanephric duct becomes polarized, forming a central lumen and a basal lamina on the outer surface. This marks the transformation of the induced mesenchymal cells into an epithelium, specifically the specialized

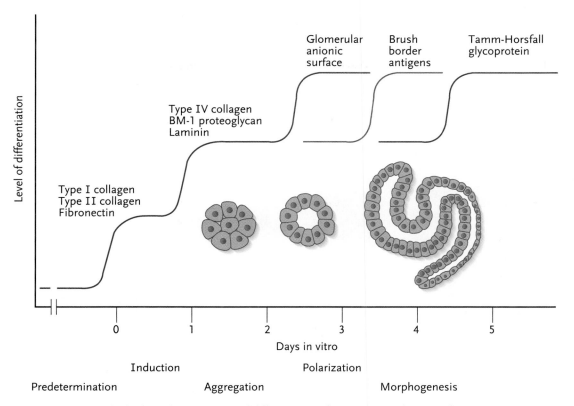

Figure 15-4 Multiphasic determination and differentiation of mouse metanephric mesoderm in vitro. (Modified from Saxén L and others: *Biology of human growth,* New York, 1981, Raven.)

podocytes, which ultimately surround the vascular endothelium of the glomerulus.

A consequence of this epithelial transformation is the formation of a slit just beneath the transforming podocyte precursors in the tubular primordium (Figure 15-5, *B*). Precursors of vascular endothelial cells grow into this slit, which ultimately forms the glomerulus. Research using interspecific hybrids has shown that the vascular endothelium migrates into the developing metanephros from outside the region of the intermediate mesoderm. Induced metanephric mesenchyme stimulates the ingrowth of endothelial cells, possibly by the release of a factor similar to FGF. Uninduced mesenchyme does not possess this capability. The endothelial cells are connected with branches from the dorsal aorta, and they form a complex looping structure that ultimately becomes the renal glomerulus. Cells of the glomerular endothelium and the adjoining podocyte epithelium form a thick basement membrane between them. This basement membrane later serves as an important component of the renal filtration apparatus.

As the glomerular apparatus of the nephron takes shape, another slit forms in the comma-shaped tubular primordium, transforming it into an S-shaped structure (Figure 15-5, *C*). Cells in the rest of the tubule primordium also undergo an ep-

ithelial transformation to form the remainder of the renal tubule. This transformation involves the acquisition of polarity by the differentiating epithelial cells. It is correlated with the deposition of laminin in the extracellular matrix along the basal surface of the cells and the concentration of the integral membrane glycoprotein **uvomorulin (E-cadherin),** which seals the lateral borders of the cells (Figure 15-6). As the differentiating tubule assumes an S shape, differing patterns of gene expression are seen along its length. Near the future glomerular end, levels of Pax-2 expression fall as WT-1 becomes strongly expressed (see Figure 15-3). At the other end of the tubule (future distal convoluted tubule), Wnt-4 and E-cadherin remain prominent, whereas in the middle (future proximal convoluted tubule) K-cadherin is a prominent cellular marker. Many of the uninduced mesenchymal cells between tubules undergo apoptosis.

Differentiation of the renal tubule progresses from the glomerulus to the proximal and then distal convoluted tubule. During differentiation of the nephron, a portion of the tubule develops into an elongated hairpin loop that extends into the medulla of the kidney as the **loop of Henle**. During differentiation, the tubular epithelial cells develop molecular features characteristic of the mature kidney (e.g., brush border antigens or the Tamm-Horsfall glycoprotein

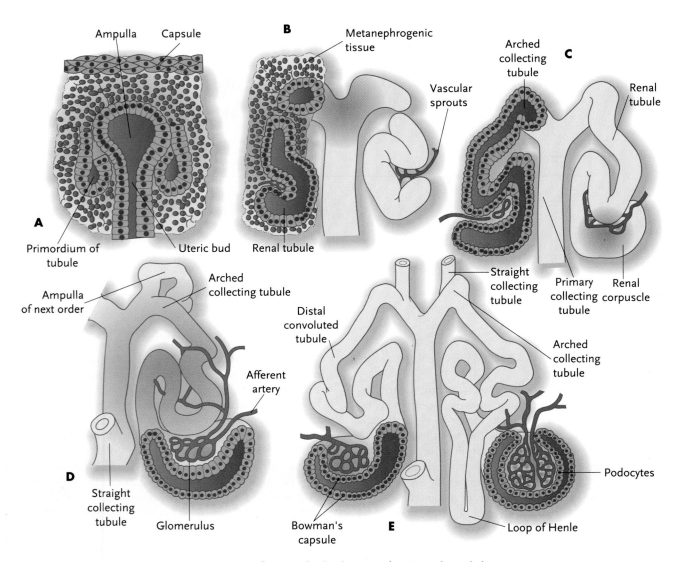

Figure 15-5 Stages in the development of a metanephric tubule.

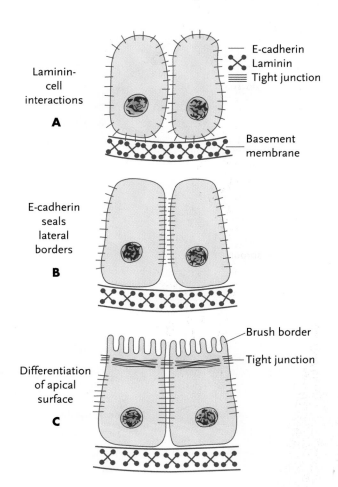

Figure 15-6 Stages in the transformation of renal mesenchyme into epithelium, with emphasis on the role of laminin and uvomorulin (E-cadherin). A, Development of polarity is triggered by interactions between laminin and the cell surface, but uvomorulin is still distributed in a nonpolar manner. B, Uvomorulin redistribution occurs, and uvomorulin interactions seal the lateral borders of the cells. C, Apical border of epithelial cells differentiates, as seen by formation of a brush border. (Based on Ekblom P: *FASEB J* 3:2141-2150, 1989.)

brush border antigens or the Tamm-Horsfall glycoprotein [see Figure 15-4]).

Growth of the kidney involves the formation of approximately 15 successive generations of nephrons in its peripheral zone, with the outermost nephrons less mature than those farther inward. Development of the internal architecture of the kidney is very complex, involving the formation of highly ordered arcades of nephrons (Figure 15-7). Details are beyond the scope of this text.

Later Changes in Kidney Development

While the many sets of nephrons are differentiating, the kidney becomes progressively larger. The branched system of ducts also becomes much larger and more complex,

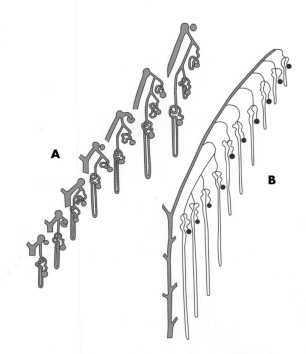

Figure 15-7 Formation of arcades of nephrons in the developing human metanephros. A, Early stages. B, Arrangement of nephrons at the time of birth. (Based on Osathanondh V, Potter EL: *Arch Pathol* 76:271-302, 1963.)

forming the pelvis and system of **calyces** of the kidney (Figure 15-8). These structures collect the urine and funnel it into the ureters. During much of the fetal period, the kidneys are divided into grossly visible lobes. By birth the lobation is already much less evident, and it disappears during the neonatal period.

When they first take shape, the metanephric kidneys are located deep in the pelvic region. During the late embryonic and early fetal period, they undergo a pronounced shift in position that moves them into the abdominal region. This shift results partly from actual migration and partly from a marked expansion of the caudal region of the embryo. Two concurrent components to the migration occur. One is a caudocranial shift from the level of the fourth lumbar to the first lumbar or even twelfth thoracic vertebra (Figure 15-9). The other is a lateral displacement. These changes bring the kidneys into contact with the adrenal glands, which form a cap of glandular tissue on the cranial pole of each kidney. During their migration, the kidneys also undergo a 90-degree rotation, with the pelves ultimately facing the midline. As they are migrating out of the pelvic cavity, the kidneys slide over the large umbilical arteries, which branch from the caudal end of the aorta. All these changes take place behind the peritoneum, since the kidneys are retroperitoneal organs. During the early phases of migration of the metanephric kidneys, the mesonephric kidneys regress. The mesonephric ducts, however, are retained as they become closely associated with the developing gonads.

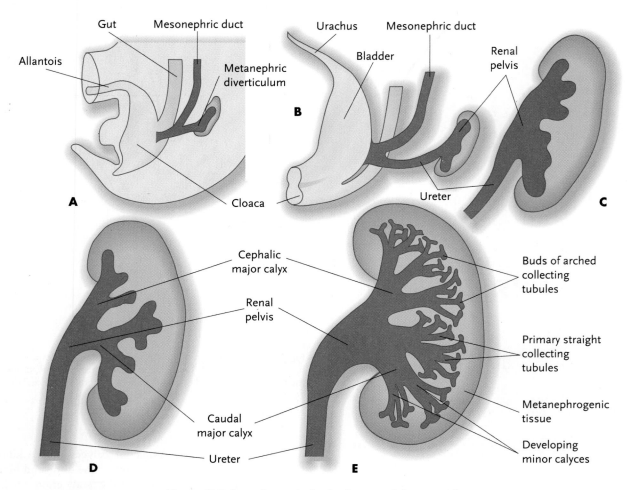

Figure 15-8 Later changes in the development of the metanephros.

Although normally supplied by one large renal artery branching directly from the aorta, the adult kidney consists of five vascular lobes. The arteries feeding each of these lobes were originally segmental vessels that supplied the mesonephros and were taken over by the migrating metanephros. Their aortic origins are typically reduced to the single pair of renal arteries, but anatomical variations are common.

Formation of the Urinary Bladder

The division of the cloaca into the rectum and urogenital sinus region was introduced in Chapter 14 (see Figure 14-9). The urogenital sinus is continuous with the allantois, which has an expanded base continuous with the urogenital sinus and an attenuated tubular process that extends into the body stalk on the other end. The dilated base of the allantois continues

to expand to form the **urinary bladder,** and its attenuated distal end solidifies into the cordlike urachus, which ultimately forms the median umbilical ligament leading from the bladder to the umbilical region (see Figure 15-18).

As the bladder grows, its expanding wall incorporates the mesonephric ducts and the ureteric buds (Figure 15-10). The result is that these structures open separately into the posterior wall of the bladder. Through a poorly defined mechanism possibly involving mechanical tension exerted by the migrating kidneys, the ends of the ureters open into the bladder laterally and cephalically to the mesonephric ducts. The region bounded by these structures is called the **trigone** of the bladder. At the entrance of the mesonephric ducts, the bladder becomes sharply attenuated. This region, originally part of the urogenital sinus, forms the **urethra,** which serves as the outlet of the bladder (see p. 389).

Text continued on p. 375

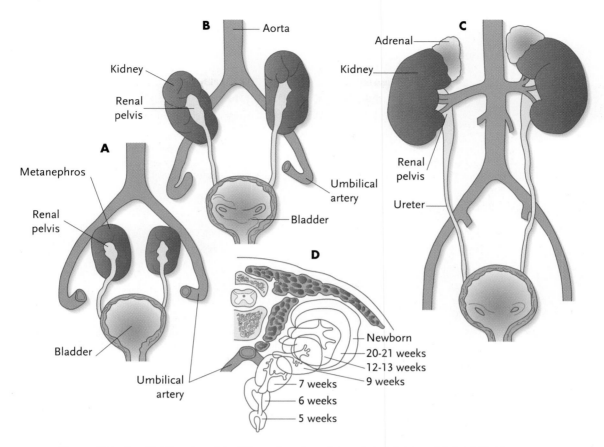

Figure 15-9 **A** to **C**, Migration of the kidneys from the pelvis to their definitive adult level. **D**, Cross section of the pathway of migration of the kidneys out of the pelvis.

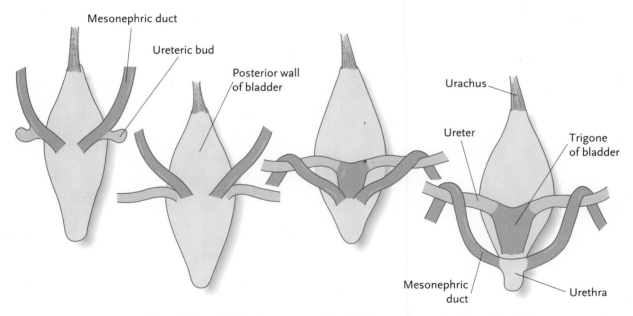

Figure 15-10 Dorsal views of the developing urinary bladder showing changing relationships of the mesonephric ducts and the ureters as they approach and become incorporated into the bladder. In the two on the right, note the incorporation of portions of the walls of the mesonephric ducts into the trigone of the bladder.

CLINICAL CORRELATION 15-1
Congenital Anomalies of the Urinary System

Anomalies of the urinary system are relatively common (3% to 4% of live births). Many are asymptomatic, and others manifest only later in life.

Figure 15-11 summarizes the locations of many of the more frequently encountered malformations of the urinary system.

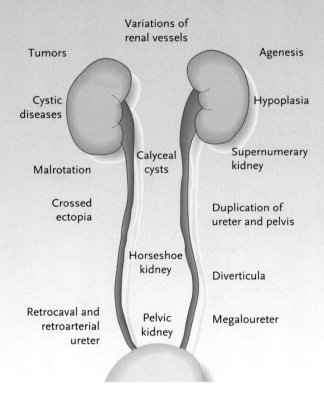

Tumors

Variations of renal vessels

Agenesis

Cystic diseases

Hypoplasia

Calyceal cysts

Supernumerary kidney

Malrotation

Crossed ectopia

Duplication of ureter and pelvis

Horseshoe kidney

Diverticula

Retrocaval and retroarterial ureter

Pelvic kidney

Megaloureter

Figure 15-11 Types and sites of anomalies of the kidneys and ureters. (Modified from Gray SW, Skandalakis JE: *Embryology for surgeons,* New York, 1972, WB Saunders.)

CLINICAL CORRELATION 15-1
Congenital Anomalies of the Urinary System—cont'd

RENAL AGENESIS

Renal agenesis is the unilateral or bilateral absence of any trace of kidney tissue (Figure 15-12, *A*). Unilateral renal agenesis is seen in roughly 0.1% of adults, whereas bilateral renal agenesis occurs in 1 in 3000 to 4000 newborns. The ureter may be present. This anomaly is usually ascribed to a faulty inductive interaction between the ureteric bud and the metanephro-genic mesenchyme. Misexpression of molecules, such as Pax-2, WT-1, or Wnt-4, which are important in early metanephric development, is a likely cause of some cases of renal agenesis. Individuals with unilateral renal agenesis are often asymptomatic, but typically the single kidney undergoes **compensatory hypertrophy** to maintain a normal functional mass of renal tissue.

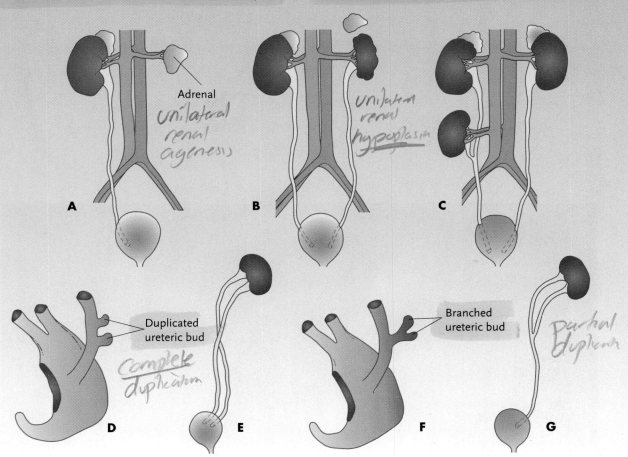

Figure 15-12 Common renal anomalies. **A,** Unilateral renal agenesis. The ureter is also missing. **B,** Unilateral renal hypoplasia. **C,** Supernumerary kidney. **D** and **E,** Complete duplication of ureter, presumably arising from two separate ureteric buds. **F** and **G,** Partial duplication of ureter, presumably arising from a bifurcated ureteric bud.

Continued

CLINICAL CORRELATION 15-1
Congenital Anomalies of the Urinary System—cont'd

An infant born with bilateral renal agenesis dies within a few days after birth. Because of the lack of urine output, reduction in the volume of amniotic fluid **(oligohydramnios)** during pregnancy is often an associated feature. Infants born with bilateral renal agenesis characteristically exhibit **Potter facies,** consisting of a flattened nose, wide interpupillary space, a receding chin, tapering fingers, and large, low-set ears (Figure 15-13). Potter facies is classified as a secondary disruption resulting from mechanical pressure of the uterus on the face of the fetus in the absence of the normal mechanical buffering of the amniotic fluid.

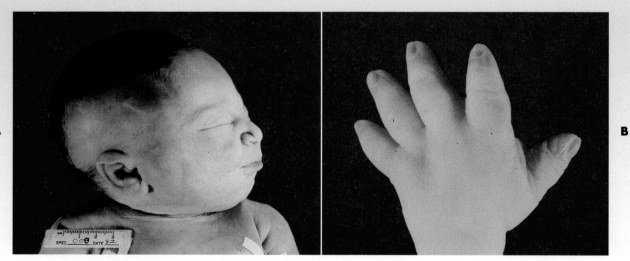

A
B

Figure 15-13 A, Potter facies, which is characteristic of a fetus who has been exposed to oligohydramnios. Note the flattened nose and low-set ears. **B,** Potter hand with thickened, tapering fingers. (Courtesy M. Barr, Ann Arbor, Mich.)

CLINICAL CORRELATION 15-1
Congenital Anomalies of the Urinary System—cont'd

RENAL HYPOPLASIA

An intermediate condition between renal agenesis and a normal kidney is **renal hypoplasia** (see Figure 15-12, *B*), in which one kidney or more rarely, both kidneys are substantially smaller than normal even though a certain degree of function may be retained. Although a specific cause for renal hypoplasia has not been identified, some cases may be related to deficiencies in growth factors or their receptors that are active during later critical phases of metanephrogenesis. As with renal agenesis, the normal counterpart to a hypoplastic kidney is likely to undergo compensatory hypertrophy.

RENAL DUPLICATIONS

Renal duplications range from a simple duplication of the renal pelvis to a completely separate **supernumerary kidney**. Like hypoplastic kidneys, renal duplications may be asymptomatic, although the inci-

dence of renal infections may be increased. Many variants of **duplications of the ureter** have also been described (see Figure 15-12). Duplication anomalies are commonly attributed to splitting or wide separation of branches of the ureteric bud.

ANOMALIES OF RENAL MIGRATION AND ROTATION

The most common disturbance of renal migration leaves a kidney in the pelvic cavity (Figure 15-14, *A*). This is usually associated with malrotation of the kidney as well, so the hilus of the **pelvic kidney** faces anteriorly instead of toward the midline. Another category of migratory malformation is **crossed ectopia**, in which one kidney and its associated ureter are found on the same side of the body as the other kidney (Figure 15-14, *B*). In this condition the ectopic kidney may be fused with the normal kidney.

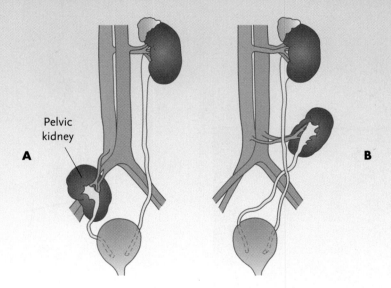

Pelvic kidney

A

B

Figure 15-14 Migration defects of the kidney. A, Pelvic kidney. B, Crossed ectopia. The right kidney has crossed the left ureter and has migrated only part of the normal distance.

Continued

CLINICAL CORRELATION 15-1
Congenital Anomalies of the Urinary System—cont'd

In the condition of **horseshoe kidney,** occurring in as many as 1 in 400 individuals, the kidneys are typically fused at their inferior poles (Figure 15-15). Horseshoe kidneys cannot migrate out of the pelvic cavity because the inferior mesenteric artery, coming off the aorta, blocks them. In most cases, horseshoe kidneys are asymptomatic, but occasionally pain or obstruction of the ureters may occur. This condition may be associated with anomalies of other internal organs. Pelvic kidneys are subject to an increased incidence of infections and obstructions of the ureters.

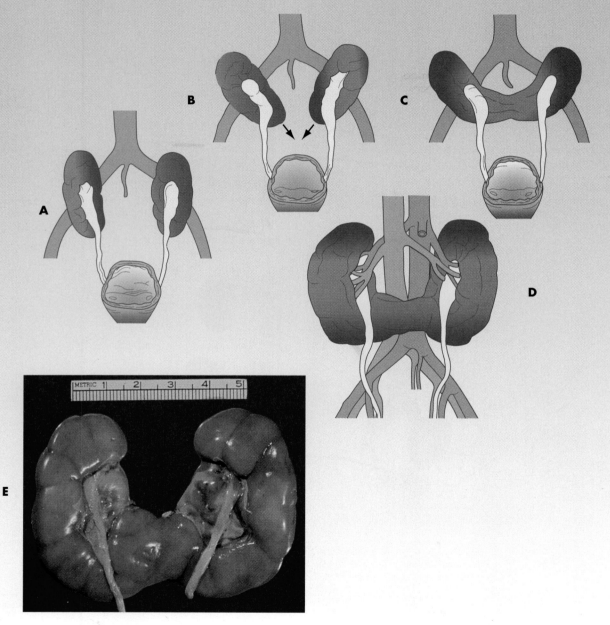

Figure 15-15 Stages in the formation of a horseshoe kidney. A to C, As the kidneys migrate out of the pelvis, their caudal poles touch and fuse. D, Pelvic kidney in an adult. Note the lack of rotation of the kidneys so that the ureters face ventrally instead of medially. E, Horseshoe kidney. (E, Photo 914E from the Arey-DaPeña Pediatric Pathology Photographic Collection, Human Developmental Anatomy Center, National Museum of Health and Medicine, Armed Forces Institute of Pathology, Washington, DC.)

CLINICAL CORRELATION 15-1
Congenital Anomalies of the Urinary System—cont'd

ANOMALIES OF THE RENAL ARTERIES

Instead of a single renal artery branching off each side of the aorta, duplications or major extrarenal branches of the renal artery are common. Because of the appropriation of segmental arterial branches to the mesonephros by the metanephros, consolidation of the major external arterial supply to the kidney occasionally does not occur.

POLYCYSTIC DISEASE OF THE KIDNEY

Congenital polycystic disease of the kidney, an autosomal recessive condition in infants, is typically manifest by the presence of large numbers of cysts of different sizes within the parenchyma of the kidney (Figure 15-16). Neither the origin nor the pathogenesis of this condition has been definitively ascertained. According to one theory, it is caused by the lack of connection between the tubular part of the nephron and the collecting duct system. The cysts have also been attributed to dilatations of the collecting duct system. Studies on mice with genetic polycystic disease have demonstrated defective expression of epidermal growth factor and high levels of certain oncogene products in the tubules of polycystic kidneys. Cysts of other organs, especially the liver and pancreas, are frequently associated with polycystic kidneys.

ECTOPIC URETERAL ORIFICES

Ureters may open into a variety of ectopic sites (Figure 15-17). Because of the continuous supply of urine flowing through them, these sites are symptomatic and usually relatively easy to diagnose. Their embryogenesis is commonly attributed to ectopic origins of the ureteric buds in the early embryo.

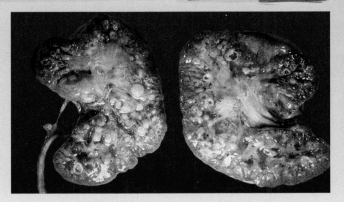

Figure 15-16 Polycystic kidneys. (Courtesy M. Barr, Ann Arbor, Mich.)

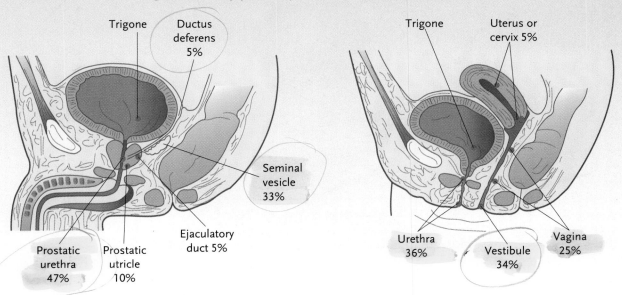

Figure 15-17 Common sites of ectopic ureteral orifices. (Modified from Gray SW, Skandalakis JE: *Embryology for surgeons,* Philadelphia, 1972, WB Saunders.)

Continued

CLINICAL CORRELATION 15-1
Congenital Anomalies of the Urinary System—cont'd

CYSTS, SINUSES, AND FISTULAS OF THE URACHUS

If parts of the lumen of the allantois fail to become obliterated, **urachal cysts, sinuses,** or **fistulas** can form (Figure 15-18). In the case of a urachal fistula, urine seeps from the umbilicus. Urachal sinuses or cysts may swell in later life if they are not evident in the infant.

EXSTROPHY OF THE BLADDER

Exstrophy of the bladder is a major defect in which the urinary bladder opens broadly onto the abdom- inal wall (Figure 15-19). Rather than being a primary defect of the urinary system, it is most commonly at- tributed to an insufficiency of mesodermal tissue of the ventral abdominal wall. Although initially the ven- tral body wall may be closed with ectoderm, it breaks down in the absence of mesoderm, and degenera- tion of the anterior wall of the bladder typically fol- lows. In males, exstrophy of the bladder commonly involves the phallus, and a condition called **epispa- dias** results (see p. 394).

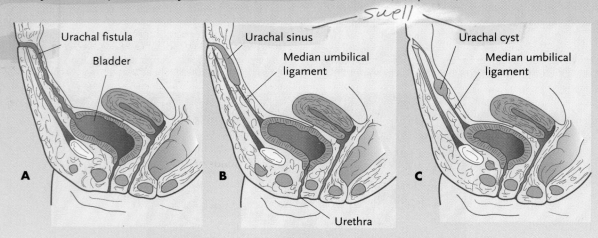

Figure 15-18 Anomalies of the urachus. **A,** Urachal fistula. **B,** Urachal sinus. **C,** Urachal cyst.

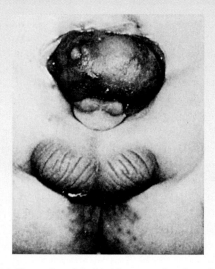

Figure 15-19 Exstrophy of the bladder in a male infant, showing pro- trusion of the posterior wall of the bladder through a defect in the lower abdominal wall. At the base of the open bladder is an abnormal, partially bifid penis with an open urethra (not seen) on its dorsal sur- face. A wide, shallow scrotum is separated from the penis. (From Crowley LV: *An introduction to clinical embryology,* St Louis, 1974, Mosby.)

GENITAL SYSTEM

Development of the genital system is one phase in the overall sexual differentiation of an individual (Figure 15-20). Sexual determination begins at fertilization, when a Y chromosome or an additional X chromosome is joined to the X chromosome already in the egg. This phase represents the genetic determination of gender. Although the genetic gender of the embryo is fixed at fertilization, the gross phenotypic gender of the embryo is not manifested until the seventh week of development. Before that time, the principal morphological indicator of the embryo's gender is the presence or absence of the **sex chromatin (Barr body)** in the female. The Barr body is the result of inactivation of one of the X chromosomes. During this morphologically **indifferent stage** of sexual development, the gametes migrate into the gonadal primordia from the yolk sac.

The phenotypic differentiation of gender is traditionally considered to begin with the gonads* and progresses with gonadal influences on the sexual duct systems. Similar influences

*Recent research, however, has shown gender differences as early as the preimplantation embryo. The Sry genes (see later section) are already transcribed before implantation. In addition, the XY preimplantation embryo develops more rapidly than the XX embryo. Male and female preimplantation embryos are antigenically distinguishable. This suggests differences in gene expression.

on the differentiation of the external genitalia and finally on the development of the secondary sexual characteristics (e.g., body configuration, breasts, hair patterns) complete the events that constitute the overall process of sexual differentiation. Sexual differentiation of the brain, which has an influence on behavior, also occurs.

Under certain circumstances an individual's genetic gender can be overridden by environmental factors so that the genotypic and phenotypic sex do not correspond. An important general principle is that the development of phenotypic maleness requires the action of substances produced by the testis. In the absence of specific testicular influences or the ability to respond to them, a female phenotype results. The female phenotype is the baseline, or default, condition, which must be acted on by male influences to produce a male phenotype.

Genetic Determination of Gender

Since 1923, scientists have recognized that the XX and XY chromosomal pairings represent the genetic basis for human femaleness and maleness. For many decades, they believed that the presence of two X chromosomes was the sex-determining factor, but in 1959, it was established that the differentiation between maleness and femaleness in humans depends on the presence of a Y chromosome. Never-

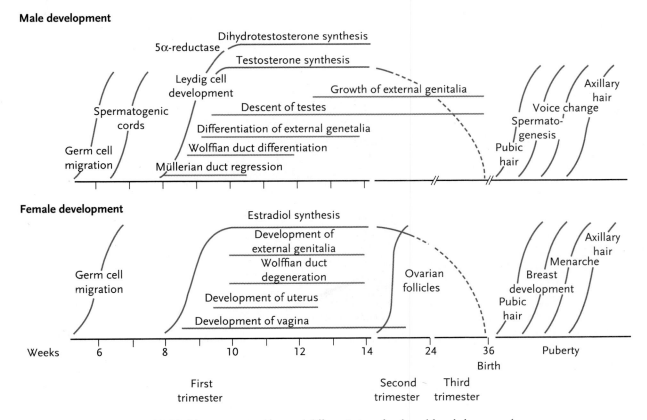

Figure 15-20 Major events in the sexual differentiation of male and female human embryos.

theless, the link between the Y chromosome and determination of the testis remained obscure. During recent decades, three candidates for the **testis-determining factor** have been proposed.

The first was the **H-Y antigen**, a minor histocompatibility antigen present on the cells of males but not females. The H-Y antigen has been mapped to the long arm of the human Y chromosome. It has been considered to be the product of the mammalian testis-determining gene. However, a strain of mice *(Sxr)* was found to produce males in the absence of the H-Y antigen. *Sxr* mice were found to have a transposition of a region of the Y chromosome onto the X chromosome, but the locus coding for the H-Y antigen was not included. In addition, certain phenotypic human males with an XX genotype were shown to be missing the genetic material for the H-Y antigen.

The next candidate was a locus on the short arm of the Y chromosome called the *zinc finger Y (ZFY)* gene. With deoxyribonucleic acid (DNA) hybridization techniques, this gene has been found in both XX male humans and in mice in which small pieces of the X and Y chromosomes were swapped during crossing-over in meiosis. Conversely, this gene was missing in some rare XY human females. However, certain XX males were found to lack the gene, and other rare cases of anomalies of sexual differentiation did not show a correspondence between sexual phenotype and the expected presence or absence of the ZFY gene.

The most recent candidate for the testis-determining gene is one called **Sry**, which is also located within a 35-kilobase region on the short arm of the Y chromosome (Figure 15-21). The *Sry* gene encodes a 223-amino acid nonhistone protein belonging to a family of proteins that contain a highly conserved 79-amino acid DNA-binding region called a **high mobility group box**. After the gene was cloned, it was detected in many cases of gender reversal, including XX males with no ZFY genes. The *Sry* gene on the human Y chromosome is located near the homologous region, making it susceptible to translocation to the X chromosome.

The *Sry* gene is also absent in a strain of XY mice that are phenotypically female. Further experimental evidence consists of producing transgenic mice with the insertion of a 14-kilobase fragment of the Y chromosome containing the *Sry* gene. Many of the transgenic XX mice developed into phenotypic males with normal testes and male behavior. In situ hybridization studies in mice have shown that expression of the *Sry* gene product occurs in male gonadal tissue at the time of sex determination, but it is not expressed in the gonads of female embryos.

Migration of Germ Cells into the Gonads

The early appearance of primordial germ cells in the lining of the yolk sac and their migration to the gonads in human embryos is briefly described in Chapter 1. Descriptive and ex-

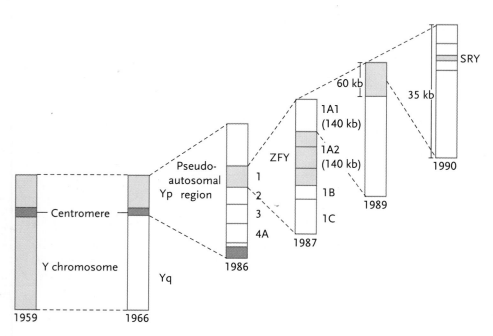

Figure 15-21 A history in the progress of localization of the sex-determining gene on the Y chromosome. (Modified from Sultan C and others: *Horm Res* 36:1-3, 1991.)

perimental studies have shown that primordial germ cells in the mouse can first be demonstrated in the epiblast. These cells pass through the early primitive streak and are next located as a small cluster of cells in the extraembryonic mesoderm near the base of the allantois. They then become associated with the endoderm of the posterior wall of the yolk sac (see Figure 1-1).

In human embryos the primordial germ cells migrate from the posterior wall of the yolk sac along the wall of the hindgut and through the dorsal mesentery until they reach the region of the newly appearing **genital ridges**. Experimental evidence suggests that the initial stages of migration of primordial germ cells at some distance from the gonads are accomplished by active ameboid movement of the cells in response to a permissive extracellular matrix substrate. Tissue displacements through differential growth of the posterior region of the embryo may also contribute. During their migration, many primordial germ cells are linked to one another through long cytoplasmic processes. How these interconnections control either migration or settling down in the gonads remains to be determined. Migrating germ cells proliferate in response to mitogenic factors such as **leukemia inhibitory factor** and **mastocyte growth factor** (stem cell factor or Steel factor).

As the germ cells approach the genital ridges late in the fifth week of development, they may be influenced by chemotactic factors secreted by the newly forming gonads. Such influences have been demonstrated by grafting embryonic tissues (e.g., hindgut, which contains dispersed germ cells) into the body cavity of a host embryo. The primordial germ cells of the graft typically concentrate on the side of the graft nearest the genital ridges of the host or sometimes migrate into the genital ridges from the graft. Approximately 1000 to 2000 primordial germ cells enter the genital ridges. Once the primordial germ cells have penetrated the genital ridges, their migratory behavior ceases.

Some primordial germ cells follow inappropriate migratory pathways, leading them to settle into extragonadal sites. These cells normally start to develop as oogonia, regardless of genotype; they then degenerate. In rare instances, however, they persist in ectopic sites, such as the mediastinum, and ultimately may give rise to **teratomas** (see Chapter 1).

Establishment of Gonadal Gender

Origin of the gonads

The gonads arise from an elongated region of steroidogenic mesoderm along the ventromedial border of the mesonephros. Cells in the cranial part of this region condense to form the **adrenocortical primordia,** and those of the caudal part become the **genital ridges,** which are identifiable midway through the fifth week. The early genital ridges consist of two major populations of cells: one derived from the **coelomic epithelium** and the other arising from the **mesonephric ridge.**

Formation of the genital ridges requires the function of at least two genes: **WT-1**, which is also important in early kidney formation (see Figure 15-3), and **SF-1** (steroidogenic factor-1), a gene required for development of both the gonads and adrenal glands.

Differentiation of the testes

When the genital ridges first appear, those of males and females are morphologically indistinguishable (indifferent stage). The general principle underlying gonadal differentiation is that under the influence of the *Sry* gene (testis-determining factor) on the Y chromosome, the indifferent gonad differentiates into a testis (Figure 15-22). In the absence of expression of products of this gene, the gonad later differentiates into an ovary.

In males, transcripts of the *Sry* gene are detected only in the genital ridge just at the onset of differentiation of the testis. Neither expression of the *Sry* gene nor later differentiation of the testis depends on the presence of germ cells. The sex-determining genes act on the somatic portion of the testis and not on the germ cells. A great deal remains to be learned about the events leading from expression of the *Sry* gene product to the overt differentiation of the testis. Current evidence suggests that the *Sry* gene product acts principally as a switch that activates other genes necessary for guiding testicular differentiation. The way the actions of specific genes relate to specific morphological events is unknown.

Timing is important in differentiation of the testis. The testis develops more rapidly than the ovary. Precursors of the Sertoli cells must be prepared to receive the genetic signals for testicular differentiation by a certain time. If not, the primordial germ cells begin to undergo meiosis and the gonad differentiates into an ovary. Early differentiation of the testis also appears to depend on a signal from the mesonephros. In the absence of the mesonephros, internal structures (testis cords) differentiate poorly.

The morphology of early gonadal differentiation has been controversial, with several scenarios of cell lineage and interactions being proposed. According to recent morphological evidence, the genital ridges first appear midway in the fifth week through the proliferation of **coelomic epithelial cells** along the medial border of the mesonephros (Figure 15-23). Later in the fifth week the primordial germ cells enter the early genital ridge, and the coelomic epithelium sends short epithelial pillars toward the interior of the gonad. Early in the sixth week a set of **primitive sex cords** takes shape in the genital ridge, and the primordial germ cells migrate into the primitive sex cords. The male gonad appears to give off a chemoattractive agent that stimulates the migration from the mesonephros of the myoid cells that surround the sex cords. In addition, endothelial cells and the myoepithelial cells that surround the vasculature migrate into the testis from the mesonephros. Ovarian tissue does not attract these cells.

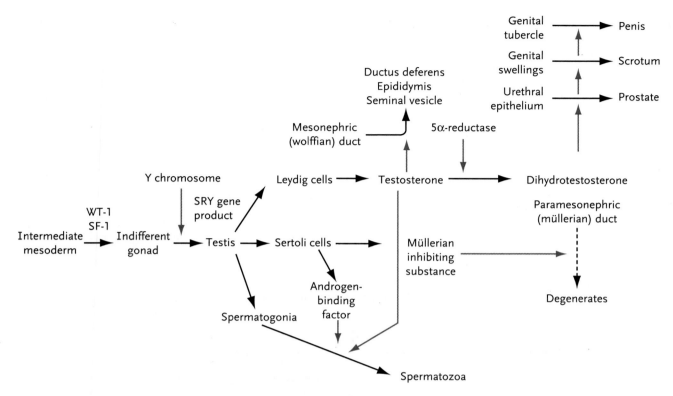

Figure 15-22 Differentiation of the male phenotype.

Late in the sixth week the testis shows evidence of differentiation. The primitive sex cords enlarge and are better defined, and their cells are thought to represent the precursors of the Sertoli cells. As the sex cords differentiate, they are separated from the surface epithelium (germinal epithelium) by a dense layer of connective tissue called the **tunica albuginea.** The deepest portions of the testicular sex cords are in contact with the fifth to twelfth sets of mesonephric nephrons. The outer portions of the testicular sex cords form the **seminiferous tubules,** and the inner portions become meshlike and ultimately form the **rete testis.** The rete testis ultimately joins the **efferent ductules,** which are derived from mesonephric tubules.

For the first 2 months of development, **Leydig cells** are not identifiable in the embryonic testis. These appear during the eighth week and soon begin to synthesize androgenic hormones (testosterone and androstenedione). This endocrine activity is important because differentiation of the male sexual duct system and the external genitalia depends on the sex hormones secreted by the fetal testis. Fetal Leydig cells secrete their hormonal products at just the period when differentiation of the hormonally sensitive genital ducts takes place (9 to 14 weeks). After weeks 17 and 18, the Leydig cells gradually involute and do not reappear until puberty, when they stimulate spermatogenesis. The fetal Leydig cells can be viewed as a cellular isoform that is later replaced by the definitive adult

form of the cells. By 8 weeks the embryonic Sertoli cells produce **müllerian inhibiting substance** (see p. 382), which also plays an important role in shaping the sexual duct system by causing involution of the precursors of the female genital ducts.

During the late embryonic and fetal periods and after birth, the primordial germ cells in the testis divide slowly by mitosis, but the fetal Sertoli cells are insensitive to androgens and fail to mature. The embryonic testis may secrete a **meiosis-inhibiting factor,** but such a factor has not been isolated or characterized. The environment of the testis does not become favorable for meiosis and spermatogenesis until puberty.

Differentiation of the ovaries

In the absence of specific testis-differentiation signals the gonads ultimately differentiate into ovaries. In contrast to the testes, the presence of viable germ cells is essential for ovarian differentiation. If primordial germ cells fail to reach the genital ridges or if they are abnormal (e.g., XO) and degenerate, the gonad regresses, and **streak ovaries** (vestigial ovaries) result.

After the primordial germ cells have entered the future ovary, they remain concentrated in the outer cortical region or near the corticomedullary border. Like the testis the ovary contains primitive sex cords in the medullary region, but these are not as well developed as those in the testis. The origin of the cells that form the ovarian follicles has not been estab-

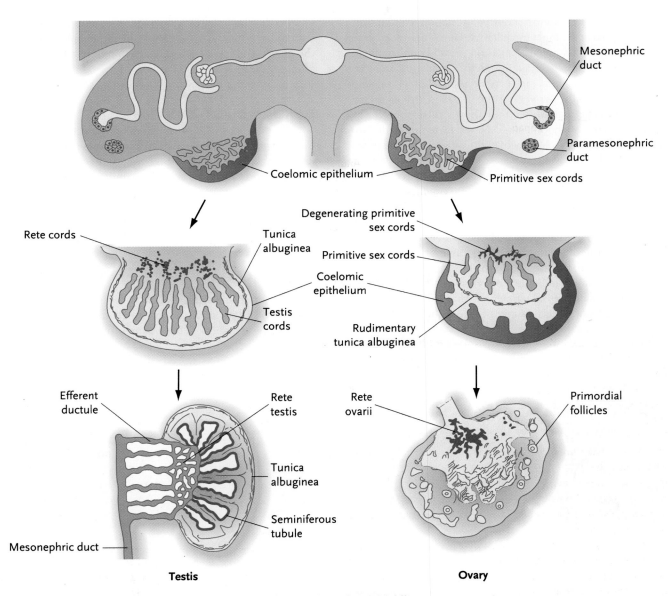

Figure 15-23 Morphology of gonadal differentiation.

lished. Three sites of origin have been proposed for the follicular epithelial cells: (1) the coelomic epithelium (secondary sex cords), (2) the primitive sex cords of mesonephric origin, and (3) a combination of the two. The last possibility is in accordance with the presence of two distinct cell types—light and dark—within the early follicular epithelium.

The primary germ cells, now properly called **oogonia**, proliferate by mitosis from the time of their entry into the gonad until the start of the fourth month of gestation. At that time, some oogonia in the inner medullary region of the ovary enter prophase of the first meiotic division, possibly under the influence of a meiosis-stimulating factor emanating from the mesonephros. This influence may be associated with clumps of mesonephrically derived epithelia called the medullary **rete ovarii**. The meiotic oogonia, now called **oocytes**, become associated with follicular cells and form **primordial follicles** (see Figure 1-5). Meanwhile, the oogonia in the cortical region of the ovary continue to divide mitotically. The oogonia and early oocytes are connected by intercellular cytoplasmic bridges that may play a role in synchronization of their development. By week 22, follicular development is well under way throughout the ovary. The oocytes continue in meiosis until they reach the diplotene stage of prophase of the first meiotic division. Meiosis is then arrested, and the oocytes remain in this stage until the block is removed. In the adult, this occurs in individual oocytes just days before ovulation. In premenopausal women, as many as 50 years may have elapsed since these oocytes entered the meiotic block in embryonic life.

In the fetal ovary an inconspicuous tunica albuginea forms at the corticomedullary junction. The cortex of the ovary is the dominant component, and it contains the majority of oocytes. The medulla fills with connective tissue and blood vessels that are derived from the mesonephros. The testis, on the other hand, is characterized by a dominance of the medullary component located inside a prominent tunica albuginea.

The developing ovary does not maintain a relationship with the mesonephros. Normally, the mesonephric tubules in the female embryo degenerate, leaving only a few remnants (Table 15-1).

SEXUAL DUCT SYSTEM

Like the gonads, the sexual ducts pass through an early indifferent stage. As the fetal testes begin to function in the male, their secretion products act on the indifferent ducts, causing some components of the duct system to develop further and others to regress. In females the absence of testicular secretory products results in the preservation of structures that regress and the regression of structures that persist in the male.

Indifferent Sexual Duct System

The indifferent sexual duct system consists of the **mesonephric (wolffian) ducts** and the **paramesonephric (müllerian) ducts** (Figure 15-24). The paramesonephric ducts appear

---

TABLE 15-1 Homologies in the Male and Female Urogenital Systems

Indifferent structure	Male derivative	Female derivative
Genital ridge	Testis	Ovary
Primordial germ cells	Spermatozoa	Ova
Sex cords	Seminiferous tubules (Sertoli cells)	Follicular cells
Mesonephric tubules	Efferent ductules	Eoophoron
	Paradidymis	Paroophoron
Mesonephric (wolffian) ducts	Appendix of epididymis	Appendix of ovary
	Epididymal duct	Gartner's duct
	Ductus deferens	
	Ejaculatory duct	
Paramesonephric (müllerian) ducts	Appendix of testis	Uterine tubes
	Prostate utricle	Uterus
		Upper vagina
Definitive urogenital sinus (lower part)	Penile urethra	Lower vagina
		Vaginal vestibule
Early urogenital sinus (upper part)	Urinary bladder	Urinary bladder
	Prostatic urethra	Urethra
Genital tubercle	Penis	Clitoris
Genital folds	Floor of penile urethra	Labia minora
Genital swellings	Scrotum	Labia majora

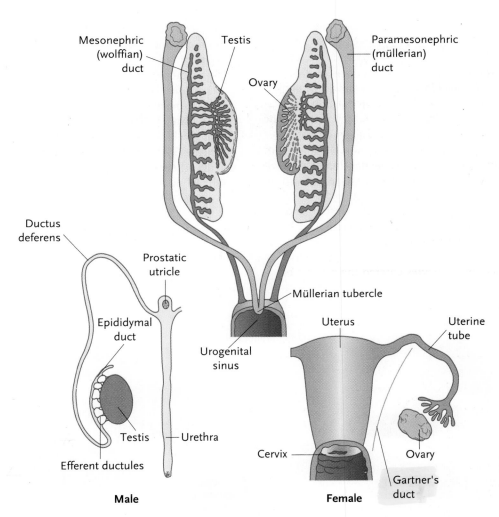

Figure 15-24 Indifferent condition of the genital ducts in the embryo at approximately **6 weeks**.

between 44 and 48 days of gestation as longitudinal invaginations of the surface epithelium along the mesonephric ridge lateral to the mesonephric ducts. The invaginations soon become epithelial cords, which grow caudally and terminate on the urogenital sinus between the ends of the mesonephric ducts without breaking into the sinus. These cords then develop a lumen in a craniocaudal direction. The cranial end of each paramesonephric duct opens into the coelomic cavity as a funnel-shaped structure. The fate of the indifferent genital ducts depends on the gender of the gonad.

Sexual Duct System of Males

Development of the sexual duct system in the male depends on secretions from the testis. Under the influence of **müllerian inhibiting substance**, a glycoprotein of the transforming growth factor-β family secreted by the Sertoli cells of the testes at 8 weeks' gestation, the paramesonephric ducts degenerate, leaving only remnants at their cranial and caudal ends (Figures 15-25 and 15-26 and Table 15-1). Müllerian inhibiting substance appears not to directly affect the epithe-

lium of the paramesonephric ducts but rather the surrounding mesenchyme. These mesenchymal cells express a gene that encodes a serine/threonine kinase membrane-bound receptor, which binds the müllerian inhibiting substance. Under its influence, the surrounding mesenchymal cells instruct the epithelial cells of the müllerian duct to regress.

Under the influence of testosterone, which is secreted by the Leydig cells of the testes, the mesonephric ducts continue to develop even though the mesonephric kidneys are degenerating. The mesonephric ducts differentiate into the paired **ductus deferens**, which constitutes the path of sperm transport from the testis to the urethra. Portions of degenerating mesonephric tubules may persist near the testis as the **paradidymis**.

Associated with development of the male genital duct system (both the ductus deferens and the urethra) is the formation of the male accessory sex glands: the **seminal vesicles**, the **prostate**, and the **bulbourethral glands** (Figure 15-27). These glands arise as epithelial outgrowths from their associated duct systems (seminal vesicles from the ductus deferens and the others from the urethra), and their formation involves epithelial-mesenchymal interactions similar to those of other

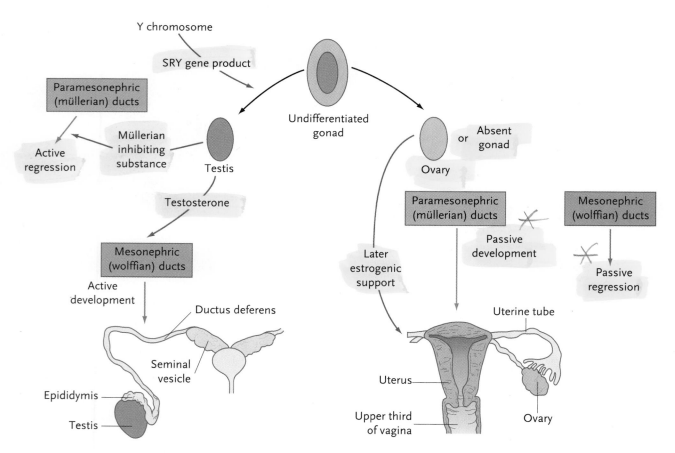

Figure 15-25 Factors involved in sexual differentiation of the genital tract. (After Hutson JM and others. In Burger H, deKrester D, eds: *The testis*, ed 2, New York, 1989, Raven, pp 143-179.)

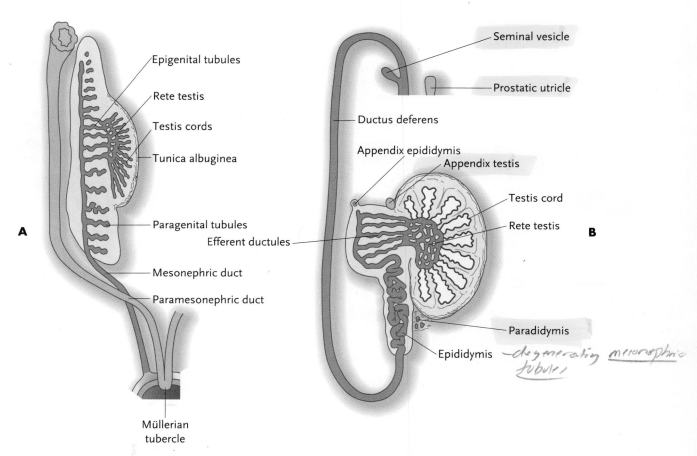

Figure 15-26 Development of the male genital duct system. **A,** At the end of the **second month. B,** In the late fetus. (Modified from Sadler T: *Langman's medical embryology,* ed 6, Baltimore, 1990, Williams & Wilkins.)

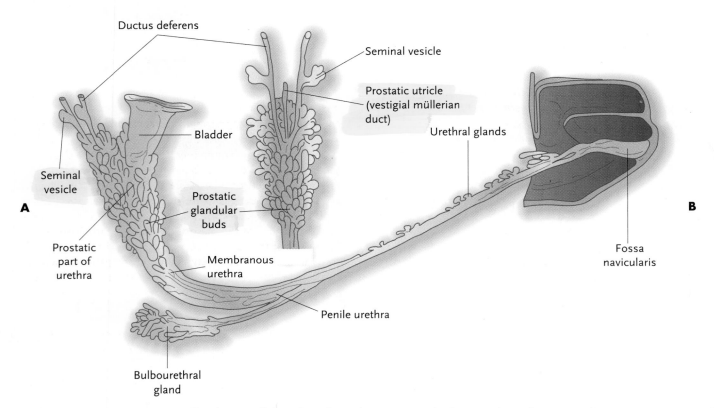

Figure 15-27 Development of the male urethra and accessory sex glands in an embryo of approximately 16 weeks. **A,** Lateral view. **B,** Dorsal view of prostatic region. (After Didusch. From Johnson FP: *J Urol* 4:447-502, 1920.)

glands. In addition, these glands depend on androgenic stimulation for their development. Specifically, the mesenchymal cells develop androgen receptors and appear to be the primary targets of the circulating androgenic hormones. (At this stage the epithelial cells do not contain androgen receptors.) After stimulation by the androgens, the mesenchymal cells act on the associated epithelium through the local paracrine effects of growth factors, causing it to differentiate with gland-specific characteristics.

In the developing prostate the urogenital mesenchyme acts on epithelial outgrowths from the urogenital sinus endoderm just below the bladder. The mesenchyme induces epithelial ducts to form, regulates proliferation of the epithelium and the expression of epithelial androgen receptors, and stimulates the synthesis of prostate-specific secretory proteins. Conversely, the developing prostatic epithelium induces the surrounding mesenchyme to differentiate into smooth muscle cells.

Tissue recombination experiments in which glandular mesoderm from mice with **testicular feminization syndrome** (lack of testosterone receptors resulting in no response to testosterone) was combined with normal epithelium demonstrated that the mesodermal component of the glandular primordia is the hormonal target. Differentiation of the epithelium did not occur. In contrast, when normal glandular mesoderm was combined with epithelium from animals with testicular feminization syndrome, normal development took place.

In the embryo the tissues around the urogenital sinus synthesize an enzyme (**5α-reductase**) that converts testosterone to dihydrotestosterone. Through the action of appropriate receptors of either form of testosterone, critical tissues of the male reproductive tract are maintained and grow (Figure 15-28).

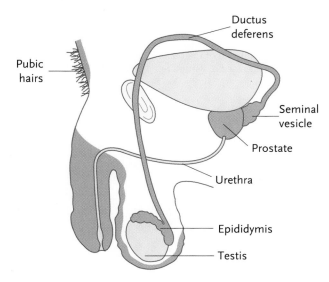

Figure 15-28 Regions of the male reproductive tract sensitive to testosterone (*brown*) and dihydrotestosterone (*blue*).

Sexual Duct System of Females

If ovaries are present or if the gonads are absent or dysgenic, the sexual duct system differentiates into a female phenotype. In the absence of testosterone secreted by the testes, the mesonephric ducts regress, leaving only rudimentary structures (see Table 15-1). In contrast, the absence of müllerian inhibitory substance allows the paramesonephric (müllerian) ducts to continue to develop into the major structures of the female genital tract (Figure 15-29).

The cranial portions of the paramesonephric ducts become the **uterine tubes,** with the cranial openings into the coelomic cavity persisting as the fimbriated ends. Toward their caudal ends the paramesonephric ducts begin to approach the midline and cross the mesonephric ducts ventrally. This crossing and ultimate meeting in the midline are caused by the medial swinging of the entire urogenital ridge (Figure 15-30). The region of midline fusion of the paramesonephric ducts ultimately becomes the uterus, and the ridge tissue that is carried along with the paramesonephric ducts forms the **broad ligament of the uterus.**

The formation of the **vagina** remains poorly understood, and several explanations for its origin have been posited. According to one commonly held hypothesis, the fused paramesonephric ducts form the upper part of the vagina, and epithelial tissue from the **müllerian tubercle (uterovaginal plate)** hollows out to form the lower part (Figure 15-31). More recently, several investigators have suggested that the most caudal portions of the mesonephric ducts participate in the formation of the vagina either by directly contributing cells to its wall or by inductively acting on the paramesonephric tissue. Full development of the female reproductive tract depends on estrogenic hormones secreted by the fetal ovaries.

Descent of the Gonads

Descent of the testes

The testes do not remain in their original site of development; they migrate from their intraabdominal location into the scrotum (Figure 15-32). Like the kidneys, the testes are retroperitoneal structures, and their descent occurs behind the peritoneal epithelium.

Control of testicular descent has been divided into three phases: The first is associated with the enlargement of the testes and the concomitant regression of the mesonephric kidneys. This causes some caudal displacement of the testes. The second phase, commonly called **transabdominal descent,** brings the testes down to the level of the inguinal ring but not into the scrotum. Control of this phase has been attributed to müllerian inhibitory substance and the regression of the paramesonephric ducts. The third phase, called **transinguinal descent,** brings the testes into the scrotum. This phase involves both the action of testosterone and the guidance of the **inguinal ligament of the mesonephros,** which in later development is called the **gubernaculum.** Whether the gubernaculum

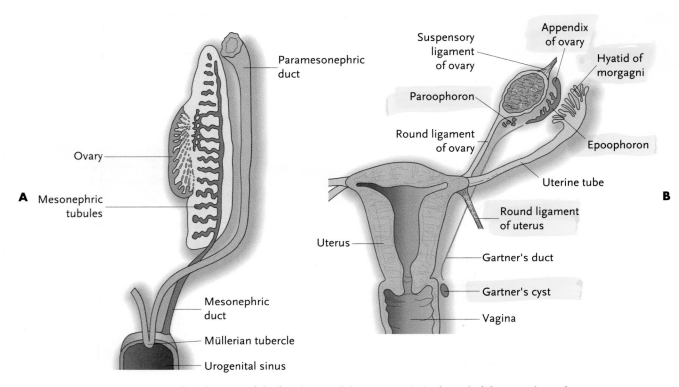

Figure 15-29 Development of the female genital duct system. **A,** At the end of the second month. **B,** Mature condition. (Modified from Sadler T: *Langman's medical embryology,* ed 6, Baltimore, 1990, Williams & Wilkins.)

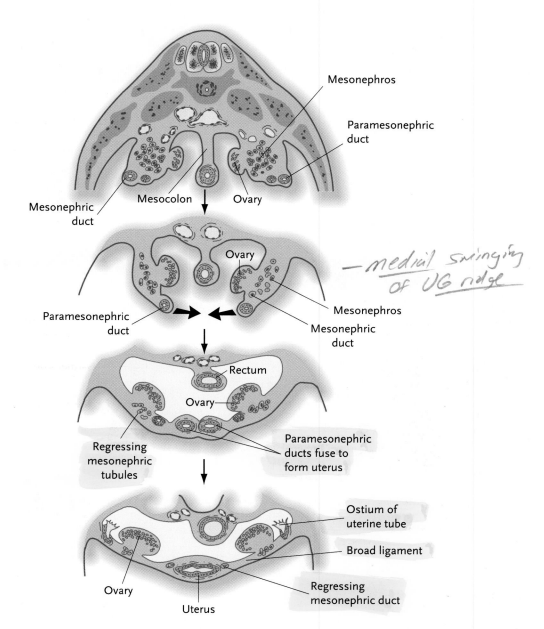

Mesonephros

Paramesonephric duct

Mesonephric duct

Mesocolon

Ovary

Ovary

— medial swinging of UG ridge

Mesonephros

Mesonephric duct

Paramesonephric duct

Rectum

Ovary

Regressing mesonephric tubules

Paramesonephric ducts fuse to form uterus

Ostium of uterine tube

Broad ligament

Regressing mesonephric duct

Ovary

Uterus

Figure 15-30 Formation of the broad ligament in the female embryo.

388

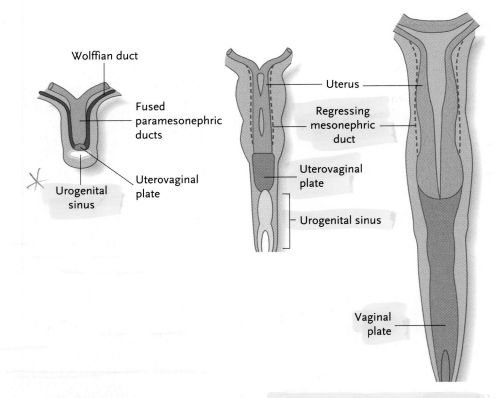

Figure 15-31 Development of the uterus and vagina. Contact between the fused müllerian ducts and urogenital sinus stimulates proliferation of the junctional endoderm to form the uterovaginal plate. Later canalization of the plate forms the lumen of the vagina.

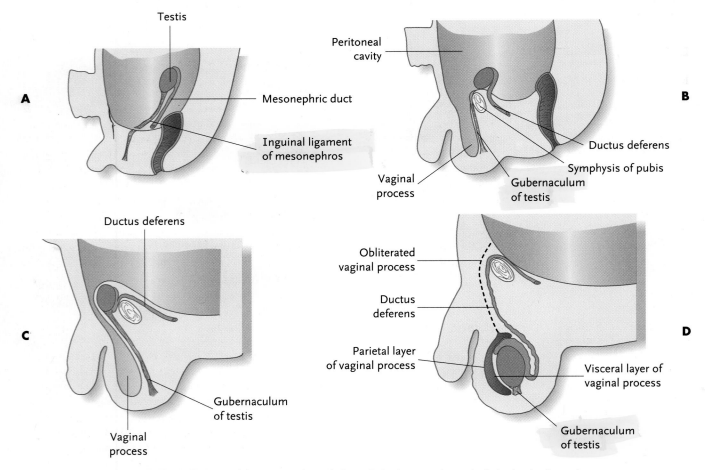

Figure 15-32 Descent of the testis in the male fetus. A, In the **second month**. B, In the **third month**. C, In the **seventh month**. D, At term.

actively pulls the testis into the scrotum or just acts as a fixed point while the other tissues grow has not been resolved. Testicular descent begins during the seventh month and may not be completed until birth. As it descends into the scrotum, the testis slides behind an extension of the peritoneal cavity: the **vaginal process** (see Figure 15-32, C). Although this cavity largely closes off with maturation of the testis, it remains as a potential mechanical weak point. With straining, it can open and permit the herniation of intestine into the scrotum.

Descent of the ovaries

Although not as dramatically as the testes, the ovaries also undergo a distinct caudal shift in position. In conjunction with their growth and the crossing over of the paramesonephric ducts, the ovaries move caudally and laterally. Their position is stabilized by two ligaments, both of which are remnants of structures associated with the mesonephros. Cranially, the **diaphragmatic ligament of the mesonephros** becomes the **suspensory ligament of the ovary.** The superior portion of the inguinal ligament (called the *caudal gonadal ligament* by some authors) develops into the **round ligament of the ovary,** and the inferior portion of the inguinal ligament becomes the **round ligament of the uterus** (see Figure 15-29). The most caudal ends of the round ligaments of the uterus become embedded in the dense fascial connective tissue of the labia majora.

EXTERNAL GENITALIA

Indifferent Stage

The external genitalia are derived from a complex of mesodermal tissue located around the cloaca. A very early midline elevation called the **genital eminence** is situated just cephalic to the proctodeal depression. This structure soon develops into a prominent **genital tubercle** (Figure 15-33), which is flanked by a pair of **genital folds** extending toward the proctodeum. Somewhat lateral to these are paired **genital swellings** (see Figure 15-34). When the genital membrane breaks down during the eighth week, the **urogenital sinus** opens directly to the outside between the genital folds. These structures, which are virtually identical in male and female embryos during the indifferent stage, form the basis for development of the external genitalia.

As with the developing limb, outgrowth of the genital tubercle depends on a continuing ectodermal-mesodermal interaction, although an apical ectodermal ridge is not present on the genital tubercle. In another similarity with the limb bud, there is a gradient of *Hoxd* gene products in the genital tubercle and genital ducts in mice; this is presumably true in humans as well. Finally, pieces of mesenchyme from the genital tubercle of mice demonstrate polarizing activity when grafted into limb buds of chick embryos (see Chapter 9).

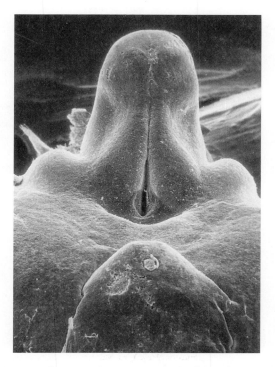

Figure 15-33 Scanning electron micrograph of the inferior aspect of the indifferent external genitalia of a human embryo at the end of the eighth week of development. (From Jirásek JE: *Atlas of human prenatal morphogenesis,* Amsterdam, 1983, Martinus Nijhoff.)

External Genitalia of Males

Under the influence of dihydrotestosterone (see Figure 15-28), the genital tubercle greatly elongates to form the penis, and the genital swellings enlarge to form the scrotal pouches (Figure 15-34, *A*). As this growth is occurring, the urogenital sinus becomes continuous with a groove that develops along the caudal face of the genital tubercle. This groove closes to become the penile part of the urethra, and the closed urogenital sinus becomes the prostatic portion of the urethra. In the most distal part of the penis a solid cord of epithelial cells grows from the glans to meet the penile urethra. When this cord canalizes, the formation of the urethra in the male is complete. The line of fusion along the urethra and passing through the scrotal swellings is the **raphe.**

External Genitalia of Females

In females the pattern of external genitalia is similar to that of the indifferent stage (Figure 15-34, *B*). The genital tubercle becomes the **clitoris,** the genital folds become the **labia minora,** and the genital swellings develop into the **labia majora.** The urogenital sinus remains open as the vestibule, into which both the urethra and vagina open. The female **urethra,** developing from the more cranial part of the urogenital sinus, is equivalent to the prostatic urethra of the male.

Text continued on p. 395

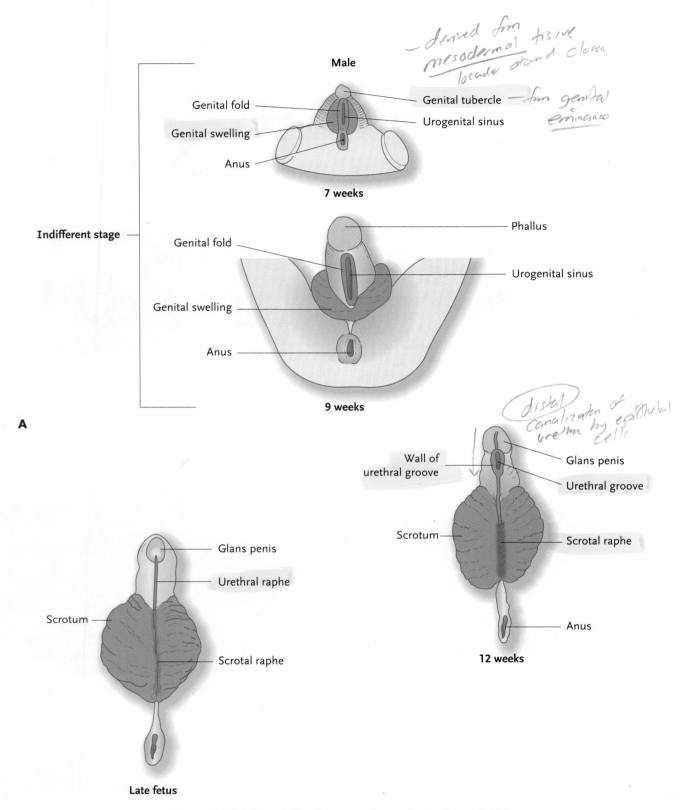

Male

Genital fold
Genital tubercle
Urogenital sinus
Genital swelling
Anus

— derived fm mesodermal tissue located aaround cloaca — fm genital eminence

7 weeks

Indifferent stage

Phallus
Genital fold
Urogenital sinus
Genital swelling
Anus

9 weeks

A

Glans penis
Urethral raphe
Scrotum
Scrotal raphe

Late fetus

distal Canalization of urethra by epithelial cells

Wall of urethral groove
Glans penis
Urethral groove
Scrotum
Scrotal raphe
Anus

12 weeks

Figure 15-34 Differentiation of the external genitalia of embryos. **A,** Male.

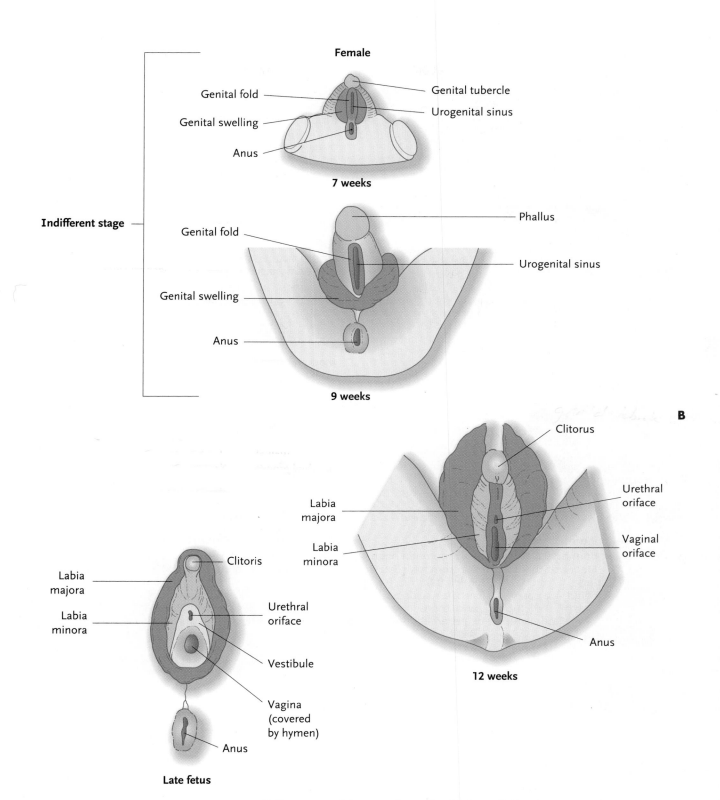

Female

Genital fold
Genital tubercle
Urogenital sinus
Genital swelling
Anus

7 weeks

Indifferent stage

Genital fold
Phallus
Genital swelling
Urogenital sinus
Anus

9 weeks

B

Clitorus
Labia majora
Urethral oriface
Labia minora
Vaginal oriface
Anus

12 weeks

Labia majora
Clitoris
Labia minora
Urethral oriface
Vestibule
Vagina (covered by hymen)
Anus

Late fetus

Figure 15-34—cont'd Differentiation of the external genitalia of embryos. **B**, Female.

CLINICAL CORRELATION 15-2
Malformations of the Genital System

ABNORMALITIES OF SEXUAL DIFFERENTIATION

Turner's syndrome (Gonadal Dysgenesis)

Turner's syndrome results from a chromosomal anomaly (45,XO) (see p. 134). Individuals with this syndrome possess primordial germ cells that degenerate shortly after reaching the gonads. Differentiation of the gonad fails to occur, leading to the formation of a **streak gonad.** In the absence of gonadal hormones the genitalia develop along female lines but remain infantile. The mesonephric duct system regresses for lack of androgenic hormonal stimulation.

True Hermaphroditism

Individuals with true hermaphroditism, which is an extremely rare condition, possess both testicular and ovarian tissue. In cases of genetic mosaicism, both an ovary and a testis may be present; in other cases, ovarian and testicular tissue are present in the same gonad **(ovotestis).** Most true hermaphrodites have a 46,XX chromosome constitution, and the external genitalia are basically female, although typically the clitoris is hypertrophied. Such individuals are usually reared as females.

Female Pseudohermaphroditism

Female pseudohermaphrodites are genetically female (46,XX) and are sex chromatin positive. The internal genitalia are typically female, but the external genitalia are masculinized, either from excessive production of androgenic hormones by the adrenal cortex **(congenital virilizing adrenal hyperplasia)** or from inappropriate hormonal treatment of pregnant women. The degree of external masculinization can vary from simple clitoral enlargement to partial fusion of the labia majora into a scrotumlike structure (see Figure 7-12).

Male Pseudohermaphroditism

Male pseudohermaphrodites are sex chromatin negative (46,XY). Because this condition commonly results from inadequate hormone production by the fetal testes, the phenotype can vary. It is often associated with hypoplasia of the phallus, and there may be varying degrees of persistence of paramesonephric duct structures.

form of

Testicular Feminization (Androgen Insensitivity) Syndrome

Individuals with testicular feminization syndrome are genetic males (46,XY) and possess internal testes, but they typically have a normal female external phenotype and are raised as females (see Figure 8-12). Often, testicular feminization is not discovered until the person seeks treatment for amenorrhea or is tested for sex chromatin before athletic events. The testes typically produce testosterone, but because of a deficiency in receptors caused by a mutation on the X chromosome, the testosterone is unable to act on the appropriate tissues. Because müllerian inhibitory substance is produced by the testes, the uterus and upper part of the vagina are absent.

VESTIGIAL STRUCTURES FROM THE EMBRYONIC GENITAL DUCTS

Vestigial structures are remnants from the regression of embryonic genital ducts, which is rarely complete. They are so common that they are not always considered to be malformations, although they can become cystic.

Mesonephric Duct Remnants

In males a persisting blind cranial end of the mesonephric duct can appear as the **appendix of the epididymis** (see Figure 15-26). Remnants of a few mesonephric tubules caudal to the efferent ductules occasionally appear as the **paradidymis.**

In females, the remains of the cranial parts of the mesonephros may persist as the **epoophoron,** or **paroophoron** (see Figure 15-29). The caudal part of the mesonephric ducts is often seen in histological sections along the uterus or upper vagina as **Gartner's ducts.** Portions of these duct remnants sometimes enlarge to form cysts.

Paramesonephric Duct Remnants

The cranial tip of the paramesonephric duct may remain as the small **appendix of the testis** (see Figure 15-26). The fused caudal ends of the paramesonephric ducts are commonly seen in the prostate gland as a small midline **prostatic utricle,** which represents the rudimentary uterine primordium. In newborn males the prostatic utricle is typically slightly enlarged because of the influence of maternal estrogenic hormones during pregnancy, but it regresses soon after birth. This structure can enlarge to form a uterus-like structure in some cases of male pseudohermaphroditism.

CLINICAL CORRELATION 15-2
Malformations of the Genital System—cont'd

In females a small part of the cranial tip of the paramesonephric duct may persist at the fimbriated end of the uterine tube as the **hydatid of Morgagni** (see Figure 15-29).

OTHER ABNORMALITIES OF THE GENITAL DUCT SYSTEM
Males
Abnormalities of the mesonephric duct system are relatively rare, but duplications or diverticula of the ductus deferens or urethra can occur. There is an interesting correlation of absent or rudimentary ductus deferens in males with cystic fibrosis. It may be the result of a defect in a gene situated along the gene causing the cystic fibrosis.

Persistent müllerian duct syndrome, characterized by the formation of a uterus and uterine tubes, has been described in a number of 46,XY phenotypic males. There is no single cause for this condition, and mutations of genes for both müllerian inhibiting substance and its receptor have been documented.

MIS gene/receptor mutations

Females
Malformations of the uterus or vagina are attributed to abnormalities of fusion or regression of the caudal ends of the paramesonephric ducts (Figure 15-35). Uterine anomalies range from a small septum extending from the dorsal wall of the uterus to complete duplication of the uterus and cervix. Numerous successful pregnancies have been recorded in women with uterine malformations. **Agenesis of the vagina** has been attributed to a failure of formation of the epithelial vaginal plate from the site of joining of the müllerian tubercle with the urogenital sinus.

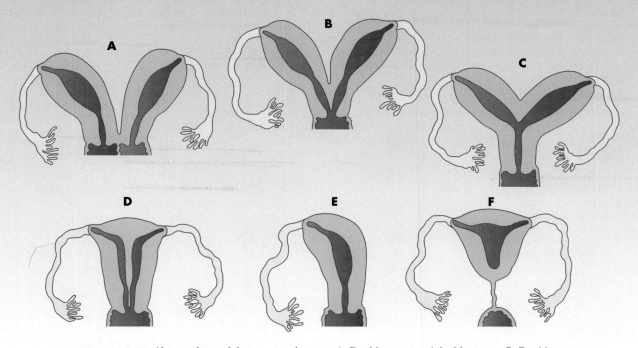

Figure 15-35 Abnormalities of the uterus and vagina. **A,** Double uterus and double vagina. **B,** Double uterus and single vagina. **C,** Bicornuate uterus. **D,** Septate uterus. **E,** Unicornuate uterus. **F,** Atresia of the cervix.

Continued

CLINICAL CORRELATION 15-2
Malformations of the Genital System—cont'd

ABNORMALITIES OF TESTICULAR DESCENT
Cryptorchidism

Undescended testes are common in premature males and are seen in about 3% of term males. Normally, the testes of these individuals descend into the scrotum within the first few months after birth. If they do not, the condition of **cryptorchidism** results. Cryptorchidism results in sterility because spermatogenesis does not normally occur at the temperature of the body cavity. There is also a fifty-fold greater incidence of malignancy in undescended testes.

Ectopic Testes

A testis occasionally migrates to some site other than the scrotum, including the thigh, perineum, and ventral abdominal wall. Because of the elevated temperature of the surrounding tissues, ectopic testes produce reduced numbers of viable spermatozoa.

Congenital Inguinal Hernia

If the peritoneal canal that leads into the fetal scrotum fails to close, a condition called **persistent vaginal process** occurs. This space may become occupied by loops of bowel that herniate into the scrotum.

MALFORMATIONS OF THE EXTERNAL GENITALIA
Males

The most common malformation of the penis is **hypospadias,** in which the urethra opens onto the ventral surface of the penis rather than at the end of the glans (Figure 15-36). The degree of hypospa-

dias can range from a mild ventral deviation of the urethral opening to an elongated opening representing an unfused portion of the urogenital sinus. In the more severe varieties the penis is often bowed ventrally **(chordee).**

Isolated **epispadias,** with the urethra opening on the dorsal surface of the penis, is very rare. A dorsal groove on the penis is commonly associated with exstrophy of the bladder (see Figure 15-19).

Duplication of the penis occurs most commonly in association with exstrophy of the bladder and appears to result from the early separation of the tissues destined to form the genital tubercle. Duplication of the penis very rarely occurs separately from exstrophy of the bladder.

Congenital absence of the penis (or clitoris in the female) is rare. With recent knowledge derived from experimental embryology, this condition might be explained on the basis of inadequate ectodermal-mesodermal interactions in the development of the genital tubercle or in mutations of Hoxa-13, Hoxd-13, or both.

Females

Anomalies of the external genitalia in females can range from hormonally induced enlargement of the clitoris to duplications. Exposure to androgens may also masculinize the genital swellings, resulting in scrotalization of the labia majora (see Figure 7-12). Depending on the degree of severity, wrinkling of the skin and partial fusion may occur.

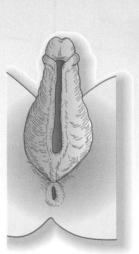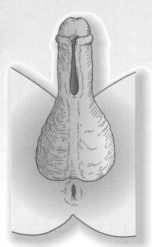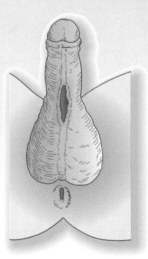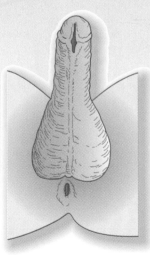

Figure 15-36 Variations in the extent of hypospadias.

UROGENITAL SYSTEM   395

CLINICAL VIGNETTE

A female athlete with amenorrhea is subjected to a routine sex chromatin test and is told that she cannot compete because she is a male.

1. What was the appearance of the cells that were tested?
2. What was the most likely basis for her female phenotype?
3. What is the likely anatomy of her gonads and genital duct systems, and why?

SUMMARY

- The urogenital system arises from the intermediate mesoderm. The urinary system arises before gonadal development begins.
- Kidney development begins with the formation of pairs of nephrotomes that connect with a pair of primary nephric ducts. Further caudally to the nephrotomes, pairs of mesonephric tubules form in a craniocaudal sequence and connect to the primary nephric ducts, which become known as *mesonephric ducts*. In the caudal part of each mesonephric duct a ureteric bud grows out and induces the surrounding mesoderm to form the metanephros.
- Within the developing metanephros, nephrons (functional units of the kidney) form from three sources: the metanephrogenic blastema, the metanephrogenic diverticulum, and ingrowing vascular endothelial cells. Nephrons continue to form throughout fetal life. The induction of nephrons involves reciprocal inductions between terminal branches of the collecting duct system (ureteric bud) and the metanephrogenic mesoderm. Many molecular interactions mediate these inductions.
- The kidneys arise in the pelvic basin, and during the late embryonic and early fetal period, they shift into the abdominal region, where they become associated with the adrenal glands. The urinary bladder arises from the base of the allantois.
- The urinary system is subject to various malformations. The most severe is renal agenesis, which is probably caused by faulty induction in the early embryo. Abnormal migration can result in pelvic kidneys, other ectopic kidneys, or horseshoe kidney. Polycystic disease of the kidney is associated with cysts in other internal organs. Faulty closure of the allantois results in urachal cysts, sinuses, or fistulas.
- Sex determination begins at fertilization by the contribution of an X or a Y chromosome to the egg by the sperm. The early embryo is sexually indifferent. Through the action of the *Sry* gene, the indifferent gonad in the male develops into a testis. In the absence of this gene the gonad becomes an ovary.
- Gonadal differentiation begins after migration of the primordial germ cells into the indifferent gonads. Under the influence of the *Sry* gene product (testis-determining factor), the testis begins to differentiate. The presence of germ cells is not required for differentiation of testis cords. In the embryonic testis, Leydig cells secrete testosterone, and Sertoli cells produce müllerian inhibitory substance. In the absence of *Sry* expression, the gonad differentiates into an ovary and contains follicles. Ovarian follicular differentiation does not occur in the absence of germ cells.

- The sexual duct system consists of the mesonephric (wolffian) and paramesonephric (müllerian) ducts. The duct system is originally indifferent. In the male, müllerian inhibitory substance causes regression of the paramesonephric duct system, and testosterone causes further development of the mesonephric duct system. In the female, the mesonephric ducts regress in the absence of testosterone, and the paramesonephric ducts persist in the absence of müllerian inhibitory substance.
- In males the mesonephric ducts form the ductus deferens and give rise to the male accessory sex glands. In females the paramesonephric ducts form the uterine tubes, the uterus, and part of the vagina.
- The testes descend from the abdominal cavity into the scrotum later in development. The ovaries also shift to a more caudal position. Faulty descent of the testes results in cryptorchidism and is associated with sterility and testicular tumors.
- The external genitalia also begin in an indifferent condition. Basic components of the external genitalia are the genital tubercle, genital folds, and genital swellings. Under the influence of dihydrotestosterone the genital tubercle elongates into a phallus, and the genital folds fuse to form the penile urethra. The genital swellings form the scrotum. In the female the genital tubercle forms the clitoris, the genital folds form the labia minora, and the genital swellings form the labia majora.
- If an individual possesses only one X chromosome (XO), Turner's syndrome results. Such individuals have a female phenotype with streak gonads. True hermaphroditism or pseudohermaphroditism can result from various causes. Testicular feminization is found in genetic males lacking testosterone receptors. Such individuals are phenotypic females. Major abnormalities of the sexual ducts are rare, but they can lead to duplications or the absence of the uterus in females.

REVIEW QUESTIONS

1. Which of the following does *not* connect directly with the primary nephric (mesonephric) duct?
   A. Metanephros
   B. Cloaca
   C. Nephrotomes
   D. Mesonephric tubules
   E. Ureteric bud
2. Which association is correct?
   A. Potter facies and hydramnios
   B. Urachal fistula and hydramnios
   C. Horseshoe kidney and superior mesenteric artery
   D. GDNF and metanephrogenic blastema
   E. Bilateral renal agenesis and compensatory hypertrophy
3. Which defect is strongly associated with oligohydramnios?
   A. Pelvic kidney
   B. Renal agenesis
   C. Horseshoe kidney
   D. Crossed ectopia
   E. Polycystic kidney
4. Which anomaly is most closely associated with exstrophy of the bladder?
   A. Epispadias
   B. Renal agenesis
   C. Anal atresia
   D. Pelvic kidney
   E. Ectopic ureteral orifice

5. The uterus arises from the
   A. Paramesonephric ducts
   B. Urogenital sinus
   C. Mesonephric tubules
   D. Pronephric ducts
   E. Mesonephric ducts

6. The floor of the penile urethra in the male is homologous to what structure in the female?
   A. Clitoris
   B. Trigone of the bladder
   C. Labia majora
   D. Labia minora
   E. Perineum

7. The metanephrogenic blastema is induced by the
   A. Pronephric duct
   B. Ureteric bud
   C. Mesonephric tubules
   D. Allantois
   E. Mesonephric duct

8. Drops of a yellowish fluid were observed around the umbilicus of a young infant. What is a likely diagnosis, and what is the embryological basis?

9. A woman who gained relatively little weight during pregnancy gives birth to an infant with large, low-set ears; a flattened nose; and a wide interpupillary space. Within hours after birth the infant is obviously in great distress and dies after 2 days. What is the diagnosis?

10. A seemingly normal woman experiences pelvic pain during the later stages of pregnancy. An ultrasound examination reveals that she has a bicornuate uterus. What is the embryological basis for this condition?

REFERENCES

Acien P: Embryological observations on the female genital tract, *Hum Reprod* 7:437-445, 1992.

Bard JBL and others: Kidney development: the inductive interactions, *Semin Cell Dev Biol* 7:195-202, 1996.

Behringer RR: The müllerian inhibitor and mammalian sexual development, *Phil Trans R Soc Lond B* 350:285-289, 1995.

Buehr M: The primordial germ cells of mammals: some current perspectives, *Exp Cell Res* 232:194-207, 1997.

Byskov AG: Differentiation of mammalian embryonic gonad, *Physiol Rev* 66:71-117, 1986.

Capel B: The role of Sry in cellular events underlying mammalian sex determination, *Curr Top Dev Biol* 32:1-37, 1996.

Cunha GR and others: The endocrinology and developmental biology of the prostate, *Endocr Rev* 8:338-363, 1987.

Cunha GR and others: Keratinocyte growth factor as mediator of mesenchymal-epithelial interactions in the development of androgen target organs, *Semin Cell Dev Biol* 7:203-210, 1996.

Dollé P and others: *Hox-4* genes and the morphogenesis of mammalian genitalia, *Genes Dev* 5:1767-1776, 1991.

Dressler GR and others: *Pax2*, a new murine paired-box-containing gene and its expression in the developing excretory system, *Development* 109:787-795, 1990.

Ekblom P: Developmentally regulated conversion of mesenchyme to epithelium, *FASEB J* 3:2141-2150, 1989.

Erickson RP: Does sex determination start at conception? *BioEssays* 19:1027-1032, 1997.

Gattone VH and others: Defective epidermal growth factor gene expression in mice with polycystic kidney disease, *Dev Biol* 138:225-230, 1990.

Ginsburg M, Snow MHL, McLaren A: Primordial germ cells in the mouse embryo during gastrulation, *Development* 110:521-528, 1990.

Godin I, Wylie C, Heasman J: Genital ridges exert long-range effects on mouse primordial germ cell numbers and direction of migration in culture, *Development* 108:357-363, 1990.

Gougeon A: Initiation of ovarian follicular growth: few facts and many hypotheses. In Filicori M, Flamigni C, eds: *The ovary: regulation, dysfunction and treatment*, Amsterdam, 1996, Elsevier Science, pp 3-12.

Greenfield A, Koopman P: SRY and mammalian sex determination, *Curr Top Dev Biol* 34:1-23, 1996.

Huhtaniemi I, Pelliniemi LJ: Fetal Leydig cells: cellular origin, morphology, life span, and special functional features, *Proc Soc Exp Biol Med* 201:125-140, 1992.

Hutson JM and others: Müllerian inhibiting substance. In Burger H, de Krester D, eds: *The testis*, ed 2, New York, 1989, Raven, pp 143-179.

Imbeaud S and others: Molecular genetics of the persistent Müllerian duct syndrome: a study of 19 families, *Hum Mol Genet* 3:125-131, 1994.

Jirásek JE: Normal sex differentiation. In Droegemueller W, Sciarra JJ, eds: *Gynecology and obstetrics*, rev ed, Philadelphia, 1991, JB Lippincott, pp 1-16.

Josso N: Anti-müllerian hormone and Sertoli cell function, *Horm Res* 38(suppl 2):72-76, 1992.

Josso N, Picard J-Y: Anti-müllerian hormone, *Physiol Rev* 66:1038-1090, 1986.

Koopman P and others: Expression of a candidate sex-determining gene during mouse testis differentiation, *Nature* 348:450-452, 1991.

Lechner MS, Dressler GR: The molecular basis of embryonic kidney development, *Mech Dev* 62:105-120, 1997.

Levy JB, Husmann DA: The hormonal control of testicular descent, *J Androl* 16:459-463, 1995.

Ludwig KS: The development of the caudal ligaments of the mesonephros and of the gonads: a contribution to the development of the human gubernaculum (Hunteri), *Anat Embryol* 188:571-577, 1993.

Makabe S and others: Migration of germ cells, development of the ovary, and folliculogenesis. In Familiari G, Makabe S, Motta PM, eds: *Ultrastructure of the ovary*, Norwell, Mass, 1991, Kluwer Academic, pp 1-27.

Martineau J and others: Male-specific cell migration into the developing gonad, *Curr Biol* 7:958-968, 1997.

Merchant-Larios H: Germ and somatic cell interactions during gonadal morphogenesis. In Van Blerkom J, Motta PM, eds: *Ultrastructure of reproduction*, Boston, 1984, Martinus Nijhoff, pp 19-30.

Mittowch U: Sex determination and sex reversal: genotype, phenotype, dogma and semantics, *Hum Genet* 89:467-479, 1992.

Miyamoto N and others: Defects of urogenital development in mice lacking Emx2, *Development* 124:1653-1664, 1997.

Muller J, Shakkebaek NE: The prenatal and postnatal development of the testis, *Bailliere Clin Endocrinol Metab* 6:251-271, 1992.

O'Rahilly RO, Muecke EC: The timing and sequence of events in the development of the human urinary system during the embryonic period proper, *Z Anat Entwickl-Gesch* 138:99-109, 1972.

Osathanondh V, Potter EL: Development of the human kidney as shown by microdissection. I. II. III. *Arch Pathol* 76:271-302, 1963.

Ramkissoon Y, Goodfellow P: Early steps in mammalian sex determination, *Curr Opin Genet Dev* 6:316-321, 1996.

Reyes FI, Winter JSD, Faiman C: Endocrinology of the fetal testis. In Burger H, de Kretser D, eds: *The testis*, ed 2, New York, 1989, Raven, pp 119-142.

Ryan G and others: Repression of Pax-2 by WT1 during normal kidney development, *Development* 121:867-875, 1995.

Sainio K and others: Differential regulation of two sets of mesonephric tubules by WT-1, *Development* 124:1293-1299, 1997.

Sainio K and others: Glial-cell-line neurotrophic factor is required for bud initiation from ureteric epithelium, *Development* 124:4077-4087, 1997.

Sariola H: Mechanisms and regulation of the vascular growth during kidney differentiation. In Feinberg RN, Sherer GK, Auerbach R, eds: *The development of the vascular system*, Basel, Switzerland, 1991, S Karger, pp 69-80.

Satoh M: Histogenesis and organogenesis of the gonad in human embryos, *J Anat* 177:85-107, 1991.

Saxén L: *Organogenesis of the kidney*, Cambridge, England, 1987, Cambridge University Press.

Schafer AJ, Goodfellow PN: Sex determination in humans, *BioEssays* 18:955-963, 1996.

Sinclair AH and others: A gene from the human sex-determining region encodes a protein with homology to a conserved DNA binding motif, *Nature* 346:240-244, 1990.

Sultan C and others: Sry and male sex determination, *Horm Res* 36:1-3, 1991.

Vainio S, Mueller U: Inductive tissue interactions, cell signaling, and the control of kidney organogenesis, *Cell* 90:975-978, 1997.

Wartenberg H: Differentiation and development of the testes. In Burger H, de Kretser D, eds: *The testis*, New York, 1989, Raven, pp 67-118.

Wartenberg H: Ultrastructure of fetal ovary including oogenesis. In Van Blerkom J, Motta PM, eds: *Ultrastructure of human gametogenesis and early embryogenesis*, Norwell, Mass, 1989, Kluer Academic, pp 61-84.

Woolf AS: Multiple causes of human kidney malformations, *Arch Dis Childhood* 77:471-473, 1997.

16

CARDIOVASCULAR SYSTEM

This chapter follows the development of the heart from a simple tubular structure to the four-chambered organ that can assume the full burden of maintaining an independent circulation at birth. Similarly, the pattern of blood vessels is traced from their first appearance to an integrated system that carries blood to all parts of the embryo and the placenta. (The early stages in the establishment of the heart and blood vessels are described in Chapter 5 [see Figures 5-20 to 5-24], and the general plan of the embryonic circulation is summarized in Figure 5-31.) Cellular aspects of blood formation are also briefly described. Clinical Correlations 16-1 and 16-2 at the end of the chapter discuss malformations of the heart and the blood vessels, respectively. Table 16-5, also at the end of the chapter, summarizes the time lines in cardiac development.

Functionally, the embryonic heart needs only to act like a simple pump that maintains the flow of blood through the body of the embryo and into the placenta, where fetal wastes are exchanged for oxygen and nutrients. An equally important function, however, is to anticipate the radical changes in the circulation that take place at birth as a consequence of the abrupt cutting off of the placental circulation and the initiation of breathing. To meet the complex requirements of the postnatal circulatory system, the embryonic heart must develop four chambers that can receive or pump the full flow of blood circulating throughout the body. The heart must also adapt to the condition of the fetal lungs, which are poorly developed and for much of the fetal period do not possess a vasculature that can accommodate a large flow of blood. This physiological dilemma is resolved by the presence of two shunts that allow each chamber of the heart to handle large amounts of blood while sparing the underdeveloped pulmonary vascular channels.

Cardiac morphogenesis involves intrinsic cellular and molecular interactions, but these must occur against a background of ongoing mechanical function. Some of these mechanisms remain elusive, but others are becoming better defined through research on normal and abnormal cardiac development.

Development of the vasculature at the level of gross patterns of arteries and veins has been well understood for many years. Only recently have new cellular and molecular markers enabled investigators to outline the cellular origins of the arteries and veins in specific organs or regions of the body. Studies on mechanisms of vascular differentiation are for the most part still in their infancy.

DEVELOPMENT OF THE VASCULAR SYSTEM

Development of the vascular system begins in the wall of the yolk sac during the third week of gestation with the formation of blood islands (see Figure 5-24). At this time the embryo has attained a size that is too large for the distribution of oxygen to all tissues by diffusion alone. This necessitates the very early development of both the heart and the vascular system. Because the tissues that normally produce blood cells in the adult have not yet begun to form, yolk sac hematopoiesis appears to be a temporary adaptation for accommodating the immediate needs of the embryo.

The founder cells of the blood islands, called **hemangioblasts,** are thought to have a bipotential developmental capacity and can give rise to either endothelial cells or hematopoietic cells. Once a commitment toward one of these two lineages has been made, daughter cells of the hemangioblasts lose the capacity to form the other type of cell.

Embryonic Hematopoiesis

Although blood cell formation (**hematopoiesis**) begins in the yolk sac, evidence from animal experimentation suggests that the yolk sac–derived cells are soon replaced by other blood cells that are independently derived from intraembryonic sites of hematopoiesis.

The blood islands contain pluripotential **hematopoietic stem cells,** which can give rise to all types of cells found in the embryonic blood. The erythrocytes produced in the yolk sac are large nucleated cells that enter the bloodstream just before the heart tube begins to beat at about 22 days' gestation. For the first 6 weeks the circulating erythrocytes are almost entirely yolk sac derived, but during that time, preparations for the next stages of hematopoiesis are taking place.

Analysis of both chicken and mouse embryos has shown that definitive **intraembryonic hematopoiesis** begins in small clusters of cells (**paraaortic clusters**) in the splanchnopleuric mesoderm associated with the ventral wall of the dorsal aorta and shortly thereafter in the **aorta/genital ridge/mesonephros region.** By 5 to 6 weeks, sites of hematopoiesis become prominent in the liver.

The erythrocytes produced by the liver are quite different from those derived from the yolk sac. Although still considerably larger-than-normal adult red blood cells, liver-derived erythrocytes are nonnucleated and contain different types of hemoglobin. By 6 to 8 weeks of gestation in humans, the liver replaces the yolk sac as the main source of blood cells. Although the liver continues to produce red blood cells until the early neonatal period, its contribution begins to decline in the sixth month of pregnancy. At this time the formation of blood cells shifts to the bone marrow, the definitive site of adult hematopoiesis. This shift is controlled by cortisol secreted by the fetal adrenal cortex. In the absence of cortisol, hematopoiesis remains confined to the liver. Before hematopoiesis becomes well established in the bone marrow, small amounts of blood formation may also occur in the omentum and possibly the spleen.

Cellular Aspects of Hematopoiesis

The first **hematopoietic stem cells** that arise in the embryo are truly pluripotential in that they can give rise to all the cell types found in the blood (Figure 16-1). These pluripotent stem cells, sometimes called **hemocytoblasts,** have great proliferative ability. They produce vast numbers of progeny, most of which are cells at the next stage of differentiation, but they also produce small numbers of their original stem cell type, which act as a reserve capable of replenishing individual lines of cells should the need arise. Very early in development, the line of active blood-forming cells subdivides into two separate lineages. **Lymphoid stem cells** ultimately form the two lines of lymphocytes: **B lymphocytes** (which are responsible for antibody production) and **T lymphocytes** (which are responsible for cellular immune reactions). **Myeloid stem cells** are precursors to the other lines of blood cells: erythrocytes, the granulocytes (neutrophils, eosinophils and basophils), monocytes, and platelets. The second-generation stem cells (lymphoid and myeloid) are still pluripotent, although their developmental potency is restricted, since neither can form the progeny of the other type.

Stemming from their behavior in certain experimental situations, the hematopoietic stem cells are often called **colony-forming units (CFUs).** The first-generation stem cell is called the *CFU-ML* because it can give rise to both myeloid and lym-

phoid lines of cells. Stem cells of the second generation are called *CFU-L* (*L,* lymphocytes) and *CFU-S* (*S,* spleen) (determined from experiments in which stem cell differentiation was studied in irradiated spleens). In all cases except one, the progeny of CFU-L and CFU-S are **committed stem cells,** which are capable of forming only one type of mature blood cell. For each lineage the forming cell types must pass through several stages of differentiation before they attain their mature phenotype.

What controls the diversification of stem cells into specific cell lines? Experiments begun in the 1970s provided evidence for the existence of specific **colony-stimulating factors (CSFs)** for each line of blood cell. CSFs are diffusible proteins that stimulate the proliferation of hematopoietic stem cells. Some CSFs act on a number of types of stem cells; others stimulate only one type. Although much remains to be learned about the sites of origin and modes of action of CSFs, many appear to be produced locally in stromal cells of the bone marrow, and some may be stored on the local extracellular matrix. CSFs are bound by small numbers of surface receptors on their target stem cells. Functionally, CSFs represent mechanisms for stimulating the expansion of specific types of blood cells when the need arises. Recognition of the existence of CSFs has prompted considerable interest in their clinical application to conditions characterized by a deficiency of white blood cells (leukopenia).

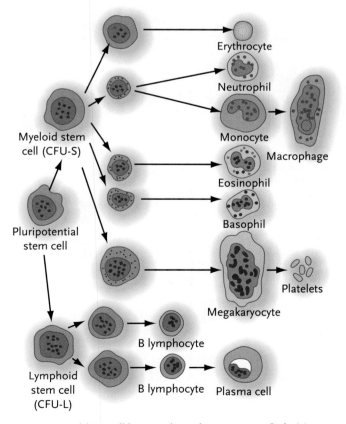

Figure 16-1 Major cell lineages during hematopoiesis. *Right,* Mature blood cells.

Certain *Hox* genes, especially those of the *Hoxa* and *Hoxb* families, play an important role in some aspects of hematopoiesis. Exposure of bone marrow to antisense oligonucleotides against specific *Hox* genes results in the suppression of specific lines of differentiation of blood cells. Conversely, engineered overexpression of genes, such as *Hoxb-8*, *Hoxa-9*, and *Hoxa-10*, causes leukemia in mice. Evidence is increasing for the involvement of *Hox* genes in the pathogenesis of human leukemias. One important function of the *Hox* genes in hematopoiesis is the regulation of proliferation.

Erythropoiesis

The erythrocyte lineage represents one line of descent from the CFU-S cells. Although the erythroid progenitor cells are restricted to forming only red blood cells, there are many generations of precursor cells (Figure 16-2). Some of these are only recently recognized, and the functions of many of the stages of precursor cells are just beginning to be understood.

The earliest stages of erythropoiesis are recognized by the behavior of the precursor cells in culture rather than by morphological or biochemical differences. These are called **ery-** throid burst-forming units (BFU-E) and **erythroid colony-forming units (CFU-E)**. Each responds to different stimulatory factors. The pluripotent CFU-S precursors (see Figure 16-1) respond to **interleukin-3**, a product of macrophages in adult bone marrow. A hormone designated as **burst-promoting activity (BPA)** stimulates mitosis of the BFU-E precursors (see Figure 16-2). A CFU-E cell, which has a lesser proliferative capacity than a BFU-E cell, requires the presence of **erythropoietin** as a stimulatory factor. Erythropoietin is a glycoprotein that stimulates the synthesis of the messenger ribonucleic acid (mRNA) for globin and is first produced in the fetal liver. Later in development, synthesis shifts to the kidney, which remains the site of erythropoietin production in the adult. Under conditions of hypoxia (e.g., from blood loss or high altitudes) the production of erythropoietin by the kidneys increases, stimulating the production of more red blood cells to compensate for the increased need. In adult erythropoiesis the CFU-E stage seems to be the one most responsive to environmental influences. The placenta appears to be impervious to erythropoietin, thereby insulating the embryo from changes in erythropoietin levels of the mother as well as eliminating the influence of fetal erythropoietin on the blood-forming apparatus of the mother.

One or two generations after the CFU-E stage, successive generations of erythrocyte precursor cells can be recognized by their morphology. The first recognizable stage is the **proerythroblast** (Figure 16-3), a large, highly basophilic cell that has not yet produced sufficient hemoglobin to be detected by cytochemical analysis. Such a cell has a large nucleolus, much uncondensed nuclear chromatin, numerous ribosomes, and a high concentration of globin mRNAs. These are classic cytological characteristics of an undifferentiated cell.

Succeeding stages of erythroid differentiation (**basophilic, polychromatophilic,** and **orthochromatic erythroblasts**) are characterized by a progressive change in the balance between the accumulation of newly synthesized hemoglobin and the decline of first the RNA-producing machinery and later the protein-synthesizing apparatus. The overall size of the cell decreases, and the nucleus becomes increasingly **pycnotic** (smaller with more condensed chromatin) until it is finally extruded at the stage of the orthochromatic erythrocyte. After the loss of the nucleus and most cytoplasmic organelles, the immature red blood cell, which still contains a small number of polysomes, is a **reticulocyte**. Reticulocytes are released into the bloodstream, where they continue to produce small amounts of hemoglobin for 1 or 2 days.

The final stage of hematopoiesis is the mature **erythrocyte**, which is a terminally differentiated cell because of the loss of its nucleus and most of its cytoplasmic organelles. Erythrocytes in embryos are larger than their adult counterparts and have a shorter life span (50 to 70 days in the fetus versus 120 days in adults).

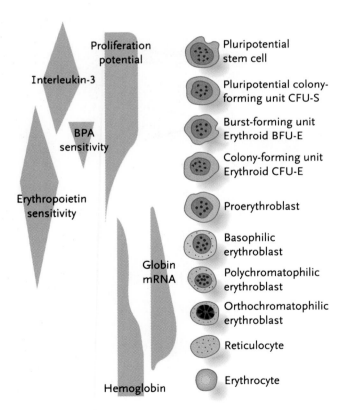

Figure 16-2 *Right,* Morphological stages in the differentiation of a red blood cell from a pluripotential stem cell. *Left,* Molecular correlates of differentiation. The thickness of the tan background is proportional to the amount at the corresponding stages of erythropoiesis. *BPA,* Burst-promoting activity; *mRNA,* messenger ribonucleic acid.

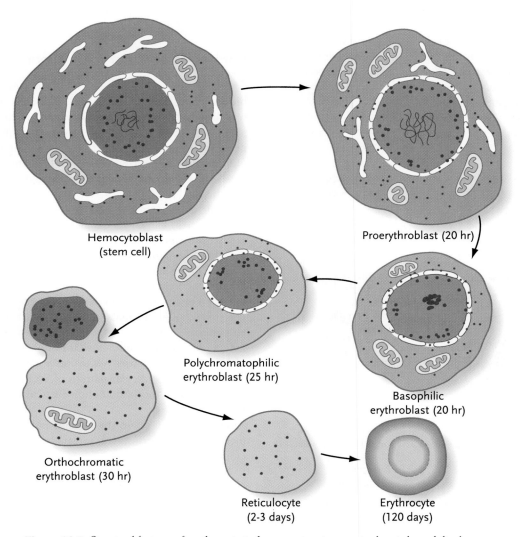

Hemocytoblast
(stem cell)

Proerythroblast (20 hr)

Polychromatophilic
erythroblast (25 hr)

Basophilic
erythroblast (20 hr)

Orthochromatic
erythroblast (30 hr)

Reticulocyte
(2-3 days)

Erythrocyte
(120 days)

Figure 16-3 Structural features of erythropoiesis. In successive stages, cytoplasmic basophilia decreases and the concentration of hemoglobin increases in the cells.

Hemoglobin Synthesis and Its Control

Both the red blood cells and the hemoglobin within them undergo isoform transitions during embryonic development. The hemoglobin molecule is a complex composed of heme and four globin chains: two α and two β chains. Both the α and β subunits are products of genes located on chromosomes 16 and 11, respectively (Figure 16-4). Different isoforms of the subunits are encoded linearly on these chromosomes.

During the period of yolk sac hematopoiesis, embryonic globin isoforms are produced. The earliest embryonic hemoglobin, sometimes called *Gower 1,* is composed of two ζ (α-type) and two ε (β-type) chains. After passing through a couple of transitional forms (Table 16-1), hemoglobin synthesis enters a fetal stage by 12 weeks, which corresponds to the shift in the site of erythropoiesis from the yolk sac to the liver. Fetal hemoglobin consists of two adult-type α chains,

which form very early in embryogenesis, and two γ chains, the major fetal isoform of the β chain. Fetal hemoglobin is the predominant form during the remainder of pregnancy. The main adaptive value of the fetal isoform of hemoglobin is that it has a higher affinity for oxygen than the adult form. This is advantageous to the fetus, which depends on the oxygen concentration of the maternal blood. Starting at about 30 weeks' gestation, there is a gradual switch from the fetal to the adult type of hemoglobin, with $\alpha_2\beta_2$ being the predominant type. A minor but functionally similar variant is $\alpha_2\delta_2$.

Formation of Embryonic Blood Vessels

The early embryo is devoid of blood vessels. Although blood islands appear in the wall of the yolk sac and extraembryonic vascular channels form in association with them (see Figure 5-24), much of the vasculature of the embryonic body is derived from intraembryonic sources. During the early period of somite formation, networks of small vessels rapidly appear in many regions of the embryonic body.

Some vascular channels coalesce to form larger vessels; others remain similar to capillaries or disappear. A fundamental principle of early vasculogenesis is dynamic change associated with growth of the structures with which the vascular channels are associated. The designation of vessels as arteries and veins is not fixed in the early embryo, since the direction of flow of blood in a given channel can easily be reversed. Although the major patterns of vascular channels are recognizable for a given species, the seemingly haphazard manner of recruiting new capillaries to become components of larger vessels primarily accounts for the frequent minor variations in the vascular pattern of an individual. The frequency of anatomical variations is particularly pronounced in the venous system.

Detailed descriptive studies and transplantation experiments involving intrinsic cellular labels or graft-specific monoclonal antibody labels have shown that **angioblasts** (endothe-

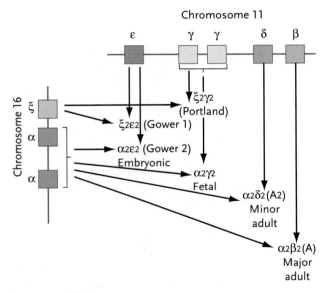

Figure 16-4 Organization of hemoglobin genes along chromosomes 11 and 16 and their sequential activation during embryonic development.

TABLE 16-1 Developmental Isoforms of Human Hemoglobin

Developmental stage	Hemoglobin type	Globin-chain composition
Embryo	Gower 1	$\zeta_2\varepsilon_2$
Embryo	Gower 2	$\alpha_2\varepsilon_2$
Embryo	Portland	$\zeta_2\gamma_2$
Embryo to fetus	Fetal	$\alpha_2\gamma_2$
Fetus to adult	A (adult)	$\alpha_2\beta_2$
Adult	A$_2$	$\alpha_2\delta_2$
Adult	Fetal	$\alpha_2\gamma_2$*

Modified from Brown MS. In Stockman J, Pochedly C, eds: *Developmental and neonatal hematology,* New York, 1988, Raven.
*The fetal hemoglobin expressed in adults differs from true fetal hemoglobin by an amino acid substitution at the 136 position of the γ chain.

lial cell precursors) arise from most mesodermal tissues of the body except notochord and prechordal mesoderm (Table 16-2). Embryonic blood vessels form from angioblasts by three main mechanisms. Many of the larger blood vessels, such as the dorsal aortae, are formed by the coalescence of angioblasts in situ. Other equally large channels, such as the endocardium, are formed by angioblasts migrating into the region from other sites. Other vessels, especially the intersegmental vessels of the main body axis and vessels of the central nervous system, arise as vascular sprouts from existing larger vessels. Many of the angioblasts of the trunk are originally associated with the splanchnic mesoderm.

The walls of blood vessels in most of the trunk and the extremities are derived from local mesoderm that becomes associated with the endothelium of the larger vessels. In the head and many areas of the aortic arch system, mesenchyme derived from neural crest ectoderm constitutes significant portions of the vascular walls (e.g., the smooth muscle cells), but neural crest does not give rise to endothelial cells.

Two-way molecular signaling appears to be involved in building up the walls of blood vessels. According to one model, perivascular mesenchymal cells produce a signaling molecule, called **angiopoietin-1**, which is bound by a tyrosine kinase receptor, **Tie-2**, on the surfaces of the endothelial cells. This stimulates the endothelial cells to release their own signaling molecules, such as **platelet-derived growth factor** (**PDGF**), which stimulate the migration of mesenchymal cells toward the vascular endothelium. Once contacted by the mesenchymal cells, the endothelial cells release transforming growth factor-β (**TGF-β**), which stimulates the differentiation of the mesenchymal cells into vascular smooth muscle or pericytes.

As with myoblasts, angioblasts appear to react to local environmental cues that determine the specific morphological pattern of a blood vessel. Tracing studies of transplanted angioblasts have shown that some can migrate long distances. Angioblasts that have migrated far from the place into which they were grafted become integrated into morphologically normal blood vessels in the areas where they settle.

Local factors also influence the initiation of vasculogenesis. In some organs (e.g., the liver) or parts of organs (e.g., the bronchi of the respiratory system), the blood vessels supplying the regions arise from local mesoderm, whereas other organs (e.g., the metanephric kidneys) or parts of organs (e.g., the alveoli of the lungs) are supplied by blood vessels that grow into the mesenchyme from other tissues. In the latter type of vascularization mechanism, evidence is increasing that the organ primordia produce **angiogenesis factors** that stimulate the growth of vascular sprouts (by promoting mitosis of endothelial cells) into the glandular mesenchyme. Many putative angiogenesis factors have not been molecularly defined, but forms of **fibroblast growth factor** and **vascular endothelial growth factor** have been shown to have angiogenic activity in a number of developing structures.

Development of the Arteries

Aortic arches and their derivatives

The system of aortic arches in early human embryos is organized along the same principles as the system of arteries supplying blood to the gills of many aquatic lower vertebrates. Blood exits from a common ventricle in the heart into a ventral aortic root, from which it is distributed through the branchial arches by pairs of aortic arches (Figure 16-5, A). In gilled vertebrates the aortic arch arteries branch into capillary beds, where the blood becomes reoxygenated as it passes through the gills. In mammalian embryos the aortic arches remain continuous vessels because gas exchange occurs in the placenta and not in the pharyngeal arches. The aortic arches empty into paired dorsal aortae where the blood enters the regular systemic circulation. In human embryos, all aortic arches are never present at the same time. Their formation and remodeling show a pronounced craniocaudal gradient. Blood from the outflow tract of the heart (the truncoconal region) flows next into an **aortic sac**, which differs from the truncoconal region in the construction of its wall. The aortic arches branch off from the aortic sac.

TABLE 16-2 Distribution of Endogenous Angioblasts in Embryonic Tissues

Tissues	Angioblasts	Tissues	Angioblasts
CEPHALIC		**TRUNK**	
Paraxial mesoderm	+	Whole somites	+
Lateral mesoderm	+	Dorsal half somites	+
Prechordal mesoderm	−	Segmental plate mesoderm	+
Notochord	−	Lateral somatic mesoderm	+
Brain	−	Lateral splanchnic mesoderm	+
Neural crest	−	Spinal cord	−

From Noden DM: *Ann NY Acad Sci* 588:236-249, 1990.

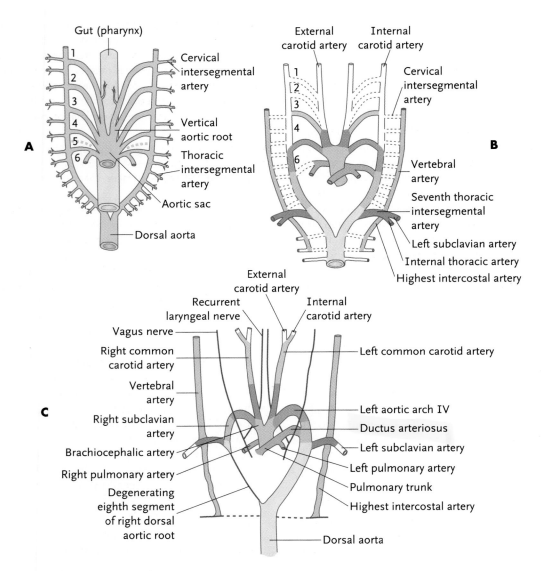

Figure 16-5 A, Schematic representation of the embryonic aortic arch system. B and C, Later steps in the transformation of the aortic arch system in the human. Disposition of the recurrent laryngeal nerve in relation to the right fourth and left sixth arch is also shown in C.

The developmental anatomy of the aortic arch system well illustrates the principle of morphological adaptation of the vascular bed during different stages of embryogenesis (Table 16-3). Continued development of the cranial and cervical regions causes components of the first three arches and associated aortic roots to be remodeled into the carotid artery system (see Figure 16-5). With the remodeling of the heart tube and the internal division of the outflow tract into aortic and pulmonary components, the fourth arches undergo an asymmetrical adaptation to the early asymmetry of the heart. The left fourth aortic arch is retained as a major channel (arch of the aorta), which carries the entire output from the left ventricle of the heart. The right fourth arch is incorporated into the right subclavian artery.

Embryology textbooks traditionally depict the aortic arch system as consisting of six pairs of vascular arches, but the fifth and sixth arches never appear as discrete vascular channels similar to the first through fourth arches. The fifth aortic arch, if it exists at all, is represented by no more than a few capillary loops. The sixth (**pulmonary arch**) arises as a capillary plexus associated with the early trachea and lung buds. The capillary plexus is supplied by ventral segmental arteries arising from the paired dorsal aortae in that region (Figure 16-6). The equivalent of the sixth arch is represented by a discrete distal segment (ventral segmental artery) connected to the dorsal aorta and a plexuslike proximal segment that establishes a connection between the aortic sac at the base of the fourth arch and the distal segmental component. As the respiratory diverticulum and early lung buds elongate, parts of the pulmonary capillary network consolidate to form a pair of discrete **pulmonary arteries** that connect to the putative sixth arch. Although the term **sixth aortic arch** is frequently used in anatomical and clinical literature, **pulmonary arch** is a more appropriate term because it does not imply equivalence to the other aortic arches.

Like the fourth aortic arch, the pulmonary arch develops asymmetrically. On the left side it becomes a large channel. Its distal segment, which was derived from a ventral segmental artery, persists as a major channel (**ductus arteriosus**) that shunts blood from the left pulmonary artery to the aorta (see Figure 16-5, C). By this shunt the lungs are protected from a flow of blood that is greater than what their vasculature can handle during most of the intrauterine period. On the right side the distal segment of the pulmonary arch regresses, and the proximal segment (the base of the right pulmonary artery) branches off from the pulmonary trunk.

The asymmetry of the derivatives of the pulmonary arch accounts for the difference between the course of the right and left **recurrent laryngeal nerves**, which are branches of the vagus nerve (cranial nerve X). These nerves, which supply the larynx, hook around the pulmonary arches. As the heart descends into the thoracic cavity from the cervical region, the branch point from the vagus of each recurrent laryngeal

TABLE 16-3 Adult Derivatives of the Aortic Arch System

	Right side	Left side
AORTIC ARCHES		
1	Disappearance of most of structure	Disappearance of most of structure
	Part of maxillary artery	Part of maxillary artery
2	Disappearance of most of structure	Disappearance of most of structure
	Hyoid and stapedial arteries	Hyoid and stapedial arteries
3	Ventral part—common carotid artery	Ventral part—common carotid artery
	Dorsal part—internal carotid artery	Dorsal part—internal carotid artery
4	Proximal part of right subclavian artery	Part of arch of aorta
5	Rarely recognizable, even in early embryo	Rarely recognizable, even in early embryo
6 (pulmonary)	Part of right pulmonary artery	Ductus arteriosus
		Part of left pulmonary artery
VENTRAL AORTIC ROOTS		
Cranial to third arch	External carotid artery	External carotid artery
Between third and fourth arches	Common carotid artery	Common carotid artery
Between fourth and sixth arches	Brachiocephalic artery	Ascending part of aorta
DORSAL AORTIC ROOTS		
Cranial to third arch	Internal carotid artery	Internal carotid artery
Between third and fourth arches	Disappearance of structure	Disappearance of structure
Between fourth and sixth arches	Central part of right subclavian artery	Descending aorta
Caudal to sixth arch	Disappearance of structure	Descending aorta

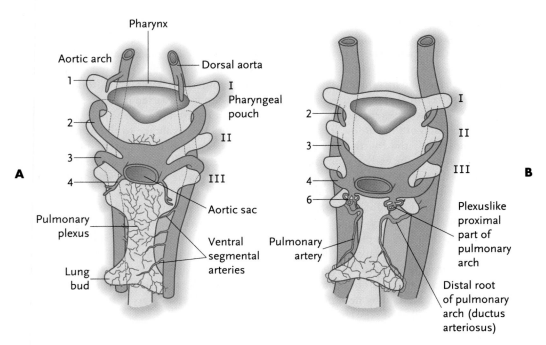

Figure 16-6 Development of the pulmonary arch, showing the early pulmonary plexus in relation to several ventral segmental arteries associated with the early respiratory diverticulum (**A**) and their consolidation into discrete vessels that establish a connection with the bases of the fourth aortic arches (**B**). (Based on DeRuiter MC and others: *Anat Embryol* 179:309-325, 1989.)

nerve is correspondingly moved. On the left side the nerve is associated with the ductus arteriosus (see Figure 16-5, C), which persists throughout the fetal period, so it is pulled deep into the thoracic cavity. On the right side, however, with the regression of much of the right pulmonary arch, the nerve moves to the level of the fourth arch, which constitutes an anatomical barrier. The positions of the right and left recurrent laryngeal nerves in the adult reflect this asymmetry, with the right nerve curving under the right subclavian artery (fourth arch) and the left nerve hooking around the **ligamentum arteriosum** (the adult derivative of the ductus arteriosus, the distal segment of the left pulmonary arch).

Major branches of the aorta

In the early embryo, when the dorsal aortae are still paired vessels, three sets of arterial branches arise from them—**dorsal intersegmental, lateral segmental,** and **ventral segmental** (Figure 16-7). These branches undergo a variety of modifications in form before assuming their adult configurations (Table 16-4). The ventral segmental arteries arise as paired vessels that course over the dorsal and lateral walls of the gut and yolk sac. With the closure of the gut

and the narrowing of the dorsal mesentery, certain branches fuse in the midline to form the celiac, superior, and inferior mesenteric arteries.

The **umbilical arteries** begin as pure ventral segmental branches supplying allantoic mesoderm, but their bases later connect with lumbar intersegmental vessels. The most proximal umbilical channels then regress, and the intersegmental branches become their main branches off the aorta. Like their subclavian counterparts in the arms, the initially small arterial branches (**iliac arteries**) supplying the leg buds appear as components of the dorsal intersegmental (lumbar) branches of the aorta. However, after the umbilical arteries incorporate the proximal segments of the intersegmental vessels, the iliac arteries appear to arise as branches off the umbilical arteries.

Arteries of the head

The arteries supplying the head arise from two sources. Ventrally, the aortic arch system (first to third arches and corresponding roots) gives rise to the arteries supplying the face (**external carotid arteries**) and the frontal part of the base of the brain (**internal carotid arteries**) (see Figure 16-5).

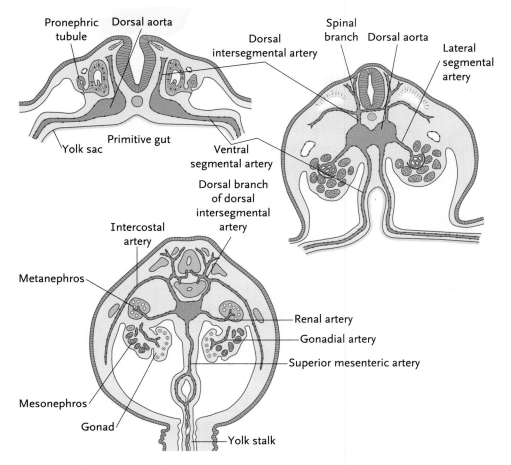

Figure 16-7 Types of segmental branches coming off the abdominal aorta at different stages of development.

At the level of the spinal cord, the **vertebral arteries**, which form through connections of lateral branches of the first six dorsal intersegmental arteries, grow toward the brain. Soon they veer toward the midline and fuse, forming the unpaired **basilar artery** (Figure 16-8). This artery runs along the ventral surface of the brainstem, supplying it with a series of paired arteries. As the basilar artery approaches the level of the diencephalon and the internal carotid arteries, sets of branches from each of these major vessels grow out and fuse, forming **posterior communicating arteries**, which join the circulations of the basilar and internal carotid arteries. Two other small branches off the internal carotid system fuse in the midline to complete a vascular ring (**circle of Willis**), which underlies the base of the diencephalon and encircles the optic chiasm and pituitary stalk. The circle of Willis is a structural adaptation that ensures a continuous blood supply in the event of occlusion of some major arteries supplying the brain.

Coronary arteries

Although intuitively one would expect the coronary arteries to arise as branches growing out from the aorta, exper-

TABLE 16-4 Major Arterial Branches of the Aorta

Embryonic vessels	Adult derivatives
DORSAL INTERSEGMENTAL BRANCHES (PAIRED)	
Cervical intersegmental (1-16)	Lateral branches joining to become vertebral arteries
Seventh intersegmentals	Subclavian arteries
Thoracic intersegmentals	Intercostal arteries
Lumbar intersegmentals	Iliac arteries
LATERAL SEGMENTAL BRANCHES	
Up to 20 pairs of vessels supplying the mesonephros	Adrenal arteries, renal arteries, gonadial (ovarian or spermatic) arteries
VENTRAL SEGMENTAL BRANCHES*	
Vitelline vessels	Celiac artery, superior and inferior mesenteric arteries
Allantoic vessels	Umbilical arteries

*Originally paired in areas where the embryonic aorta itself consists of paired components.

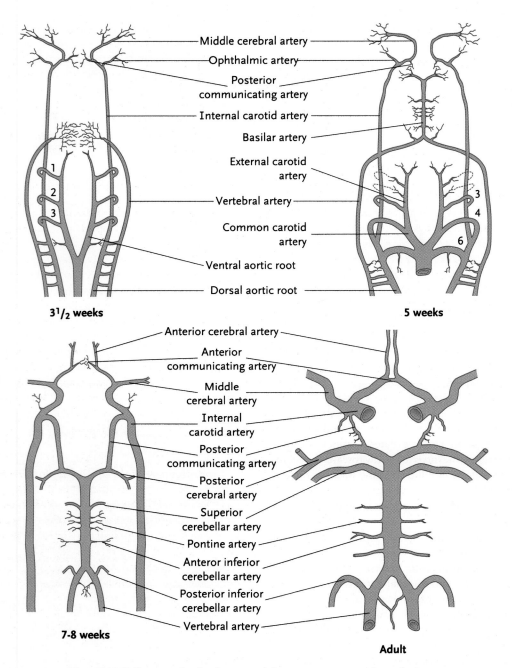

Figure 16-8 Stages in the development of the major arteries supplying the brain.

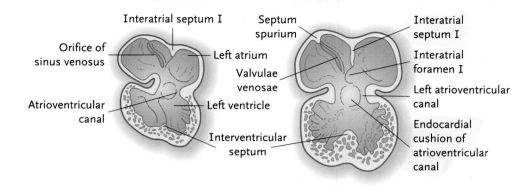

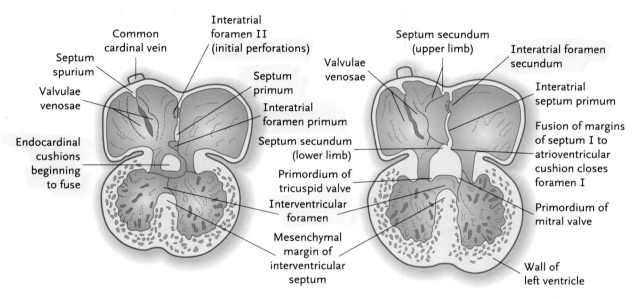

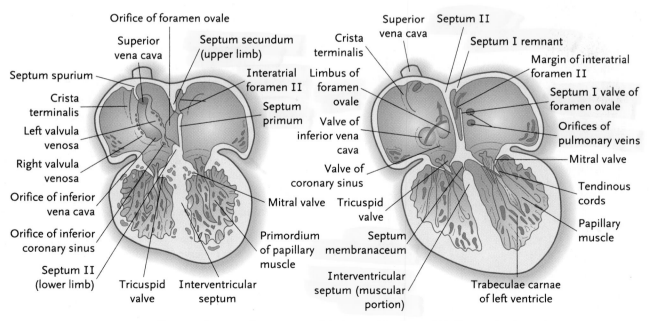

Figure 16-18 Stages in the internal partitioning of the heart. (After Patten BM: *Human embryology*, ed 3, New York, 1988, McGraw-Hill.)

Repositioning of the sinus venosus and the venous inflow into the right atrium

During the stage of the straight tubular heart, the sinus venosus is a bilaterally symmetrical chamber into which the major veins of the body empty (see Figure 16-11). As the heart undergoes looping and the interatrial septa form, the entrance of the sinus venosus shifts completely to the right atrium (see Figures 16-15 and 16-18). As this occurs, the right horn of the sinus venosus becomes increasingly incorporated into the wall of the right atrium, so the much reduced left horn, the **coronary sinus** (which is the common drainage channel for the coronary veins), opens directly into the right atrium (see Figure 16-12). Also in the right atrium, valvelike flaps of tissue (**valvulae venosae**) form around the entrances of the superior and inferior venae cavae. Because of the orientation of the orifice and its pressure, blood entering the right atrium from the inferior vena cava passes mostly through the interatrial shunt and into the left atrium, whereas blood entering from the superior vena cava and the coronary sinus flows through the tricuspid valve into the right ventricle.

Partitioning of the ventricles

When the interatrial septa are first forming, a muscular **interventricular septum** begins to grow from the apex of the common ventricle toward the atrioventricular endocardial cushions. The early division of the common ventricle is also reflected by the presence of a groove on the outer surface of the heart (Figure 16-19). Although an **interventricular foramen** is initially present, it is ultimately obliterated. This

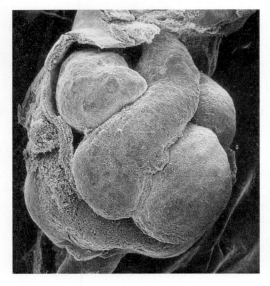

Figure 16-19 Scanning electron micrograph showing a right oblique view of the heart of a human embryo **early in the sixth week.** The pericardium has been dissected free from the heart. (From Jirásek J: *Atlas of human prenatal morphogenesis,* Boston, 1983, Martinus Nijhoff.)

is accomplished by (1) further growth of the muscular interventricular septum, (2) a contribution by truncoconal ridge tissue that divides the outflow tract of the heart, and (3) a membranous component derived from endocardial cushion connective tissue.

Partitioning of the outflow tract of the heart

In the very early tubular heart the outflow tract is a single tube, the bulbus cordis. By the time the interventricular septum begins to form, the bulbus elongates and can be divided into a proximal conus arteriosus and a distal truncus arteriosus (see Figure 16-14). Although initially a single channel, the outflow tract is partitioned into separate aortic and pulmonary channels through the appearance of two spiral **truncoconal ridges,** which are derived largely from neural crest mesenchyme. These ridges bulge into the lumen and finally meet, separating it into two channels. The aortic sac, which is located distal to the truncoconal region, does not contain ridges. Partitioning of the outflow tract begins near the ventral aortic root between the fourth and sixth arches and extends toward the ventricles, spiraling as it goes (Figure 16-20). This accounts for the partial spiraling of the aorta and the pulmonary artery in the adult heart.

Before and during the partitioning process, the neural crest–derived cells of the wall of the outflow tract begin to produce elastic fibers, which provide the resiliency required of the aorta and other great vessels. Elastogenesis follows a gradient, first through the outflow tract, then into the aorta itself, and ultimately into the smaller arterial branches off the aorta.

At the base of the conus, where endocardial cushion tissue is formed in the same manner as in the atrioventricular canal, two new sets of **semilunar valves** form (Figure 16-21). These valves, each of which has three leaflets, prevent ejected blood from washing back into the ventricles. Cranial neural crest cells and cardiac mesoderm are said to contribute to the formation of the semilunar valves, although not all investigators agree on the neural crest contribution. As previously stated, the most proximal extensions of the truncoconal ridges contribute to the formation of the interventricular septum. Just past the aortic side of the aortic semilunar valve, the two coronary arteries join the aorta to supply the heart with blood.

Innervation of the Heart

Although initial heart development occurs independently of nerves, three sets of nerve fibers ultimately innervate the heart (Figure 16-22). Sympathetic (adrenergic) nerve fibers, which act to speed up the heart beat, arrive as outgrowths from sympathetic ganglia of the trunk. These nerve fibers are derived from trunk neural crest. Parasympathetic (cholinergic) innervation is derived from the cardiac component of the cranial neural crest. Neurons of the cardiac ganglia, which are the second-order parasympathetic neurons, migrate directly to

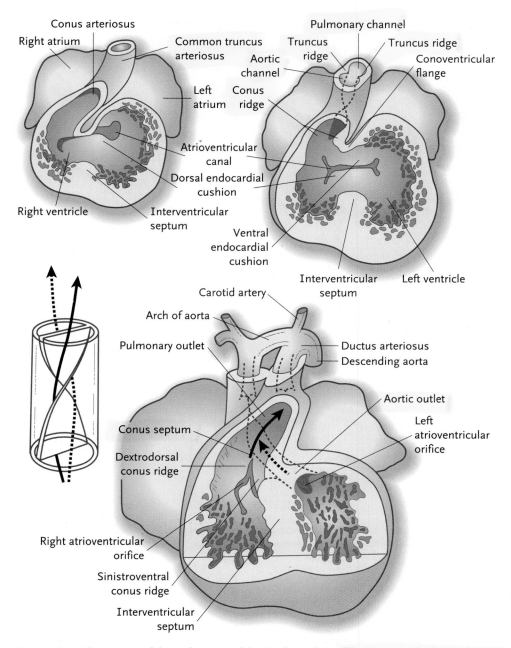

Figure 16-20 Partitioning of the outflow tract of the developing heart. The truncoconal ridges undergo a 180-degree spiraling. (After Kramer TC: *Am J Anat* 71:343-370, 1942.)

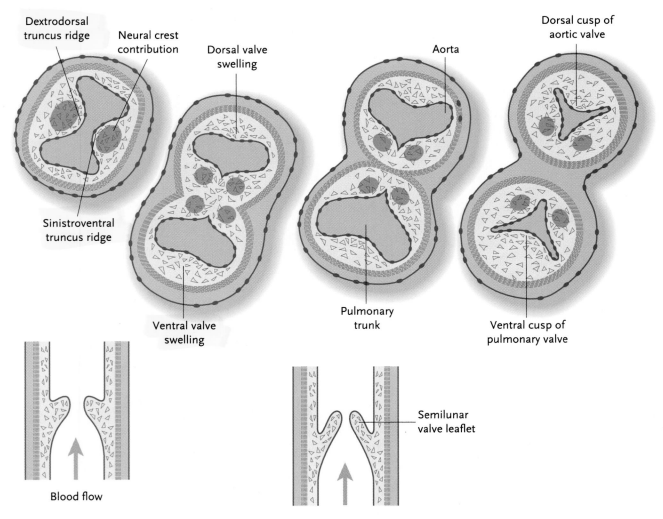

Figure 16-21 Formation of the semilunar valves in the outflow tract of the heart. Neural crest cells (*green areas*) may contribute in part to the formation of the valvular leaflets.

the heart from the neural crest. These synapse with axons of first-order parasympathetic neurons that gain access to the heart via the vagus nerve. Sensory innervation of the heart is also supplied via the vagus nerve, but the sensory neurons originate from placodal ectoderm (nodose placode) (see Figure 5-14). Thus the innervation of the heart has three separate origins.

If the cardiac neural crest is removed in the early chick embryo, cholinergic cardiac ganglia still form. Experiments have determined that the nodose placodes compensate for the loss of neural crest by supplying neurons that take the place of the normal parasympathetic ones.

Conducting System of the Heart

The normal heart beat is a reflection of a complex of internal pacemakers and a conducting system that rapidly dis-

tributes the contractile stimulus throughout the heart. The input of the autonomic nerves, which modulate the heart beat to a faster (sympathetic) or slower (parasympathetic) rate, is also involved.

In very early heart development the location of the pacemaker shifts from the caudalmost end of the left tube of the unfused heart to the sinus venosus. As the sinus venosus is incorporated into the right atrium, the pacemaker, now called the **sinoatrial node**, becomes situated high in the right atrium, close to the entrance of the superior vena cava. Somewhat later, an **atrioventricular node** forms in the interatrial septal area just above the endocardial cushion tissue. These two nodes are connected by several strands of highly modified cardiac muscle cells that conduct the contractile stimulus from the sinoatrial node to the atrioventricular node. From the atrioventricular node a well-defined **atrioventricular bundle** passes from the atrium into the ventricle and splits

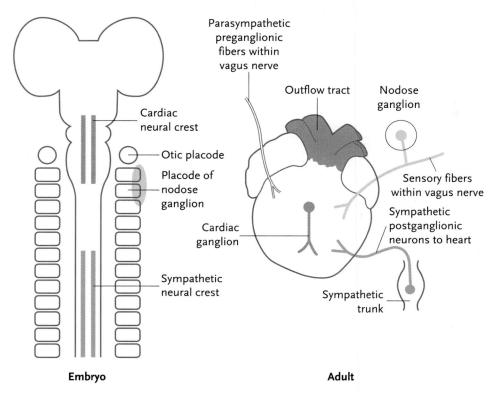

Figure 16-22 Contributions of the cranial and trunk neural crest and the nodose placode to the innervation of the avian heart. (Modified from Kirby ML: *Cell Tissue Res* 252:17-22, 1988.)

into right and left branches. These branches then distribute conducting tissue (**Purkinje fibers**) throughout the ventricular myocardium.

Many aspects of the embryology of the conduction system remain poorly understood. Mature conducting bundles consist of highly modified cardiac myocytes that contain large amounts of glycogen. There is evidence that cells of the atrioventricular bundle differentiate from separate precursor cells, possibly from the rings of tissue ultimately forming the cardiac skeleton, and that Purkinje cells are derived from a separate lineage that branches off from the cells that give rise to ventricular myocytes. These same cells express the transcription factor Msx-2 throughout much of their developmental history. Although the conducting system is richly innervated, it forms before nerves enter the heart. Thus the innervation is eliminated as a causative factor in their development.

INITIATION OF CARDIAC FUNCTION

Because of its accessibility, the chick embryo has taught scientists most of what is known about the earliest functions of the embryonic heart. In recent years the application of ultrasound techniques has allowed the investigation of some aspects of cardiac function in human embryos as young as 4 1/2 to 5 weeks of age.

Bilateral regions of precardiac mesoderm in the chick embryo differentiate into right and left cardiac tubes with functional ventricular, atrial, and sinoatrial regions. Contraction of the embryonic heart begins as the right and left heart tubes begin to fuse, and circulation of the blood begins soon thereafter. In the human embryo, this occurs between 21 and 23 days' gestation.

Different parts of the tubular heart have different intrinsic beats, and experimental transplantation studies have shown that the functional characteristics of the regions of the heart depend on extracellular cues. For example, if preatrial tissue is grafted into a preventricular area, it acquires the functional characteristics of ventricular tissue.

As the heart tubes of the chick embryo first fuse in the ventricular region, the fused ventricles have an intrinsic beat of 25 per minute, and the unfused atria do not beat. A few hours later, when the atrial parts of the cardiac tubes have fused, the atrial region beats at a rate of 62 per minute. The atrial beat acts as a pacemaker, causing the ventricle to beat at the same rate. However, if the atrium is separated from the ventricle, the beat of the ventricle slows to an intrinsic rate of only 24 per minute. Finally, when the sinus venosus takes shape, its intrinsic beat of 140 per minute drives the overall heart beat.

In the early fusing heart a distinct pacemaker region is located in the left sinus venosus region. The pacemaker consists of an aggregation of approximately 60 to 150 cells rather than a signal arising from a single cell. The pacemaker initiates an excitation wave that is propagated through the early heart in about 0.5 second. As the heart matures and gets larger, the rate of propagation increases proportionally to the size of the heart. Thus the conduction velocity of the excitation stimulus increases by 100-fold, but the actual conduction time does not greatly change despite a 1000-fold increase in the mass of the heart in the chick embryo. Increasing numbers of gap junctions between developing cardiac myocytes may partly account for the increasing conduction velocity in the developing heart.

The mechanism by which the tubular heart is able to pump blood in the absence of valves is still not well understood. Once the atrium fills with blood from the sinus venosus, it contracts and sends the blood into the ventricle. A peristalsis-like contraction then moves the blood to the truncus region, from which it leaves the heart and enters the aortic sac. Active contraction of the truncus region prevents the reflux of blood into the heart from the aortic root. Even in the early heart the endocardial cushions of the atrioventricular canal and the outflow tract have a valvelike function. At times the patterns of blood flow in the early heart have been considered to be responsible for the patterns of internal septation of the heart. However, careful studies have shown that many aspects of cardiac morphogenesis are separate from its function.

The blood pressure of an early embryo is very low (0.61/0.43 mm Hg in the 3-day-old chick embryo). As the embryo grows, the blood pressure rises exponentially and then tapers off before birth.

FETAL CIRCULATION

In many respects the overall plan of the embryonic circulation seems to be inefficient and more complex than needed to maintain the growth and development of the fetus. How-ever, the embryo must prepare for the moment when it suddenly shifts to a totally different pattern of oxygenation of blood through the lungs rather than the placenta, making the modifications of the fetal plan of circulation essential.

Highly oxygenated blood from the placenta enters the umbilical vein in a large stream that is sometimes under increased pressure because of uterine contractions. Within the substance of the liver, blood from the umbilical vein under higher pressure passes directly into the ductus venosus, which allows it to bypass the small circulatory channels of the liver and flow directly into the inferior vena cava (Figure 16-23). Once in the vena cava, it has immediate access to the heart. Poorly oxygenated blood flowing in the inferior vena cava can be somewhat backed up because of the strength of the umbilical blood flow.

Functional evidence exists for a physiological sphincter in the ductus venosus, which forces much of the umbilical blood to pass through hepatic capillary channels and enter the inferior vena cava through hepatic veins when it tightens. This considerably reduces the pressure of the umbilical blood and allows poorly oxygenated systemic blood from the inferior vena cava to enter the right atrium at a lower pressure. Higher-pressure blood entering the umbilical vein from the placenta also tends to prevent blood from the hepatic portal vein from entering the ductus venosus. When the uterus is relaxed and the umbilical venous blood is under low pressure, poorly oxygenated portal blood mixes with the umbilical blood in the ductus venosus. More mixing of umbilical and systemic blood occurs in the inferior vena cava as well.

In the right atrium the orientation of the entrance of the inferior vena cava allows a stream of blood under slightly increased pressure to pass directly through the foramen ovale and foramen secundum into the left atrium (see Figure 16-23). This is the route normally taken by highly oxygenated umbilical blood entering the body under increased pressure. Because the interatrial shunt of the fetus is smaller than the opening of the inferior vena cava, some of the highly oxygenated caval blood eddies in the right atrium and enters the right ventricle. When low-pressure blood (typically poorly oxygenated systemic blood) enters the right atrium, it joins with the venous blood draining the head through the superior vena cava and the heart through the coronary sinus and is mostly directed through the tricuspid valve into the right ventricle.

All blood entering the fetal right ventricle leaves through the pulmonary artery and passes toward the lungs. Even in the relatively late fetus, the pulmonary vasculature is not ready to handle the full volume of blood that enters the pulmonary artery. The blood that cannot be accommodated by the pulmonary arteries is shunted to the aorta via the ductus arteriosus. This structure protects the lungs from circulatory overload, yet allows the right ventricle to exercise in preparation for its functioning at full capacity at birth. The control of patency of the ductus arteriosus has been subject to considerable speculation. Patency of both the ductus arte-

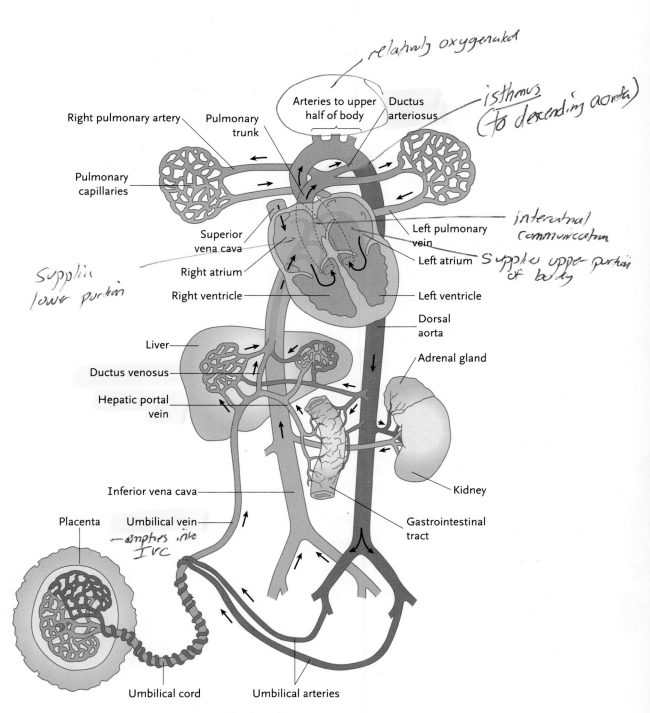

Figure 16-23 Fetal circulation at term.

Handwritten annotations:
- relatively oxygenated
- isthmus (to descending aorta)
- interatrial communication
- Supplies upper portion of body
- Supplies lower portion
- empties into IVC

Labels:
Right pulmonary artery
Pulmonary trunk
Arteries to upper half of body
Ductus arteriosus
Pulmonary capillaries
Superior vena cava
Left pulmonary vein
Right atrium
Left atrium
Right ventricle
Left ventricle
Dorsal aorta
Liver
Adrenal gland
Ductus venosus
Hepatic portal vein
Inferior vena cava
Kidney
Placenta
Umbilical vein
Gastrointestinal tract
Umbilical cord
Umbilical arteries

riosus and ductus venosus in the fetus is maintained actively through the action of prostaglandins (prostaglandin E_2 and prostaglandin I_2, respectively).

The left atrium receives a stream of highly oxygenated umbilical blood through the interatrial shunt and a small amount of poorly oxygenated blood from the pulmonary veins. This blood, which in aggregate is relatively highly oxygenated, passes into the left ventricle and leaves the heart through the aorta. Some of the first arterial branches leaving the aorta supply the heart and brain, organs that require a high concentration of oxygen for normal development.

Where the aortic arch begins to descend, the ductus arteriosus empties poorly oxygenated blood into it. This mixture of well-oxygenated and poorly oxygenated blood is then distributed to the tissues and organs that are supplied by the thoracic and abdominal branches of the aorta. Near its caudal end the aorta gives off two large umbilical arteries, which carry blood to the placenta for renewal.

TABLE 16-5 Timelines in Normal and Abnormal Cardiac Development

Normal time	Developmental events	Malformations arising during period
18 days	Horseshoe-shaped cardiac primordium appears.	Lethal mutants
20 days	Bilateral cardiac primordia fuse.	Cardia bifida (experimental)
	Cardiac jelly appears.	—
	Aortic arch is forming.	—
22 days	Heart is looping into S shape.	Dextrocardia
	Heart begins to beat.	—
	Dorsal mesocardium is breaking down.	—
	Aortic arches I and II are forming.	—
24 days	Atria are beginning to bulge.	—
	Right and left ventricles act like two pumps in series.	—
	Outflow tract is distinguishable from right ventricle.	—
Late fourth week	Sinus venosus is becoming incorporated into right atrium.	Venous inflow malformations
	Endocardial cushions appear.	Persistent atrioventricular canal
	Early septum I appears between left and right atria.	Common atrium
	Muscular interventricular septum is forming.	Common ventricle
	Truncoconal ridges are forming.	Persistent truncus arteriosus
	Aortic arch I is regressing.	—
	Aortic arch III is formed.	—
	Aortic arch IV is forming.	—
Early fifth week	Endocardial cushions are coming together, forming right and left atrioventricular canals.	Persistent atrioventricular canal
	Further growth of interatrial septum I and muscular interventricular septum occurs.	Muscular ventricular septal defects
	Truncus arteriosus is dividing into aorta and pulmonary artery.	Transposition of great vessels Aortic and pulmonary stenosis or atresia
	Atrioventricular bundle is forming; there is possible neurogenic control of heart beat.	—
	Pulmonary veins are becoming incorporated into left atrium.	Aberrant pulmonary drainage
	Aortic arches I and II have regressed.	—
	Aortic arches III and IV have formed.	—
	Aortic arch VI is forming.	—
Late fifth to early sixth week	Endocardial cushions fuse.	—
	Interatrial foramen II is forming.	—
	Interatrial septum I is almost contacting endocardial cushion.	Low atrial septal defects
	Membranous part of interventricular septum starts to form.	Membranous interventricular septal defects
	Semilunar valves begin to form.	Aortic and pulmonary valvular stenosis
Late sixth week	Interatrial foramen II is large.	High atrial septal defects
	Interatrial septum II starts to form.	—
	Atrioventricular valves and papillary muscles are forming.	Tricuspid or mitral valvular stenosis or atresia
	Interventricular septum is almost complete.	Membranous interventricular septal defects
	Coronary circulation is becoming established.	—
Eighth to ninth week	Membranous part of interventricular septum is completed.	Membranous interventricular septal defects

With an incidence of almost 1 per 100 live births, heart defects represent the most common class of congenital malformations. Because of the close physiological balance of the circulation, most malformations produce symptoms. Clinically, heart malformations are typically classified as those that are associated with cyanosis **(cyanotic defects)** in postnatal life and those that are not **(acyanotic defects).**

Cyanosis results when the blood contains more than 5 g/dl of reduced hemoglobin. Cyanosis is readily recognizable by a purplish to bluish tinge to the skin in areas with a dense superficial capillary circulation. It is associated with **polycythemia,** an increased concentration of erythrocytes in the blood resulting from the overall decreased oxygen saturation of the blood. Long-term cyanosis is associated with a prominent clubbing of the ends of the fingers and decreased growth. In severe cases of cyanosis, children often assume a squatting posture that may facilitate re-oxygenation of the blood.

Postnatally, cyanosis is associated with the presence of a right-to-left shunt in which venous blood mixes with systemic blood. Some heart defects are acyanotic for many years but then become cyanotic. These defects are initially characterized by a left-to-right shunt in which oxygenated systemic blood re-fluxes into the right atrium or ventricle. The net result is an increased pumping load on the right ventricle, ultimately leading to right ventricular hypertrophy. Over a long period the increased blood flow through the lungs provokes a hypertensive re-action in the pulmonary vasculature, which effectively increases the pressure in the right ventricle and atrium. When the blood pressure on the right side of the heart exceeds that in the corresponding left chamber, the shunt reverses, and poorly oxygenated blood passes to the systemic circulation, leading to cyanosis. At this point the condition of the patient who has the cardiac lesion often rapidly worsens.

CHAMBER-TO-CHAMBER SHUNTS
Interatrial Septal Defects
Several types of anatomical defects in the interatrial septum can result in a persisting shunt between the two atria. The most common varieties are caused by excessive resorption of tissue around the foramen secundum or hypoplastic growth of the septum secundum (Figure 16-24, *A*). A less common variety is a low septal defect, which is usually caused by the lack of union between the leading edge of the septum primum and the endocardial cushions (Figure 16-24, *B*). If the defect is the result of a deficiency of endocardial cushion tissue, associated defects of the atrioventricular valves can considerably complicate the lesion. Lack of septation of the atrium results in a **common atrium,** a serious defect that is usually associated with other heart defects. Atrial septal defects are among the most common heart malformations. Increasingly, atrial septal defects are being associated with chromosome 21. Individuals with Down syndrome (trisomy of chromosome 21) have a high incidence of defects of both the atrial and ventricular septa.

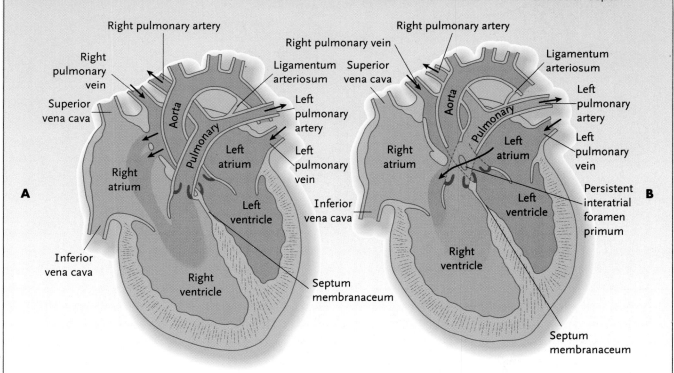

Figure 16-24 High (A) and low (B) atrial septal defects in the heart. Red denotes well-oxygenated arterial blood, blue denotes poorly oxygenated venous blood, and purple denotes a mixture of arterial and venous blood.

Continued

CLINICAL CORRELATION 16-1
Malformations of the Heart—cont'd

Individuals with autosomal dominant mutations of the *Nkx2-5* gene (see p. 416) have a high incidence of abnormalities of the septum secundum, resulting in atrial septal defects. Associated with the atrial septal defects is an equally high incidence of atrioventricular block, which can lead to sudden death in affected individuals whose hearts are not assisted by pacemakers. Before the discovery of this mutation, it was suspected that many of the cases of atrioventricular block were due to disruption of the atrioventricular bundle by the repair procedure. During the early days of cardiac surgery, before the anatomy of the atrioventricular bundle was precisely determined, surgically induced bundle branch block was a problem in the repair of low atrial septal defects.

Uncomplicated atrial septal defects are usually compatible with many years of symptom-free life. Even during the symptom-free period, blood from the left atrium, which is under slightly higher pressure than that in the right atrium, passes into the right atrium. This additional blood causes right atrial hypertrophy and results in increased blood flow into the lungs. Over many years, pulmonary hypertension can develop. This increases the blood pressure of the right ventricle and ultimately that of the right atrium. Only a few millimeters of increased right atrial pressure reverses the blood flow in the interatrial shunt and causes cyanosis.

A more serious condition is **premature closure of the foramen ovale.** In this situation the entire input of blood into the right atrium passes into the right ventricle, causing massive hypertrophy of the right side of the heart. The left side is severely hypoplastic because of the reduced blood that the left chambers carry. Although this defect is usually compatible with intrauterine life, infants typically die shortly after birth because the hypoplastic left heart cannot handle a normal circulatory load.

Persistent Atrioventricular Canal

The usual basis for persistent atrioventricular canal is underdevelopment of the endocardial cushions that results in a lack of division of the early atrioventricular canal into right and left channels. A number of specific causes of atrioventricular canal defects may exist, ranging from inappropriate expression of Msx-1 to defects in the production or reception of inductively active extracellular matrix components (e.g., subunits of adherons) by the endocardial cells (see Figure 16-16).

A persistent atrioventricular canal is often associated with major interatrial and interventricular septal defects (Figure 16-25). This severe defect leads to

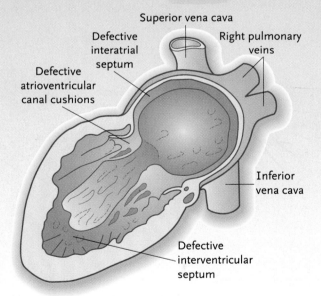

Figure 16-25 Dissection of a heart with a persistent atrioventricular canal in a **12-day-old boy**. (After Patten BM: *Human embryology*, ed 3, New York, 1988, McGraw-Hill.)

CLINICAL CORRELATION 16-1
Malformations of the Heart—cont'd

poor growth and a considerably shortened life. Interestingly, despite the potential for mixing of blood, the predominant shunt direction is left to right, and some patients have little cyanosis.

Tricuspid Atresia

In tricuspid atresia, the etiology of which is poorly understood, the normal valvular opening between the right atrium and right ventricle is completely occluded

(Figure 16-26, *B*). Such a defect alone causes death because the blood cannot gain access to the lungs for oxygenation. However, children can survive with this malformation, illustrating an important point in cardiac embryology. Often a primary lesion is accompanied by one or more secondary lesions (usually shunts) that permit survival, although frequently at a poor functional level.

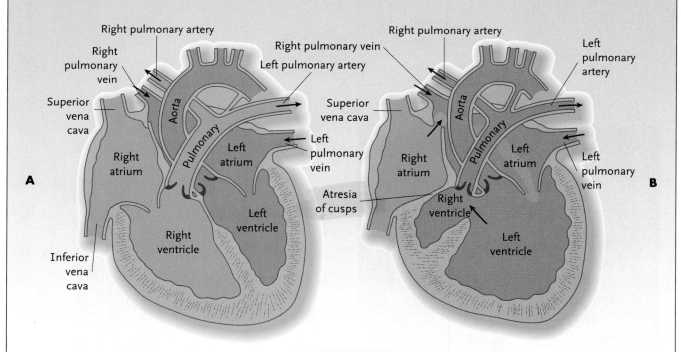

Figure 16-26 A, Normal postnatal heart. B, Tricuspid atresia, with compensating defects in the interatrial septum and interventricular septum *(arrows)*, which allow this patient to survive.

Continued

CLINICAL CORRELATION 16-1
Malformations of the Heart—cont'd

In this condition, secondary shunts must accomplish two things. First, a persisting atrial septal defect must shunt the blood that cannot pass through the atretic tricuspid valve into the left atrium. The left atrial blood then flows into the left ventricle. Second, one or more secondary shunts must allow blood to gain access to the lungs so that it can become oxygenated. Left ventricular blood could enter the right ventricle and pulmonary arterial system if a defect is present in the interventricular septum. Another possibility is for the blood in the left ventricle to pass into the systemic circulation, where it can gain access to the lungs by passing from the aorta through a patent ductus arteriosus into the pulmonary arteries. From the lungs the oxygenated blood enters the left atrium, perhaps to be recycled through the lungs again before entering the systemic circulation.

Mitral atresia can also occur, but it is much rarer than tricuspid atresia. Secondary compensating defects again have to be present for survival. Infants with these lesions typically survive only a few months or years.

Interventricular Septal Defect

Defects in the interventricular septum, which are not as common as atrial septal defects, typically occur in the membranous portion of the septum where several embryonic tissues converge (Figure 16-27). Because the pressure of the blood in the left ventricle is higher than that in the right, this lesion is initially associated with a left-to-right acyanotic shunting of blood flow (Figure 16-28). However, the increased blood flow into the right ventricle causes right ventricular hypertrophy and can lead to pulmonary hypertension, ultimately causing reversal of the shunt. The basic pathological dynamics are similar to those for atrial septal defects.

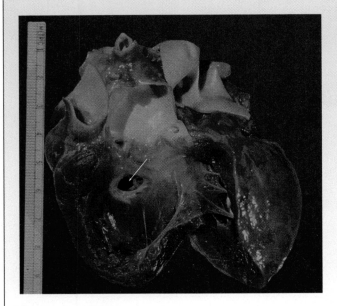

Figure 16-27 Ventricular septal defect (*arrow*) associated with tricuspid atresia. (Photo 147 from the Arey-DaPeña Pediatric Pathology Photographic Collection, Human Developmental Anatomy Center, National Museum of Health and Medicine, Armed Forces Institute of Pathology, Washington, DC.)

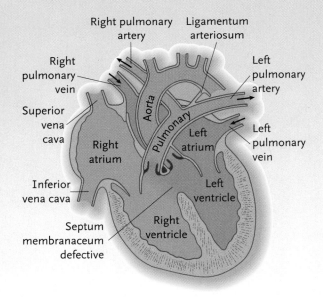

Figure 16-28 Interventricular septal defect (membranous portion). Mixing of arterial and venous blood occurs in both outflow tracts but especially in the pulmonary artery.

CLINICAL CORRELATION 16-1
Malformations of the Heart—cont'd

MALFORMATIONS OF THE OUTFLOW TRACT

The outflow tract of the heart (truncoconal region) is subject to a variety of malformations. Experimental studies have shown a prominent contribution of neural crest cells to this region. Extirpation and transplantation experiments have shown specific requirements for cardiac neural crest cells in the normal development of the cardiac outflow tract, (Figure 16-29). If the cardiac neural crest is removed, ectodermal cells from the nodose placode populate the outflow tract, but septation of the outflow tract does not occur, leading to a persistent truncus arteriosus. If mesencephalic or truncal neural crest is grafted in place of cardiac neural crest or if foreign neural crest is grafted lateral to the cardiac neural crest, persistent truncus arteriosus consistently results. The last experiment shows that foreign neural crest interferes with the normal migration or function of the cardiac neural crest.

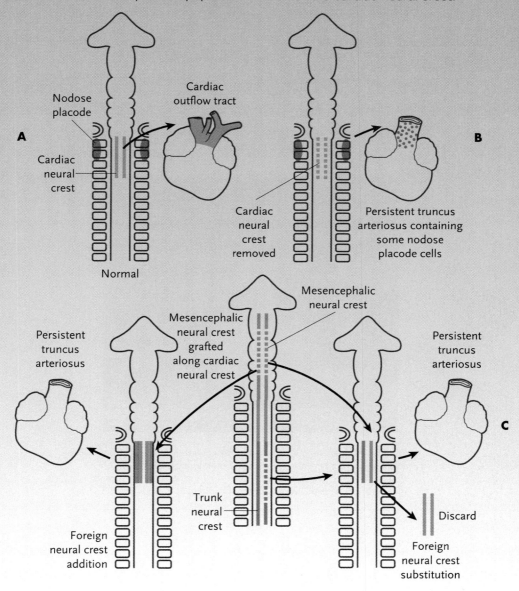

Figure 16-29 Neural crest and morphogenesis of the outflow tract of the heart. A, Normal structure, showing cardiac neural crest contributing to the formation of the outflow tract in the avian heart. B, Removal of the cardiac neural crest leads to the formation of a persistent truncus arteriosus containing cells derived from the nodose placode. C, Experiments illustrating the importance of cardiac neural crest in the morphogenesis of the outflow tract. (Based on Kirby ML, Waldo KL: *Circulation* 82:332-340, 1990.)

Continued

CLINICAL CORRELATION 16-1
Malformations of the Heart—cont'd

Although all malformations of this area cannot be attributed to defective neural crest development, circumstantial evidence suggests that this may be a significant factor. A number of defects of the outflow tract are associated with translocations or deletions in chromosome 22, and most of these involve the neural crest. Lesions of the outflow tract can be produced experimentally by interfering with the function of specific genes, often genes located on chromosome 22 and genes that affect properties of cranial neural crest cells. For example, outflow tract abnormalities are seen in mice deficient in **neurotrophin-3 (NT-3)**, a member of the nerve growth factor family.

Persistent Truncus Arteriosus

Persistent truncus arteriosus is caused by the lack of partitioning of the outflow tract by the truncoconal ridges (Figures 16-30 and 16-31, *A*). Because of the

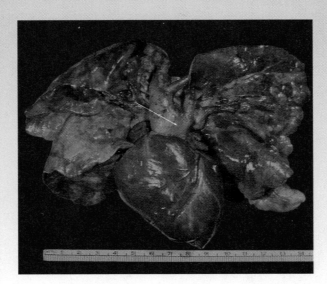

Figure 16-30 Persistent truncus arteriosus *(arrow)*. (Photo 117 from the Arey-DaPeña Pediatric Pathology Photographic Collection, Human Developmental Anatomy Center, National Museum of Health and Medicine, Armed Forces Institute of Pathology, Washington, DC.)

CLINICAL CORRELATION 16-1
Malformations of the Heart—cont'd

contribution of the truncoconal ridges to the membranous part of the interventricular septum, this malformation is almost always accompanied by a ventricular septal defect. A large arterial outflow vessel overrides the ventricular septum and re-

ceives blood that exits from each ventricle. As may be predicted, individuals with a persistent truncus arteriosus are highly cyanotic. Without treatment, 60% to 70% of infants born with this defect die within 6 months.

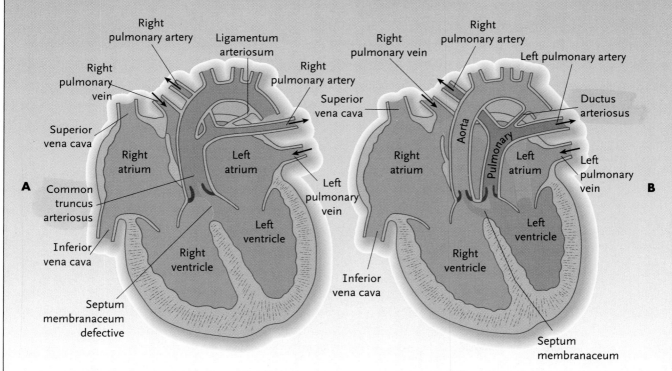

Figure 16-31 A, Persistent truncus arteriosus. A single outflow tract is fed by blood entering from both the right and left ventricles. The membranous part of the interventricular septum is commonly defective. **B,** Transposition of the great vessels caused by lack of spiraling of the truncoconal ridges in the early embryo. The aorta arises from the right ventricle and the pulmonary artery from the left ventricle.

Continued

CLINICAL CORRELATION 16-1
Malformations of the Heart—cont'd

Transposition of the Great Vessels

On rare occasions the truncoconal ridges fail to spiral as they divide the outflow tract into two channels. This results in two totally independent circulatory arcs, with the right ventricle emptying into the aorta and the left ventricle emptying into the pulmonary artery (Figure 16-31, *B*). If the condition were uncorrected, the left circulatory arc would continue pumping highly oxygenated blood through the left side of the heart and the lungs, whereas the right side of the heart would pump venous blood through the aorta into the systemic circulatory channels and back into the right atrium. This lesion, which is the most common cause of cyanosis in newborns, is compatible with life only if an atrial and a ventricular septal defect and an associated patent ductus arteriosus accompany it. Even with these anatomical compensations, the quality of blood reaching the body is poor.

Aortic and Pulmonary Stenosis

If the septation of the outflow tract by the truncoconal ridges is asymmetrical, either the aorta or pulmonary artery is abnormally narrowed, resulting in **aortic** and **pulmonary stenosis** (Figures 16-32 and 16-33). The severity of symptoms is related to the degree of stenosis. In the most extreme case, the stenosis is so severe that the lumen of the vessel is essentially obliterated. This condition is known as **aortic** or **pulmonary atresia**. A lesion reminiscent of pulmonary stenosis has been produced in mice bearing a null mutant of the gene for **connexin43**, which encodes a protein component of the gap junction channel. Why such a genetic lesion would affect principally the pulmonary outlet of the heart is not yet known.

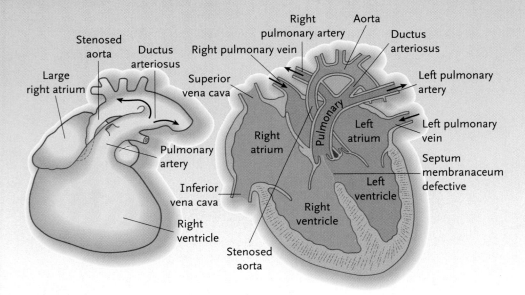

Figure 16-32 Aortic stenosis. In severe cases the ductus arteriosus commonly remains patent. *Right,* Mixed arterial and venous blood in the pulmonary artery is shown in purple. Initially, blood from the pulmonary trunk *(purple)* goes through the ductus arteriosus into the aorta, often leading to cyanosis.

CLINICAL CORRELATION 16-1
Malformations of the Heart—cont'd

One of the best-known lesions of this type is the **tetralogy of Fallot,** which is characterized by (1) pulmonary stenosis, (2) a membranous interventricular septal defect, (3) a large aorta (overriding aorta, the opening of which extends into the right ventricle), and (4) right ventricular hypertrophy. The basic defect in tetralogy of Fallot is an asymmetrical fusion of the truncoconal ridges and a malalignment of the aortic and pulmonary valves. Because of the pulmonary stenosis and the wider-than-normal aortic opening, some poorly oxygenated right ventricular blood leaves via the enlarged aorta, causing cyanosis. Tetralogy of Fallot is the most common cyanotic heart lesion.

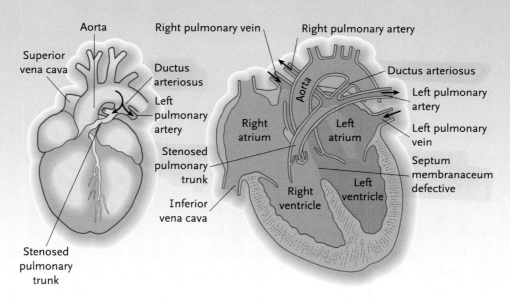

Figure 16-33 Pulmonary stenosis. *Right,* Patterns of blood flow. In severe cases the ductus arteriosus remains patent, with blood flowing from the aorta into the pulmonary circulation (*arrows*).

Continued

Because of their mode of formation, in which one vascular channel is favored within a dense network, blood vessels (especially veins) are subject to numerous variations from normal. Most variations seen in the dissecting laboratory are of little functional significance. Animal experiments suggest that disturbances in the neural crest may be involved in the genesis of certain anomalies of the major arteries. When the cardiac neural crest is removed from early avian embryos, malformations involving the carotid arteries and arch of the aorta result. Certain malformations of the larger vessels can cause serious symptoms or be significant during surgery.

DOUBLE AORTIC ARCH

Rarely, the segment of the right dorsal aortic arch between the exit of the right subclavian artery and its point of joining with the left aortic arch persists instead of degenerating. This results in a complete vascular ring surrounding the trachea and esophagus (Figures 16-34, *A*, and 16-35). A double aortic arch can cause **dyspnea** (difficulty breathing) in infants while they feed. Even if the condition is asymptomatic early in life, later growth typically narrows the diameter of the ring in relation to the size of the trachea and esophagus, causing symptoms in later years.

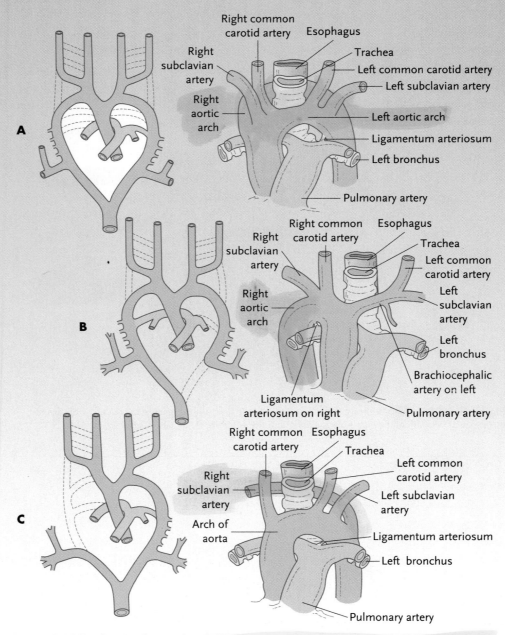

Figure 16-34 Aortic arch anomalies. **A,** Double aortic arch. **B,** Right aortic arch. **C,** Right subclavian artery from the arch of the aorta.

CLINICAL CORRELATION 16-2
Malformations of the Blood Vessels—cont'd

RIGHT AORTIC ARCH

A right aortic arch arises from the persistence of the complete embryonic right aortic arch and the disappearance in the left arch of the segment caudal to the exit of the left subclavian artery (Figure 16-34, *B*). This condition is essentially a mirror image of normal development of the aortic arch, and it can occur as an isolated anomaly or as part of complete situs inversus of the individual. Symptoms are typically mild or absent unless an aberrant left subclavian artery presses against the esophagus or trachea.

RIGHT SUBCLAVIAN ARTERY ARISING FROM THE ARCH OF THE AORTA

If the right fourth aortic arch degenerates between the common carotid artery and the exit of the right seventh thoracic intersegmental artery (see Figure 16-5, *B* and *C*) and if the segment between the exit of the right subclavian artery and the more distal segment of the right aortic arch (which normally disappears) persists, the right subclavian artery arises from the left aortic arch and passes behind the esophagus and trachea to reach the right arm (Figure 16-34, *C*). As with a double aortic arch, this condition can cause difficulties in breathing and swallowing.

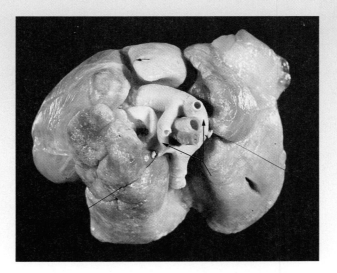

Figure 16-35 Double aortic arch *(arrow).* (Photo 5992 from the Arey-DaPeña Pediatric Pathology Photographic Collection, Human Developmental Anatomy Center, National Museum of Health and Medicine, Armed Forces Institute of Pathology, Washington, DC.)

Continued

INTERRUPTION OF THE LEFT AORTIC ARCH

Interruption of the left aortic arch is a relatively uncommon vascular malformation that usually results in a break distal to the exit of the left subclavian artery (Figure 16-36). To be compatible with life, this lesion is usually accompanied by a patent ductus arteriosus, which allows blood flow to the lower part of the body. This lesion has been produced in mice that are lacking in the winged helix transcription factor **MFH-1** (mesenchyme fork head-1).

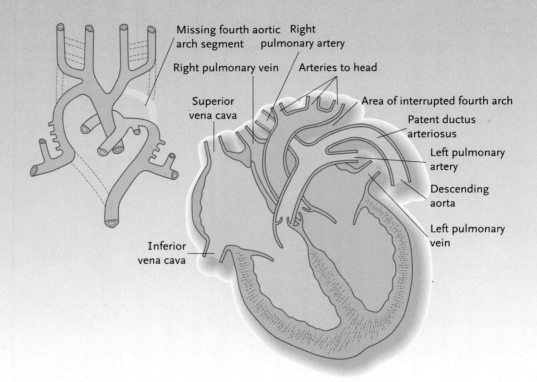

Figure 16-36 Interruption of the left aortic arch. This lesion is associated with a deficiency in the MFH-1 winged helix transcription factor.

CLINICAL CORRELATION 16-2
Malformations of the Blood Vessels—cont'd

PATENT DUCTUS ARTERIOSUS

One common vascular anomaly is failure of the ductus arteriosus to close after birth (Figure 16-37). At least half of infants with this condition experience no symptoms, but over many years the strong flow of blood from the higher-pressure systemic (aortic) circulation into the pulmonary circulation overloads the vasculature of the lungs, resulting in pulmonary hypertension and ultimately heart failure.

COARCTATION OF THE AORTA

Another relatively common, nonlethal malformation of the vascular system is coarctation of the aorta, which occurs in two main variants. One consists of an abrupt narrowing of the descending aorta caudal to the entrance of the ductus arteriosus (Figure 16-38, *B*). The other variant, called **preductal coarctation**, occurs upstream from the ductus (Figure 16-38, *A*). The former variety **(postductal coarctation)** is by far the most common, accounting for over 95% of all cases. The embryogenesis of coarctation is still not clear. Several underlying causes may lead to the same condition. In patients with both Down and Turner's syndromes, the incidence of coarctation of the aorta is increased.

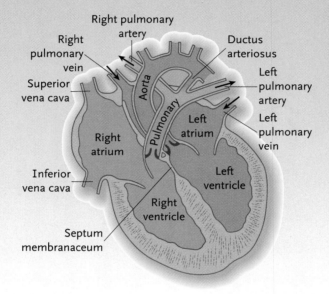

Figure 16-37 Patent ductus arteriosus showing the flow of blood from the aorta into the pulmonary circulation. Later in life, pulmonary hypertension may result, causing the reversal of blood flow through the shunt and cyanosis.

Continued

CLINICAL CORRELATION 16-2
Malformations of the Blood Vessels—cont'd

In preductal coarctation of the aorta, which may be related to inadequate expression of MFH-1, the ductus arteriosus typically remains patent after birth. The blood supplying the trunk and limbs reaches the descending aorta through the ductus. This can lead to **differential cyanosis,** in which the head and upper trunk and arms have a normal color, but the lower trunk and limbs are cyanotic because of the flow of venous blood into the aorta through the patent ductus arteriosus.

The vasculature must compensate for a postductal coarctation in a different manner, since the location of the narrowing in this case effectively cuts off the arterial circulation of the head and arms from that of the trunk and legs. The body responds by opening up collateral circulatory channels and connections through normally relatively small arteries that lead from the upper to the lower body (Figure 16-38, *C*). Such channels are the internal thoracic arteries, the arteries associated with the scapula, and the anterior spinal artery. The unusually large flow of blood through these arteries passes through segmental branches (e.g., intercostal arteries) into

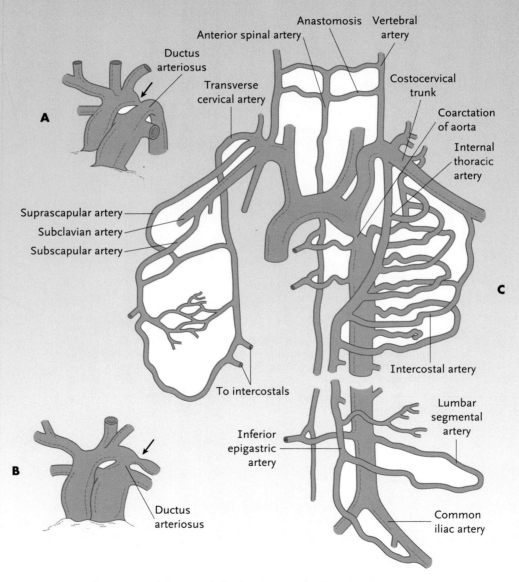

Figure 16-38 Coarctation of the aorta. **A,** Preductal coarctation (*arrow*) with accompanying patent ductus arteriosus. **B,** Postductal coarctation (*arrow*) with an accompanying patent ductus arteriosus. **C,** Collateral circulation in postductal coarctation, with enlarged peripheral vessels carrying blood to the lower part of the body.

CLINICAL CORRELATION 16-2
Malformations of the Blood Vessels—cont'd

the descending aorta caudal to the coarctation. The increased blood flow in the intercostal arteries causes a distinct notching in the ribs that can be readily seen in radiological images. Despite these compensatory circulatory adaptations the blood pressure in patients with a postductal coarctation is much higher in the arms than in the legs.

MALFORMATIONS OF THE VENAE CAVAE

As might be expected from their complex mode of formation (see Figure 16-9), the superior and inferior venae cavae are subject to a wide range of malformations. Common variants are duplications of the superior and inferior venae cavae or persistence of the left instead of the right segments of these vessels along with the absence of the normal vessel. In most cases, these malformations are asymptomatic.

ANOMALOUS PULMONARY RETURN

Because of the way the individual pulmonary veins are joined and the later absorption of the distal part of the pulmonary venous system into the left atrial wall, inappropriate connections of pulmonary veins

to the heart can occur (Figure 16-39). One of the more common is for one or more branches of the pulmonary vein to enter the right instead of the left atrium. In other cases **(total anomalous pulmonary return)**, all pulmonary veins empty into the right atrium or superior vena cava. Such a case must be accompanied by an associated shunt (e.g., interatrial shunt) to bring oxygenated blood into the systemic circulation.

MALFORMATIONS OF THE LYMPHATIC SYSTEM

Although minor anatomical variations of lymphatic channels are common, anomalies that cause symptoms are rare. These typically present as swelling caused by dilatation of major lymphatic vessels. By far the most common major lymphatic anomaly seen in fetuses is **cystic hygroma**, which manifests as large swellings, sometimes even collarlike, in the region of the neck (see Figure 7-1, *A*). Although the embryological basis for cystic hygroma is not certain, excessive local production and growth of lymphatic tissue, possibly originating as pinched off buds from the jugular lymph sacs, is probably the cause.

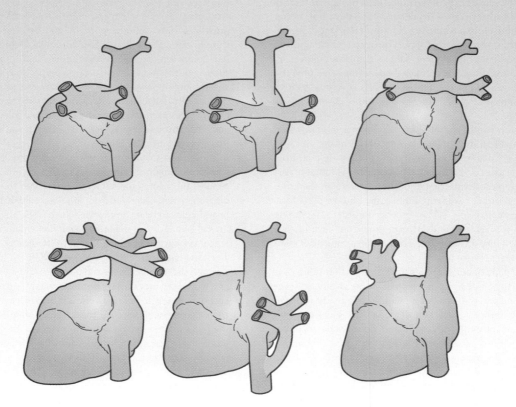

Figure 16-39 Variants of anomalous pulmonary drainage.

CLINICAL VIGNETTE

An 8-year-old boy is brought to the doctor with a complaint of excessive fatigue and uncomfortable legs when walking or running. On physical examination, the doctor notes a reduced dorsalis pedis pulse and some signs of cyanosis of the toes. The boy's hands showed no signs of cyanosis.

On the basis of the physical examination the doctor suspected the presence of what malformation? Why?

SUMMARY

- The vascular system arises from mesodermal blood islands in the wall of the yolk sac. Hemangioblasts give rise to either blood cells or vascular endothelial cells. Nucleated red blood cells produced in the blood islands are the first blood cells found in the embryo. Later, hematopoiesis shifts to the embryonic body, beginning in the paraaortic bodies, and then to the liver, and finally to the bone marrow.

- During hematopoiesis, hemocytoblasts give rise to lymphoid and myeloid stem cells. Each of these stem cells further differentiates into the definitive lines of blood cells. Erythropoiesis involves the passage of precursor cells of red blood cells through a number of stages. The earliest stages are defined by behavioral, rather than morphological, characteristics. During later stages of differentiation, the precursor cells of erythrocytes gradually lose their RNA-producing machinery and accumulate increasing amounts of hemoglobin in their cytoplasm; at the same time the nucleus becomes more condensed and is eventually lost. Hemoglobin also undergoes isoform transitions during embryonic development.

- The earliest blood and associated extraembryonic blood vessels arise from blood islands in the mesodermal wall of the yolk sac. Much of the vasculature of the embryonic body is derived from intraembryonic sources. Endothelial cell precursors (angioblasts) arise from most mesodermal tissues of the body except the notochord and prechordal mesoderm. Embryonic blood vessels form by three main mechanisms: (1) coalescence in situ, (2) migration of angioblasts into organs, and (3) sprouting from existing vessels. Ingrowth of blood vessels into some organ primordia is stimulated by angiogenetic factors.

- The first three pairs of aortic arches form arteries that supply the head. The fourth pair of arches develops asymmetrically, with the left arch forming part of the aortic arch of the adult. The fifth pair of arches never forms. A sixth pair of arches arises as a capillary plexus that connects with the fourth arch. The distal part of the left sixth arch forms the ductus arteriosus, a shunt that allows blood to bypass the immature lungs and directly enter the aorta. Many of the larger arteries of the adult arise from three sets of aortic branches: the dorsal intersegmental, the lateral segmental, and the ventral segmental. The coronary arteries arise from capillary plexuses associated with the epicardium. These plexuses are secondarily connected with the aorta.

- The venous system arises from very complex capillary networks that initially develop into components of the cardinal vein system.

Anterior and posterior cardinal veins drain the head and trunk, respectively. They then empty into the paired common cardinal veins and ultimately into the sinus venosus of the heart. Paired subcardinal veins are associated with the developing mesonephros. Paired extraembryonic umbilical and vitelline veins pass through the developing liver and directly into the sinus venosus. The pulmonary veins arise as separate structures and empty into the left atrium. The lymphatic system first appears as six primary lymph sacs. These become connected by lymphatic channels. Lymphatics from most of the body collect into the thoracic duct, which empties into the venous system at the base of the left internal jugular vein.

- The heart arises from splanchnic mesoderm as a horseshoe-shaped primordium. Originally, bilateral endocardial tubes fuse in the midline. The fused cardiac tube then undergoes an S-shaped looping, and soon, specific regions of the heart can be identified. Starting with the inflow tract, these regions are the sinus venosus, the atria, the ventricles, and the outflow tract (bulbus cordis). The outflow tract later divides into the conus arteriosus and the truncus arteriosus.

- Atrial endocardial cushions are thickenings between the atria and ventricles. The underlying myocardium induces cells from the endothelial lining of the endocardial cushion to leave the endocardial layer and transform into mesenchymal cells that invade the cardiac jelly. These events serve as the basis for the formation of the atrioventricular valves.

- Internal partitioning of the heart begins with the separation of the atria from the ventricles and formation of the mitral and tricuspid valves. The left and right atria become separated by growth of the septum primum and septum secundum, but throughout embryonic life a shunt remains from the right to the left atrium via the foramen secundum and foramen ovale. The sinus venosus and the venae cavae empty into the right atrium, and the pulmonary veins drain into the left atrium. The ventricles are divided by the interventricular septum. Spiral truncoconal ridges partition the common outflow tract into pulmonary and aortic trunks. Semilunar valves prevent the reflux of blood in these vessels into the heart.

- In addition to sensory innervation, the heart receives sympathetic and parasympathetic innervation. The conduction system distributes the contractile stimulus throughout the heart. The conduction system is derived from modified cardiac muscle cells. The heart begins to beat early in the fourth week of gestation. Physiological maturation of the heart beat follows maturation of the pacemaker system and the innervation of the heart.

- The fetal circulation brings oxygenated blood from the placenta through the umbilical vein and into the right atrium, where much of it is shunted into the left atrium. Other blood entering the right atrium passes into the right ventricle. Blood leaving the right ventricle enters the pulmonary trunk, which supplies some blood to the lungs and the majority to the aorta via the ductus arteriosus. Blood in the left atrium empties into the left ventricle and aorta, where it supplies the body. Poorly oxygenated blood enters the umbilical arteries and is carried to the placenta for renewal.

- Common malformations of the heart consist of atrial septal defects, which in postnatal life allow blood to pass from the left to the right atrium. Ventricular septal defects, which also result in a left-right shunting of blood, are more serious. Defects that block a channel for blood flow (e.g., tricuspid atresia) must be accompanied by secondary shunt defects to be compatible with life. A persistent atrioventricular canal can be attributed to a defect in the formation or further development of the atrioventricular endocardial cushions. Most malformations of the outflow tract of the heart appear to be related to inappropriate partitioning by the truncoconal ridges. The basis for this is frequently found in neural crest abnormalities.

- Malformations of the major arteries often result from the inappropriate appearance or disappearance of specific components of the aortic arch system. Some, such as double aortic arch or right aortic arch, can interfere with swallowing or breathing because of pressure. Patent ductus arteriosus is caused by the failure of the ductus arteriosus to close properly after birth. Coarctation of the aorta must be compensated by either a patent ductus arteriosus or the opening of collateral vascular channels that allows blood to bypass the site of coarctation.

- Because of their complex mode of origin, veins are commonly subject to considerable variation, but these malformations are frequently asymptomatic. Anomalous pulmonary return, which brings oxygenated blood into the right atrium, must be accompanied by a right-to-left shunt to be compatible with life. Malformations of the lymphatic system can cause local swellings such as cystic hygroma, which results in a collarlike swelling in the neck.

REVIEW QUESTIONS

1. Nucleated erythrocytes found circulating in the embryo are produced in the:
   A. Yolk sac
   B. Paraaortic clusters
   C. Liver
   D. Bone marrow
   E. None of the above
2. In a 7-month-old fetus, blood draining the left temporalis muscle enters the heart via the:
   A. Left anterior cardinal vein
   B. Coronary sinus
   C. Left common cardinal vein
   D. Superior vena cava
   E. None of the above
3. Adherons are inductive particles released by what structure in the endocardial cushion area?
   A. Endocardium
   B. Cardiac jelly
   C. Myocardium
   D. Epicardium
   E. None of the above
4. Neural crest contributes to the structure of which of the following?
   A. Truncus arteriosus
   B. Ascending aorta
   C. Pulmonary trunk
   D. All of the above
   E. None of the above
5. For which of these cardiovascular malformations is a patent ductus arteriosus necessary for survival of the individual?
   A. Atrial septal defect
   B. Ventricular septal defect
   C. Double aortic arch
   D. Right subclavian artery from arch of aorta
   E. None of the above

6. Five days after birth, an infant becomes cyanotic during a prolonged crying spell. The cyanosis is most likely caused by venous blood entering the systemic circulation through the:
   A. Interatrial septum
   B. Ductus arteriosus
   C. Ductus venosus
   D. Umbilical vein
   E. Interventricular septum
7. The internal carotid artery arises from aortic arch number:
   A. 1
   B. 2
   C. 3
   D. 4
   E. 5
8. A 12-year-old boy tells his doctor that over the past few months he has noticed some difficulty in swallowing when eating meat. The doctor performs a physical examination and then orders an upper gastrointestinal x-ray series. After examining the films, the doctor refers the boy for some vascular studies. What is the reasoning behind this decision?
9. An individual with atresia of the mitral valve could not survive after birth without other defects of the cardiovascular system that could compensate for the primary defect, in this case a complete blockage between the left atrium and ventricle. Construct at least one set of associated defects that could physiologically compensate for the disruption caused by the mitral atresia.
10. What is the embryological basis for a duplication of the inferior vena cava caudal to the kidneys?

REFERENCES

Anderson RH: Simplifying the understanding of congenital malformations of the heart, *Int J Cardiol* 32:131-142, 1991.

Bartelings MM, Gittenberger-de Groot AC: Morphogenetic considerations on congenital malformations of the outflow tract. I. Common arterial trunk and tetralogy of Fallot, *Int J Cardiol* 32:213-230, 1991.

Bartelings MM, Gittenberger-de Groot AC: Morphogenetic considerations on congenital malformations of the outflow tract. II. Complete transposition of the great arteries and double outlet right ventricle, *Int J Cardiol* 33:5-26, 1991.

Biben C, Harvey RP: Homeodomain factor Nkx2-5 controls left/right asymmetric expression of *bHLH* gene eHand during murine heart development, *Genes Dev* 11:1357-1369, 1997.

Bockman DE, Kirby ML, eds: Embryonic origins of defective heart development, *Ann NY Acad Sci* 588:1-464, 1990.

Bristow J: The search for genetic mechanisms of congenital heart disease, *Cell Mol Biol Res* 41:307-319, 1995.

Celoria GC, Patton RB: Congenital absence of the aortic arch, *Am Heart J* 58:407-413, 1959.

Chan-Thomas PS and others: Expression of homeobox genes *Msx-1* (*Hox-7*) and *Msx-2* (*Hox-8*) during cardiac development in the chick, *Dev Dyn* 197:203-216, 1993.

Clark EB, Takao A, eds: *Developmental cardiology: morphogenesis and function,* Mount Kisco, NY, 1990, Futura.

Coceani F, Olley PM: The control of cardiovascular shunts in the fetal and perinatal period, *Can J Physiol Pharmacol* 66:1129-1134, 1988.

Congdon ED: Transformation of the aortic-arch system during the development of the human embryo, *Carnegie Contr Embryol* 14:47-110, 1922.

Conte G, Pellegrini A: On the development of the coronary arteries in human embryos, stages 14-19, *Anat Embryol* 169:209-218, 1984.

Crossin KL, Hoffman S: Expression of adhesion molecules during the formation and differentiation of the avian endocardial cushion tissue, *Dev Biol* 145:277-286, 1991.

DeHaan RL: Cardia bifida and the development of pacemaker function of the early chick heart, *Dev Biol* 1:586-602, 1959.

DeRuiter MC and others: The special status of the pulmonary arch artery in the branchial arch system of the rat, *Anat Embryol* 179:309-325, 1989.

Dettman RW and others: Common epicardial origin of coronary vascular smooth muscle, perivascular fibroblasts, and intermyocardial fibroblasts in the avian heart, *Dev Biol* 193:169-181, 1998.

Dieterlen-Lièvre F: Intraembryonic hematopoietic stem cells, *Hematol Oncol Clin North Am* 11:1149-1171, 1997.

Dieterlen-Lièvre F and others: Sites of hemopoietic stem cell production in early embryogenesis, *Colloque INSERM* 235:5-11, 1995.

Edwards JE and others: *Congenital heart disease: correlation of pathologic anatomy and angiocardiography*, vols 1 and 2, Philadelphia, 1965, WB Saunders.

Eichmann A and others: Ligand-dependent development of the endothelial and hematopoietic lineages from embryonic mesodermal cells expressing vascular endothelial growth factor receptor 2, *Proc Natl Acad Sci USA* 94:5141-5146, 1997.

Eisenberg LM, Markwald RR: Molecular regulation of atrioventricular valvuloseptal morphogenesis, *Circ Res* 77:1-6, 1995.

Evans SM and others: *Tinman*, a *Drosophila* homeobox gene required for heart and visceral mesoderm specification, may be represented by a family of genes in vertebrates: *Xnkx-2.3*, a second vertebrate homologue of tinman, *Development* 121:3889-3899, 1995.

Feinberg RN, Sherer GK, Auerbach R: *The development of the vascular system*, Basel, Switzerland, 1991, Karger.

Fisher SA and others: Forced expression of the homeodomain protein Gax inhibits cardiomyocyte proliferation and perturbs heart morphogenesis, *Development* 124:4405-4413, 1997.

Fishman MC, Chien KR: Fashioning the vertebrate heart: earliest embryonic decisions, *Development* 124:2099-2117, 1997.

Fukiishi Y, Morris-Kay GM: Migration of cranial neural crest cells to the pharyngeal arches and heart in rat embryos, *Cell Tissue Res* 268:1-8, 1992.

Gillum RF: Epidemiology of congenital heart disease in the United States, *Am Heart J* 127:919-927, 1994.

Goor DA, Lillehei CW: *Congenital malformations of the heart: embryology, anatomy and operative considerations*, New York, 1975, Grune & Stratton.

Heuser CH: The branchial vessels and their derivatives in the pig, *Carnegie Contr Embryol* 15:121-139, 1923.

Ho E, Shimada Y: Formation of the epicardium studied with the scanning electron microscope, *Dev Biol* 66:579-585, 1978.

Icardo JM: Developmental biology of the vertebrate heart, *J Exp Zool* 275:144-161, 1996.

Iida K and others: Essential roles of the winged helix transcription factor MFH-1 in aortic arch patterning and skeletogenesis, *Development* 124:4627-4638, 1997.

Kanjuh VI, Edwards JE: A review of congenital anomalies of the heart and great vessels according to functional categories, *Pediatr Clin North Am* 11:55-105, 1964.

Kern MJ, Argao EA, Potter SS: Homeobox genes and heart development, *Trends Cardiovasc Med* 5:47-54, 1995.

Kirby ML: Nodose placode provides ectomesenchyme to the developing chick heart in the absence of cardiac neural crest, *Cell Tissue Res* 252:17-22, 1988.

Kirby ML: Role of extracardiac factors in heart development, *Experientia* 44:944-951, 1988.

Kirby ML, Waldo KL: Role of neural crest in congenital heart disease, *Circulation* 82:332-340, 1990.

Kramer TC: The partitioning of the truncus and conus and the formation of the membranous portion of the interventricular septum of the human heart, *Am J Anat* 71:343-370, 1942.

Lyons GE: Vertebrate heart development, *Curr Opin Genet Dev* 6:454-460, 1996.

Maenner J: Experimental study on the formation of the epicardium in chick embryos, *Anat Embryol* 187:281-289, 1993.

Magovern JH, Moore GW, Hutchins GM: Development of the atrioventricular valve region in the human embryo, *Anat Rec* 215:167-181, 1986.

Markwald RR and others: Epithelial-mesenchymal transformations in early avian heart development, *Acta Anat* 156:173-186, 1996.

McClure CFW, Butler EG: The development of the vena cava inferior in man, *Am J Anat* 35:331-383, 1925.

Mikawa T, Fischman DA: Retroviral analysis of cardiac morphogenesis, *Proc Natl Acad Sci* 89:9504-9508, 1992.

Mikawa T, Gourdie RG: Pericardial mesoderm generates a population of coronary smooth muscle cells migrating into the heart along with ingrowth of the epicardial organ, *Dev Biol* 174:221-232, 1996.

Mohun T, Sparrow D: Early steps in vertebrate cardiogenesis, *Curr Opin Genet Dev* 7:628-633, 1997.

Nakajima Y and others: An autocrine function for transforming growth factor (TGF)-β3 in the transformation of atrioventricular canal endocardium into mesenchyme during chick heart development, *Dev Biol* 194:99-113, 1998.

Noden DM: Development of craniofacial blood vessels. In Feinberg RN, Sherer GK, Auerbach R, eds: *The development of the vascular system*, Basel, Switzerland, 1991, Karger, pp 1-24.

Noden DM: Origins and assembly of avian embryonic blood vessels, *Ann NY Acad Sci* 588:236-249, 1990.

Noden DM: Origins and patterning of avian outflow tract endocardium, *Development* 111:867-876, 1991.

Olson EN, Srivastava D: Molecular pathways controlling heart development, *Science* 272:671-676, 1996.

Pardanaud L and others: Two distinct endothelial lineages in ontogeny, one of them related to hemopoiesis, *Development* 122:1363-1371, 1996.

Patten BM: The development of the sinoatrial conduction system, *Univ Mich Med Bull* 22:1-21, 1956.

Pexieder T: The tissue dynamics of heart morphogenesis. I. The phenomena of cell death, *Z Anat Entwickl-Gesch* 138:241-253, 1972.

Pexieder T and others: A suggested nomenclature for the developing heart, *Int J Cardiol* 25:255-264, 1989.

Reaume AG and others: Cardiac malformations in neonatal mice lacking connexin43, *Science* 267:1831-1834, 1995.

Robbins J: Regulation of cardiac gene expression during development, *Cardiovasc Res* 31:E2-E16, 1996.

Sabin FR: The origin and development of the lymphatic system, *Johns Hopkins Hosp Rep* 17:347-440, 1916.

Schott J-J and others: Congenital heart disease caused by mutations in the transcription factor NKX2-5, *Science* 108-111, 1998.

Sherer GK: Vasculogenic mechanisms and epitheliomesenchymal specificity in endodermal organs. In Feinberg RN, Sherer GK, Auerbach R, eds: *The development of the vascular system*, Basel, Switzerland, 1991, Karger, pp 37-57.

Sissman NJ: Developmental landmarks in cardiac morphogenesis: comparative chronology, *Am J Cardiol* 25:141-148, 1970.

Srivastava D, Olson EN: Knowing in your heart what is right, *Trends Cell Biol* 7:447-453, 1997.

Srivastava D, Olson EN: Neurotrophin-3 knocks heart off Trk, *Nature Med* 2:1069-1071, 1996.

Steding G and others: Developmental aspects of the sinus valves and the sinus venosus septum of the right atrium in human embryos, *Anat Embryol* 181:469-475, 1990.

Takamura K and others: Association of cephalic neural crest cells with cardiovascular development, particularly that of the semilunar valves, *Anat Embryol* 182:263-272, 1990.

Thorsteinsdottir U, Sauvageau G, Humphries RK: *Hox* homeobox genes as regulators of normal and leukemic hematopoiesis, *Hematol Oncol Clin North Am* 11:1221-1237, 1997.

Tomanek RJ: Formation of the coronary vasculature: a brief review, *Cardiovasc Res* 31: E46-E51, 1996.

Wilting J, Christ B: Embryonic angiogenesis: a review, *Naturwissenschaften* 83:153-164, 1996.

FETAL PERIOD AND BIRTH

After the eighth week of pregnancy the period of organogenesis (embryonic period) is largely completed, and the fetal period begins. By the end of the embryonic period, almost all the organs of the body are present in a grossly recognizable form. The external contours of the embryo show a very large head in proportion to the rest of the body and greater development of the cranial than of the caudal part of the body (Figures 17-1 and 17-2).

The fetal period has often been considered a time of growth and physiological maturation of organ systems, and it has not received much attention in traditional embryology courses. However, recent advances in imaging and other diagnostic techniques have provided considerable access to the fetus. Determining the fetus' pattern of growth and state of well-being with remarkable accuracy is now possible. Improved surgical techniques and the realization that surgical wounds in the fetus heal without scarring have led to a new field of fetal surgery.

This chapter emphasizes the functional development of the fetus and the adaptations that ensure a smooth transition to independent living once the fetus has passed through the birth canal and the umbilical cord is cut. Techniques that are used to monitor the functional state of the fetus are also described in Clinical Correlation 17-1 later in the chapter.

GROWTH AND FORM OF THE FETUS

Despite the intense developmental activity that occurs during the embryonic period (3 to 8 weeks), the absolute growth of the embryo in both length and mass is not great (Figure 17-3). The fetal period (9 weeks to birth), however, is characterized by intense growth. The change in proportions of the various regions of the body during the prenatal and postnatal growth periods is as striking as the absolute growth of the embryo. The early dominance of the head is reduced as development of the trunk becomes a major factor in the growth of the early fetus. Even later, a relatively greater growth of the limbs

changes the proportions of various regions of the body. During the early fetal period, the entire body is hairless and very thin because of the absence of subcutaneous fat (Figure 17-4). By midpregnancy the contours of the head and face approach those of the neonate, and the abdomen begins to fill out. Beginning at around week 27, the deposition of subcutaneous fat causes the body to round out. (Some of the major developmental landmarks during the fetal period are summarized in the table on pp. xvi and xvii.)

FETAL PHYSIOLOGY

Circulation

The circulation of the human embryo can be first studied at about 5 weeks by means of ultrasound. At that time the heart beats at a rate of approximately 100 beats per min. This probably represents an inherent atrial rhythm. The pulse rate rises to about 160 beats per min by 8 weeks and then drops to 150 beats per min in the 15-week-old fetus, with a further slight decline near term. The pulse rate in utero is remarkably constant, and embryos exhibiting **bradycardia** (slow pulse rate) often die before term. Near term the pulse rate varies to some extent if conditions in the uterus change or if the embryo is stressed. This is probably the result of the functional establishment of the autonomic innervation of the heart (Figure 17-5).

The heart of the fetus has gross physiological properties quite different from those of the postnatal heart. For example, the myocardial force, the velocity of shortening, and the extent of shortening are all less in the fetal heart. Some gross functional characteristics of the fetal heart are related to the presence of fetal isoforms of contractile proteins in the cardiac myocytes. For example, in fetal heart cells the β-myosin heavy chain isoform predominates. This is advantageous because a lower oxygen requirement and less adenosine triphosphate are needed to develop the same amount of force as the α-myosin isoform in the adult heart.

The **stroke volume** (blood expelled with one heart beat) of the early (18 to 19 weeks' gestation) fetus is very small (less

Text continued on p. 452

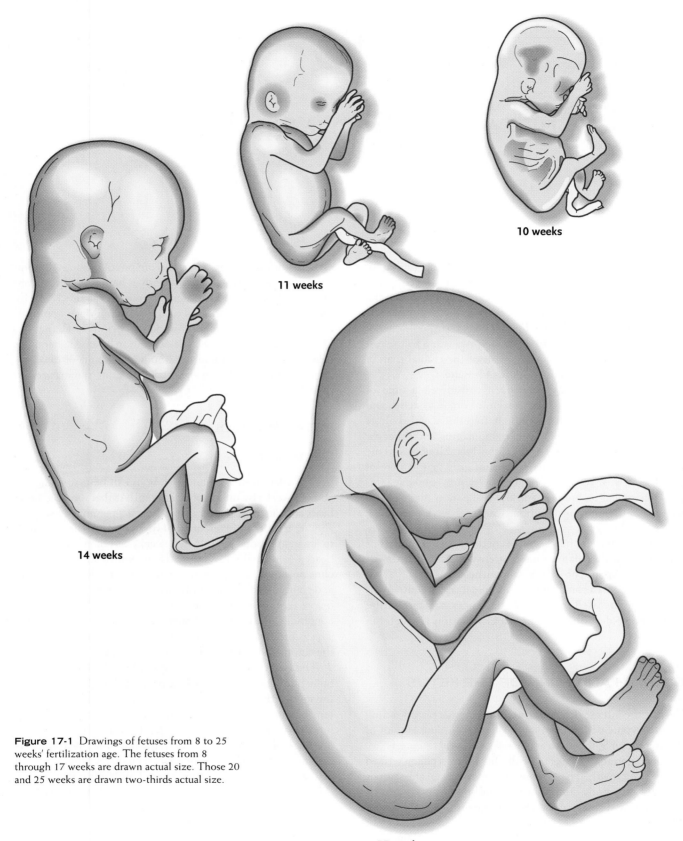

10 weeks

11 weeks

14 weeks

17 weeks

Figure 17-1 Drawings of fetuses from 8 to 25 weeks' fertilization age. The fetuses from 8 through 17 weeks are drawn actual size. Those 20 and 25 weeks are drawn two-thirds actual size.

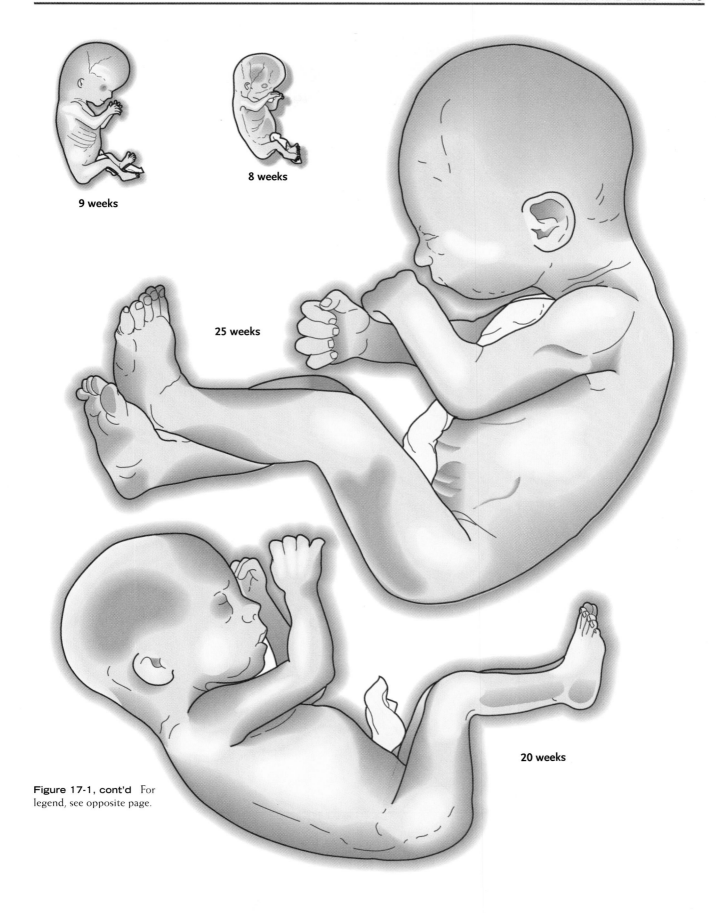

9 weeks

8 weeks

25 weeks

20 weeks

Figure 17-1, cont'd For legend, see opposite page.

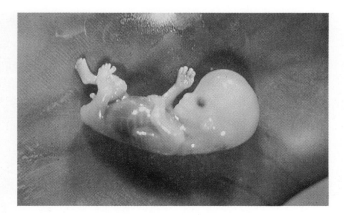

Figure 17-2 A 37-mm crown-rump length human fetus, approximately **9 weeks** old. (Courtesy A. Burdi, Ann Arbor, Mich.)

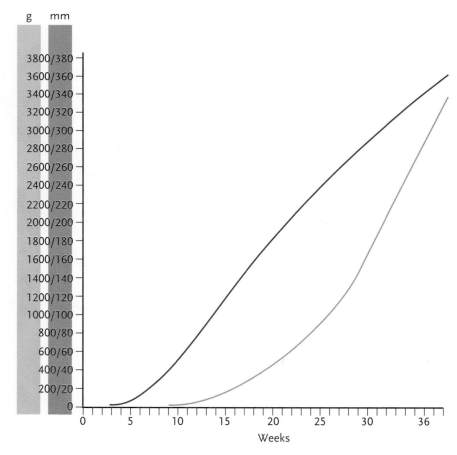

Figure 17-3 Growth in crown-rump length (*green*) and weight (*orange*) of the human fetus. (Data from Patten BM: *Human embryology*, New York, 1968, McGraw-Hill.)

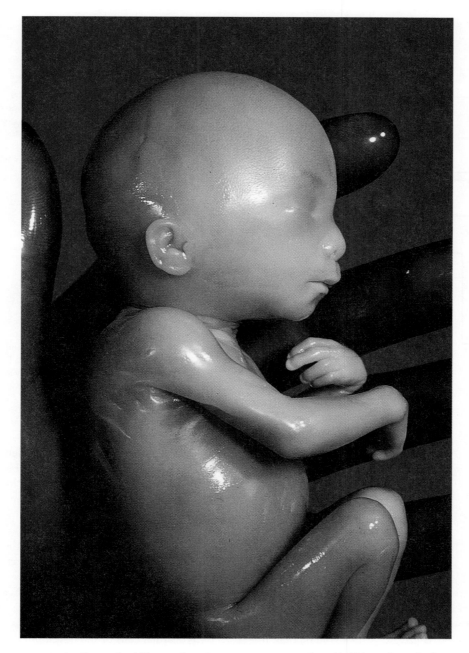

Figure 17-4 A 3³/₄-month-old human fetus (130-mm crown-rump length). EH 902 from the Patten Embryological Collection at the University of Michigan. (Courtesy of A. Burdi, Ann Arbor, Mich.)

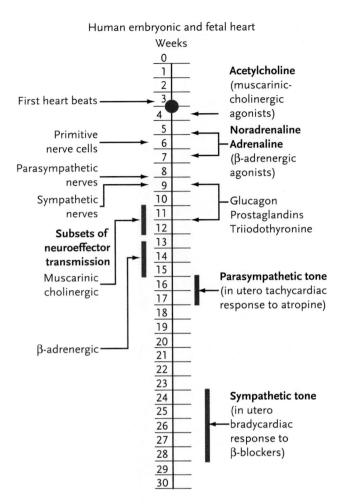

Human embryonic and fetal heart

Weeks

First heart beats ⟶

Acetylcholine (muscarinic-cholinergic agonists)

Primitive nerve cells ⟶

Noradrenaline Adrenaline (β-adrenergic agonists)

Parasympathetic nerves ⟶

Sympathetic nerves

Subsets of neuroeffector transmission

Muscarinic cholinergic

Glucagon Prostaglandins Triiodothyronine

Parasympathetic tone (in utero tachycardiac response to atropine)

β-adrenergic

Sympathetic tone (in utero bradycardiac response to β-blockers)

Figure 17-5 Sequence of events in the autonomic innervation of the heart. (Based on Papp JG: *Basic Res Cardiol* 83:2-9, 1988.)

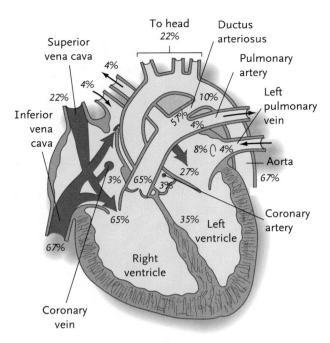

Figure 17-6 Percentages of blood entering and leaving the fetal heart via various channels. (From Teitel DF. In Polin R, Rox W, eds: *Fetal and neonatal physiology*, vol 1, Philadelphia, 1992, WB Saunders, pp 609-619.)

than 1 ml), but it increases rapidly with continued growth of the fetus. In the term human fetus the combined ventricular output is about 450 ml/kg/min. The right ventricle of the human fetus has a somewhat greater stroke volume than the left. This is correlated with an 8% greater diameter of the pulmonary artery than of the fetal aorta.

Quantitative studies have shown a good correlation between blood flow and functional needs of various regions of the embryo. Approximately 40% of the combined cardiac output goes to the head and upper body, thus supplying the relatively great needs of the developing brain. Another 30% of the combined cardiac output goes to the placenta via the umbilical arteries for replenishment. Figure 17-6 shows the relative amounts of blood that enter and leave the heart via various vascular channels. (The general qualitative pattern of blood flow in the human fetus is presented in Chapter 16.)

Differential streaming of blood within the heart results in different concentrations of oxygen in the chambers of the

fetal heart. For example, blood in the left ventricle is 15% to 20% more saturated with oxygen than blood in the right ventricle (see Figure 16-23). This and the high volume of blood supplying the head via branches of the ascending aorta ensure that the developing heart and brain receive an adequate supply of oxygen.

A key factor in the maintenance of the fetal pattern of circulation is the patency of the ductus arteriosus and the ductus venosus. Patency of the fetal ductus venosus is maintained through the actions of prostaglandins E_2 and I_2, whereas only prostaglandin E_2 is involved in maintaining patency of the ductus arteriosus.

Myocardial cells of the developing atrium gradually produce and store granules containing **atrial natriuretic peptide**, a hormone that has pronounced vasodilatory, natriuretic, and diuretic properties. This hormone is released after the atrial walls are stretched, normally a sign of increased blood volume. It has been detected in atrial cardiomyocytes as early as 8 to 9 weeks' gestation. After intrauterine blood transfusions during midgestation or later, blood levels of atrial natriuretic peptide increase significantly in response to the increased blood volume.

Fetal Lungs and Respiratory System

The lungs develop late in the embryo and are not involved in respiratory gas exchange during fetal life. However, they must be prepared to assume the full burden of gas exchange as soon as the umbilical cord is cut.

The fetal lungs are filled with fluid, and the blood circulation to them is highly reduced. To perform normal postnatal breathing, the lungs must grow to an appropriate size, respiratory movements must be carried out continuously, and the air sacs (**alveoli**) must become appropriately configured for air exchange.

Normal growth of the fetal lungs depends on their containing an adequate amount of fluid. During the last trimester of pregnancy, fluid constitutes 90% to 95% of the total weight of the lung. The fluid filling the fetal lungs differs in composition from amniotic fluid, and it has been shown to be secreted by the pulmonary epithelial cells. Secretion begins with a net movement of chloride ions into the lumens of the pulmonary passages. Water movement then follows the chloride ions. A number of studies have shown a relationship between total fluid volume in the lungs and fetal breathing movements, with dilatation and constriction of the larynx serving a valvelike function. In vitro studies have shown that proliferation of lung epithelial cells is stimulated by mechanical stretching. In vivo the internal pressure of the lung fluid serves as the stretching agent. A reduced volume of lung fluid is associated with **pulmonary hypoplasia**.

Ultrasound analysis has shown that the fetus begins to make gross breathing movements as early as 11 weeks. These movements are periodic rather than continuous, and they take on two forms. One type of movement is rapid and irregular, with varying rate and amplitude. The other form is represented by isolated, slow movements, almost like gasps. The former type is by far the most prominent and is associated with conditions of rapid eye movement (REM) sleep. Periods of rapid breathing (often for about 10 minutes) alternate with periods of **apnea** (cessation of breathing).

Much remains to be learned about the control of fetal breathing, but the breathing movements are known to be responsive to maternal factors, many of which remain to be identified. The amount of breathing (minutes of breathing per hour) is highest in the evening and lowest in the early morning. The fetal breathing rate increases after the mother has eaten. This is related to the concentration of glucose in the maternal blood. Maternal smoking causes a rapid decrease in the rate of fetal breathing for up to an hour.

Fetal breathing movements are essential for postnatal survival. One obvious function of fetal breathing is to condition the respiratory muscles so that they can perform regular postnatal contractions. Another important function is to stimulate the growth of the embryonic lungs. If intrauterine breathing movements are suppressed in fetal lambs, lung growth is retarded.

An important developmental adaptation of the fetal respiratory system is growth of the upper airway. Although a newborn is about 4% the weight of an adult, the diameter of its trachea is one third that of the adult trachea. Other components of the airway are similarly proportioned. If the trachea were narrower, the physical resistance to air flow would be so great that movement of air would be almost impossible. Even with these adaptations, the resistance of the neonate's airway is 5 to 6 times greater than that of the adult.

A functionally important aspect of fetal lung development is the secretion of **pulmonary surfactant** by the newly differentiating type II alveolar cells of the lung starting around 24 weeks' gestation. Surfactant is a mixture of phospholipids (about two-thirds phosphatidylcholine) and protein that lines the surface of the alveoli and lowers the surface tension. This reduces the inspiratory force required to inflate the alveoli and prevents the collapse of the alveoli during expiration.

Despite the relatively early initiation of surfactant synthesis, large amounts are not synthesized until a few weeks before birth. At this time the production of surfactant by the type II alveolar cells is higher than at any other period in an individual's life, an adaptation that is an important preparation for the newborn's first breath. A number of hormones and growth factors are involved in the synthesis of surfactant, and the effects of thyroid hormone and glucocorticoids are particularly strong.

Prematurely born infants are often afflicted with **respiratory distress syndrome**, which is manifested by rapid, labored breathing shortly after birth. This condition is related to a deficiency in pulmonary surfactant and can be ameliorated by the administration of glucocorticoids, which stimulate the production of surfactant by the alveolar epithelium.

Fetal Movements and Sensations

Ultrasound analysis has revolutionized the analysis of fetal movements and behavior because the fetus can be examined virtually undisturbed (except for an increase in vascular activity induced by the ultrasound) for extended periods. Earlier studies of fetal movements were principally concerned with the development of reflex responses, and the information was obtained largely by the analysis of newly aborted fetuses (see Chapter 10). Although valuable information on maturation of reflex arcs was obtained in this manner, many of the movements elicited were not those normally made by the fetus in utero.

The undisturbed embryo does not show any indication of movement until about 7½ weeks. The first spontaneous movements consist of slow flexion and extension of the vertebral column, with the limbs being passively displaced. Within a short time, a relatively large repertoire of fetal movements evolves. After study by a number of investigators, a classification of fetal movements has been suggested (Box 17-1). The first fetal movements are followed in a few days by startle and general movements. Shortly thereafter, isolated limb movements are added (Figure 17-7). Late in appearance are movements associated with the head and jaw (Figure 17-7).

BOX 17-1   Major Types of Fetal Movements

Anteflexion of the head Normally slow, forward bending of the head

Fetal breathing movements Paradoxical movements in which the thorax moves inward and the abdomen outward with each contraction of the diaphragm

General movements Slow gross movements involving the whole body lasting several seconds to a minute

Hand-face contact Contact that occurs any time the moving hand touches the face or mouth

Hiccups Repetitive phasic contractions of the diaphragm (A bout may last several minutes.)

Isolated arm or leg movements Movements of extremities that occur without movement of the trunk

Lateral rotation of the head Movement that involves isolated turning of the head from side to side

Opening of mouth Isolated movement that may be accompanied by protrusion of the tongue

Retroflexion of the head Slow to jerky backward bending of the head

Startle movements Quick (1 second), generalized movements that always start in the limbs and may spread to the trunk and neck

Stretch Complex movement that involves overextension of the spine, retroflexion of the head, and elevation of the arms

Sucking Burst of rhythmical jaw movements that is sometimes followed by swallowing (With this movement the fetus may be drinking amniotic fluid.)

Yawn Movement in which the mouth is slowly opened and rapidly closed after a few seconds

Based on studies by Prechtl HFR. In Hill A, Volpe J, eds: *Fetal neurology*, New York, 1989, Raven, pp 1-16.

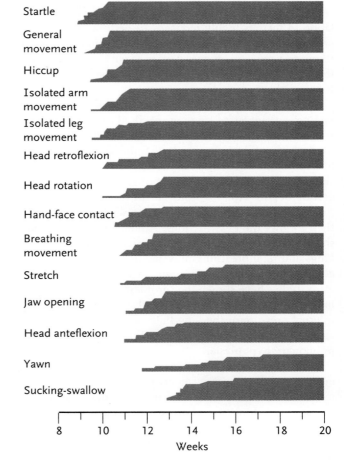

Figure 17-7 Time of appearance of specific patterns of fetal motor movements. Each corner on the jagged edge at the left of the broad lines represents one fetus. (From Prechtl HFR. In Hill A, Volpe J, eds: *Fetal neurology*, New York, 1989, Raven, pp 1-16.)

Continuous ultrasound monitoring for extended periods reveals patterns involving many types of movements (Figure 17-8). At different weeks of pregnancy, some movements are predominant, whereas others are in decline or are just beginning to take shape. Analysis of anencephalic fetuses has shown that although many movements take place, they are poorly regulated. They start abruptly, are maintained at the same force, and then stop abruptly. These abnormal patterns of movements are considered evidence for strong supraspinal modulation of movement in the fetus.

Human fetal activities, as reflected in breathing or general activity level, show distinct diurnal rhythms beginning at about 20 to 22 weeks' gestation. There is a strong negative correlation between maternal plasma glucocorticoid levels and fetal activity. Fetal activity is highest in the early evening, when maternal blood glucocorticoid levels are lowest, and lowest in the early morning, when the concentration of maternal hormone peaks. Studies of women who have been given additional glucocorticoids or inhibitors have shown increased fetal activity when maternal corticoid levels are low. Usually when the overall fetal activity is low, the fetus is in a state of REM sleep, but definitions of sleep and wakefulness in the fetus need further clarification.

A number of sensory systems also begin to function during the fetal period. (Reflex responses to tactile stimulation are outlined in Chapter 10.) Near-term fetuses are responsive to 2000-Hz stimuli when in a state of wakefulness, but they are unresponsive during periods of sleep. Loud vibroacoustic stimuli applied to the maternal abdomen produce a fetal response consisting of an eye blink, a startle reaction, and an increase in heart rate. Although the fetus is constantly in the dark, the **pupillary light reflex** can usually be elicited by 30 weeks.

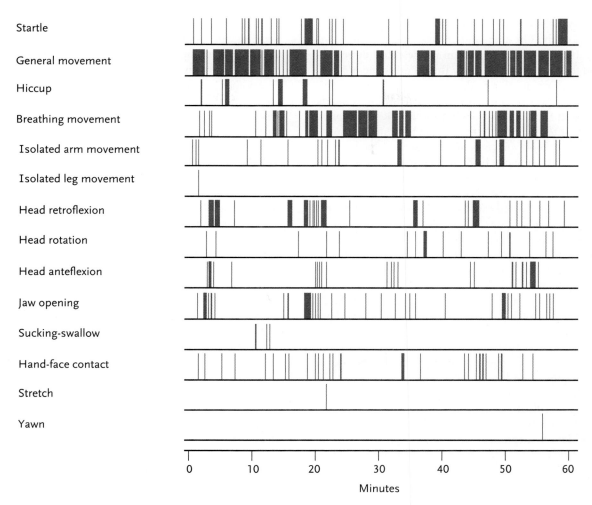

Startle

General movement

Hiccup

Breathing movement

Isolated arm movement

Isolated leg movement

Head retroflexion

Head rotation

Head anteflexion

Jaw opening

Sucking-swallow

Hand-face contact

Stretch

Yawn

0   10   20   30   40   50   60

Minutes

Figure 17-8 Actogram record of types of movements of a **14-week-old** fetus taken over 60 minutes. (Modified from Prechtl HFR: *Fetal neurology,* New York, 1989, Raven.)

Fetal Digestive Tract

The fetal digestive tract is not functional in the standard sense because the fetus obtains its nutrition from the maternal blood via the placenta. However, the digestive tract must be prepared to assume the full responsibility for nutritional intake after birth. Once the basic digestive tube and glands have formed in the early embryo, the remainder of the intrauterine period is devoted to cellular differentiation of the epithelia of the gut and preparation of the numerous cells involved for their specific roles in the digestive process. Below the epithelium the walls of the digestive tube must become capable of propelling ingested food and liquid. Analysis of development of the fetal digestive tract has concentrated on (1) the biochemical adaptations of the epithelium of the various regions for digestive function and (2) the development of motility of the digestive tube.

The development and differentiation of epithelia or specific regional characteristics of the gut lining typically follow gradients along the length of the segment of the gut specifically involved. In both the esophagus and stomach, differentiation of the mucosal epithelium is well underway starting around 4 months. Although **parietal cells** (hydrochloric acid producing) and **chief cells** (pepsinogen producing) are first seen at 11 and 12 weeks, respectively, there is little evidence of their secretions during fetal life. In fact, the contents of the stomach have a near-neutral pH until after birth, but then gastric acid production increases greatly within a few hours.

In the small intestine, villi begin to form in the upper duodenum at the end of the second month, and crypts appear 1 to 2 weeks later. The formation of villi and crypts spreads along the length of the intestine in a spatiotemporal gradient.

By approximately 16 weeks, villi have formed along the entire length of the intestine, and crypts appear in the lower ileum by 19 weeks. Villi even form in the colon during the third and fourth months, but they then regress and are gone by the seventh or eighth month.

Individual epithelial cell types, including **Brunner's glands,** which protect the duodenal lining from gastric acid, appear in the small intestine early in the second trimester. Although the presence of most enzymes or proenzymes characteristic of the intestinal lining can be demonstrated histochemically during the midfetal period, their amounts are generally quite small. Activity of a number of the enzymes secreted by the exocrine pancreatic tissue can also be demonstrated between 16 and 22 weeks' gestation.

Meconium, a greenish mixture of desquamated intestinal cells, swallowed lanugo hair, and various secretions, begins to fill the lower ileum and colon late in the fourth month (Figure 17-9).

Differentiation of the neuromuscular complex of the digestive tract also follows a gradient, with the circular layer of smooth muscle forming in the esophagus at 6 weeks. **Myenteric plexuses** (parasympathetic neurons) take shape after the inner circular muscle layer is present but before the formation of the outer longitudinal layer of muscle a couple weeks later in any given region. Starting in the esophagus at 6 weeks, the final formation of myenteric plexuses throughout the length of the digestive tract is complete at 12 weeks. The first spontaneous rhythmical activity in the small intestine is seen in the seventh week at approximately the time of formation of the inner circular muscular layer. Recognizable peristaltic movements, however, do not begin until the fourth month. Fetuses older than 34 weeks are able to pass meconium in utero.

Another intrauterine preparation for feeding is the development of swallowing and the sucking reflex. Swallowing is first detected at 11 weeks, and then its incidence gradually increases. The function of fetal swallowing is unclear, but by term, fetuses swallow 200 to 750 ml or more of amniotic fluid per day. The swallowed amniotic fluid may contain growth factors that facilitate the differentiation of epithelial cells in the digestive tract. To a certain extent, taste seems to regulate fetal swallowing. Taste buds are seemingly mature by 12 weeks, and the amount of swallowing increases if saccharin is introduced into the amniotic fluid. Conversely, swallowing is reduced if noxious chemicals are added.

Sucking movements appear late in fetal development. Before 32 weeks, there is no sucking. From 32 to 36 weeks the fetus undertakes short bursts of sucking, but these are not associated with effective swallowing movements. Ineffective sucking is the main reason why premature infants of this age must be fed through a nasogastric tube. Mature sucking capability appears after 36 weeks.

Fetal Kidney Function

Although the placenta carries out most excretory functions characteristic of the kidney during prenatal life, the developing kidneys also function by producing urine. As early as the fifth week of gestation, the mesonephric kidneys produce small amounts of very dilute urine, but the mesonephros degenerates late in the third month, after the metanephric kidneys have taken shape. Tubules of the metanephric kidneys begin to function between 9 and 12 weeks, and resorptive functions involving the loop of Henle occur by 14 weeks, even though new nephrons continue to form until birth. The urine produced by the fetal kidney is hypotonic to plasma throughout most of pregnancy. This is a reflection of immature resorptive mechanisms, which are manifested morphologically by short loops of Henle. As the neural lobe of the hypophysis produces antidiuretic hormone beginning at the eleventh week, another mechanism for the concentration of urine begins to be established.

Intrauterine renal function is not necessary for fetal life because embryos with bilateral renal agenesis survive in utero. Bilateral renal agenesis, however, is commonly associated with oligohydramnios (see Chapter 6), indicating that the overall balance of amniotic fluid requires a certain amount of fetal renal function.

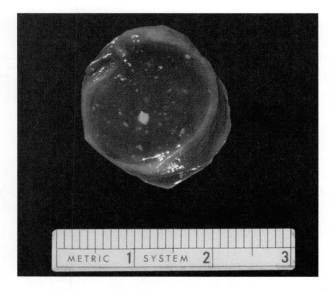

Figure 17-9 Meconium ileus (accumulation of fetal meconium [the greenish material]) in the fetal small intestine. (Photo 2536 from the Arey-DaPeña Pediatric Pathology Photographic Collection, Human Developmental Anatomy Center, National Museum of Health and Medicine, Armed Forces Institute of Pathology, Washington, DC.)

Endocrine Function in the Fetus

The development of prenatal endocrine function occurs in several phases. Most peripheral endocrine glands (e.g., thyroid, pancreatic islets, adrenals, gonads) form early in the second month as the result of epithelial-mesenchymal interactions. As these glands differentiate late in the second month or early in the third, they develop the intrinsic capacity to synthesize their specific hormonal products. In most cases the amount of hormone secreted is initially very small; increased secretion often depends on the stimulation of the gland by a higher-order hormone produced in another gland.

The anterior pituitary gland develops like many other endocrine glands. Its hormonal products generally stimulate more peripheral endocrine glands such as the thyroid, adrenals, and gonads to produce or release their specific hormonal products. Pituitary hormones can be demonstrated immunocytochemically within individual pituitary epithelial cells as early as 8 weeks (adrenocorticotrophic hormone) or 10 weeks (luteinizing hormone and follicle-stimulating hormone). However, most pituitary hormones are typically not present in the blood in detectable quantities until a couple of months after they can be demonstrated in the cells that produce them. An exception is growth hormone, which can be detected in plasma as early as 10 weeks.

While the anterior pituitary is developing its intrinsic synthetic capacities, the hypothalamus also takes shape and develops its capacity to produce the various releasing and inhibitory factors that modulate the function of the pituitary gland. Regardless of its intrinsic capacities, the hypothalamus is limited in its influence on the embryonic pituitary gland until about 12 weeks, when the neurovascular links between the hypothalamus and pituitary become established.

At each level in the control hierarchy a generally low intrinsic level of hormone production can be stimulated by the actions of hormones produced by the next higher-order gland. For example, the amount of thyroid hormone released is considerably increased when thyroid-stimulating hormone, released by the anterior pituitary, acts on the thyroid gland. The release of this hormone by the pituitary is regulated by thyrotropin-releasing hormone, which is produced in the hypothalamus. Regardless of the nature of the upstream stimulation of the thyroid, the forms of thyroid hormone released by the fetal thyroid are largely biologically inactive because of enzymatic modifications or through sulfation. Studies on anencephalic fetuses have shown that the anterior pituitary can produce and release most of its hormones in the absence of hypothalamic input, although plasma concentrations of some are reduced.

Among the fetal endocrine glands the adrenal remains the most enigmatic. By 6 to 8 weeks of development, the inner cortex enlarges greatly to form a distinct fetal zone, which later in pregnancy occupies about 80% of the gland. By the end of pregnancy, the adrenal glands weigh 4 g each, the same mass as that of the adult glands (Figure 17-10). The fetal adrenal cortex produces 100 to 200 mg of steroids each day, an amount several times higher than that of the adult adrenal glands. The main hormonal products of the fetal adrenal are Δ^5-3β-hydroxysteroids such as dehydroepiandrosterone, which are inactive alone but are converted to biologically ac-

tive steroids (e.g., estrogens, especially estrone) by the placenta and liver. The fetal adrenal cortex depends on the presence of pituitary adrenocorticotrophic hormone; in its absence the fetal adrenal cortex is small. Conversely, if exogenous adrenocorticotrophic hormone is administered, the fetal adrenal cortex persists after birth.

Despite the prominence of the fetal adrenal cortex, its specific functions during pregnancy are still not clear. Fetal adrenal hormones influence maturation of the lungs (as prolactin has also been postulated to do), liver, and epithelium of the digestive tract. In sheep, products of the adrenal cortex prepare the fetus for independent postnatal life and influence the initiation of parturition, but the situation in primates is considerably less clear. Shortly after birth the fetal adrenal cortex rapidly involutes (see Figure 17-10). Within a month after birth the weight of each gland is reduced by 50%, and by 1 year of age each gland weighs only 1 g. Not until adulthood does the mass of the adrenal glands return to that of the late fetus.

Fetal endocrinology is complicated by the presence of the placenta, which can synthesize and release many hormones, convert hormones released from other glands to active forms, and potentially exchange other hormones with the maternal circulation. By 6 to 7 weeks, hormone production (e.g., progesterone) by the placenta is enough to maintain pregnancy even if the ovaries are removed.

Text continued on p. 463

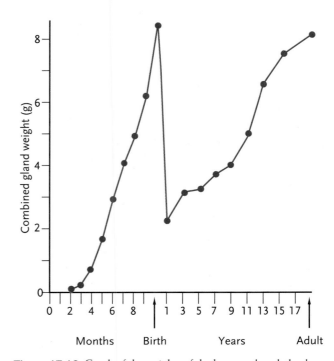

Figure 17-10 Graph of the weights of the human adrenal glands during prenatal and postnatal development. After birth, the weight of the gland decreases dramatically with the reorganization of the cortex of the gland. (Based on data from Neville AM, O'Hare MJ: *The human adrenal cortex*, Berlin, 1982, Springer-Verlag.)

CLINICAL CORRELATION 17-1
Clinical Study and Manipulation of the Fetus

New imaging and diagnostic techniques have revolutionized the study of the living fetus. Many congenital malformations can be diagnosed in utero with considerable accuracy. On the basis of this information the surgeon can treat some congenital malformations through fetal surgery much more efficiently than by traditional surgery on infants or older children.

FETAL DIAGNOSTIC PROCEDURES
Imaging Techniques
Because of its safety, cost, and ability to look at the fetus in real time, **ultrasonography** is currently the most widely used obstetrical imaging technique (Figures 17-11 and 17-12). It is useful for the simple diagnosis of structural anomalies and can be used in real time to guide fetal invasive procedures such as chorionic villus sampling and intrauterine transfusions. The major uses of ultrasonography are summarized in Box 17-2.

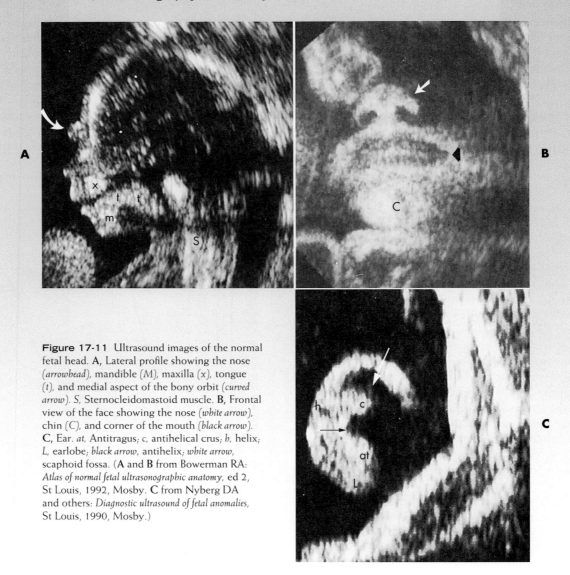

Figure 17-11 Ultrasound images of the normal fetal head. **A,** Lateral profile showing the nose (*arrowhead*), mandible (*M*), maxilla (*x*), tongue (*t*), and medial aspect of the bony orbit (*curved arrow*). *S,* Sternocleidomastoid muscle. **B,** Frontal view of the face showing the nose (*white arrow*), chin (*C*), and corner of the mouth (*black arrow*). **C,** Ear. *at,* Antitragus; *c,* antihelical crus; *h,* helix; *L,* earlobe; *black arrow,* antihelix; *white arrow,* scaphoid fossa. (**A** and **B** from Bowerman RA: *Atlas of normal fetal ultrasonographic anatomy,* ed 2, St Louis, 1992, Mosby. **C** from Nyberg DA and others: *Diagnostic ultrasound of fetal anomalies,* St Louis, 1990, Mosby.)

CLINICAL CORRELATION 17-1
Clinical Study and Manipulation of the Fetus—cont'd

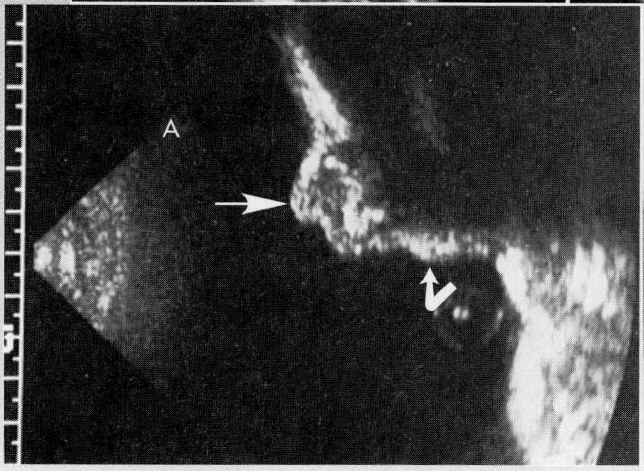

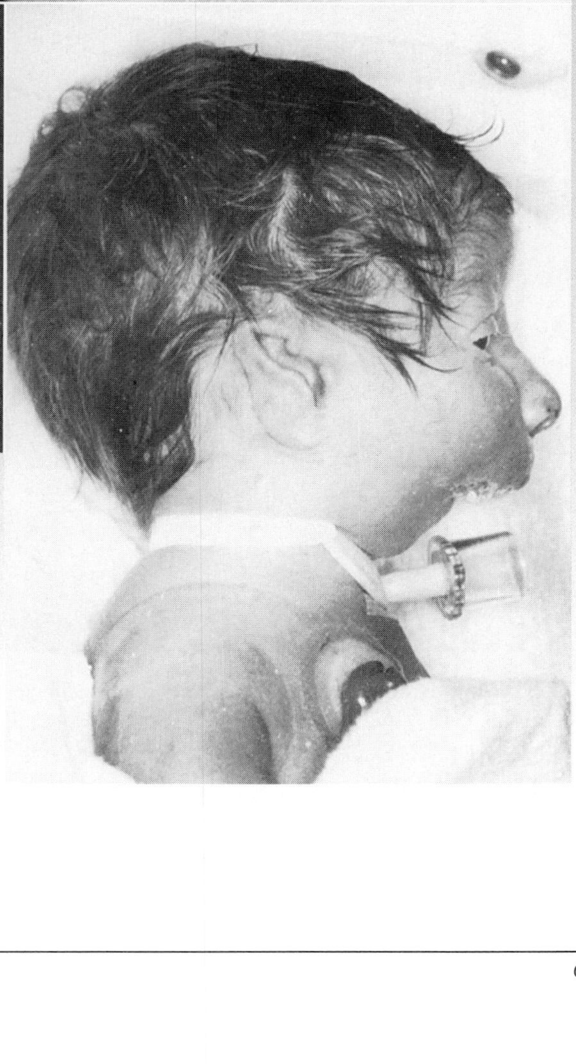

Figure 17-12 A, Ultrasound image of a fetus with trisomy 13 and a midline cleft lip (L) and palate. *N,* Nose; *curved arrow,* tongue. **B,** Postnatal photograph confirming the diagnosis. *L,* Lip; *N,* nose. **C,** Ultrasound image of facial profile showing marked micrognathia *(curved arrow). A,* Anterior; *straight arrow,* nose. **D,** Postnatal photograph confirming the diagnosis. (A and B from Nyberg D, Mahony B, Pretorius D: *Diagnostic ultrasound of fetal anomalies,* St Louis, 1990, Mosby. **C** and **D** from Benson CB and others: *Ultrasound Med* 7:163-167, 1988.)

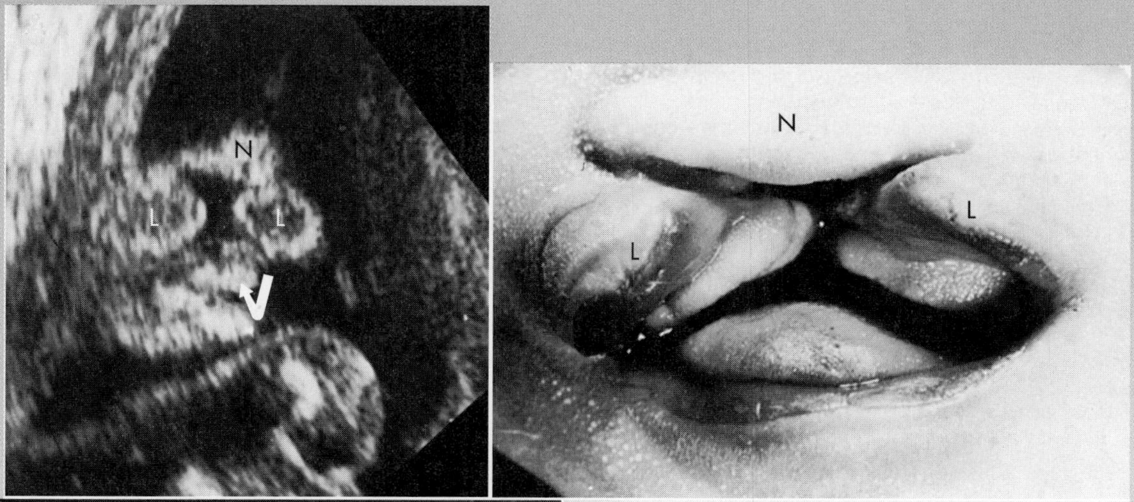

Continued

CLINICAL CORRELATION 17-1
Clinical Study and Manipulation of the Fetus—cont'd

Conventional **x-ray** testing continues to be used in certain circumstances, but because of the potential for radiation damage to the fetal and maternal gonads, its use is less common than in previous years. The use of x-ray testing is relatively limited by its inability to discriminate the details of soft tissues, including cartilaginous components of the skeleton. By injecting radiopaque substances into the amniotic cavity **(amniography, fetography)**, clinicians can obtain outlines of the fetus and amniotic cavity. Other imaging techniques, such as **magnetic resonance imaging (MRI), computed tomographic (CT) scans,** and **xeroradiography,** produce useful images of the fetus, but their use is limited because of factors such as cost and availability (Figures 17-13 and 17-14).

Fetoscopy is the direct visualization of the fetus through a tube inserted into the amniotic cavity.

This is accomplished principally through the use of fiberoptic technology. Because of the risk of spontaneous abortion and infection, this technique is not normally used for purely diagnostic purposes but rather as an aid to intrauterine sampling procedures. Its use has been largely supplanted by other techniques that rely on ultrasonic guidance.

Sampling Techniques

The classical sampling technique is **amniocentesis,** which involves the insertion of a needle into the amniotic sac and removal of a small amount of amniotic fluid for analysis. Amniocentesis is normally not performed before the thirteenth week because of the relatively small amount of amniotic fluid.

Amniocentesis was originally used for detecting chromosomal anomalies (e.g., Down syndrome) in fetal cells found in the amniotic fluid and for the de-

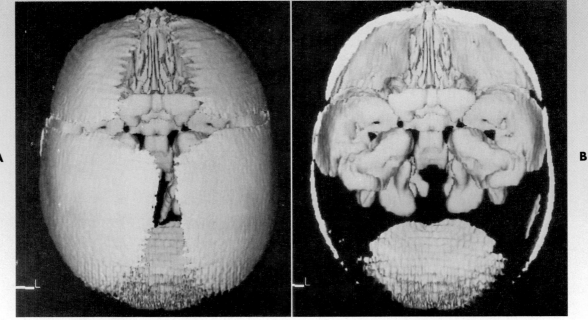

Figure 17-13 High-resolution computed tomographic reconstructions of the skull of an **18-week-old** fetus. **A,** Focus on superficial bones of the skull. **B,** Deeper bones from the same skull. (Courtesy R.A. Levy, H. Maher, and A.R. Burdi, Ann Arbor, Mich.)

CLINICAL CORRELATION 17-1
Clinical Study and Manipulation of the Fetus—cont'd

termination of levels of α-**fetoprotein**, a marker for closure defects of the neural tube and certain other malformations. Analysis of the fetal cells in amniotic fluid is also the basis for determining the gender of embryos. This is typically accomplished by the use of a fluorescent dye that intensely stains the Y chromosome. At present, various analytic procedures on amniotic fluid and cells cultured from the fluid are used to detect many enzymatic and biochemical defects in embryos and to monitor the condition of the fetus.

Another widely used diagnostic technique is **chorionic villus sampling.** In this technique, ultrasonography is used as a guide to insert a biopsy needle into the placenta, where a small sample of the villi is removed for diagnostic purposes. This technique is typically used at earlier periods of pregnancy (6 to 9 weeks) than amniocentesis.

With increasing sophistication of fetal imaging techniques, especially ultrasonography, sampling fetal tissues directly is possible. Ultrasonography-guided sampling of fetal blood, mainly from umbilical vessels, is now relatively common for the diagnosis of hereditary and pathological conditions such as immunodeficiencies, coagulation defects, hemoglobin abnormalities, and fetal infections. It is also possible to biopsy fetal skin and even the fetal liver for organ-specific abnormalities.

THERAPEUTIC MANIPULATIONS ON THE FETUS

Some conditions are better treated in the fetal period than after birth (Box 17-3). In some cases involving blockage, severe structural damage to the fetus can be prevented. In other cases the buildup of toxic waste products can be reduced. The recognition that fetal surgery produces essentially scarless results has stimulated some surgeons to consider corrective surgery in utero rather than waiting until after birth.

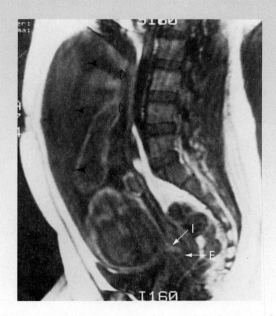

Figure 17-14 Magnetic resonance image of a normal third-trimester fetus inside the uterus. The head of the fetus is near the point of the arrow from *I* (internal cervical os). *E,* External cervical os; *closed arrowheads,* placenta; *open arrowheads,* uterine wall. (From Friedman AC and others: *Clinical pelvic imaging,* St Louis, 1990, Mosby.)

Continued

CLINICAL CORRELATION 17-1
Clinical Study and Manipulation of the Fetus—cont'd

Fetal shunts can be applied to correct specific conditions in which major permanent damage would result before the time of birth. One such situation is a shunt into the urinary bladder to relieve the pressure and subsequent kidney damage caused by anatomical obstructions of the lower urinary tract. Figure 17-15 shows the consequence of nontreatment of a persistent cloacal plate, which results in **megacystitis** (enlarged bladder). Fetal shunts have also been used in attempts to relieve the cerebrospinal pressures that result in hydrocephaly (see Figure 10-36), but the results of these procedures have been equivocal.

Fetal blood transfusions are used for the treatment of fetal anemia and severe erythroblastosis fetalis (see Chapter 6). Earlier, the blood was introduced intraperitoneally. With the increasing sophistication of umbilical cord blood sampling techniques, direct intravascular transfusions are now possible.

Open fetal surgery can now be performed because of the diagnostic procedures that allow an accurate assessment of the condition of the fetus. This is still a very new and highly experimental procedure, and its application has been confined to cases of fetal anomalies that would cause grave damage to the fetus if left uncorrected before birth. Currently, the principal indications for open fetal surgery are blockage of the urinary tract, severe diaphragmatic hernia, and some cases of hydrocephalus. Open fetal surgery entails a risk to the mother as well, and the advisability of such a procedure must be carefully considered. With future improvements in procedures, correcting other malformations such as cleft lip and palate or limb deformities in utero may be possible.

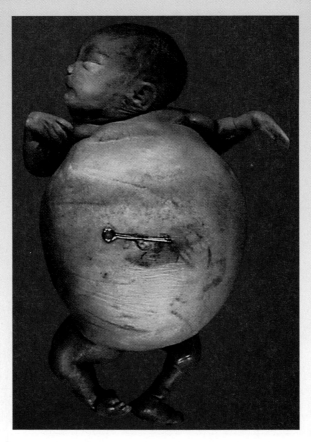

Figure 17-15 Fetus with great abdominal distention as a result of megacystis (large bladder) caused by a cloacal plate. (Courtesy M. Barr, Ann Arbor, Mich.)

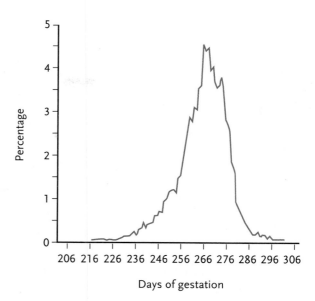

Figure 17-16 Graph showing the distribution in days of normal pregnancy in 1336 spontaneous, full-term deliveries. (Modified from Wigglesworth J, Singer D: *Textbook of fetal and perinatal pathology*, London, 1991, Blackwell Scientific.)

PARTURITION

Parturition, the process of childbirth, occurs approximately 38 weeks after fertilization (Figure 17-16). The process of childbirth consists of three distinct stages of labor. The first, the **stage of dilatation,** begins with the onset of regular, hard contractions of the uterus and ends with complete dilatation of the cervix. Although the contractions of the uterine smooth muscle may appear to be the dominant process in the first stage of labor, the most important component is the effacement and dilatation of the cervix. During the entire pregnancy the cervix functions to retain the fetus in the uterus. For the childbirth process to proceed, the cervix must change consistency from a firm, almost tubular structure to one that is soft, distendible, and not like a canal. This change involves a reconfiguration and possibly removal of much of the cervical collagen. Although many of the factors underlying the reconfiguration of the cervix during the first stage of labor remain undefined, considerable evidence exists for an important role of prostaglandin $F_2\alpha$ in the process. Although variation is great, the average length of the first stage of labor is approximately 12 hours.

The second stage of labor (**stage of expulsion**) begins with complete dilatation of the cervix and ends with the passage of the baby from the birth canal. During this stage, which typically lasts 30 to 60 minutes depending on the number of previous deliveries of the mother, the baby still depends on a functioning umbilical circulation for survival.

The third stage of labor (**placental stage**) represents the period between delivery of the baby and expulsion of the placenta. Typically, the umbilical cord is cut within minutes of delivery, and the baby must then quickly adapt to independent living. During the next 15 to 30 minutes, continued con-

One of the earliest placental hormones produced is **chorionic gonadotropin (HCG)** (see Chapter 6). One later function of HCG is to stimulate steroidogenesis by the placenta. The synthesis of HCG by the syncytiotrophoblast of the placenta is regulated by the production of **gonadotropin-releasing hormone** by cells of the cytotrophoblast. Synthesis of this hormone by the placenta supplants its normal production by the hypothalamus and is probably an adaptation that allows earlier and more local control of HCG than could be accomplished by the hypothalamus.

tractions of the uterus separate the placenta from the maternal decidua and the intact placenta is delivered. After delivery of the placenta, major hemorrhage from the spiral uterine arteries is prevented naturally by continued contraction of the myometrium. In actual clinical practice the third stage is commonly abbreviated by the intramuscular injection of synthetic oxytocin and external manipulation of the uterus to reduce the amount of uterine blood loss.

The mechanisms underlying the initiation and progression of parturition in humans remain remarkably poorly understood, even though considerable progress has been made in uncovering the stimuli for parturition in certain domestic animals. In sheep, parturition is initiated by a sharp increase in the cortisol concentration in the fetal blood. As a result, placental enzyme activity changes, resulting in the conversion of placental progesterone to estrogen synthesis. This increase in estrogen stimulates the formation and release of prostaglandin $F_2\alpha$.

In humans, there is less dependence on activity of the pituitary-adrenal cortical axis for the initiation of parturition. In fact, spontaneous labor occurs in cases of pituitary or adrenal hypoplasia of the fetus or even in anencephaly, but the timing of parturition typically has a considerably wider range than normal. As in sheep, the local release of prostaglandin $F_2\alpha$ may be important in the initiation of labor in humans. A significant question is whether the initiation of parturition depends on fetal or maternal factors. The evidence favors a dominant fetal stimulus in human parturition, although maternal factors exert a modulating influence. In rare cases of human twins implanted in different horns of a double uterus, one member of the pair may not be born until several days or even weeks after the first delivery.

ADAPTATIONS TO POSTNATAL LIFE

When the umbilical cord is clamped after birth, the neonate is suddenly thrust into a totally independent existence. The respiratory and cardiovascular systems must almost instantaneously assume a type and level of function quite different from those during the fetal period. Within hours or days of birth, the digestive system, immune system, and sense organs must also adapt to a much more complex environment.

Circulatory Changes at Birth

Two major events drive the functional adaptations of the circulatory system immediately at birth. The first is the cutting of the umbilical cord, and the second is the changes in the lungs after the first breaths of the newborn. These events stimulate a series of sweeping changes that not only alter the circulatory balance but also result in major structural changes in the circulatory system of the infant.

Cutting the umbilical cord results in an immediate cessation of blood entering the body via the umbilical vein. This eliminates the major blood flow through the ductus venosus and greatly reduces the amount of blood that enters the right atrium via the inferior vena cava. A consequence of this is a reduction of the stream of blood that was directly shunted from the right to the left atrium via the foramen ovale during fetal life.

After just a few breaths, the pulmonary circulatory bed expands and can accommodate much greater blood flow than during the fetal period. Consequences of this change are a reduced flow of blood through the ductus arteriosus and a correspondingly greater return of blood into the left atrium via the pulmonary veins. Within minutes after birth, the ductus arteriosus undergoes a reflex closure. This shunt, which in prenatal life is actively kept open in great part through the actions of prostaglandin E_2, rapidly constricts after the oxygen concentration in the blood increases. The mechanism for constriction appears to involve the action of cytochrome P-450, but the way it is translated into contraction of the smooth musculature of the ductus is not entirely clear. The principal tissue involved in closure of the ductus is smooth muscle, and the shunt also experiences a breakdown of elastic fibers and a thickening of the inner intimal layer.

Because of closure of the ductus arteriosus, increased pulmonary venous flow, and loss of 25% to 50% of the peripheral vasculature (placental circulation) when the umbilical cord is cut, the blood pressure in the left atrium becomes slightly increased over that in the right atrium. This results in a physiological closure of the interatrial shunt, with the result that all the blood entering the right atrium empties into the right ventricle (Figure 17-17). Structural closure of the valve at the foramen ovale is prolonged, occurring over several months after birth. Before complete structural obliteration of the interatrial valve, it possesses the property of "probe patency," which allows a catheter inserted into the right atrium to pass freely through the foramen ovale into the left atrium. As structural fusion of the valve to the interatrial septum progresses, the property of probe patency is gradually reduced and ultimately disappears. In approximately 20% of individuals, structural closure of the interatrial valve is not completed, leading to the normally asymptomatic condition of **probe patent foramen ovale**.

Although the ductus venosus also loses its patency after birth, its closure is more prolonged than that of the ductus arteriosus. The tissue of the wall of the ductus venosus is not as responsive to increased oxygen saturation of the blood as that of the ductus arteriosus.

After the postnatal pattern of the circulation is fully established, obliterated vessels or shunts that were important circulatory channels in the fetus are either replaced by connective tissue strands, forming ligaments, or are represented by relatively smaller vessels (Figures 17-17 and 17-18). These changes are summarized in Table 17-1. In early postnatal life, the umbilical vein can still be used for exchange transfusions (in cases of hemolytic disease resulting from erythroblastosis fetalis) before its lumen becomes obliterated.

Lung Breathing in the Perinatal Period

Immediately after birth, the baby must begin to breathe regularly and effectively with the lungs to survive. The initial breaths are difficult because the lungs are filled with fluid and

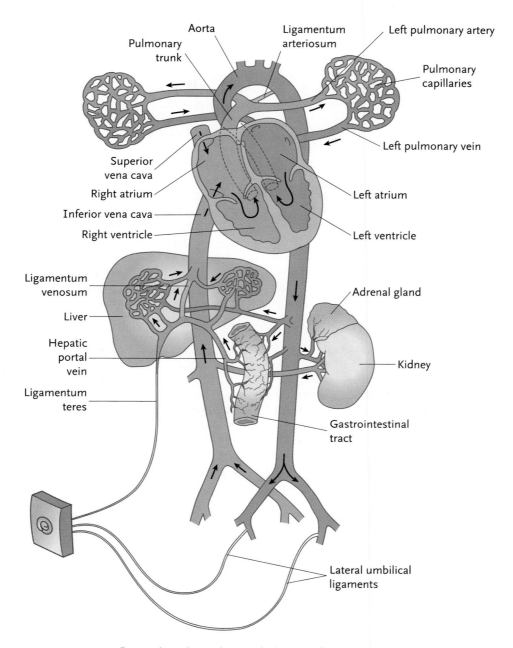

Figure 17-17 Postnatal circulation showing the location of remnants of embryonic vessels.

the alveoli are collapsed at birth. On a purely mechanical basis, air breathing is facilitated by a proportionally large diameter of the trachea and major airways. This reduces resistance to airflow, which would be insurmountable if these passageways were proportionally as small as the lungs.

Just before birth, increased levels of both **arginine vasopressin** and **adrenalin** suppress the secretion of fetal lung fluid and stimulate its resorption. At birth the lungs contain about 50 ml of alveolar fluid, which must be removed for adequate air breathing. Approximately half of that volume enters the lymphatic system. Of the remainder, perhaps half may be expelled during birth. The remainder enters the bloodstream.

The alveolar sacs in the lungs begin to inflate on the first inspiration. The pulmonary surfactant, which was secreted in increasing amounts during the last few weeks of a term pregnancy, reduces the surface tension that would otherwise be present at the air-fluid interface on the alveolar surfaces and facilitates inflation of the lungs. With the rush of air into the lungs, the pulmonary vasculature opens, allowing a greatly increased flow of blood through the lungs. This results in an increased oxygen saturation of the blood; the color of the newborn changes from a dusky purple to pink.

Breathing movements in the fetus are intermittent and irregular even after birth. Many factors can affect the frequency of breathing, but those responsible for the transition

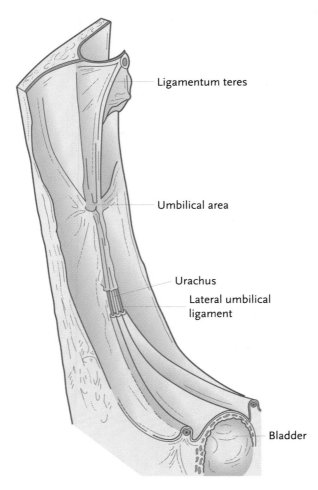

- Ligamentum teres
- Umbilical area
- Urachus
- Lateral umbilical ligament
- Bladder

Figure 17-18 Posterior view of the umbilical region of the abdominal wall showing the two obliterated umbilical arteries flanking the urachus leading from the bladder to the umbilicus. The single strand at the top is the ligamentum teres (remnant of the umbilical vein) leading from the umbilicus to the liver.

from intermittent to regular breathing remain poorly understood. Factors such as cold, touch, chemical stimuli, sleep patterns, and signals emanating from the carotid and aortic bodies have been implicated. During periods of wakefulness, breathing of the neonate soon stabilizes, but for several weeks after birth, short periods of apnea (5 to 10 seconds) are common during REM sleep.

OVERVIEW

The story of prenatal development is complex but fascinating. Many generalizations can be extracted from the study of embryology, but one dominant theme is that of an overall coordination of a large number of very complex integrative processes that range from the translation of information encoded in structural genes, such as the homeobox-containing genes, to the influence of physical factors, such as pressure and tension, on the form and function of the developing embryo.

Sometimes, things go wrong. Studies on spontaneous abortions show that nature has provided a screening mechanism that eliminates many of the embryos least capable of normal development or independent survival. A simple base substitution in the deoxyribonucleic acid of an embryo can produce a defect that may be highly localized or have far-reaching consequences on the development of a variety of systems.

With ever greater insight into the molecular and cellular mechanisms underlying normal and abnormal development and with increasingly sophisticated technology, biomedical scientists and physicians can manipulate the embryo in ways that were unimaginable not long ago. It is an exciting era that is rapidly increasing in technological complexity and uncertain in many social and ethical aspects. It also has an economic impact that is difficult to predict.

SUMMARY

- The fetal period is characterized by intense growth in length and mass of the embryo. With time, the trunk grows relatively faster

TABLE 17-1   Postnatal Derivatives of Prenatal Circulatory Shunts or Vessels

Prenatal structure	Postnatal derivative
Ductus arteriosus	Ligamentum arteriosum
Ductus venosus	Ligamentum venosum
Interatrial shunt	Interatrial septum
Umbilical vein	Ligamentum teres
Umbilical arteries	Distal segments, lateral umbilical ligaments; proximal segments, superior vesical arteries

CLINICAL VIGNETTE

A routine ultrasound examination of a woman in her eighth month of pregnancy showed a swelling of the abdomen of the fetus. A repeat examination a week later showed a further progression of the swelling. The woman was referred to an academic medical center and was told that without intrauterine surgery, there was a very good chance that the fetus would undergo irreversible pathological changes before it was born. She was informed that the condition affecting her fetus was one in which fetal surgery has produced a good record of success.

From this history, what is the likely type of condition, and what would be the nature of the surgical procedure?

than the head, and later the limbs show the greatest growth. The early fetus is thin because of the absence of subcutaneous fat. By midpregnancy, subcutaneous fat is deposited.

- At 5 weeks, the heart beats at 100 beats per min; the heart rate rises to 160 beats per min by 8 weeks and then declines slightly during the remainder of pregnancy. Some different physiological properties of the fetal heart can be explained by the presence of fetal isozymes in the cardiac muscle. The patency of the ductus arteriosus in the fetus is actively maintained through the actions of prostaglandin E_2.

- The fetal lungs are filled with fluid, but they must be prepared for full respiratory function within moments after birth. The fetus begins to make anticipatory breathing movements as early as 11 weeks. Fetal breathing is affected by maternal physiological conditions such as eating and smoking. Disproportionate growth in diameter of the upper airway is important in allowing the newborn to take the first breath. The secretion of pulmonary surfactant begins at about 24 weeks, but large amounts are not synthesized until just a few weeks before birth. Premature infants with a deficiency of pulmonary surfactant often suffer from respiratory distress syndrome.

- Fetal movements begin at about 7½ weeks and increase in complexity thereafter. The maturation of fetal movements mirrors the structural and functional maturation of the nervous system. Diurnal rhythms in fetal activity appear at 20 to 22 weeks. The fetus has alternating periods of sleep and wakefulness. Near term the fetus responds to vibroacoustic stimuli, and by 30 weeks the pupillary light reflex can be elicited.

- The fetal digestive tract is nonfunctional in the usual sense, but maturation of enzyme systems for digestion and absorption occurs. Spontaneous rhythmical movements of the small intestine begin as early as 7 weeks. Meconium begins to fill the lower intestinal tract by midpregnancy. By term the fetus typically swallows over ½ L of amniotic fluid per day.

- Fetal kidneys produce small amounts of dilute urine. Fetal endocrine glands produce small amounts of hormones that can be histochemically demonstrated in glandular tissue early in the fetal period, but several months often pass before the same hormones can be measured in the blood. The fetal adrenal cortex is very large and produces 100 to 200 mg of steroids per day. The exact functions of the fetal adrenal gland remain poorly understood, but fetal cortisol appears to prepare a number of organ systems for the transition to independent life after birth. The placenta continues to produce a variety of hormones throughout most of pregnancy.

- Many new diagnostic techniques have considerably improved access to the fetus. Among the imaging techniques, ultrasonography has emerged as the most widely used in obstetrics. Through sampling techniques such as amniocentesis and chorionic villus sampling, fluids or cells of the embryo and fetus can be removed for analysis. These techniques allow certain manipulations on the fetus (e.g., fetal blood transfusions, fetal surgery for certain anomalies).

- Parturition occurs in three stages of labor. The first is the stage of dilatation, which culminates with effacement of the cervix. The second stage culminates with expulsion of the baby. The third stage represents the period between delivery of the baby and expulsion of the placenta. The mechanisms underlying the initiation of parturition in the human remain poorly understood.

- After birth and cutting of the umbilical cord, the newborn must quickly adapt to an independent existence in terms of breathing and

cardiac function. After the first breaths and severing of the umbilical cord, the pulmonary circulation opens. In response to increased flow into the left atrium, the interatrial shunt undergoes physiological closure, and the ductus arteriosus undergoes a reflex closure. Closure of the ductus venosus in the liver is more prolonged.

REVIEW QUESTIONS

1. The ligamentum teres is the postnatal remains of the:
   A. Ductus arteriosus
   B. Ductus venosus
   C. Umbilical vein
   D. Umbilical artery
   E. Urachus
2. Insufficient production of which of the following is a major cause of poor viability of infants born 24 to 26 weeks after conception?
   A. Pulmonary surfactant
   B. α-Fetoprotein
   C. Meconium
   D. Lanugo
   E. Urine
3. Meconium is formed in the fetal:
   A. Liver
   B. Ileum
   C. Lungs
   D. Amniotic fluid
   E. Kidneys
4. Which organ is much larger in the fetus than it is shortly after birth?
   A. Kidneys
   B. Heart
   C. Liver
   D. Urinary bladder
   E. Adrenal gland
5. Fetal movements can usually first be detected by ultrasound at how many weeks?
   A. 6
   B. 8
   C. 10
   D. 12
   E. 14
6. What blood vessel is commonly used for exchange transfusions in newborn infants?
   A. Umbilical artery
   B. Jugular vein
   C. Femoral artery
   D. Umbilical vein
   E. None of the above
7. A premature infant develops labored breathing and dies within a few days. What is the likely cause?
8. A rare condition that can persist even into adulthood is "caput medusae" (Medusa's head), in which a dark vascular ring with irregular radiations appears around the umbilicus with straining of the abdomen. What is an embryological basis for this condition?
9. A pregnant woman typically first feels fetal movements about 15 weeks into pregnancy. The movements become more noticeable during succeeding weeks but are commonly reduced during the last couple of weeks before parturition. What is the explanation for this?
10. List some recent medical advances that have allowed fetal surgery to become a reality.

REFERENCES

Adzick NS, Harrison MR: Fetal surgical therapy, *Lancet* 343:897-902, 1994.

Avery ME, Wang N-S, Taeusch HW: The lung of the newborn infant, *Sci Am* 228:75-85, 1973.

Barclay AE, Franklin KJ, Prichard MML: *The foetal circulation and cardiovascular system, and the changes that they undergo at birth*, Oxford, England, 1944, Blackwell Scientific.

Barcroft J: *Researches on prenatal life*, vol 1, Oxford, 1946, Blackwell Scientific.

Barron DH: The changes in the fetal circulation at birth, *Physiol Rev* 24:277-295, 1944.

Bowerman RA: *Atlas of normal fetal ultrasonographic anatomy*, ed 2, St Louis, 1992, Mosby.

Busnel MC, Granier-Deferre C, LeCanuet JP: Fetal audition, *Ann NY Acad Sci* 662:118-134, 1992.

Coceani F, Olley PM: The control of cardiovascular shunts in the fetal and perinatal period, *Can J Physiol Pharmacol* 66:1129-1134, 1988.

D'Alton ME, DeCherney AH: Prenatal diagnosis, *N Engl J Med* 328:114-120, 1993.

Dawes GS: The development of fetal behavioural patterns, *Can J Physiol Pharmacol* 66:541-548, 1988.

Duenhoelter JH, Pritchard JA: Fetal respiration, *Am J Obstet Gynecol* 129:326-338, 1977.

Fuchs A-R, Fuchs F: Endocrinology of human parturition: a review, *Br J Obstet Gynecol* 91:948-967, 1984.

Fuse Y: Development of the hypothalamic-pituitary-thyroid axis in humans, *Reprod Fertil Dev* 8:1-21, 1996.

Grannum PA, Copel JA: Invasive fetal procedures, *Radiol Clin North Am* 28:217-226, 1990.

Hooper SB, Harding R: Fetal lung liquid: a major determinant of the growth and functional development of the fetal lung, *Clin Exp Pharmacol Physiol* 22:235-247, 1995.

Johnson P: The development of breathing. In Jones C, Nathanielsz P, eds: *The physiological development of the fetus and newborn*, London, 1985, Academic, pp 201-210.

Jones CT, Nathanielsz PW, eds: *The physiological development of the fetus and newborn*, London, 1985, Academic.

Kitterman JA: Physiological factors in lung growth, *Can J Physiol Pharmacol* 66:1122-1128, 1988.

Lagercrantz H, Slotkin TA: The "stress" of being born, *Sci Am* 254:100-107, 1986.

Larsen T and others: Normal fetal growth evaluated by longitudinal ultrasound examinations, *Early Hum Dev* 24:37-45, 1990.

Lavery JP: *The human placenta: clinical perspectives*, Rockville, Md, 1987, Aspen.

Liggins GC: Initiation of parturition, *Br Med Bull* 35:145-150, 1979.

Liggins GC: The role of cortisol in preparing the fetus for birth, *Reprod Fertil Dev* 6:141-150, 1994.

Liu M and others: Stimulation of fetal rat lung cell proliferation in vitro by mechanical stretch, *Am J Physiol* 263:L376-L383, 1992.

Manning FA: Fetal breathing movements, *Postgrad Med* 61:116-122, 1977.

Mastroiacovo P and others: Limb anomalies following chorionic villus sampling: a registry based case-control study, *Am J Med Genet* 44:856-864, 1992.

Naeye RL: *Disorders of the placenta, fetus, and neonate: diagnosis and clinical significance*, St Louis, 1992, Mosby.

Norgaard-Pedersen B, Christiansen M, Jensen SP: α-Fetoprotein in fetal pathology. In Pasqualini JR, Scholler R, eds: *Hormones and fetal pathophysiology*, New York, 1992, Marcel Dekker, pp 369-412.

Nyberg DA, Mahony BS, Pretorius DH: *Diagnostic ultrasound of fetal anomalies: text and atlas*, St Louis, 1990, Mosby.

Polin RA, Fox WW, eds: *Fetal and neonatal physiology*, vols 1 and 2, Philadelphia, 1992, WB Saunders.

Prechtl HFR: Fetal behavior. In Hill A, Volpe J, eds: *Fetal neurology*, New York, 1989, Raven, pp 1-16.

Rigatto H: Control of breathing in fetal life and onset and control of breathing in the neonate. In Polin, R, Fox W, eds: *Fetal and neonatal physiology*, vol 1, Philadelphia, 1992, WB Saunders, pp 790-801.

Semmekrot B, Guignard J-P: Atrial natriuretic peptide during early human development, *Biol Neonate* 60:341-349, 1991.

Siler-Khodr TM: Endocrine and paracrine function of the placenta. In Polin R, Fox W, eds: *Fetal and neonatal physiology*, vol 1, Philadelphia, 1992, WB Saunders, pp 74-86.

St. John Sutton M, Gill T, Plappert T: Functional anatomic development in the fetal heart. In Polin R, Fox W, eds: *Fetal and neonatal physiology*, vol 1, Philadelphia, 1992, WB Saunders, pp 598-609.

Stahlman MT, Gray ME, Whitsett JA: The ontogeny and distribution of surfactant protein B in human fetuses and newborns, *J Histochem Cytochem* 40:1471-1480, 1992.

Teitel DF: Physiologic development of the cardiovascular system in the fetus. In Polin R, Fox W, eds: *Fetal and neonatal physiology*, vol 1, Philadelphia, 1992, WB Saunders, pp 609-619.

Van Golde LMG and others: Synthesis of surfactant lipids in the developing lung. In Jones C, Nathanielsz P, eds: *The physiological development of the fetus and newborn*, London, 1985, Academic, pp 191-200.

Wetzel GT, Klitzner TS: Developmental cardiac electrophysiology. Recent advances in cellular physiology, *Cardiovasc Res* 31:E52-E60, 1996.

Winter JSD: Fetal and neonatal adrenocortical physiology. In Polin R, Fox W, eds: *Fetal and neonatal physiology*, vol 2, Philadelphia, 1992, WB Saunders, pp 1829-1841.

Answers to Clinical Vignettes and Review Questions

CHAPTER 1

Clinical Vignette

C. Although most tissues of the body are affected to some extent, the heart is not a primary target tissue of ovarian steroid hormones.

Review Questions

1. D
2. E
3. B
4. A mediastinal teratoma, which is likely to have arisen from an aberrant primordial germ cell that became lodged in the connective tissue near the heart.
5. In the female, meiosis begins during embryonic life; in the male, meiosis begins at puberty.
6. At prophase (diplotene stage) of the first meiotic division and at metaphase of the second meiotic division.
7. Chromosomal abnormalities, such as polyploidy or trisomies of individual chromosomes.
8. Spermatogenesis is the entire process of sperm formation from a spermatogonium. It includes the two meiotic divisions and the period of spermiogenesis. Spermiogenesis, or sperm metamorphosis, is the process of transformation of a postmeiotic spermatid, which looks like an ordinary cell, to a highly specialized spermatozoon.
9. Estrogens, secreted by the ovary, support the preovulatory proliferative phase. From the time of ovulation, progesterone is secreted in large amounts by the corpus luteum and is responsible for the secretory phase, which prepares the endometrium for implantation of an embryo.
10. FSH produced by the anterior lobe of the pituitary gland and testosterone produced by the Leydig cells of the testis.

CHAPTER 2

Clinical Vignette

1. Before the plane crash, the issue is who is the "real" mother. After the crash, the issue is who gets the money—the surrogate mother who claims that she is the real mother or the aunt who claims a blood affinity. Although these present as legal issues that would likely be decided in a court, the concept of what is meant by surrogacy also involves psychological and religious issues.
2. This is a very important issue that hasn't been resolved. If the parents had been of a religion that strongly supports the rights of embryos to life, should the remaining embryos also be implanted into someone, and if so, whom? In a case where a considerable inheritance is involved, the financial implications could considerably cloud the issue. On the other hand, if there were no parental money, who would undergo both the risk and expense to prevent the frozen embryos from being simply thrown out? In many cases of in vitro fertilization and embryo transfer, the question of what to do with the "extra" frozen embryos when the first transfer is successful is a real one. Many frozen embryos are being stored at various sites around the world.

Review Questions

1. E
2. D
3. The sharp surge of luteinizing hormone produced by the anterior lobe of the pituitary gland.
4. Capacitation is a poorly understood interaction between a spermatozoon and female reproductive tissues that increases the ability of the sperm to fertilize an egg. In some mammals, capacitation is obligatory, but in humans the importance of capacitation is less well established.

5. Fertilization usually occurs in the upper third of the uterine tube.
6. The ZP3 protein acts as a specific sperm receptor through its O-linked oligosaccharides; much of its polypeptide backbone must be exposed to stimulate the acrosomal reaction.
7. Polyspermy is the fertilization of an egg by more than one spermatozoon. It is prevented through the fast electrical block on the plasma membrane of the egg and by the later zona reaction, by which products released from the cortical granules act to inactivate the sperm receptors in the zona pellucida.
8. She had probably taken clomiphene for the stimulation of ovulation. Natural septuplets are almost never seen.
9. The introduction of more than one embryo into the tube of the woman is commonly done because the chance of any single implanted embryo surviving to the time of birth is quite small. The reasons for this are poorly understood. Extra embryos are frozen because if a pregnancy does not result from the first implantation, the frozen embryos can be implanted without the inconvenience and expense of obtaining new eggs from the mother and fertilizing them in vitro.
10. In cases of incompatibility between the sperm and egg, poor sperm motility, or deficient sperm receptors in the zona, introducing the sperm directly into or near the egg can bypass a weak point in the reproductive sequence of events.

CHAPTER 3

Clinical Vignette

1. The woman had complete situs inversus. When her appendix, which was located in her lower left instead of right abdominal quadrant, became inflamed and ruptured, this unusual pattern of pain resulted.
2. She had an ectopic pregnancy in her left uterine tube. With the rapidly increasing size of the embryo and its extraembryonic structures, her left uterine tube had ruptured.

Review Questions

1. D
2. E
3. A
4. C
5. The embryonic body proper arises from the inner cell mass.
6. The presence of activation promoting factor, which is a complex of cdc2 protein and cyclin, stimulates mitosis.
7. Trophoblastic tissues.
8. Regulation.
9. Cells derived from the cytotrophoblast fuse to form the syncytiotrophoblast.

10. In addition to the standard causes of lower abdominal pain such as appendicitis, the doctor should consider ectopic pregnancy (tubal variety) as a result of stretching and possible rupture of the uterine tube containing the implanted embryo.

CHAPTER 4

Clinical Vignette

Because of the respiratory problems associated with his situs inversus, this man probably has a mutation of a dynein gene. Commonly such individuals also have immotile spermatozoa, a condition that would lead to infertility.

Review Questions

1. D
2. A
3. B
4. B
5. C
6. The epiblast.
7. The primitive node acts as the organizer of the embryo. Through it pass the cells that will become the notochord. The notochord induces the formation of the nervous system. The primitive node is also the site of synthesis of morphogenetically active molecules such as retinoic acid. If a primitive node is transplanted to another embryo, it stimulates the formation of another embryonic axis.
8. Hyaluronic acid and fibronectin.
9. Vg1 and activin.
10. Cell adhesion molecules are lost in a migratory phase. When the migratory cells settle down, they may reexpress cell adhesion molecules.

CHAPTER 5

No Clinical Vignette.

Review Questions

1. B
2. C
3. E
4. C
5. A
6. A homeobox is a highly conserved region consisting of 183 nucleotides that is found in many morphogenetically active genes. Homeobox gene products act as transcription factors.
7. A change in cell shape at the median hinge point and pressures of the lateral ectoderm acting to push up the lateral walls of the neural plate.

8. Neuromeres provide the fundamental organization of parts of the brain in which they are present. Certain homeobox genes are expressed in a definite sequence along the neuromeres.

9. The somites. Axial muscles form from cells derived from the medial halves of the somites, and limb muscles arise from cellular precursors located in the lateral halves of the somites.

10. In blood islands that arise from mesoderm of the wall of the yolk sac.

CHAPTER 6

Clinical Vignette

D. α-Fetoprotein, which is produced principally by the fetal liver, is found in many tissues of the body, but normally, only small amounts are excreted into the amniotic fluid. With open neural tube defects, large quantities of α-fetoprotein escape through the opening and enter the amniotic fluid.

Review Questions

1. A
2. E
3. B
4. D
5. E
6. C
7. Because the placental villi (specializations of the chorion) are directly bathed in maternal blood.
8. This depends on the age of the embryo. In an early fetus the molecule may have to pass through as many layers as the following: syncytiotrophoblast, cytotrophoblast, basal lamina underlying cytotrophoblast, villous mesenchyme, basal lamina of a fetal capillary, and endothelium of the fetal capillary. In a mature placenta the same molecule may pass from the maternal to the fetal circulation by traversing as few layers as syncytiotrophoblast, a fused basal lamina of trophoblast and capillary endothelium, and the endothelium of a fetal capillary.
9. Human chorionic gonadotropin. This is the first distinctive embryonic hormone to be produced by the trophoblastic tissues. Early pregnancy tests involved injecting small amounts of urine of a woman into female African clawed toads (Xenopus laevis). If the woman was pregnant, the chorionic gonadotropin contained in the urine stimulated the frogs to lay eggs the next day. Contemporary pregnancy tests, which can be done using kits bought over the counter, give almost instantaneous results.
10. Many substances that enter a woman's blood are now known to cross the placental barrier. These include alcohol, many drugs (both prescribed and illicit), steroid hormones, and other low-molecular-weight substances.

In general, molecules with molecular weights below 5000 daltons should be assumed to cross the placental barrier with little difficulty.

CHAPTER 7

Clinical Vignette

Although this woman's history suggests a number of risk factors, none of her children's problems could be definitely attributed to any specific cause. Nevertheless, there is a good likelihood that the spina bifida in the first child and the anencephaly of the third child could be related to overall poor nutrition and a specific deficiency in folic acid, since poor nutrition is not uncommon in alcoholics. The small stature of the middle child could possibly result from the mother's heavy smoking, but the behavior problem could be a consequence of the mother's cocaine use, smoking, or alcohol consumption. On the other hand, there could be no relation between any of the mother's risk factors and a prenatal influence on the child's later behavior. An important point is that despite a number of well-known risk factors, it is very difficult, if not impossible, to assign a given congenital anomaly to a specific cause. Realistically, one can only speak in terms of probabilities.

Review Questions

1. E
2. C
3. E
4. B
5. A
6. B
7. The conditions that result in cleft palate occur during the second month of pregnancy. By the fourth month the palate is normally completely established. It is almost certain that this malformation had already been established by the time of the accident.
8. Although there may be a connection between the drug and the birth defect, proving a connection between an individual case and any drug, especially a new one, is very difficult. The woman's genetic background, other drugs that she may have taken during the same period, her history of illnesses during early pregnancy, her nutritional status, and so on should be investigated. Even in the best of circumstances, the probability of a specific malformation being caused by a particular factor can only be estimated in many cases.
9. A common cause of such malformations is an insufficiency of amniotic fluid (oligohydramnios), which can place exposed parts of fetuses under excessive mechanical pressure from the uterine wall and lead to deformations of this type.
10. Dysplasia of ectodermal derivatives is a likely cause.

CHAPTER 8

Clinical Vignette

1. B
2. A

Review Questions

1. D
2. E
3. D
4. B
5. C
6. B
7. The dermis. Recombination experiments have clearly shown that the dermis confers regional morphogenetic information on the epidermis, instructing it to form, for example, cranial hair or abdominal hair.
8. They may be supernumerary nipples located along the caudal ends of the embryonic milk lines.
9. In the early embryo, brain tissue induces the formation of the surrounding membranous skeletal elements. If a significant region of the brain is missing, the inductive interaction does not occur.
10. In experiments involving the use of the quail nuclear marker, quail somites were grafted in place of the original somites in chick embryos. The muscles in the developing limbs all contained quail and not chick nuclei.

CHAPTER 9

Clinical Vignette

At a descriptive level, the mirror image asymmetry of the duplicated foot and digits is a classic example of Bateson's rule of symmetry in duplicated structures (see p. 52). The best explanation for this malformation would be the presence of a duplicated zone of polarizing activity (ZPA) in the anterior margin of the affected limb. Through the actions of sonic hedgehog, secreted by the duplicated ZPA, a secondary gradient of morphogenetic activity could have instructed the anterior mesoderm of the leg bud to form an additional set of posterior structures. This rare defect in humans parallels almost exactly the formation of supernumerary wing structures produced by ZPA transplant experiments on chickens (see Figure 9-14), and the possible mechanism for the duplication is illustrated in Figure 9-21, B.

Review Questions

1. B
2. D
3. A
4. C

5. E
6. D
7. A tear of the amnion during the chorionic villus sampling procedure could have resulted in an amniotic band wrapping around the digits and strangulating their blood supply, causing the tips to degenerate and fall off.
8. This defect is unlikely to be related to the amniocentesis procedure because the morphology of the digits is well established by the time such a procedure is undertaken (usually around 15 to 16 weeks). The most likely cause is a genetic mutation.
9. Muscle-forming cells arise from the somites.
10. The immediate cause is likely the absence of programmed cell death in the interdigital mesoderm. The cause of the disturbance in cell death is currently not understood.

CHAPTER 10

Clinical Vignette

The most immediate problems are surgery to deal with (1) the open spinal cord and (2) the developing hydrocephalus. The surgery for the rachischisis must first be directed toward closing the open lesion to prevent infection and to prevent the leakage of cerebrospinal fluid. Later, surgery will likely be necessary for problems associated with traction on the spinal cord and spinal nerves as the child grows. The hydrocephalus is typically treated by implantation of a shunt to lead excess cerebrospinal fluid from the ventricular system of the brain. Patency of the shunt must be maintained.

In addition to surgery, this infant will face many problems associated with impaired function of the lower spinal nerves. Impaired urinary bladder function is common among such infants, as is impaired mobility of the lower extremities. Infection is a constant threat because of the problem with both containment and circulation of the cerebrospinal fluid in the spinal cord lesion. Children with various forms of spina bifida typically require intensive physical therapy for a variety of problems. Clogging of the shunt leading from the ventricular system is a recurring threat. In this patient the thinning of the walls of the brain indicates that the brain tissue itself has been compromised. Some element of mental retardation and the associated educational and socialization problems represent another component of the problem.

In short, even relatively simple cases of spina bifida pose many chronic problems. The total annual medical, rehabilitation, and education costs of treatment for one individual are often significant. In addition to these are the stresses in the family, which is faced with a continuing need to care for the affected individual. There is a significantly higher than normal divorce rate among parents of children with chronic problems resulting from congenital malformations. A strong support network is important for successfully dealing with children with spina bifida conditions.

Review Questions

1. E
2. A
3. D
4. B
5. D
6. C
7. C
8. B
9. Congenital megacolon (Hirschsprung's disease), in which a segment of large intestine develops without parasympathetic ganglia. Intestinal contents cannot actively move through such an aganglionic segment.
10. The nerves would be hypoplastic (much smaller than normal), and the spinal cord would be thinner than normal in the area from which the nerves supplying the affected limb arise. The likely cause is excessive neuronal cell death because of the absence of an end organ for many of the axons that normally supply the limb.

CHAPTER 11

Clinical Vignette

With the diagnosis of immune deficiency along with the infant's outflow tract defect of the heart, the pediatrician's differential diagnosis included the DiGeorge syndrome. This was confirmed when the blood levels of parathyroid hormone were found to be low. The cause of the infant's problem probably goes back to the fourth week of pregnancy or possibly earlier, when the cranial neural crest supplying the outflow tract of the heart and pharynx was migrating or preparing to migrate into the affected regions.

Review Questions

1. E
2. B
3. C
4. D
5. A
6. B
7. C
8. D
9. Along the length of the spinal cord, migrating neural crest cells are funneled into the anterior sclerotomal region of the somites and are excluded from the posterior half. This results in the formation of a pair of ganglia for each vertebral segment and space between ganglia in the craniocaudal direction.
10. Cranial crest cells can form skeletal elements; trunk crest cells cannot. Migrating cranial neural crest cells have more morphogenetic information encoded in them than trunk crest cells do. (For example, craniocaudal

levels are specified in cranial crest, whereas they are not fixed in trunk crest cells.) Cranial crest cells form large amounts of dermis and other connective tissues, whereas trunk crest cells do not.

CHAPTER 12

Clinical Vignette

The common embryological denominator is a deficit in neural crest associated with the first pharyngeal arch. The first arch gives rise to the lower jaw, much of the middle ear complex, and a significant part of the external ear. Because of the statistical association between abnormalities of the external ear and kidney defects, the doctor wants to be sure that there are no underlying abnormalities of the urinary system.

Review Questions

1. D
2. B
3. A
4. D
5. C
6. Coloboma of the iris is caused by failure of the choroid fissure to close during the sixth week of pregnancy. Because the area of the defect remains open when the rest of the iris constricts in bright light, excessive unwanted light can enter the eye through the defect.
7. Some of the secretions of the lacrimal glands enter the nasolacrimal ducts, which carry the lacrimal fluid into the nasal cavity.
8. Hyaluronic acid. Migration of neural crest cells into the developing cornea occurs during a period when large amounts of hyaluronic acid have been secreted into the primary corneal stroma.
9. During the fetal period the middle ear cavity is filled with a loose connective tissue that dampens the action of the middle ear ossicles. After birth the connective tissue is resorbed.
10. Like the lower jaw, much of the external ear arises from tissue of the first arch bordering the first pharyngeal cleft.

CHAPTER 13

Clinical Vignette

The woman had a hormone-secreting thyroid adenoma that gave her the symptoms of hyperthyroidism. Because the radioactivity was concentrated at the base of her tongue, its location suggested that the tumor formed within a remnant of thyroid tissue left behind at the beginning of the pathway of thyroid tissue migration from its site of origin at the midline base of the future tongue.

Review Questions

1. B
2. B
3. C
4. E
5. A
6. One option is simply acne. Another more significant possibility is a branchial cyst. Branchial cysts are typically located along the anterior border of the sternocleidomastoid muscle. One possible reason for its late manifestation is that the same conditions that resulted in the boy's acne caused a simultaneous reaction in the epidermis lining the cyst.
7. First, all epithelium lining the cyst must be removed, or the remnants could reform into a new cyst and the symptoms could recur. The surgeon must also determine that the cyst is isolated and not connected to the pharynx via a sinus, which would result from an accompanying persistence of the corresponding pharyngeal pouch.
8. Some of the secretions of the lacrimal glands enter the nasolacrimal ducts, which carry the lacrimal fluid into the nasal cavity.
9. By 10 weeks, all the processes of fusion of facial primordia have already been completed. The cause of the defects could almost certainly be attributed to something that influenced the embryo long before the time when the anticonvulsant therapy was initiated, probably before the seventh week of pregnancy.
10. These defects could be a manifestation of fetal alcohol syndrome. They would represent a relatively mild form of holoprosencephaly, which in this case would relate to defective formation of the forebrain (prosencephalon). The defects in olfaction and in the structure of the upper lip could be secondary effects of a primary defect in early formation of the prosencephalon.

CHAPTER 14

Clinical Vignette

The girl had a Meckel's diverticulum that contained ectopic endometrial tissue. When she had menstrual periods, the reaction of the ectopic endometrial tissue gave her upper abdominal cramps. After surgery, her symptoms disappeared.

Review Questions

1. E
2. A
3. C
4. C
5. B
6. A

7. Esophageal atresia or a tracheoesophageal fistula. In the former, the milk fills the blind esophageal pouch and then spills into the trachea via the laryngeal opening. In the latter, milk may pass directly from the esophagus into the trachea depending on the type of fistula.
8. Congenital pyloric stenosis. Projectile vomiting is a common symptom of this condition, and palpation of the knotted pyloric opening of the stomach confirmed the diagnosis.
9. The most likely diagnosis is a vitelline duct fistula connecting the midgut with the umbilicus. This allows some contents of the small intestine to escape through the umbilicus. Another possibility is a urachal fistula (see Chapter 15), which connects the urinary bladder to the umbilicus through a persistent allantoic duct. In this case, however, the escaping fluid would be urine and would likely not be accompanied by mucus.
10. Imperforate anus. When examining a newborn, clinicians must ensure that there is an anal opening.

CHAPTER 15

Clinical Vignette

1. To be diagnosed as a male by the sex chromatin test, none of the cells that were examined should have exhibited Barr bodies (condensed X-chromosomes).
2. The most likely cause for her female phenotype is a lack of testosterone receptors (androgen insensitivity syndrome).
3. Her gonads would be male (internal testes). Because in the embryo her testes produced müllerian inhibitory substance, her paramesonephric ducts regressed. Hence, she formed no uterus, uterine tubes, or upper vagina. This, of course, is also the reason for her amenorrhea, although amenorrhea is common in female athletes who train intensively. Although her testes produce abundant testosterone, the lack of receptors resulted in the lack of differentiation of male genital duct structures or external genitalia that would normally be dependent on testosterone.

Review Questions

1. A
2. D
3. B
4. A
5. A
6. D
7. B
8. The most likely cause is a urachal fistula connecting the urinary bladder to the umbilicus and allowing the leakage of urine. This is caused by the persistence of the lumen in the distal part of the allantois.

9. Bilateral renal agenesis. The first clue was the mother's low weight gain, which could have been the result of oligohydramnios (although this is not the only cause for low weight gain during pregnancy). The infant's appearance showed many of the characteristics of Potter's syndrome, which is caused by intrauterine pressures on the fetus when the amount of amniotic fluid is very low.

10. In normal development the caudal ends of the paramesonephric ducts swing toward the midline and fuse. In this patient's case the point of fusion probably occurred more caudally than normal. This condition is not incompatible with a normal pregnancy and delivery, although in some cases, pain or problems with delivery can occur.

CHAPTER 16

Clinical Vignette

The doctor suspected a high coarctation of the aorta with an accompanying patent ductus arteriosus. In both high and low coarctation of the aorta, the pulse in the lower part of the body is commonly reduced. The cyanosis of the feet resulted from the spillage of venous blood into the systemic circulation through the patent ductus arteriosus.

Review Questions

1. A
2. D
3. C
4. D
5. E
6. A
7. C
8. The doctor suspected that the boy had a double aortic arch or a right aortic arch, either of which can cause difficulty in swallowing (dysphagia) during childhood, especially when growth spurts are occurring. Another possibility for an embryologically based dysphagia is esophageal stenosis.
9. To survive, an individual with this defect would have to have a means for draining blood entering the left atrium and a means of getting blood into the left ventricle or the systemic circulation. One combination that would compensate is an atrial septal defect, which allows incoming blood to escape from the left atrium, and an associated ventricular septal defect, which allows blood from the right ventricle to pass into the left ventricle. A patent ductus arteriosus added to the first two compensatory defects could also help to balance the circulation by adding blood to the systemic side of the circulation. This would not be very helpful in the phys-

iological sense, however, because the added blood would be unoxygenated blood entering the aorta from the pulmonary artery.

10. Persistence of the caudal segment of the left supracardinal vein. Normally the caudal segment of the right supracardinal vein persists and becomes incorporated into the inferior vena cava, and the corresponding segment of the left supracardinal vein disappears (see Figure 16-9). A wide variety of anomalous patterns of the abdominal veins exists.

CHAPTER 17

Clinical Vignette

The fetus likely had an obstruction of the lower urinary tract (perhaps urethral valves) leading to megacystis (see Figure 17-15). This condition is treated by inserting a shunt into the bladder, allowing the urine to escape into the amniotic fluid. If the shunt functions during the remainder of pregnancy, the actual problem with the urinary outlet can be treated surgically after birth. The placement of shunts into the fetal bladder is one of the more successful types of intrauterine surgery practiced to date.

Review Questions

1. C
2. A
3. B
4. E
5. B
6. D
7. Hyaline membrane disease of the newborn. If the baby was born prematurely, the fetal lungs had not produced sufficient pulmonary surfactant to support normal breathing.
8. This condition is the result of persistence of a patent ductus venosus and umbilical vein. When the individual strains, venous blood fills these vessels and small venous branches radiating from the umbilical area. This is reminiscent of the head of Medusa, with snakes taking the place of hairs.
9. One simple explanation is that with continued growth of the fetus the extremities become so tightly packed in the uterus that there is little room for movement.
10. More refined imaging techniques, such as ultrasonography, that allow more accurate diagnosis in utero of congenital malformations; recognition of the exceptional healing powers of the fetus; improved intrauterine and extrauterine surgical techniques, some assisted by ultrasonographic visualization, that allow direct surgery on the fetus; and increased ability to forestall or prevent premature labor after surgery on the uterus.

Index

Page references in *italics* indicate figures; page references followed by *t* indicate tables.